Netter's Integrated Review of Medicine

Pathogenesis to Treatment

Editor

BRYAN C. LEPPERT, MD
Assistant Professor of Clinical Medicine
Weill Cornell Medical College
Cornell University;
Assistant Attending Physician
New York-Presbyterian Hospital
New York, New York

Associate Editor

CHRISTOPHER R. KELLY,
MD, MS, RPVI
Cardiologist
North Carolina Heart and Vascular
UNC Health Care
Raleigh, North Carolina

Illustrations by

FRANK H. NETTER, MD

Contributing Illustrators
Carlos A. G. Machado, MD
Kristen Wienandt Marzejon, MS, MFA
James A. Perkins, MS, MFA
John A. Craig, MD
Paul Kim, MS

ELSEVIER

Elsevier
1600 John F. Kennedy Blvd.
Ste 1800
Philadelphia, PA 19103-2899

NETTER'S INTEGRATED REVIEW OF MEDICINE ISBN: 978-0-323-47938-7

Notice

Practitioners and researchers must always rely on their own experience and knowledge in evaluating and using any information, methods, compounds or experiments described herein. Because of rapid advances in the medical sciences, in particular, independent verification of diagnoses and drug dosages should be made. To the fullest extent of the law, no responsibility is assumed by Elsevier, authors, editors or contributors for any injury and/or damage to persons or property as a matter of products liability, negligence or otherwise, or from any use or operation of any methods, products, instructions, or ideas contained in the material herein.

International Standard Book Number: 978-0-323-47938-7

Publisher: Elyse O'Grady
Senior Content Development Specialist: Marybeth Thiel
Publishing Services Manager: Catherine Jackson
Specialist: Kristine Feeherty
Design Direction: Patrick Ferguson

Printed in China

Last digit is the print number: 9 8 7 6 5 4 3 2

Working together
to grow libraries in
developing countries

www.elsevier.com • www.bookaid.org

To the educators of the next generation of physicians—the experienced practitioners, committed residents, enthusiastic students, and most importantly, the patients whose understanding and trust provide the opportunity to refine our craft.

Preface

As I entered medical school, the number of available resources overwhelmed me. Books, podcasts, online videos, flashcards, interactive quiz books—a seemingly endless collection explaining anatomy, physiology, pathophysiology, diagnosis, and treatment. All sought to help me assimilate the massive amount of information that lay ahead, but choosing a few was daunting. I turned to the upperclassmen for their advice, and though they had individual preferences, one was constant: "Netter cards." Dr. Frank Netter, with over 20,000 illustrations in his lifetime, was the go-to study aid for students to learn anatomy, and I promptly purchased my own box of flashcards. That box, depicting virtually every organ and organ system in different angles, reflections, and sections, followed me from medical school to residency and beyond.

In the first edition of *Netter's Integrated Review of Medicine*, we sought to create a reference for students in the first phase of their medical career. Our goal was not to create an exhaustive review of a topic—the pace of medical advancement is far too quick to allow for that. Rather, we hope to highlight a continuous thread, building on the underlying pathophysiology and biochemical mechanisms to introduce the practical concerns of evaluation, diagnosis, and treatment. Augmented by Dr. Netter's illustrations, as accurate today as ever, each chapter provides a firm foundation that can be expanded and developed with deeper inquiry.

It is a particular point of pride that, when work on this book began, the majority of the authors were themselves residents and fellows, still actively training and seeking to better perfect their own practice of medicine. Who better to instruct learners using this book than those who could best relate to the student experience? We want to extend our sincerest thanks to our devoted authors who, with the guidance of our associate editors, produced the text before you. Just as medical school upperclassmen directed me to Netter cards, so too do we hope that our experience, put into this book alongside Dr. Netter's work, serves as a valuable and accessible resource.

Bryan C. Leppert, MD
New York, New York

About the Editor

Bryan Leppert is an Assistant Professor of Clinical Medicine at Weill Cornell Medical College in New York City. Hailing from small-town Iowa, he received his BS in Biology from the University of Iowa before heading east to North Carolina and Duke University School of Medicine. After receiving his MD, he moved with his wife to New York City to complete an internal medicine residency at Columbia University Medical Center. He is heavily involved in undergraduate medical education, with special interests in simulation, remediation, and interprofessional learning.

Our thanks to the staff at Elsevier for their tireless faith in this book, to all of our authors and associate editors for their dedication, and to our families for their love and boundless support.

About the Artists

FRANK H. NETTER, MD

Frank H. Netter was born in 1906, in New York City. He studied art at the Art Students' League and the National Academy of Design before entering medical school at New York University, where he received his MD degree in 1931. During his student years, Dr. Netter's notebook sketches attracted the attention of the medical faculty and other physicians, allowing him to augment his income by illustrating articles and textbooks. He continued illustrating as a sideline after establishing a surgical practice in 1933, but he ultimately opted to give up his practice in favor of a full-time commitment to art. After service in the US Army during World War II, Dr. Netter began his long collaboration with the CIBA Pharmaceutical Company (now Novartis Pharmaceuticals). This 45-year partnership resulted in the production of the extraordinary collection of medical art so familiar to medical professionals worldwide.

In 2005, Elsevier, Inc., purchased the Netter Collection and all publications from Icon Learning Systems. Over 50 publications featuring the art of Dr. Netter are available through Elsevier, Inc. (in the United States: https://www.us.elsevierhealth.com/; outside the United States: www.elsevierhealth.com).

Dr. Netter's works are among the finest examples of the use of illustration in the teaching of medical concepts. The 13-book *Netter Collection of Medical Illustrations*, which includes the greater part of the more than 20,000 paintings created by Dr. Netter, became and remains one of the most famous medical works ever published. *The Netter Atlas of Human Anatomy*, first published in 1989, presents the anatomical paintings from the Netter Collection. Now translated into 16 languages, it is the anatomy atlas of choice among medical and health professions students the world over.

The Netter illustrations are appreciated not only for their aesthetic qualities, but, more important, for their intellectual content. As Dr. Netter wrote in 1949, "… clarification of a subject is the aim and goal of illustration. No matter how beautifully painted, how delicately and subtly rendered a subject may be, it is of little value as a *medical illustration* if it does not serve to make clear some medical point." Dr. Netter's planning, conception, point of view, and approach are what inform his paintings and make them so intellectually valuable.

Frank H. Netter, MD, physician and artist, died in 1991.

Learn more about the physician-artist whose work has inspired the Netter Reference collection: https://netterimages.com/artist-frank-h-netter.html.

CARLOS MACHADO, MD

Carlos Machado was chosen by Novartis to be Dr. Netter's successor. He continues to be the main artist contributing to the Netter collection of medical illustrations.

Self-taught in medical illustration, cardiologist Carlos Machado has meticulously updated some of Dr. Netter's original plates and has created many original paintings of his own in the style of Netter as an extension of the Netter collection. Dr. Machado's photorealistic expertise and keen insight into the physician-patient relationship inform his vivid and unforgettable visual style. His dedication to researching each topic and subject he paints places him among the premier medical illustrators at work today.

Learn more about his background and see more of his art at: https://netterimages.com/artist-carlos-a-g-machado.html.

Section Editors

Justin M. Belcher, MD, PhD
Assistant Professor of Medicine
Section of Nephrology
Yale University School of Medicine
VA Connecticut Healthcare System
New Haven, Connecticut
Section 8: Renal Diseases

Talal Dahhan, MD, MSEd, FACP, FCCP
Assistant Professor of Medicine
Education Lead and Faculty
Division of Pulmonary, Allergy, and Critical Care
    Medicine
Department of Medicine
Duke University
Durham, North Carolina;
Assistant Professor
College of Medicine
Alfaisal University
Riyadh, Saudi Arabia;
Director of Quality and Consultant
Adult Critical Care Medicine Department
King Faisal Specialist Hospital and Research Center
    (KFSHRC)
Riyadh, Saudi Arabia
Section 7: Pulmonary Diseases

David J. Engel, MD
Associate Professor of Medicine
Columbia University Irving Medical Center
New York, New York
Section 5: Cardiovascular Diseases

Christopher R. Kelly, MD, MS, RPVI
Cardiologist
North Carolina Heart and Vascular
UNC Health Care
Raleigh, North Carolina
*Section 1: Common Symptoms, Section 2: Common
    Examination Findings, Section 3: Common
    Abnormalities in Blood Tests*

Alfred Lee, MD, PhD
Associate Professor of Medicine (Hematology)
Associate Program Director, Internal Medicine
    Traditional Residency Program
Yale School of Medicine
New Haven, Connecticut
Section 12: Diseases of Blood Cells

Bryan C. Leppert, MD
Assistant Professor of Clinical Medicine
Weill Cornell Medical College
Cornell University;
Assistant Attending Physician
New York-Presbyterian Hospital
New York, New York
*Section 4: Performance and Interpretation of Common
    Tests and Procedures*

Benjamin A. Miko, MD, MSc
Assistant Professor of Medicine
Division of Infectious Diseases
Columbia University Medical Center
New York, New York
Section 10: Infectious Diseases

Katherine G. Nickerson, MD
Professor of Medicine
Vagelos College of Physicians and Surgeons
Columbia University Irving Medical Center
New York, New York
Section 9: Rheumatologic Diseases

Tara Sanft, MD
Associate Professor of Medicine
Yale University School of Medicine
Director of Survivorship Program
Yale Cancer Center
New Haven, Connecticut
Section 13: Solid Organ Tumors

Jessica R. Starr, MD
Assistant Attending Physician
Hospital for Special Surgery
New York, New York
Section 6: Endocrine Diseases

David W. Wan, MD
Assistant Professor of Medicine
Department of Medicine
Division of Gastroenterology and Hepatology
New York-Presbyterian/Weill Cornell Medicine
New York, New York
Section 11: Gastrointestinal Diseases

Contributors

Justin G. Aaron, MD
Assistant Professor of Medicine
Columbia University Irving Medical Center
New York, New York
Infective Endocarditis, Clostridioides *(Formerly* Clostridium*) difficile Colitis*

Zaid I. Almarzooq, MBBCh
Fellow in Cardiovascular Medicine
Brigham and Women's Hospital
Harvard Medical School
Boston, Massachusetts
Adventitial Lung Sounds

Isabelle Amigues, MD, MS, RhMSUS
Assistant Professor
National Jewish Health
University of Colorado
Denver, Colorado
Rheumatoid Arthritis

Rachel Arakawa, MD
Endocrinology Fellow
Columbia University Medical Center
New York, New York
Thyroid Cancer and Thyroid Nodules

Dianne M. Augelli, MD
Assistant Professor of Medicine
Medicine and Neurology
Weill Medical College of Cornell University;
Attending Physician
New York-Presbyterian Hospital
New York, New York
Sleep Apnea

Ahmad Najdat Bazarbashi, MD
Gastroenterology and Hepatology Fellow
Brigham and Women's Hospital
Harvard Medical School
Boston, Massachusetts
Ascites

Jason M. Beckta, MD, PhD
Resident Physician
Therapeutic Radiology
Yale School of Medicine
New Haven, Connecticut
Hepatocellular Carcinoma (HCC)

Ankeet S. Bhatt, MD, MBA
Clinical Fellow
Cardiovascular Disease
Brigham and Women's Hospital
Harvard Medical School
Boston, Massachusetts
Hyperlipidemia

Manisha Bhattacharya, MD, MBA
Neuro-Oncology Hospitalist
Medical Instructor
Duke University School of Medicine
Durham, North Carolina
Chronic Myelogenous Leukemia (CML)

Victor P. Bilan, MD
Hematology and Medical Oncology
Thomas Jefferson University
Philadelphia, Pennsylvania
Sickle Cell Disease, Thalassemia

Eric J. Burnett, MD, MBS
Instructor of Medicine
Department of Medicine, Section of Hospital Medicine
Associate Program Director, Internal Medicine Residency Program
Columbia University Medical Center
New York, New York
HIV/AIDS: Common Opportunistic Infections

Mary Elizabeth Card, MD
Pulmonary and Critical Care Medicine Postdoctoral Fellow
Johns Hopkins University
Baltimore, Maryland
Diffuse Parenchymal Lung Disease

Bina Choi, MD
Resident
Department of Medicine
Columbia University Medical Center
New York, New York
Respiratory System Anatomy Review

Mohsin Chowdhury, MD
Cardiovascular Medicine Fellow
Beth Israel Deaconess Medical Center
Harvard Medical School
Boston, Massachusetts
Aortic Stenosis

Tariq Chukir, MD
Endocrinology Fellow
New York-Presbyterian Hospital/Weill Cornell
New York, New York
Hyperthyroidism and Thyrotoxicosis

Margot E. Cohen, MD
Assistant Professor of Clinical Medicine
Department of Medicine
Section of Hospital Medicine
University of Pennsylvania
Philadelphia, Pennsylvania
Endoscopy and Colonoscopy

Sarah P. Cohen, MD
Fellow Physician
Adult Pulmonary and Critical Care, and Pediatric
    Pulmonary
Ohio State University and Nationwide Children's
    Hospital
Columbus, Ohio
Mechanical Ventilation

Shirley Cohen-Mekelburg, MD, MS
Clinical Lecturer and Research Scientist
University of Michigan;
VA Center for Clinical Management Research
VA Ann Arbor Health System
Ann Arbor, Michigan
Celiac Disease, Inflammatory Bowel Disease

Jigar Contractor, MD
Assistant Professor of Medicine
Weill Cornell Medicine
New York, New York
Anemia

Joshua R. Cook, MD, PhD
Endocrinology, Diabetes, and Metabolism Fellow
New York-Presbyterian Hospital
Columbia University Medical Center
New York, New York
Diabetic Ketoacidosis and Hyperosmolar Hyperglycemic State

Joséphine A. Cool, MD
Instructor in Medicine
Beth Israel Deaconess Medical Center
Harvard Medical School
Boston, Massachusetts
Irritable Bowel Syndrome

Sara J. Cromer, MD
Clinical and Research Fellow
Endocrinology, Diabetes, and Metabolism
Massachusetts General Hospital
Boston, Massachusetts
*Pancreas Anatomy and Physiology Review,
Adrenal Glands Anatomy and Physiology Review*

Talal Dahhan, MD, MSEd, FACP, FCCP
Assistant Professor of Medicine
Education Lead and Faculty
Division of Pulmonary, Allergy, and Critical Care
    Medicine
Department of Medicine
Duke University
Durham, North Carolina;
Assistant Professor
College of Medicine
Alfaisal University
Riyadh, Saudi Arabia;
Director of Quality and Consultant
Adult Critical Care Medicine Department
King Faisal Specialist Hospital and Research Center
    (KFSHRC)
Riyadh, Saudi Arabia
*Hypoxemia, Adventitial Lung Sounds, Pulmonary
    Function Tests (PFTs), Thoracentesis*

Madison Dennis, MD
Weill Cornell Medicine
New York, New York
Alcohol-Associated Liver Disease

Catherine DeVoe, MD
Infectious Diseases Fellow
University of California, San Francisco
San Francisco, California
Osteomyelitis

Robert Diep, MD
Internal Medicine Resident
Duke University Medical Center
Durham, North Carolina
Nephrotic Syndrome

Mia Djulbegovic, MD
Postdoctoral Fellow
National Clinician Scholars Program
Yale University School of Medicine
New Haven, Connecticut;
Veterans Affairs Connecticut Healthcare System
West Haven, Connecticut
Hypercoagulable States and Deep Venous Thrombosis

Megan M. Dupuis, MD, PhD
Hematology/Oncology Fellow
MD Anderson Cancer Center
Houston, Texas
Bladder Cancer

Daniel Edmonston, MD
Medical Instructor
Department of Medicine
Division of Nephrology
Duke University
Durham, North Carolina
Hyponatremia and Hypernatremia

Chidiebube C. Egwim, MD, MPH
Clinical Fellow in Nephrology
Vanderbilt University Medical Center
Nashville, Tennessee
Acute Kidney Injury

Pierre Elias, MD
Fellow in Cardiovascular Disease
Columbia University
New York, New York
Hypoxemia

David J. Engel, MD
Associate Professor of Medicine
Columbia University Irving Medical Center
New York, New York
Hypertensive Crisis, Tachycardia, Bradycardia

Sasha A. Fahme, MD
Assistant Professor of Medicine
Global Health Research Fellow
Weill Cornell Medicine
New York, New York
Tuberculosis

Fahad Faruqi, MD, MPH
Hematology and Medical Oncology Fellow
Mayo Clinic
Rochester, Minnesota
Hemophilia, Disseminated Intravascular Coagulation

Rachel Feder, MD
Gastroenterology Fellow
University of Washington
Seattle, Washington
Abnormal Liver Function Tests

Kelly J. Fitzgerald, MD, PhD
Radiation Oncology Resident
Memorial Sloan Kettering Cancer Center
New York, New York
Prostate Cancer

Benjamin D. Gallagher, MD
Instructor
Section of General Internal Medicine
Department of Internal Medicine
Yale School of Medicine
New Haven, Connecticut
Cushing Syndrome

Cecily J. Gallup, MD, MPH
Assistant Clinical Professor of Internal Medicine and
    Pediatrics
University of California, Los Angeles
Los Angeles, California
Fever

Gaurav Ghosh, MD
Gastroenterology and Hepatology Fellow
New York-Presbyterian/Weill Cornell Medical Center
New York, New York
Peptic Ulcer Disease and Helicobacter pylori

Stephanie L. Gold, MD
Gastroenterology Fellow
Mount Sinai Hospital
New York, New York
Celiac Disease, Inflammatory Bowel Disease

Maryam Gondal, MD
Nephrology Fellow
Yale New Haven Hospital
New Haven, Connecticut
Polycystic Kidney Disease

Armand Gottlieb, MD
Internal Medicine Resident
New York-Presbyterian/Columbia University Irving
   Medical Center
New York, New York
*Cardiovascular System Anatomy Review, Cardiovascular
   System Physiology Review*

Michael J. Grant, MD
Internal Medicine Resident
Department of Medicine
Duke University Medical Center
Durham, North Carolina
Lymphoma

Vikas Gupta, MD, PhD
Instructor
Division of Gastroenterology and Hepatology
Department of Medicine
Weill Cornell Medical College
New York, New York
*Irritable Bowel Syndrome, Cirrhosis and Portal
   Hypertension*

Leila Haghighat, MPhil, MD
Chief Resident
Internal Medicine
Yale New Haven Hospital
New Haven, Connecticut
Hypertensive Crisis, Echocardiography

Emilia A. Hermann, MD, MPH
Instructor
Clinical Medicine
Vagelos College of Physicians and Surgeons
Columbia University Irving Medical Center
New York, New York
Pulmonary Embolism

Will Hindle-Katel, MD
Cardiology Fellow
Yale School of Medicine
New Haven, Connecticut
Aortic Dissection

Tara Holder, MD
Cardiovascular Fellow
Vanderbilt University Medical Center
Nashville, Tennessee
Hypercalcemia and Hypocalcemia

Margaret Infeld, MD, MS
Fellow in Cardiovascular Disease
University of Vermont Medical Center
Burlington, Vermont
Bradycardia

Gina P. Jabbour, MD
Adjunct Assistant Professor of Clinical Medicine
Weill Cornell Medicine
New York, New York
Abnormal Coagulation Studies

Jeremy B. Jacox, MD, PhD
Hematology/Oncology Fellow
Yale New Haven Hospital
New Haven, Connecticut
Pancreatic Cancer

Debbie Jiang, MD
Hematology/Oncology Fellow
University of Washington
Seattle, Washington
Microangiopathic Hemolytic Anemia (MAHA)

Elena K. Joerns, MD
Rheumatology Fellow
UT Southwestern Medical Center
Dallas, Texas
Vasculitides

Christopher R. Kelly, MD, MS, RPVI
Cardiologist
North Carolina Heart and Vascular
UNC Health Care
Raleigh, North Carolina
*Headache, Dizziness, Cough, Sore Throat, Syncope, Chest
   Pain, Dyspnea, Nausea and Vomiting, Jaundice,
   Abdominal Pain, Gastrointestinal Bleeding, Acute
   Coronary Syndromes, Aortic Dissection*

Judith Kim, MD
Gastroenterology Fellow
New York-Presbyterian Hospital
New York, New York
Adrenal Masses

Richard K. Kim, MD, MSc
Clinical Instructor
Department of Anesthesiology, Perioperative, and
   Pain Medicine
Stanford University School of Medicine
Stanford, California
Adrenal Insufficiency

Emily N. Kinsey, MD
Hematology/Oncology Fellow
Duke University
Durham, North Carolina
Esophageal Cancer

Jonathan R. Komisar, MD
Internal Medicine/Psychiatry Resident
Duke University Hospital
Durham, North Carolina
Urinary Tract Infection

Eugene C. Kovalik, MD, CM, FRCP(C), FACP, FASN
Professor of Medicine
Duke University Medical Center
Durham, North Carolina
Acid-Base Disturbances

Govind M. Krishnan, MD
Internal Medicine/Pediatrics, PGY-4
Duke University Hospital
Durham, North Carolina
Tachycardia

Balakumar Krishnarasa, MD
Assistant Professor of Medicine
Department of Medicine
Weill Cornell Medicine
New York, New York
Hematuria, Aplastic Anemia (AA)

Steffne Kunnirickal, MD
Cardiovascular Fellow
Yale University
New Haven, Connecticut
Arterial Blood Gas

Matthew K. Labriola, MD
PGY4 Hematology/Oncology Fellow
Duke University Hospital
Durham, North Carolina
Multiple Myeloma

Amit Lakhanpal, MD, PhD
Rheumatology Fellow
Hospital for Special Surgery
New York, New York
Spondyloarthridities

Perola Lamba, MD
Nephrology Fellow
New York-Presbyterian Hospital/Weill Cornell Medicine
New York, New York
Urinary System Anatomy Review

Joshua Lampert, MD
Cardiology Fellow
Mount Sinai Hospital
New York, New York
Coronary Artery Disease and Stable Angina

Justin C. Laracy, MD
Infectious Diseases Fellow
Columbia University Medical Center/New
    York-Presbyterian
New York, New York
Urethritis

Monika Laszkowska, MD
Physician
Division of Digestive and Liver Diseases
Department of Medicine
Columbia University
New York, New York
Paracentesis

Alfred Lee, MD, PhD
Associate Professor of Medicine (Hematology)
Associate Program Director, Internal Medicine
    Traditional Residency Program
Yale School of Medicine
New Haven, Connecticut
Thrombocytopenia, Peripheral Blood Smear

Ruediger W. Lehrich, MD
Associate of Professor of Medicine
Department of Medicine
Division of Nephrology
Duke University
Durham, North Carolina
Hyponatremia and Hypernatremia

Bryan C. Leppert, MD
Assistant Professor of Clinical Medicine
Weill Cornell Medical College
Cornell University;
Assistant Attending Physician
New York-Presbyterian Hospital
New York, New York
Joint Pain

Hana I. Lim, MD
Clinical Fellow
Hematology and Oncology
New York-Presbyterian
Weill Cornell Medical Center
New York, New York
Peripheral Blood Smear

Ying L. Liu, MD, MPH
Assistant Attending
Memorial Sloan Kettering Cancer Center
New York, New York
Constipation, Pituitary Gland Anatomy and Physiology Review

Zoë Lysy, MDCM, FRCPC, MPH
Adjunct Assistant Professor
University of Toronto
Toronto, Ontario, Canada
Hyperparathyroidism

Melissa S. Makar, MD
Assistant Professor of Clinical Medicine
Indiana University School of Medicine
Indianapolis, Indiana
Acid-Base Disturbances

Divyanshu Malhotra, MBBS
Clinical Instructor
Department of Medicine/Nephrology
Yale University
New Haven, Connecticut
Acute Tubular Necrosis

Waqas A. Malick, MD
Cardiology Fellow
Mount Sinai Hospital
New York, New York
Pericarditis and Pericardial Effusions, Amyloidosis

Paul B. Martin, MD, MPH
Assistant Professor of Clinical Medicine
Weill Cornell Medicine
New York, New York
Diarrhea

Elizabeth Mathew, MD
Rheumatologist
King's Daughters Medical Center
Ashland, Kentucky
Polymyositis and Dermatomyositis

Anne M. Mathews, MD
Medical Instructor/Faculty
Division of Pulmonary, Allergy, and Critical Care Medicine
Duke University Medical Center
Durham, North Carolina
Cystic Fibrosis

Matthew R. McCulloch, MD
Internal Medicine and Pediatrics Resident
Duke University
Durham, North Carolina
Cellulitis

Julia E. McGuinness, MD
Hematology/Oncology Fellow
Columbia University Irving Medical Center
New York, New York
Renal Cell Carcinoma (RCC)

William C. McManigle, MD
Fellow
Division of Pulmonary, Allergy, and Critical Care Medicine
Department of Medicine
Duke University Medical Center
Durham, North Carolina
Respiratory System Physiology Review

Karishma K. Mehra, MD
Hematologist/Medical Oncologist
Smilow Cancer Hospital at Saint Francis Cancer Center
Hartford, Connecticut
Breast Cancer

Amit Mehta, MD
Gastroenterology Fellow
New York-Presbyterian/Weill Cornell Medical Center
New York, New York
Nonalcoholic Fatty Liver Disease (NAFLD)

Dennis G. Moledina, MD, PhD
Assistant Professor
Medicine (Nephrology)
Yale School of Medicine
New Haven, Connecticut
Acute Tubulointerstitial Nephritis

Jeffrey Mufson, MD
Clinical Fellow
Section of Medical Oncology
Department of Medicine
Yale School of Medicine
New Haven, Connecticut
Lung Cancer

Michael Murn, MD
Pulmonary and Critical Care Medicine Fellow
New York-Presbyterian Hospital
Columbia University Medical Center
New York, New York
Chronic Obstructive Pulmonary Disease

Marina Mutter, MD
Clinical Instructor of Medicine
University of Pittsburgh School of Medicine
Pittsburgh, Pennsylvania
Nephrolithiasis

Abhinav Nair, MD
Cardiology Fellow
Jefferson Heart Institute
Thomas Jefferson University Hospital
Philadelphia, Pennsylvania
Hypothyroidism

Yunseok Namn, MD
Gastroenterology Fellow
Stony Brook University Hospital
Stony Brook, New York
*Gastroesophageal Reflux Disease (GERD) and Barrett
    Esophagus, Biliary Disease*

Neelima Navuluri, MD, MPH
Pulmonary, Critical Care, and Global Health Fellow
Division of Pulmonary, Allergy, and Critical Care
    Medicine
Department of Medicine
Duke University
Durham, North Carolina
Thoracentesis, Acute Respiratory Distress Syndrome

Saman Nematollahi, MD
Infectious Diseases Fellow
Johns Hopkins University
School of Medicine
Baltimore, Maryland
Cholangitis

G. Titus K. Ngeno, MD
Global Health Fellow
Duke University
Durham, North Carolina
Lower Extremity Edema

Aleksey Novikov, MD
Advanced Endoscopy Fellow
Thomas Jefferson University Hospital
Philadelphia, Pennsylvania
*Gastroesophageal Reflux Disease (GERD) and Barrett
    Esophagus, Biliary Disease*

John I. O'Reilly, MD, MPH
Infectious Diseases Fellow
University of California, Los Angeles
Los Angeles, California
Osteoarthritis

Vedran Oruc, MD
Cardiology Fellow
Division of Cardiovascular Medicine
University of Alabama at Birmingham
Birmingham, Alabama
Atrial Fibrillation

Kinjan Parikh, MD
Cardiology Fellow
NYU Langone Health
New York, New York
Acute Myeloid Leukemia (AML)

Alexandra C. Perel-Winkler, MD
Provincial Health Services Authority
Vancouver, British Columbia
Systemic Lupus Erythematosus

Theodore T. Pierce, MD
Instructor of Radiology
Massachusetts General Hospital
Harvard Medical School
Boston, Massachusetts
*Chest Radiography, CT Scan of the Head, CT Scan
    of the Chest, CT Scan of the Abdomen and Pelvis,
    Abdominal Ultrasound*

Lauren Pischel, MD
Infectious Disease Fellow
Yale University
New Haven, Connecticut
Meningitis

Christopher A. Pumill, MD
Cardiology Fellow
Mount Sinai Hospital
New York, New York
Pulmonary Function Tests (PFTs)

Kartik N. Rajagopalan, MD, PhD
Pulmonary and Critical Care Fellow
New York-Presbyterian Hospital
Columbia University Medical Center
New York, New York
Sleep Apnea

Hannah Roeder, MD, MPH
Neurology Resident
Columbia University Irving Medical Center
New York, New York
Shock

Evan Rosenbaum, MD
Medical Oncology Fellow
Department of Medicine
Memorial Sloan Kettering Cancer Center
New York, New York
Gastric Cancer

Russell Rosenblatt, MD, MS
Assistant Professor of Medicine
Weill Cornell Medicine
New York, New York
Acute Liver Failure, Nonalcoholic Fatty Liver Disease (NAFLD)

Paula Roy-Burman, MD, MPH, DTM&H
Assistant Professor
Department of Medicine
Weill Cornell Medical College
New York, New York
Electrocardiogram (ECG), Pituitary Masses

Jonah Rubin, MD
Internal Medicine Resident
Columbia University Medical Center
New York, New York
Aortic Aneurysm

Monica Saumoy, MD, MS
Assistant Professor
Clinical Medicine
Hospital of the University of Pennsylvania
Philadelphia, Pennsylvania
Gastrointestinal System Anatomy Review, Gastrointestinal System Physiology Review, Achalasia, Acute Pancreatitis

Yecheskel Schneider, MD, MS
Clinical Assistant Professor
Medicine
St Luke's University Health Network
Bethlehem, Pennsylvania
Gastrointestinal System Anatomy Review, Gastrointestinal System Physiology Review, Achalasia, Acute Pancreatitis

Chindhuri Selvadurai, MD
Neurology Resident Physician
Yale New Haven Hospital
New Haven, Connecticut
Altered Mental Status

Shawn L. Shah, MD
Gastroenterology Attending Physician
New York-Presbyterian/Weill Cornell Medical Center
New York, New York
Peptic Ulcer Disease and Helicobacter pylori

Nicole T. Shen, MD
Gastroenterology and Hepatology Fellow
New York-Presbyterian/Weill Cornell Medical Center
New York, New York
Viral Hepatitis, Alcohol-Associated Liver Disease

Zachary Sherman, MD
Chief Medical Resident
Instructor of Medicine
New York-Presbyterian/Weill Cornell Medical College
New York, New York
Irritable Bowel Syndrome

Eliezer Shinnar, MD
Internal Medicine Resident
Columbia University Irving Medical Center
New York, New York
Gastroenteritis

Pranay Sinha, MD
Infectious Diseases Fellow
Boston University
Boston, Massachusetts
Septic Arthritis and Bursitis, Pneumonia

Colin M. Smith, MD
Internal Medicine/Psychiatry Resident
Duke University Hospital
Durham, North Carolina
HIV/AIDS: Infection and Treatment

David B. Snell, MD
Gastroenterology Fellow
NYU Langone Health
New York, New York
Acute Liver Failure

Ashley L. Spann, MD
Research Fellow
Division of Gastroenterology, Hepatology and Nutrition
Department of Medicine
Clinical Informatics Fellow
Department of Biomedical Informatics
Vanderbilt University
Nashville, Tennessee
Pulmonary Hypertension

Toi N. Spates, MD
Fellow in Cardiovascular Disease, PGY-4
Duke University Medical Center
Durham, North Carolina
Elevated Troponin

Maximilian Stahl, MD
Hematology/Oncology Fellow
Memorial Sloan Kettering Cancer Center;
Visiting Fellow
Rockefeller University
New York, New York
*Myelodysplastic Syndromes (MDS), Myeloproliferative
    Neoplasms*

Tyler F. Stewart, MD
Hematology/Oncology Fellow
Yale Cancer Center
New Haven, Connecticut
Thyroid Cancer and Thyroid Nodules

Martin S. Tallman, MD
Leukemia Service
Department of Medicine
Division of Hematologic Malignancies
Memorial Sloan Kettering Cancer Center
New York, New York
*Myelodysplastic Syndromes (MDS), Myeloproliferative
    Neoplasms*

Alice J. Tang, MD
Assistant Professor of Clinical Medicine
Weill Cornell Medical College
New York, New York
Thrombocytopenia

Stephanie J. Tang, MD
Assistant Professor of Medicine
Weill Cornell Medicine
New York, New York
Thrombocytopenia

Beverly G. Tchang, MD
Instructor of Medicine
Division of Endocrinology, Diabetes, and Metabolism
New York-Presbyterian Hospital
Weill Cornell Medical College
New York, New York
Diabetes Mellitus

Sunena Tewani, MD
Assistant Professor
Clinical Medicine
New York-Presbyterian Hospital
Weill Cornell Medical College
New York, New York
Polymyalgia Rheumatica and Temporal Arteritis

Christopher Bentley Traner, MD
Resident Physician
Department of Neurology
Yale School of Medicine
New Haven, Connecticut
Lumbar Puncture

Carol Traynor, MB, BCh BAO
Medical Instructor
Division of Nephrology
Duke University
Durham, North Carolina
Chronic Kidney Disease

Nidhi Tripathi, MD
Cardiovascular Disease Fellow
New York University Langone Health
New York, New York
Mitral Regurgitation

Lauren K. Truby, MD
Cardiovascular Disease Fellow
Duke University Medical Center
Durham, North Carolina
Heart Failure

Bryan M. Tucker, DO, MS
Assistant Professor of Medicine
Department of Medicine
Section of Nephrology
Baylor College of Medicine
Houston, Texas
Glomerulonephritis

Jesse Tucker, MD, MPH
Pulmonary and Critical Care Physician
CHI Memorial Buz Standefer Lung Center
Chattanooga, Tennessee
Asthma

Daniel J. Turner, MD
Pulmonary and Critical Care Fellow
Duke University Medical Center
Durham, North Carolina
Sepsis

Natalie F. Uy, MD
Internal Medicine Resident
Yale New Haven Hospital
New Haven, Connecticut
Acute Myeloid Leukemia (AML)

Anthony Valeri, MD
Professor of Medicine
Department of Medicine
Columbia University
Medical Director
DaVita-Haven Dialysis Center
New York, New York;
Medical Director
Workman's Circle Multicare Center Dialysis
Bronx, New York
Hyperkalemia and Hypokalemia, Urinalysis, Renal Replacement Therapy

Merilyn S. Varghese, MD
Cardiology Fellow
Beth Israel Deaconess Medical Center
Boston, Massachusetts
Hypertension

Abhirami Vivekanandarajah, MD
Attending Physician
Hematology/Oncology
Advantage Care Physicians
Staten Island University Hospital
Richmond University Medical Center
New York, New York
Hematuria, Chronic Lymphocytic Leukemia (CLL)

Hao Xie, MD, PhD
Instructor of Medicine and Oncology
Division of Medical Oncology
Mayo Clinic
Rochester, Minnesota
Melanoma

Jessica Yang, MD
Assistant Attending
Memorial Sloan Kettering Cancer Center
New York, New York
Colorectal Cancer (CRC)

George S. A. Yankey, Jr., MD
Cardiology Fellow
Duke University Medical Center
Durham, North Carolina
Cardiac Murmurs

Michele Yeung, MD
Instructor of Medicine
Division of Endocrinology, Diabetes, and Metabolism
Weill Cornell Medicine
New York, New York
Thyroid and Parathyroid Glands Anatomy and Physiology Review

Pauline B. Yi, MD
Clinical Instructor
University of California, Los Angeles
Los Angeles, California
Gout

Jae Hee Yun, MD
Assistant Professor
University of Virginia School of Medicine
Charlottesville, Virginia
Systemic Sclerosis

Fangfei Zheng, MD
Assistant Professor of Clinical Medicine
Weill Cornell Medical College
New York, New York
Urinary System Physiology Review

Sharon Zhuo, MD
Assistant Professor of Medicine
New York-Presbyterian/Columbia University Irving Medical Center
New York, New York
Central Venous Catheterization

Kahli E. Zietlow, MD
Clinical Assistant Professor
Division of Geriatric and Palliative Medicine
Department of Medicine
Michigan Medicine
University of Michigan
Ann Arbor, Michigan
Osteoporosis

Contents

CHAPTER 1

Headache

CHRISTOPHER R. KELLY

INTRODUCTION

Headache is a common symptom that can take many forms and occurs either as a primary phenomenon or secondary to an underlying medical condition. Headache is considered chronic when it occurs during more than 15 days per month for at least 3 consecutive months.

According to the *International Classification of Headache Disorders,* Third Edition, **primary headaches** include tension-type headaches, migraine headaches, and trigeminal autonomic cephalalgias (e.g., cluster headaches). **Secondary headaches,** meanwhile, occur in the setting of trauma (e.g., whiplash injury, epidural or subdural hematoma), vascular disorders (e.g., ischemic stroke, subarachnoid or intracerebral hemorrhage, aneurysm, arteritis), nonvascular disorders (e.g., abnormal intracranial pressure, tumor, seizure), substance use, infection (e.g., meningitis), metabolic disorder, disease of cranial structures (e.g., rhinosinusitis, glaucoma, temporomandibular joint disorder), psychiatric disorder, or painful cranial neuropathies and other facial pains (e.g., trigeminal neuralgia).

EVALUATION

The principal focus of an effective headache history and exam is determining the likelihood that a patient has a primary versus secondary headache syndrome.

Obtain a history that includes the timing and speed of headache onset, chronicity, location and laterality, nature (e.g., throbbing or steady, sharp or dull), severity, associated symptoms (e.g., weakness, vision loss, nausea, photophobia, phonophobia, osmophobia [aversion to strong smells], and scalp allodynia/hypersensitivity), presence of aura (e.g., sensory disturbances preceding/heralding headache onset), exacerbating/mitigating factors (psychosocial stressors, irregular habits [including sleep patterns and caffeine intake]), and use of any analgesic medications (especially NSAIDs, caffeine, and opiates). Check vital signs and perform a complete neurological exam.

If the patient reports the headache is the worst ever experienced and that it reached maximum intensity within 60 seconds of onset (i.e., "thunderclap" headache), then intracranial hemorrhage should be ruled out with an emergent CT scan. If the CT scan is negative but concern for hemorrhage remains high, a lumbar puncture should be performed to assay the cerebrospinal fluid (CSF) for abnormal erythrocyte counts and/or xanthochromia (discoloration of centrifuged CSF by lysed erythrocytes).

Patients with the following alarm features or "red flags" also generally warrant neuroimaging (with MRI preferred over CT): alteration or loss of consciousness, exacerbation of symptoms with Valsalva maneuver, immunosuppression (e.g., HIV, cancer), abnormal neurological examination findings (e.g., papilledema, cranial neuropathy, or focal weakness/numbness), pain severe enough to awaken the patient from sleep, significant change from prior headaches, age over 50 years, and new daily persistent headache.

DIFFERENTIAL DIAGNOSIS AND TREATMENT

If alarm features are absent or neuroimaging is unremarkable, diagnose the headache subtype according to its clinical features. A review of the many causes of secondary headache is beyond the scope of this chapter; however, some of the common conditions that present with headache as the predominant symptom are reviewed here.

Primary Headaches (Fig. 1.1)

Migraine headache is the most common type of primary headache among those seeking medical attention. Its numerous clinical features (see Fig. 1.1) can be severe

1

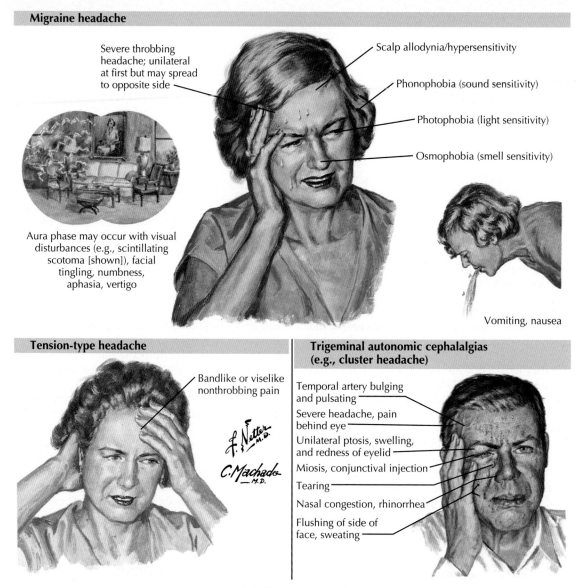

Migraine headache

Severe throbbing headache; unilateral at first but may spread to opposite side

Scalp allodynia/hypersensitivity

Phonophobia (sound sensitivity)

Photophobia (light sensitivity)

Osmophobia (smell sensitivity)

Aura phase may occur with visual disturbances (e.g., scintillating scotoma [shown]), facial tingling, numbness, aphasia, vertigo

Vomiting, nausea

Tension-type headache

Bandlike or viselike nonthrobbing pain

Trigeminal autonomic cephalalgias (e.g., cluster headache)

Temporal artery bulging and pulsating

Severe headache, pain behind eye

Unilateral ptosis, swelling, and redness of eyelid

Miosis, conjunctival injection

Tearing

Nasal congestion, rhinorrhea

Flushing of side of face, sweating

FIG. 1.1 **Primary Headaches.**

and debilitating. About one-third of patients experience **aura,** a sensory experience that precedes or accompanies the headache, typically developing over at least 5 minutes but not lasting more than 60 minutes. Some patients with migraine may experience aura without headache. Migraines generally begin in adolescence and recur with variable frequency. They are more common in women and may occur more frequently during or around menstruation (**catamenial** migraines). Fatigue, stress,

certain foods, strong smells, and even changes in weather can also trigger attacks.

Patients should treat migraines as early as possible with abortive therapies—the most effective being acetaminophen, NSAIDs, and/or triptans. Patients with intractable vomiting can use nasal or subcutaneous triptans. Patients with the most severe symptoms or with refractory symptoms (termed **status migrainosus** when lasting more than 72 hours) should receive intravenous metoclopramide (given with diphenhydramine to avoid dystonic reactions), valproic acid, or ketorolac. Intravenous dihydroergotamine is effective if these initial medications fail. Opioids and barbiturates are usually avoided. Of note, frequent use (>8–10 days per month) of acetaminophen or NSAIDs can lead to **medication overuse headache.**

Patients who have 5 or more days with migraines per month, at least 1 day of debilitating symptoms leading to loss of productivity, or a poor response to abortive therapies should be offered preventative therapies. Hundreds of medications have been proposed for migraine prophylaxis, but few have been sufficiently studied to definitively determine efficacy. Nonetheless, first-line options include β-blockers (propranolol, metoprolol, timolol), antidepressants (amitriptyline, nortriptyline, venlafaxine, duloxetine), calcium channel blockers (verapamil), and antiepileptics (topiramate, valproic acid, gabapentin, and zonisamide). Other nutraceuticals have been proposed as having a role in migraine prevention, including riboflavin. Patients with chronic migraine (>15 episodes per month) may also benefit from botulinum toxin injections around the head and neck.

Tension-type headache (TTH) causes steady, nonthrobbing, bandlike, and bilateral pain, often improving with activity and not associated with other symptoms. TTH is the most common type of headache; however, many patients do not seek medical attention. Fatigue and stress are common triggers. Treat with NSAIDs and/or acetaminophen; multimodal therapies focusing on stress reduction and physical therapy (including massage) should be considered in patients with chronic TTH, which can be debilitating.

Finally, **trigeminal autonomic cephalalgias** cause unilateral pain and autonomic phenomena (including lacrimation, ptosis, miosis, rhinorrhea, and/or diaphoresis). The various types—which include cluster headaches, paroxysmal hemicranias, hemicranias continua, and short unilateral neuralgiform headache with conjunctival irritation and tearing (SUNCT)—are generally distinguished from one another based on episode duration and frequency.

Cluster headaches last between 15 and 180 minutes and can recur up to eight times per day, with pain-free intervals. As the name suggests, attacks occur in temporal clusters, sometimes remitting for months or years. They are much more common in men than in women. In rare cases cluster headaches occur secondary to an underlying tumor or vascular anomaly; therefore affected patients should undergo MRI. See Chapter 109 for further details. If imaging is normal, patients can take medications to both abort and prevent headaches. Acute attacks should be aborted with 100% inhaled oxygen and/or subcutaneous sumatriptan. Preventative medications include verapamil and lithium. Patients with refractory, debilitating cluster headache may benefit from intravenous dihydroergotamine, suboccipital steroid injections, or an occipital nerve stimulator.

Paroxysmal hemicrania causes attacks that are shorter (2–30 minutes) and more frequent (5–40 times per day) than cluster headache. Hemicrania continua causes milder but more continuous symptoms without pain-free intervals. SUNCT causes even briefer attacks (seconds to minutes) that recur frequently, sometimes over 100 times per day. Paroxysmal hemicrania and hemicrania continua can be aborted and prevented using indomethacin. SUNCT is more difficult to treat but may respond to lamotrigine.

Secondary Headaches

Pseudotumor cerebri (idiopathic intracranial hypertension [IIH]) (Fig. 1.2) refers to increased intracranial pressure in the absence of a structural cause, such as tumor or venous sinus thrombosis, or another predisposing condition (e.g., acute hepatic failure, hypercarbia, hypertensive crisis). The headache lacks specific features, but some patients also have retrobulbar, neck, and/or back pain. Most cases occur in obese women. Because of compression of the optic and abducens nerves, some patients report visual disturbances (blurred vision, transient shadows, or black spots) and/or diplopia. On examination nearly all patients have papilledema (bilateral disc swelling, as opposed to papillitis, which is typically inflammatory and unilateral). All patients suspected of having IIH should be urgently referred to a neurologist and ophthalmologist, as well as undergo MRI with MR venography to assess for secondary causes. Increased opening pressure on lumbar puncture (≥25 cm H_2O), coupled with normal CSF composition, is diagnostic. Treatment is essential to prevent vision loss. Weight loss is the best way to alleviate symptoms but is often unsuccessful; bariatric surgery has been successful when conservative nutritional approaches fail. Acetazolamide decreases CSF production and intracranial pressure. Patients with persistent symptoms may require invasive management, such as optic nerve defenestration and/or a ventricular shunt.

Temporal arteritis (giant cell arteritis) causes unilateral, temporal headache associated with pain while eating or talking (**jaw** or **tongue claudication**), marked scalp tenderness (e.g., when combing hair), and eventually vision loss. It almost always occurs in patients older than 50 years and can be a systemic, life-threatening

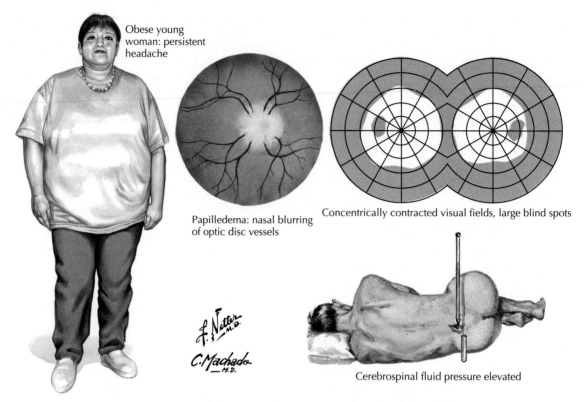

Obese young woman: persistent headache

Papilledema: nasal blurring of optic disc vessels

Concentrically contracted visual fields, large blind spots

Cerebrospinal fluid pressure elevated

FIG. 1.2 **Pseudotumor Cerebri (Idiopathic Intracranial Hypertension).**

disease. Patients may also have constitutional symptoms, such as fever or weight loss, and/or ipsilateral vision disturbances. The underlying disease process is inflammation of the temporal artery and other branches of the external carotid artery, as well as the extracranial branches of the internal carotid artery (including the ophthalmic artery). Diagnosis and treatment must be prompt to prevent irreversible vision loss. Recent pathological studies suggest substantial overlap with varicella zoster infections, although the role of antiviral treatments remains uncertain.

Trigeminal neuralgia (not to be confused with the trigeminal autonomic cephalalgias described earlier) causes severe, stabbing/electric, unilateral attacks of facial pain in the trigeminal nerve distribution, usually the maxillary (V2) or mandibular (V3) branches, provoked by touching or moving the face (e.g., talking, eating, shaving). Attacks last only seconds but can occur in rapid succession. Remissions are unpredictable but can last for days or even months. Some cases can be attributed to a specific disorder of the trigeminal nerve root causing demyelination (i.e., multiple sclerosis) or compression (i.e., vascular abnormality). Thus patients with trigeminal neuralgia should undergo MRI, including vascular imaging, to assess for secondary causes. If none is found, treat with carbamazepine. If symptoms do not remit, add a second-line agent (e.g., lamotrigine, gabapentin, baclofen, clonazepam). If there is still no response, ablative gamma-knife radiosurgery or surgical microvascular decompression of the trigeminal nerve may provide relief.

CHAPTER 2

Dizziness

CHRISTOPHER R. KELLY

INTRODUCTION

Dizziness is a nonspecific term generally used by patients to refer to one of three phenomena: presyncope, vertigo, or disequilibrium (Fig. 2.1). **Presyncope** is the sensation of lightheadedness that occurs secondary to cerebral hypoperfusion. **Vertigo** is the hallucination of movement secondary to vestibular dysfunction. It can reflect peripheral vestibular dysfunction or, far less often, a brain or brainstem lesion. **Disequilibrium** is an unstable gait secondary to many possible causes, such as impaired proprioception or vision. In some cases, a specific cause for dizziness will not be apparent despite a thorough evaluation.

EVALUATION

Attempt to clarify if the patient has presyncope, vertigo, or disequilibrium, then inquire about associated symptoms and perform a physical examination.

Patients with presyncope usually describe nearly fainting, or feeling lightheaded or weak. Determine if the symptoms are positional (e.g., when getting up from a chair) or situational (e.g., after physical exertion). Inquire about palpitations, including whether they precede or follow other symptoms. Measure heart rate and blood pressure in the supine, sitting, and then erect positions. Following each change in position, check the blood pressure at least once per minute until it nadirs. Auscultate the heart and obtain a 12-lead electrocardiogram (ECG). If the cardiac examination is abnormal, or if the patient reports that symptoms worsen with physical exertion, obtain an echocardiogram. If the patient has frequent symptoms but there is no evidence of structural disease and the resting ECG is normal, screen for arrhythmias using an outpatient ECG event recorder.

Patients with vertigo, meanwhile, describe a spinning or tilting sensation often associated with nausea and an unstable posture. Head movement exacerbates this sensation; unlike with orthostatic hypotension, however, symptoms occur even when head movement is in a supine plane and cerebral perfusion is unchanged. Perform a complete review of symptoms, asking specifically about hearing loss, tinnitus, and any other neurological symptoms. Perform a complete neurological exam. Look carefully for the presence of nystagmus (a rhythmic beating of the eyes during gaze movement). Horizontal nystagmus that extinguishes with visual fixation supports a peripheral cause of vertigo. Nystagmus that changes directions with gaze or has a primarily vertical or torsional component is more suggestive of a central cause.

Provocative head movements can help establish the cause of vertigo. An abnormal head thrust test (i.e., the patient cannot maintain visual fixation after sudden head movement) indicates peripheral vestibular dysfunction. Nystagmus during the Dix-Hallpike maneuver (Fig. 2.2) supports benign paroxysmal positional vertigo (BPPV) related to the posterior semicircular canal (the most commonly affected of the three semicircular canals). If there is concern for a central cause of vertigo, or the patient has multiple risk factors for stroke, obtain an MRI. Additional tests, such as electronystagmography, audiometry, and caloric testing, may be helpful in patients with chronic, unexplained vertigo.

Finally, patients with disequilibrium experience symptoms only when ambulating, standing, and in some cases sitting, and sometimes only with more challenging maneuvers, such as turning or navigating stairs. There are many possible causes; therefore perform a complete neurological and joint examination that includes a careful assessment of gait. Patients with dizziness associated with disequilibrium may demonstrate wide-based gait, listing, or leaning to one side.

Patients with subjective dizziness but no other specific symptoms should be assessed for other potential causes, such as medication side effects, psychiatric/somatic symptoms, or toxic ingestions, including of alcohol.

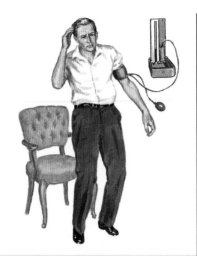 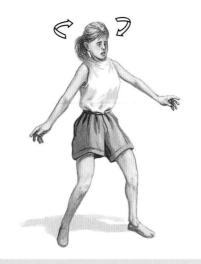 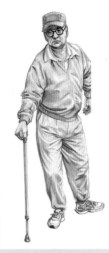

Presyncope (cerebral hypoperfusion)	Vertigo	Disequilibrium
Orthostatic hypotension	Peripheral	Neuropathy
Tachyarrhythmia	Benign paroxysmal positional vertigo (BPPV)	Joint disease
Bradyarrhythmia	Meniere disease	Weakness
Severe aortic stenosis	Vestibular neuritis	Impaired vision
Hypertrophic cardiomyopathy	Perilymphatic fistula	Movement disorder
Myocardial infarction	Herpes zoster oticus	
Severe heart failure	Otitis media	
Pulmonary embolus	Central	
Vasovagal reaction	Migraine	
Bilateral carotid or basilar artery stenosis	Multiple sclerosis	
	Temporal lobe epilepsy	
	Stroke	
	Acoustic neuroma	

FIG. 2.1 **Major Causes of Dizziness.**

DIAGNOSIS AND TREATMENT

The most common cause of presyncope is **orthostatic hypotension,** or failure of the autonomic system to augment cardiac output when rising to a standing position. It can be diagnosed when the systolic blood pressure (BP) falls by ≥20 mm Hg, or the diastolic BP by ≥10 mm Hg, within 3 minutes of an upright posture. Orthostatic hypotension can occur secondary to volume depletion (e.g., poor oral intake, excessive diuretic use, gastrointestinal bleeding) or autonomic dysfunction (e.g., diabetic neuropathy, parkinsonian disorders, β-blocker use). The best strategy is to address the underlying cause. If no fixable cause can be identified, some patients experience relief with supportive measures, such as compression stockings or abdominal binders. Medication options include midodrine, which increases vascular tone, and/or fludrocortisone, which can expand intravascular volume. The other causes of presyncope usually become evident during the cardiac evaluation and are discussed in detail in separate chapters.

A detailed review of the many causes of vertigo is outside the scope of this book; however, the most common diagnoses are BPPV, Meniere disease, and vestibular neuritis.

BPPV, the most common cause of vertigo overall, is confirmed if the patient briefly experiences vertigo and nystagmus during provocative head movements, such as the Dix-Hallpike maneuver. It is caused by a process known as canalithiasis (or cupulolithiasis), in which otoconia (calcium carbonate crystals) become dislodged and deposit in the cupulae of the semicircular canals or in the utricle. The process can occur spontaneously or after head trauma. The otoconia have a higher specific gravity than endolymph; thus, when head motion occurs, the otoconia cause tonic stimulation of the affected structure, which is perceived as continued movement (usually rotational).

The primary treatment is a repositioning maneuver that steers the otoconia out of the affected structure (Fig. 2.3). Such manipulations are so simple and effective

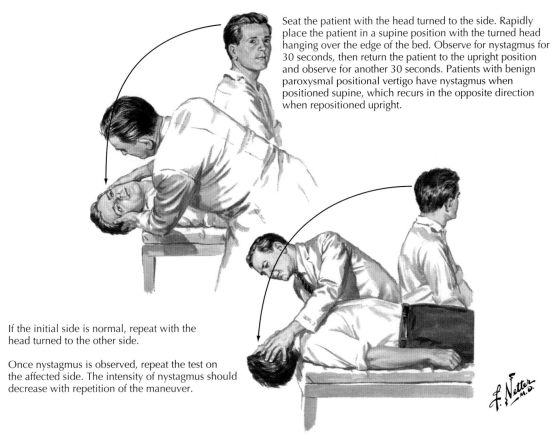

Seat the patient with the head turned to the side. Rapidly place the patient in a supine position with the turned head hanging over the edge of the bed. Observe for nystagmus for 30 seconds, then return the patient to the upright position and observe for another 30 seconds. Patients with benign paroxysmal positional vertigo have nystagmus when positioned supine, which recurs in the opposite direction when repositioned upright.

If the initial side is normal, repeat with the head turned to the other side.

Once nystagmus is observed, repeat the test on the affected side. The intensity of nystagmus should decrease with repetition of the maneuver.

FIG. 2.2 **Dix-Hallpike Maneuver (for Benign Paroxysmal Positional Vertigo of the Posterior Semicircular Canal).**

that they may be performed even when the diagnosis of BPPV is uncertain. For many patients, these maneuvers substantially accelerate resolution of symptoms. Even without them, however, patients often achieve spontaneous remission within weeks. A small number have persistent symptoms and may require more advanced interventions, such as surgical occlusion of the affected semicircular canal.

Meniere disease is the likely diagnosis in a patient with intermittent vertigo, fluctuating low-frequency sensorineural hearing loss, and tinnitus. Many patients also describe the sensation of aural fullness. Vestibular and audiometric testing should be performed to assess the severity of the deficits. An MRI should be obtained to rule out lesions of the vestibulocochlear nerve (e.g., multiple sclerosis, acoustic neuroma). If Meniere disease is the likely diagnosis, treat with salt restriction and diuretics to reduce endolymphatic pressure.

Vestibular rehabilitation is often helpful. In refractory cases, refer to an otolaryngologist for consideration of more advanced therapies (e.g., surgical endolymphatic decompression).

Vestibular neuritis causes severe, continuous vertigo and is thought to represent viral infection of the vestibular system. It is sometimes preceded by or associated with symptoms of upper respiratory infection and thus may be a postinfectious inflammatory process. There is no specific diagnostic test, and neuroimaging is often obtained to rule out central disease. The condition improves on its own, though steroids may shorten the time to recovery.

Acute attacks of vertigo, regardless of the cause, can be treated with meclizine (an antihistamine) and/or scopolamine (an anticholinergic). More severe attacks can be treated with diazepam and antiemetics (e.g., promethazine, metoclopramide).

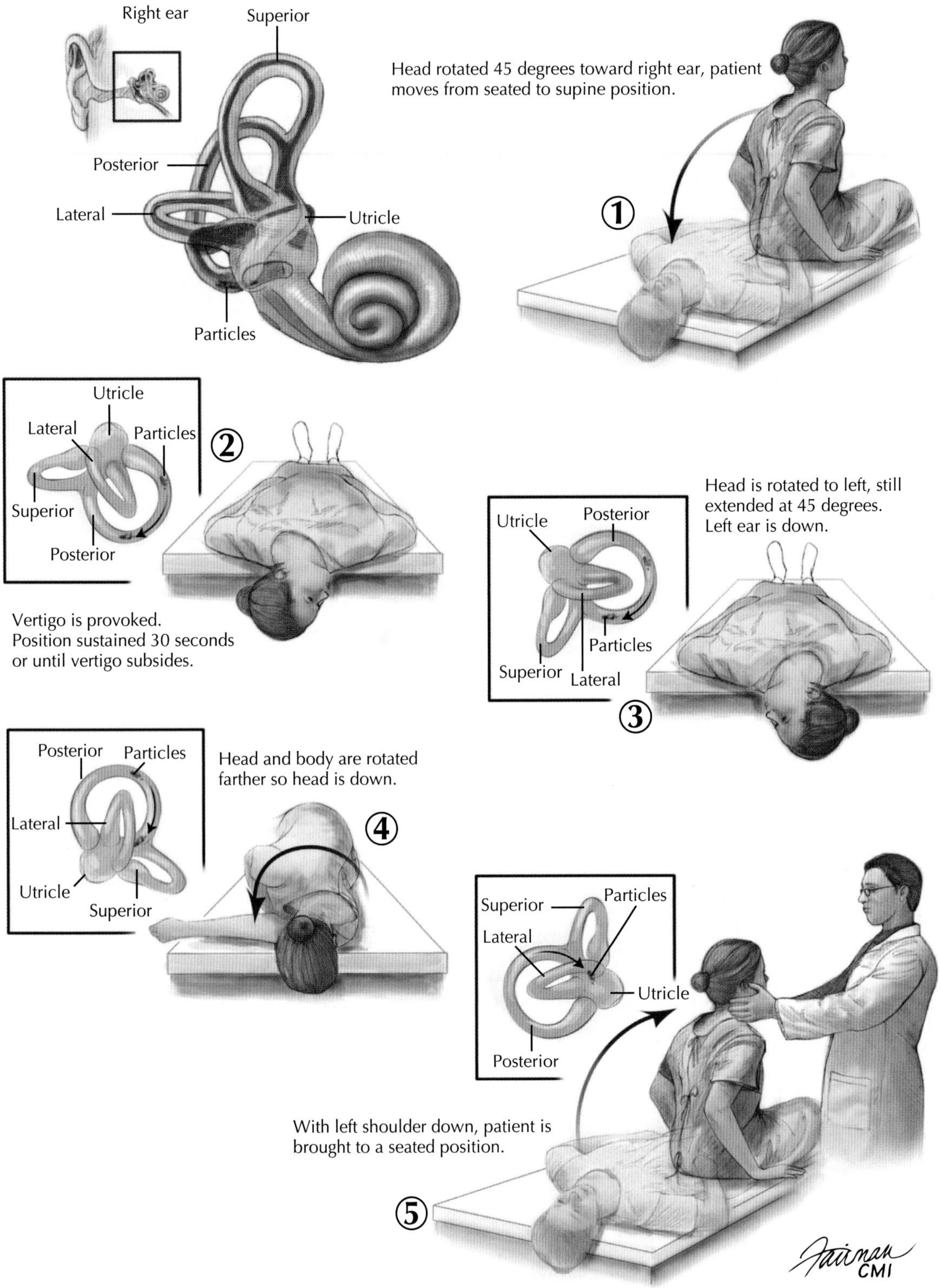

Right ear   Superior

Head rotated 45 degrees toward right ear, patient moves from seated to supine position.

Posterior

Lateral   Utricle

Particles

①

Utricle

Lateral   Particles

②

Superior

Posterior

Vertigo is provoked.
Position sustained 30 seconds or until vertigo subsides.

Head is rotated to left, still extended at 45 degrees. Left ear is down.

Utricle   Posterior

Particles

Superior   Lateral

③

Posterior   Particles

Head and body are rotated farther so head is down.

Lateral

④

Utricle   Superior

Superior   Particles

Lateral

Utricle

Posterior

With left shoulder down, patient is brought to a seated position.

⑤

Jairman
CMI

FIG. 2.3 **Canalith Repositioning (Epley Maneuver).**

CHAPTER 3

Cough

CHRISTOPHER R. KELLY

INTRODUCTION

Cough is a common symptom with many potential causes. The differential diagnosis begins with a determination of symptom chronicity. Cough is considered **acute** when it has been present for less than 3 weeks. Major causes of acute cough include viral or bacterial respiratory tract infections, such as rhinosinusitis, pharyngitis, bronchitis, and pneumonia; acute exacerbations of chronic diseases, such as chronic obstructive pulmonary disease (COPD), asthma, heart failure, and bronchiectasis; and environmental exposures (e.g., pollen, fumes).

Cough is considered **subacute** when it has been present for 3 to 8 weeks. Most cases are postinfectious, occurring in the context of a recent upper respiratory infection. In this setting cough results primarily from postnasal mucous drip, also known as upper airway cough syndrome (UACS); other contributing factors may include bronchial hyperresponsiveness and impaired mucociliary clearance.

Cough is considered **chronic** when it lasts for more than 8 weeks (Fig. 3.1). Causes include UACS, gastroesophageal reflux disease (GERD)/laryngopharyngeal reflux (LPR), ACE inhibitor use, asthma, nonasthmatic eosinophilic bronchitis (NAEB), bronchiectasis, COPD, chronic lung infection (e.g., tuberculosis), chronic microaspiration, lung cancer, and irritation of the external auditory canal.

EVALUATION

Determine the timeline along with any precipitants (e.g., cold air, pollen); symptoms, including constitutional symptoms (fever, chills, night sweats), upper respiratory symptoms (rhinorrhea, congestion, frequent throat-clearing), heart failure symptoms (orthopnea, paroxysmal nocturnal dyspnea, lower extremity edema), chest pain, dyspnea, wheezing, and dyspepsia/heartburn; whether family members of coworkers have had similar symptoms; smoking history; use of ACE inhibitors; and all medical comorbidities.

Measure vital signs, including peripheral oxygen saturation. Examine the nares and mouth for signs of inflammation, such as enlarged nasal turbinates, enlarged tonsils, nasopharyngeal secretions, and pharyngitis. Auscultate the heart and lungs. Evaluate the extremities for clubbing and edema.

Consider chest imaging in cases of chronic cough, immune compromise, signs of lower respiratory tract infection (i.e., fever, tachypnea, tachycardia, adventitious breath sounds), or signs of malignancy (i.e., digit clubbing, hemoptysis). Start with posteroanterior (PA) and lateral chest x-rays. If the x-rays raise concern for serious illness—such as malignancy, opportunistic infection, or interstitial lung disease—or if the patient does not respond to treatment for a presumptive diagnosis, obtain a noncontrast CT scan of the chest.

DIAGNOSIS AND TREATMENT
Acute Cough

A patient with acute cough, no underlying history of chronic heart or lung disease, and no identifiable trigger (e.g., pollen, fumes) likely has **acute viral rhinosinusitis** or **bronchitis.** Supportive treatment with a combination first-generation antihistamine and decongestant (e.g., pseudoephedrine) may improve cough symptoms. Newer generation (nonsedating) antihistamines are less effective. NSAIDs (e.g., naproxen) may help with overall symptoms, but the evidence for an effect on cough specifically is uncertain. Patients with significant wheezing may benefit from inhaled short-acting β_2 agonists (e.g., albuterol).

Antibiotics are generally not indicated for acute upper respiratory infections in the absence of chronic lung disease, even in the minority of patients with bacterial infection, since symptoms usually resolve on their own. An exception to this rule is patients with a likely *Bordetella pertussis* infection, also known as whooping cough. Patients can be presumptively diagnosed with whooping cough when they have paroxysms of coughing associated with posttussive vomiting and an inspiratory whooping sound. A nasopharyngeal culture confirms the diagnosis. Macrolides are the treatment of choice.

A patient with acute cough, signs of systemic infection (fever, tachypnea, tachycardia), and/or an abnormal chest

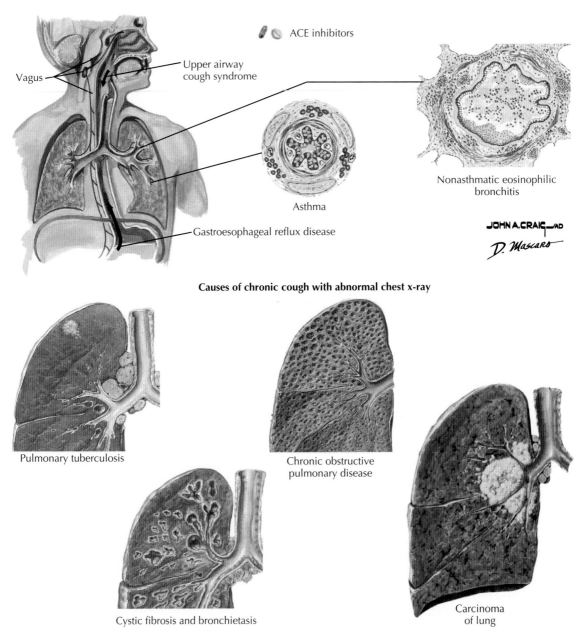

ACE inhibitors

Upper airway cough syndrome

Vagus

Nonasthmatic eosinophilic bronchitis

Asthma

Gastroesophageal reflux disease

JOHN A. CRAIG—AD

D. Mascaro

Causes of chronic cough with abnormal chest x-ray

Pulmonary tuberculosis

Chronic obstructive pulmonary disease

Cystic fibrosis and bronchietasis

Carcinoma of lung

FIG. 3.1 **Major Causes of Chronic Cough.**

x-ray should be presumptively treated for pneumonia (see Chapter 114). If the symptoms do not improve within 1 week of antibiotic therapy, obtain a noncontrast CT scan of the chest to assess for infectious complications (e.g., lung abscess) or noninfectious etiologies (e.g., malignancy).

Subacute or Chronic Cough

A patient with subacute cough and no other evidence of systemic illness should initially be treated for UACS with a combination of first-generation antihistamines and decongestants. Patients with symptoms of rhinitis (i.e., rhinorrhea, sneezing) should receive intranasal glucocorticoids.

Patients with chronic cough, normal chest imaging, and no ongoing smoking or ACE inhibitor use most likely have UACS, asthma, NAEB, or GERD (see Fig. 3.1). The clinical history and physical examination often help differentiate one condition from another. For example, a patient with cough and wheeze, especially if associated with specific triggers (e.g., cold air, animal dander, exhaust fumes), most likely has asthma. Meanwhile a patient with cough that is worse after meals or when supine likely has GERD.

If one diagnosis appears no more likely than the others, however, the general strategy is to pursue them in sequence until the cough resolves. First, treat UACS for at least 2 to 3 weeks, as described earlier. If the cough does not improve, obtain spirometry prebronchodilators and postbronchodilators to assess for asthma. If spirometry is unremarkable, consider a methacholine inhalational challenge test, which can demonstrate bronchial hyperresponsiveness that would be consistent with asthma. If these tests are abnormal or unobtainable, treat empirically with an inhaled, short-acting β_2 agonist (e.g., albuterol).

If cough persists and asthma is unlikely, next assess for NAEB by inducing sputum for eosinophils. If the sputum eosinophil count is elevated, prescribe oral steroids. If cough still persists, then NAEB is unlikely, and the next step is to attempt empirical therapy for GERD using a proton-pump inhibitor (e.g., omeprazole or esomeprazole). If cough still persists, obtain 24-hour esophageal pH monitoring to definitively rule out GERD (since empirical therapy may have been ineffective). If UACS, asthma, NAEB, and GERD are all effectively ruled out, evaluate for uncommon causes of cough by obtaining a noncontrast CT scan of the chest and referring to a specialist.

CHAPTER 4

Sore Throat

CHRISTOPHER R. KELLY

INTRODUCTION

Sore throat is a common symptom that almost always reflects infection of the pharynx (i.e., pharyngitis). In adults, pharyngitis is usually from viral infection, but it is important to consider other possible causes (Fig. 4.1).

EVALUATION

Inquire about the chronicity and laterality of the pain, including any radiation to the ears or neck; other symptoms of upper respiratory tract infection, including fever, conjunctivitis, rhinorrhea, nasal congestion, sinus pain, and cough; changes in voice; excessive drooling; difficulty swallowing (dysphagia); and dyspnea. Determine if the patient has had sick household or work contacts.

Measure the respiratory rate and check peripheral oxygen saturation. Carefully examine the oropharynx and tonsils for erythema, ulceration, swelling, deformation, and pooling of secretions. Palpate the lymph nodes of the head and neck. Auscultate the lungs for stridor (a high-pitched inspiratory breath sound), which would indicate partial airway obstruction.

DIAGNOSIS AND MANAGEMENT

In rare cases, sore throat can be the first sign of or precursor to a life-threatening condition. Patients with sore throat and signs of systemic infection (e.g., fever, tachycardia, hypotension, tachypnea) may have a **deep neck space** (e.g., **retropharyngeal, parapharyngeal, submandibular**) infection, which mandates intravenous antibiotics and emergent, contrast-enhanced CT imaging of the neck. These patients may require exploration or drainage of the infectious collection. Meanwhile patients with sore throat who have a muffled voice and respiratory distress may have **severe epiglottitis** and require emergency evaluation by an otolaryngologist.

A patient who is more clinically stable can generally be diagnosed based on the history and physical examination. Most patients will describe sore throat associated with other features suggestive of upper respiratory infection, such as fever, nasal congestion, and cough; these patients have viral pharyngitis and require only reassurance, symptom control, and follow-up. Menthol-containing lozenges are popular and readily available; however, lidocaine or benzocaine lozenges are more effective. Acetaminophen and/or NSAIDs can be used alongside lozenges.

In stable patients without evidence of upper respiratory infection, the main task is determining the likelihood of bacterial pharyngitis. Most cases of bacterial pharyngitis are due to **group A streptococcus** (GAS). The likelihood of GAS infection is determined using the **Centor score**, which assigns 1 point for each of the following features: fever (including by report), absence of cough, tender anterior cervical lymphadenopathy, and tonsillar exudates.

Patients with 0 to 2 points are not likely to have GAS infection and should not receive antibiotics. Patients with 3 or 4 points are more likely to have GAS infection and should undergo a rapid antigen detection test (if available) and/or throat culture. If microbiological data support GAS infection, antibiotics are generally prescribed to reduce both contagion and the risk of poststreptococcal complications, such as peritonsillar abscess and acute rheumatic fever. Penicillin or amoxicillin is effective.

Most other cases of pharyngitis will resolve without intervention or end up being treated with antibiotics because of symptoms resembling GAS infection. A minority of patients will have persistent symptoms, or symptoms that point to a specific cause.

Peritonsillar abscess (also known as quinsy) may complicate bacterial pharyngitis and cause fever, sore throat, muffled voice, and a markedly enlarged, fluctuant tonsil. Some patients also experience trismus (i.e., lockjaw, secondary to inflammation of the internal pterygoid muscle), neck swelling/pain, and/or ear pain. Patients require prompt antibiotics and abscess drainage.

Epiglottitis can result from infection with many different pathogens, the most common being *Haemophilus influenzae*. It can present with respiratory distress, as mentioned, or with more subacute symptoms, including fever, sore throat, muffled voice, drooling, and stridor. Patients may also have tenderness on palpation around

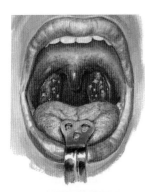

Infectious Pharyngitis

Viral
- Adenovirus
- Rhinovirus
- Coronavirus
- Herpes simplex virus
- Coxsackievirus
- Influenza
- Epstein-Barr virus
- Human immunodeficiency virus
  (acute infection)

Bacterial
- *Streptococcus* spp. (especially group A)
- *Corynebacterium diphtheriae*
- *Fusobacterium necrophorum*
- *Chlamydia pneumoniae*
- *Mycoplasma pneumoniae*
- *Neisseria gonorrhoeae*

Fungal
- *Candida*

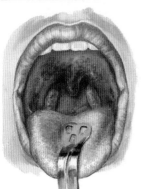

Noninfectious Pharyngitis

- Dehumidified air
- Laryngopharyngeal reflux
- Allergies
- Smoking

Malignancy

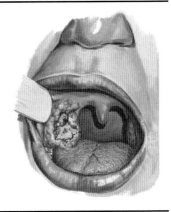

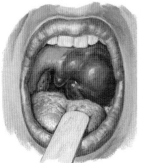

Infections/Abscessess of Adjacent Structures

- Peritonsillar abscess *(shown)*
- Epiglottitis
- Submandibular infection
- Retropharyngeal infection

FIG. 4.1 Differential Diagnosis of Sore Throat.

---

the hyoid bone. If the diagnosis seems possible, obtain blood cultures, administer antibiotics, and obtain an emergent lateral neck radiograph to assess for swelling of the epiglottis and aryepiglottic folds. Consult an otolaryngologist to assess the degree of airway obstruction and potential need for intubation. Steroids may reduce airway inflammation, though the evidence is mixed. Admit the patient to a closely monitored setting even if the airway is not initially compromised.

Diphtheria, or infection with *Corynebacterium diphtheriae,* is an uncommon infection in the era of vaccination but may still be encountered, especially in travelers to developing countries or patients who have not been vaccinated. Symptoms include fever, cervical lymphadenopathy, sore throat, pharyngeal erythema, and gray tonsillopharyngeal exudates that coalesce to form so-called pseudomembranes, which adhere to the mucosa and bleed when scraped. In some patients the pseudomembranes may extend to (or be located primarily in) the larynx, causing cough and dysphonia. In severe cases the bacteria release a toxin that can cause myocarditis and neuropathy. Treat with antibiotics (usually erythromycin or penicillin) and, in severe cases, antitoxin.

Fusobacterium necrophorum pharyngitis can cause septic thrombophlebitis of the internal jugular vein by local extension, a phenomenon known as **Lemierre syndrome.** Affected patients are typically septic and may have tenderness or overt inflammation overlying the jugular vein. Respiratory symptoms may occur secondary to septic pulmonary thromboemboli. The diagnosis is established by demonstrating bacteremia and thrombosis of the jugular vein (using ultrasound or contrast-enhanced CT). Treat with ampicillin-sulbactam or piperacillin-tazobactam. The role of anticoagulation is uncertain.

Candida pharyngitis, or **thrush,** is not inherently dangerous but can signal the presence of an underlying immunocompromising state, such as HIV or uncontrolled diabetes; however, it can also result from more benign phenomena, such as inhaled corticosteroid use, antibiotic use, or xerostomia (dry mouth). Affected patients have white pseudomembranes on their palate, tongue, pharynx, and/or tonsils; in more severe cases the larynx and esophagus are affected. Treat with oral nystatin solution for mild cases and fluconazole for more severe or refractory cases.

Laryngopharyngeal reflux (LPR), or reflux of gastric contents into the laryngopharynx, is similar to gastroesophageal reflux disease (GERD) in that there is abnormal passage of material from the stomach through the lower esophageal sphincter; however, unlike in GERD, the material also passes through the upper esophageal sphincter and into the laryngopharynx, where very small quantities of acid can cause symptoms. LPR should be considered in patients with subacute sore throat associated with hoarseness (from inflammation of the vocal cords) and cough (a reflexive effort to clear the airway of acid).

Oropharyngeal cancer should be considered in older patients with risk factors (e.g., tobacco abuse, heavy alcohol consumption) who present with subacute, persistent throat pain associated with dysphagia, weight loss, referred pain (e.g., to the ear), and/or unilaterality. Some patients may have overt masses on exam. All such patients should be promptly referred to an otolaryngologist for a complete examination.

CHAPTER 5

Syncope

CHRISTOPHER R. KELLY

INTRODUCTION

Syncope occurs when transient cerebral hypoperfusion causes a brief, sudden loss of consciousness (LOC), followed by a prompt and spontaneous return to normal mental status. Syncope affects 2 to 4 per 100 individuals per year, with a bimodal age distribution peaking at 10 to 30 years and >75 years.

The etiologies of syncope are categorized as reflex (or neurally mediated), orthostatic, and cardiogenic, in decreasing order of frequency (Fig. 5.1). **Reflex syncope** occurs when a specific stimulus triggers an inappropriate withdrawal of sympathetic tone that results in bradycardia and/or systemic vasodilation. **Syncope related to orthostatic hypotension** occurs when normal autonomic mechanisms fail to preserve venous return to the heart (and therefore cardiac output) upon standing. **Cardiogenic syncope** occurs when cardiac output falls in response to arrhythmias, obstructive disease, or severe heart failure.

EVALUATION

It is important to first rule out conditions that cause LOC but are not true syncope. Patients with generalized seizures, for example, often experience sudden LOC accompanied by abnormal movements of the extremities, tongue biting, and/or loss of bladder continence. The return to normal consciousness may be slow, and focal neurological deficits may persist (i.e., Todd paresis). Meanwhile, patients with pseudoseizures or psychogenic syncope may have atypical symptoms, such as purposeful movements, eye closure, and prolonged LOC (e.g., >10 minutes). Finally, patients with drop attacks experience a sudden loss of postural tone without LOC (e.g., due to vestibular dysfunction).

Patients with true syncope, in contrast, often report lightheadedness, blurred/tunneled vision, generalized warmth or cold, nausea, and/or palpitations prior to complete, brief LOC. Cerebral hypoperfusion may sometimes cause jerking motions of the extremities, mimicking a seizure, but normal consciousness should return within a few minutes (usually <1 minute), and persistent neurological deficits should not occur.

Obtain a detailed description of the LOC event (or events), speaking to a witness if possible. Ask about preceding symptoms or activities, whether complete LOC occurred, the duration of LOC, the appearance of the patient before and during the attack (e.g., diaphoresis, pallor, abnormal movements), and the time course of recovery. Ask about symptoms that could suggest intrinsic heart disease, such as palpitations, dyspnea, orthopnea, and edema. Document the past medical history and all active medications. Perform a physical examination that includes an assessment of orthostatic vital signs and a neurological examination. Obtain a 12-lead surface electrocardiogram (ECG). Assess the patient's risk for pulmonary embolism (see Chapter 89) and obtain further testing if appropriate.

In many cases, this assessment will yield a presumptive diagnosis. If the diagnosis remains uncertain, however, the patient should be risk stratified to determine the need for further workup or hospitalization. Several decision-making tools have been developed to help triage patients with syncope (Table 5.1). Patients who are high risk or have had recurrent events require an inpatient workup consisting of continuous ECG monitoring, an echocardiogram, and additional studies as indicated:

- Diagnostic carotid sinus massage (with continuous monitoring of blood pressure and heart rate) may be undertaken in patients who are >40 years old and do not have carotid bruits or recent stroke. The diagnosis of carotid sinus syncope is established if the patient experiences asystole lasting more than 3 seconds or a fall in systolic blood pressure of more than 50 mm Hg.
- A wearable or implantable event monitor may be used to assess for arrhythmias in patients with infrequent episodes.
- Tilt table testing can help establish the diagnosis of reflex syncope in patients with atypical but recurrent episodes if other causes of syncope have been ruled out.

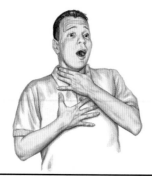

Reflex (neurally mediated) syncope

- Vasovagal syncope
  - Emotional stressors (fear, pain)
  - Prolonged standing

- Situational syncope
  - Related to micturition, defecation, coughing, sneezing, swallowing, laughing, exercise

- Carotid sinus syncope

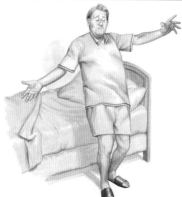

Syncope related to orthostatic hypotension
(defined as fall in systolic BP by ≥20 mm Hg or diastolic BP by ≥10 mm Hg when changing from supine to standing position)

- Volume depletion
  - Overdiuresis
  - Vomiting
  - Diarrhea
  - Hemorrhage

- Primary autonomic failure
  - Parkinson disease
  - Multiple system atrophy

- Secondary autonomic failure
  - Diabetes
  - Amyloidosis

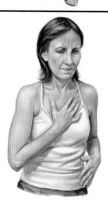

Cardiogenic syncope

- Bradyarrhythmia

- Tachyarrhythmia

- Obstruction
  - Severe aortic stenosis
  - Hypertrophic cardiomyopathy
  - Pulmonary embolus
  - Aortic dissection
  - Cardiac tumor

- Heart failure

F. Netter M.D.

C. Machado M.D.

FIG. 5.1 **Causes of Syncope.** *BP*, Blood pressure.

DIFFERENTIAL DIAGNOSIS AND MANAGEMENT

All patients with syncope should take precautions to avoid fall-related injuries and may need to avoid driving or engaging in other high-risk activities until symptoms abate, especially if symptoms occur without warning or while seated. Further therapy depends on the specific diagnosis.

Reflex syncope can be diagnosed when there is a typical trigger and/or prodrome. Patients should be reassured that their condition is not intrinsically dangerous, so long as they take appropriate precautions to avoid fall-related injuries. Patients should be advised to perform physical counterpressure maneuvers (PCMs), such as hand grip and leg crossing, during prodrome events to raise their blood pressure and try to prevent syncope. Patients with continued events despite PCMs can try using medications that raise blood pressure, though their efficacy is unclear. Midodrine is an α-adrenergic agonist that increases vascular tone, but it can cause

TABLE 5.1
Risk Scoring Systems for Patients With Syncope

Scoring System	Components and Points	Results
San Francisco Syncope Rule	• Abnormal ECG (+1) • Congestive heart failure (+1) • Shortness of breath (+1) • Hematocrit <30% (+1) • Systolic blood pressure <90 mm Hg (+1)	Score ≥1 indicates high risk for serious outcome within 7 days, defined as "death, myocardial infarction, arrhythmia, pulmonary embolism, stroke, subarachnoid hemorrhage, significant hemorrhage, or any condition causing a return ED visit and hospitalization" (sensitivity 98%, specificity 56%)
EGSYS Score	• Palpitations preceding syncope (+4) • Heart disease, abnormal ECG, or both (+3) • Syncope during effort (+3) • Syncope while supine (+2) • Precipitating or predisposing factors (warm, crowded place; prolonged orthostasis; fear/pain/emotion) (–1) • Autonomic prodrome (nausea/vomiting) (–1)	Score ≥3 indicates increased risk of 2-year mortality (21% vs 2%) and greater probability of cardiac syncope (sensitivity 92%, specificity 69%)

ECG, Electrocardiogram; *ED,* emergency department; *EGSYS,* Evaluation of Guidelines in Syncope Study.
Data from Quinn J, McDermott D, Stiell I, et al: Prospective validation of the San Francisco Syncope Rule to predict patients with serious outcomes, *Ann Emerg Med* 47(5):448–454, 2006; and Del Rosso A, Ungar A, Maggi R, et al: Clinical predictors of cardiac syncope at initial evaluation in patients referred urgently to a general hospital: the EGSYS score, *Heart* 94(12):1620–1626, 2008.

urinary obstruction in older men. Fludrocortisone is a mineralocorticoid that increases intracellular volume, but it can cause hypokalemia and volume overload. Patients with documented severe bradycardia or pauses during reflex syncope events may benefit from cardiac pacing.

Orthostatic syncope can be diagnosed when a patient has syncope associated with symptomatic orthostatic hypotension. Patients taking antihypertensives, especially β-blockers and diuretics, should have their dosages reduced or discontinued. Patients without contraindications should increase their sodium and water intake (to 5–10 g and 2–3 L per day, respectively). PCMs, compression stockings, and abdominal binders help eliminate venous pooling. Midodrine and/or fludrocortisone can also be helpful.

Cardiogenic syncope requires therapy directed at the specific abnormality; see the relevant chapters in the cardiovascular diseases section for more details.

CHAPTER 6

Chest Pain

CHRISTOPHER R. KELLY

INTRODUCTION

Chest pain is a common symptom that can reflect many different conditions of the heart, great vessels, lungs, digestive system, and chest wall (Fig. 6.1). All clinicians should be able to perform a basic evaluation that rapidly assesses for life-threatening conditions.

EVALUATION

Obtain a history of the pain that includes the timing of onset, the circumstances immediately preceding onset, the tempo of onset (gradual vs. sudden), quality (e.g., crushing vs. stabbing), severity, location (including sites of radiation), any maneuvers that may modify the pain (e.g., exertion, sitting upright or assuming some other position, taking a deep breath), and any medications that relieve the pain (e.g., NSAIDs, nitroglycerin). Determine if the pain has occurred before and, if so, with what frequency and under which circumstances.

An electrocardiogram (ECG) should be promptly obtained unless the pain is readily explained by non-cardiac causes and is benign, such as point tenderness following a chest wall injury.

Determine the patient's past medical history. Note any major risk factors for coronary artery disease, including male gender, advanced age, other known vascular disease (e.g., carotid or peripheral arterial disease), hypertension, hypercholesterolemia, diabetes mellitus, family history of premature coronary artery disease, and tobacco abuse.

Perform a focused physical examination that includes a measurement of vital signs (including blood pressure in both arms), assessment of the height of the jugular venous pulsation, examination of the neck and chest (including palpation for focal tenderness), and auscultation of the heart and lungs.

DIFFERENTIAL DIAGNOSIS AND MANAGEMENT

Patients with pressurelike, crushing, nonpleuritic, nonpositional chest pain that radiates to the arms or neck, is worse with exertion, and is relieved with rest have typical angina (Fig. 6.2), consistent with myocardial ischemia from coronary artery disease.

Patients with chronic angina that occurs with a predictable amount of exertion have **stable angina** (see Chapter 57 for more details). In contrast, patients with angina at rest or with minimal exertion likely have an **acute coronary syndrome (ACS).**

ST-segment elevation myocardial infarction (STEMI) is diagnosed when the ECG demonstrates ST-segment elevations that are not readily explained by other causes (e.g., pericarditis, left ventricular hypertrophy, bundle branch block). STEMI is a medical emergency that requires immediate evaluation by a cardiologist and, in nearly all cases, emergent percutaneous coronary intervention (see Chapter 58 for more details).

Non–ST-segment elevation acute coronary syndrome (NSTEACS) is diagnosed when a patient has angina at rest or with minimal exertion, but the ECG lacks ST-segment elevations. The ECG may feature ST-segment depression or T-wave abnormalities, or it may be normal. The term NSTEACS encompasses both non-STEMI and unstable angina (UA), distinguished based on the presence of biochemical evidence of myocardial infarction (MI) (e.g., elevated serum troponin concentration) in the former but not the latter (see Chapter 58 for more details).

Patients with chest pain that is worse when recumbent, improved when sitting upright, and associated with diffuse PR-segment depression and/or ST-segment elevation likely have **acute pericarditis.** An echocardiogram should be performed to assess for pericardial effusion and/or associated myocarditis (see Chapter 61 for more details).

Patients with sudden-onset sharp, ripping, or tearing chest pain that radiates to the back should be emergently evaluated for **aortic dissection,** especially if the pain is associated with a diminished systolic blood pressure in one upper extremity and/or focal neurological deficits (indicating extension of the dissection into the subclavian and carotid arteries, respectively). The diagnosis is established using contrast-enhanced CT scan or, if unavailable, transesophageal echocardiogram (see Chapter 64 for more details).

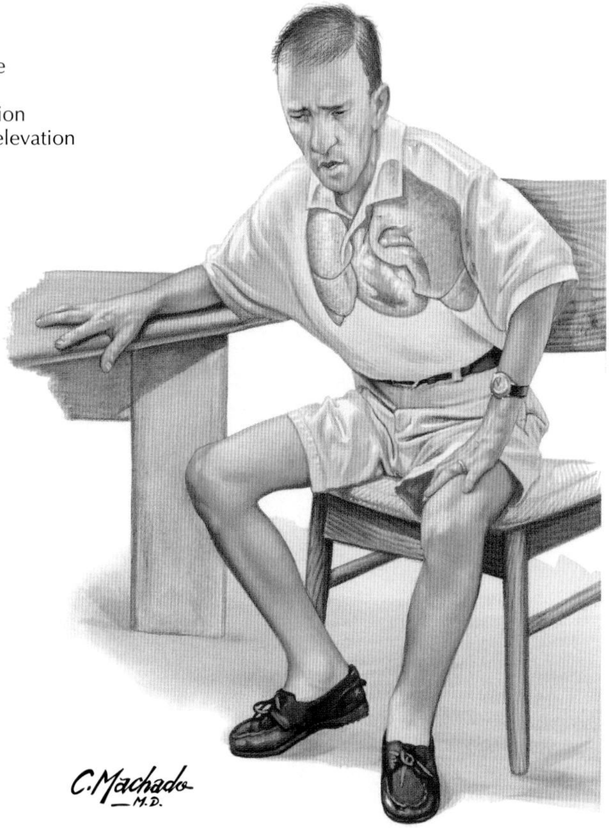

Cardiac
- Acute coronary syndrome
  - Myocardial infarction
    - ST-segment elevation
    - Non–ST-segment elevation
  - Unstable angina
- Acute pericarditis
- Aortic dissection

Pulmonary
- Pulmonary embolus
- Pneumothorax
- Pneumonia
- Asthma

Gastrointestinal
- Gastroesophageal reflux
- Esophageal spasm
- Esophageal rupture

Musculoskeletal
- Costochondritis
- Intercostal muscle spasm
- Chest wall injury

Miscellaneous
- Mediastinitis
- Herpes zoster

FIG. 6.1 **Differential Diagnosis for Chest Pain.**

Patients with tachycardia, dyspnea, and either evidence of deep venous thrombosis (e.g., painful, unilateral leg swelling) or its risk factors (malignancy, immobilization, prior history of thrombus) should be evaluated for **pulmonary embolism (PE).** Several clinical prediction rules have been devised to help determine the likelihood of PE (see Chapter 89 for more details).

A patient with sudden-onset chest pain associated with dyspnea should be evaluated for **pneumothorax.** Men are affected more often than women, and patients may not have prior known lung disease. If the pneumothorax is large enough, physical exam reveals decreased breath sounds, hyperresonant percussion, and/or reduced chest wall excursion on the affected side. Hypotension and/or tachycardia may occur if pressure accumulates around the collapsed lung and compromises venous return to the heart (tension pneumothorax). Chest x-ray is diagnostic. All patients with pneumothorax should receive supplemental oxygen to accelerate the reabsorption of pleural air. If the pneumothorax is small (<2–3 cm of

space between the lung and chest wall), the patient is stable, and there is no other evidence of lung disease, observation is reasonable. In other cases, decompression is generally required.

A patient with progressive pleuritic chest pain associated with fever, cough, and dyspnea likely has **pneumonia.** Chest x-ray can usually establish the diagnosis (see Chapter 114 for more details). A patient who experiences progressive dyspnea, tachypnea, and generalized chest tightness following exposure to various precipitants (e.g., cold air, allergens, prolonged exercise) is likely experiencing an **asthma exacerbation.** The patient may have a history of similar episodes. Lung auscultation reveals wheezing or, in severe cases, poor air movement (see Chapter 84 for more details).

If the chest pain is worse after eating and in a supine position, **gastroesophageal reflux disease (GERD)** is a plausible diagnosis. Patients may also report regurgitation and dysphagia. Symptoms usually improve with antacids. Patients with **diffuse esophageal spasm** report chest

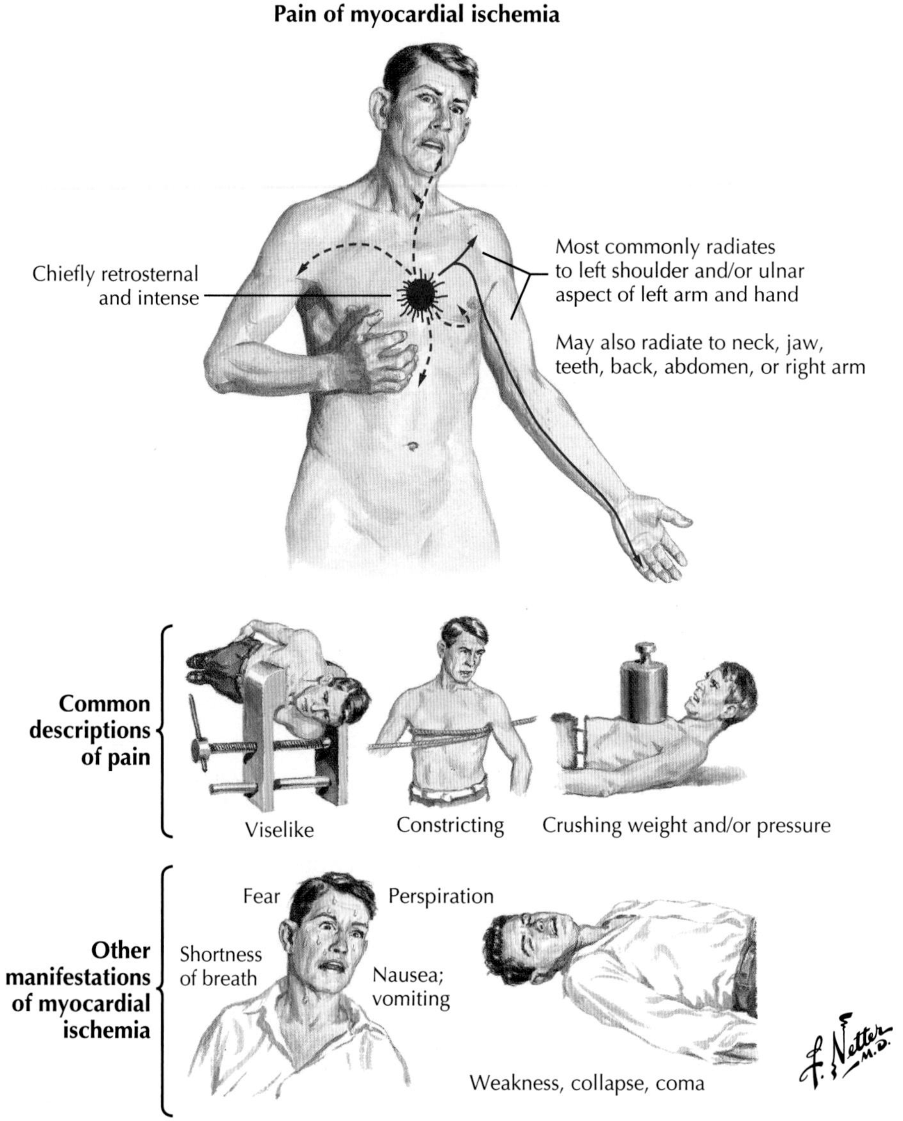

Pain of myocardial ischemia

Chiefly retrosternal and intense

Most commonly radiates to left shoulder and/or ulnar aspect of left arm and hand

May also radiate to neck, jaw, teeth, back, abdomen, or right arm

Common descriptions of pain

Viselike Constricting Crushing weight and/or pressure

Other manifestations of myocardial ischemia

Fear Perspiration

Shortness of breath Nausea; vomiting

Weakness, collapse, coma

FIG. 6.2 **Typical Angina.**

pain accompanied by dysphagia and a sensation of food becoming stuck in the chest. Patients with **esophageal rupture,** also known as Boerhaave syndrome, experience severe chest pain that is often (but not always) associated with a recent history of vomiting or retching. The extension of air into and beyond the mediastinum may cause audible crackling during cardiac auscultation and/or crepitus over the chest wall. Chest x-ray may reveal free mediastinal or pleural air along with a pleural effusion. If the diagnosis is suspected, obtain a CT scan of the chest with water-soluble oral contrast. Prohibit all other oral intake. Administer prompt intravenous antibiotics, bolus with an intravenous proton-pump inhibitor, and consult with a general surgeon.

Finally, patients with pain that is sharp, worse with movement, and reproducible with palpation of specific points on the chest wall likely have **musculoskeletal pain,** such as costochondritis. Note that the presence of reproducible chest pain lowers but does not eliminate the probability of more serious conditions (such as acute myocardial infarction [AMI]) in patients with multiple risk factors.

CHAPTER 7

Dyspnea

CHRISTOPHER R. KELLY

INTRODUCTION

Dyspnea is defined by the American Thoracic Society as "a subjective experience of breathing discomfort, comprised of qualitatively distinct sensations that derives from interactions among multiple physiological, psychological, social, and environmental factors." It can encompass several different sensations, including increased work of breathing, chest tightness, and air hunger. A patient with dyspnea may avoid physical exertion, resulting in deconditioning and a further reduction in exercise tolerance.

Dyspnea can reflect primary disorders of the airways, lungs, and respiratory muscles, or it can occur secondary to diseases originating in other organ systems. The differential diagnosis should begin with a distinction between acute dyspnea (over hours to days, with previously normal breathing), chronic dyspnea, and an acute exacerbation of chronic dyspnea.

DIFFERENTIAL DIAGNOSIS

Acute and chronic dyspnea may result from several different pathophysiological disturbances (Table 7.1 and Box 7.1). Acute exacerbations of chronic dyspnea frequently occur in patients with chronic pulmonary or cardiac diseases.

EVALUATION

Patients with moderate or severe respiratory distress (rapid and labored breathing, inability to speak in full sentences), cyanosis, and/or altered mental status must be promptly transferred to an emergency or intensive care setting for resuscitation, including oxygen supplementation and likely mechanical ventilation.

If the patient is clinically stable, obtain a focused history to further characterize the dyspnea. First, determine if the patient has known lung disease or has had similar episodes of dyspnea in the past. Inquire about the time course of the dyspnea and the presence of any associated symptoms, such as fever, night sweats, cough, hemoptysis, chest pain, edema, and/or muscle weakness. Identify any recurring precipitants (e.g., cold air, allergens, certain locations such as the workplace) that would suggest asthma. Review risk factors for deep venous thrombosis (DVT) and pulmonary embolism (PE), such as hypercoagulable disorder, malignancy, recent immobilization or injury to the leg, and estrogen use. Ask if the dyspnea becomes worse when supine (orthopnea) and if it wakes the patient from sleep (paroxysmal nocturnal dyspnea), which would indicate a volume-overload state, such as heart failure. Inquire about the use of cigarettes and inhaled drugs, such as crack cocaine.

Observe the patient as he or she breathes, noting the rate, pattern, and depth of breathing. Examine the shape of the chest wall to determine if it appears hyperinflated or barrel shaped (consistent with chronic obstructive pulmonary disease [COPD]), or if it is kyphoscoliotic or has a pectus deformity (which could cause restrictive lung disease). Note if the patient is using accessory muscles of respiration (such as the suprasternal and intercostal muscles), a sign of respiratory distress. Finally, note if the patient's lips are pressed together (pursed) during exhalation. This maneuver is common among patients with COPD, as it generates back pressure and thereby maintains the patency of smaller airways so that air is not trapped.

Listen for dysphonia and stridor, which could indicate upper airway obstruction. Assess whether the trachea is midline or deviated, which could indicate tension pneumothorax or massive pleural effusion. Measure the height of the jugular venous pulsations, which become elevated in right heart failure. Auscultate the heart for murmurs or gallops that would suggest significant valvular disease and/or heart failure. Assess tactile fremitus over the lungs; increases suggest consolidation of lung tissue (e.g., from airway-filling processes such as pneumonia), while decreases suggest hyperinflation (e.g., from COPD) or pneumothorax. Percuss the lung fields for dullness (consolidation) or hyperresonance (hyperinflation or pneumothorax). Auscultate for crackles or wheezes (see Chapter 24 for additional details). Examine the extremities for clubbing, cyanosis, and edema.

TABLE 7.1
Causes of Acute Dyspnea

Narrowing or obstruction of the airways	Asthma, anaphylaxis, angioedema, croup, epiglottitis, bronchitis, organophosphate poisoning, foreign-body aspiration
Filling of the alveolar airspaces	Pneumonia, acute respiratory distress syndrome, cardiogenic pulmonary edema, pulmonary hemorrhage
External compression of the lung, with restriction of lung expansion	Pleural effusion, pneumothorax
Pulmonary arterial insufficiency	Pulmonary embolus, pulmonary arterial hypertension
Impairment of the muscles of respiration	Neuromuscular disease, ascites, pregnancy, flail chest
Increase in blood carbon dioxide from metabolic acidosis	Kussmaul breathing secondary to diabetic ketoacidosis (common example)
Decrease in blood oxygen-carrying capacity	Anemia, carbon monoxide poisoning
Pathological stimulation of the respiratory center	Salicylate overdose, panic attack

BOX 7.1
Causes of Chronic Dyspnea

- Pulmonary disease
  - Asthma
  - Chronic obstructive pulmonary disease
  - Cystic fibrosis
  - Diffuse parenchymal lung disease
- Cardiovascular disease
  - Coronary artery disease
  - Cardiomyopathy
  - Valvular disease
  - Pulmonary hypertension
  - Chronic pulmonary thromboembolic disease
- Chest deformities
  - Kyphoscoliosis
  - Pectus excavatum
  - Anemia
  - Obesity
  - Physical deconditioning

If the cause of dyspnea is not readily apparent from the history and physical exam, obtain a chest x-ray, electrocardiogram, and basic blood tests, including a comprehensive metabolic panel and complete blood count. A patient with a significant smoking history or chronic cough should be referred for pulmonary function testing to assess for COPD (see Chapters 46 and 85). A patient with a severe chest wall abnormality or generalized weakness should also undergo pulmonary function testing to better quantify breathing mechanics. A patient who reports exercise-induced dyspnea and orthopnea should be referred for echocardiography to assess for heart failure and pulmonary hypertension (see Chapter 59).

If the history, physical, and basic workup do not point to a particular cause, and dyspnea persists, additional diagnostic tests can be empirically pursued in a less selective manner, including echocardiography, chest CT, pulmonary function testing, and/or cardiopulmonary exercise testing.

Patients with chronic dyspnea should grade their symptoms using questionnaires, such as the Borg and modified Medical Research Council (mMRC) scales. These indices can help establish a baseline, categorize the severity of disease (e.g., in COPD), and help measure the efficacy of various interventions.

CHAPTER 8

Nausea and Vomiting

CHRISTOPHER R. KELLY

INTRODUCTION

Nausea is a common symptom that may culminate in **retching,** in which the gastric and abdominal musculature contract but the glottis remains closed, or **vomiting,** in which the glottis opens and gastric contents are expelled through the mouth. **Regurgitation** refers to the effortless passage of food from the stomach back into the esophagus and possibly the mouth.

The area postrema, located at the base of the fourth ventricle, lies outside of the blood-brain barrier and can sense drugs and toxins; information from this site and visceral afferents converge in the nucleus tractus solitarius, located in the medulla, which can initiate the motor sequence that culminates in vomiting.

The many different causes of nausea and vomiting are shown in Fig. 8.1.

EVALUATION

Determine the onset and chronicity along with any precipitants. Ask the patient to describe the vomitus (e.g., its consistency, color, and smell). The recurrent vomiting of partially digested food, for example, may indicate a gastric outlet obstruction. Feculent vomitus may indicate a distal small bowel or colonic obstruction.

Ask about the relationship between symptoms and oral intake. Perform a complete review of systems, asking specifically about headache, vertigo, heartburn, abdominal pain, and diarrhea. Obtain a current list of medications, including supplements, and ask about alcohol intake and illicit drug use. During physical exam, look for signs of dehydration, including dry mucous membranes, decreased skin turgor, and decreased axillary sweat.

All women of childbearing age should have a pregnancy test. If the patient appears dehydrated or symptoms are chronic, obtain a basic laboratory workup (complete metabolic panel, complete blood count, pancreatic enzymes). If the pain localizes to the right upper quadrant or is associated with jaundice, obtain an abdominal ultrasound to assess for biliary obstruction. If symptoms are chronic or significant abdominal pain is present, obtain an abdominal CT; if imaging is normal but symptoms persist, refer for endoscopy.

DIFFERENTIAL DIAGNOSIS AND MANAGEMENT

Patients with **acute-onset vomiting,** a negative pregnancy test, no new medications, and no findings to suggest a specific cause (e.g., bowel obstruction, pancreatitis, biliary obstruction, vestibular disorder) usually have **infectious gastroenteritis,** which may also be associated with diffuse, mild-to-moderate abdominal pain and/or diarrhea (see Chapter 117 for more details).

Patients with more **chronic vomiting** have a broader differential diagnosis. Many of the underlying conditions will be discovered on history and physical (e.g., migraine), laboratory workup (e.g., metabolic disorders), abdominal imaging (e.g., gastric outlet obstruction), and/or endoscopy (e.g., peptic ulcer disease); however, some conditions can be more difficult to detect.

Those who report early satiety and bloating but lack evidence of gastric outlet obstruction may have **gastroparesis,** or abnormally slow gastric emptying. It is usually idiopathic or the result of diabetes mellitus–associated autonomic neuropathy. A splashing sound may be heard over the stomach if the patient is rocked side to side (succussion splash). Scintigraphy establishes the diagnosis by demonstrating prolonged gastric emptying time. Affected patients should eat frequent, small meals with low-residue foods that are low in fat (which can further slow gastric emptying). Erythromycin and metoclopramide are also helpful.

Patients with recurrent episodes of vomiting separated by symptom-free intervals may have **cyclic vomiting syndrome.** Cycles of recurrent vomiting generally occur in response to certain triggers (stress, infection), last for hours to days, and recur 5 to 10 times per year. The pathogenesis is unclear. The Rome III criteria include stereotypical episodes of vomiting regarding onset and duration, three or more discrete episodes in the past year, and the absence of nausea and vomiting between episodes. Many patients have a personal or family history

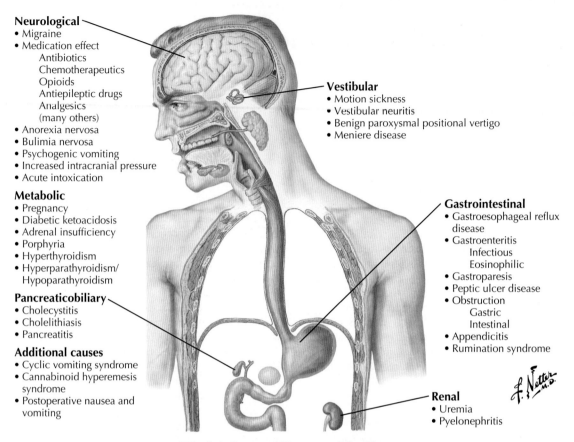

Neurological
- Migraine
- Medication effect
  Antibiotics
  Chemotherapeutics
  Opioids
  Antiepileptic drugs
  Analgesics
  (many others)
- Anorexia nervosa
- Bulimia nervosa
- Psychogenic vomiting
- Increased intracranial pressure
- Acute intoxication

Metabolic
- Pregnancy
- Diabetic ketoacidosis
- Adrenal insufficiency
- Porphyria
- Hyperthyroidism
- Hyperparathyroidism/
  Hypoparathyroidism

Pancreaticobiliary
- Cholecystitis
- Cholelithiasis
- Pancreatitis

Additional causes
- Cyclic vomiting syndrome
- Cannabinoid hyperemesis
  syndrome
- Postoperative nausea and
  vomiting

Vestibular
- Motion sickness
- Vestibular neuritis
- Benign paroxysmal positional vertigo
- Meniere disease

Gastrointestinal
- Gastroesophageal reflux
  disease
- Gastroenteritis
  Infectious
  Eosinophilic
- Gastroparesis
- Peptic ulcer disease
- Obstruction
  Gastric
  Intestinal
- Appendicitis
- Rumination syndrome

Renal
- Uremia
- Pyelonephritis

FIG. 8.1 **Causes of Nausea and Vomiting.**

of migraine headaches. Treatment consists of supportive care and antiemetic agents. Antimigraine medications are used in severe or refractory cases, or when there is a personal or family history of migraines.

Finally, patients who report frequent marijuana use may have **cannabinoid hyperemesis syndrome,** which occurs in a small number of regular (daily or weekly) users. The overall duration of cannabis use is less important than the frequency. Many patients report that a hot bath or shower mitigates their symptoms. Cannabis cessation leads to complete resolution of symptoms.

Antiemetics

Many different medications effectively treat nausea. Metoclopramide is a D2 dopamine receptor antagonist that acts in both the central and peripheral (enteric) nervous system; in higher doses it also acts as a serotonin receptor antagonist and exerts a prokinetic effect by stimulating cholinergic receptors on gastric smooth muscle cells. Its gastric effects make it a frequent choice for the treatment of gastroparesis. Unfortunately, its central effects can

result in anxiety and restlessness, with some patients experiencing irreversible tardive dyskinesia. In addition, QT-segment prolongation can occur, predisposing to arrhythmia. Diphenhydramine is often given to help reduce (but not eliminate) the central side effects. Domperidone is a related dopamine receptor antagonist that does not cross the blood-brain barrier but is not currently available in the United States.

Prochlorperazine is a different type of D2 dopamine receptor antagonist that acts primarily at the area postrema of the brain; however, it can also cause dystonia and tardive dyskinesia. Ondansetron is a 5-hydroxytryptamine (5HT3) serotonin receptor antagonist that is widely used to prevent or treat chemotherapy-associated nausea but may cause QT prolongation and, in rare cases, headache and/or dizziness. Scopolamine, a muscarinic receptor antagonist, is used primarily to prevent nausea associated with motion sickness but often causes dry mouth and/or fatigue. Erythromycin, a macrolide antibiotic, activates the gastrointestinal motilin receptor and can be used as a prokinetic agent for gastroparesis.

CHAPTER 9

Jaundice

CHRISTOPHER R. KELLY

INTRODUCTION

Jaundice is the term for the yellowish discoloration of skin, mucous membranes, and sclerae that occurs when serum bilirubin concentrations exceed 2.5 to 3 mg/dL. Discoloration of the mucous membranes and sclerae often precedes that of the skin. The term **jaundice** comes from the French word *jaune,* for yellow. Although there are some benign genetic syndromes that cause jaundice, new-onset jaundice in an adult often indicates a serious underlying medical disorder and always warrants a comprehensive evaluation.

DIFFERENTIAL DIAGNOSIS

The creation and metabolism of bilirubin provide a framework for the differential diagnosis of jaundice (Fig. 9.1).

The average person generates about 4 mg of bilirubin per kilogram of body weight per day. The initial substrate is heme, which is converted by heme oxygenase to biliverdin, which is then converted by biliverdin reductase to bilirubin. In healthy individuals most bilirubin is produced during the catabolism of hemoglobin in red blood cells. A smaller amount is generated by the metabolism of heme found in other proteins (e.g., myoglobin, cytochromes).

The bilirubin generated by biliverdin reductase is **unconjugated,** or not conjugated to glucuronic acids; it is insoluble in blood and mostly bound to albumin. In the liver, unconjugated bilirubin dissociates from albumin and is transported into hepatocytes, which conjugate bilirubin to glucuronic acid. Conjugated bilirubin is transported alongside bile salts into canaliculi. Bile is conveyed through these canaliculi into the extrahepatic biliary tree for eventual release into the duodenum. Intestinal bacteria reduce bilirubin to urobilinogen, which is largely reabsorbed into the portal blood, then reprocessed into conjugated bilirubin (enterohepatic recirculation) or excreted into urine.

Abnormalities at each stage of this process can result in abnormally high bilirubin levels and the clinical appearance of jaundice (Fig. 9.2).

EVALUATION

Inquire about the timing of jaundice onset and perform a complete review of symptoms, asking specifically about fever, chills, and abdominal pain. Ask about stool color, as patients with complete **biliary obstruction** have acholic (pale, clay-colored) stools. Determine if the patient has recently been exposed to any new medications or supplements. Quantify alcohol intake. Assess risk factors for hepatitis C infection, such as blood transfusions before 1992 or intravenous drug use. Obtain a complete medical history, asking specifically about any prior hepatobiliary disorders. Determine if there is any family history of jaundice or liver disease.

Measure vital signs and perform a complete physical examination. Check for signs of anemia (pale conjunctiva, nail beds, and palmar creases) or advanced hepatic dysfunction (i.e., spider angiomata, palmar erythema, evidence of portal hypertension [e.g., splenomegaly, caput medusae, ascites]).

Obtain a comprehensive metabolic panel, complete blood count, and prothrombin time. Most laboratories report direct and indirect bilirubin measurements in the metabolic panel. These values refer to a laboratory assay (van den Bergh reaction) in which a diazo reagent is used to convert bilirubin to azobilirubin, which is easier to measure. Conjugated bilirubin converts to azobilirubin within 1 minute and constitutes the direct fraction. Unconjugated bilirubin has a configuration that is resistant to the diazo reaction; therefore a catalyst must be added (such as ethanol) and the total bilirubin measured 30 minutes later. The indirect fraction, representing unconjugated bilirubin, is the difference between the total and the direct fractions. Of note, about 10% of unconjugated bilirubin will rapidly react with the diazo reagent; thus the direct fraction slightly overestimates conjugated bilirubin.

Prolonged high levels of conjugated bilirubin can result in its covalent binding to albumin, which forms delta bilirubin. Delta bilirubin cannot be filtered into urine and is metabolized more slowly than unbound bilirubin. It reacts rapidly with the diazo reagent and therefore contributes to the direct fraction. As a result,

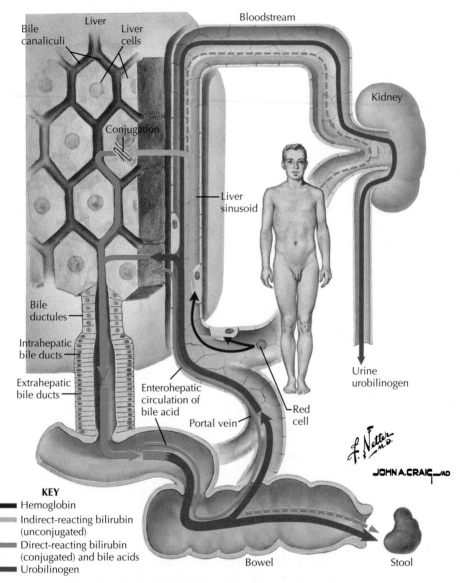

FIG. 9.1 Normal Bilirubin Production and Metabolism.

KEY
- Hemoglobin
- Indirect-reacting bilirubin (unconjugated)
- Direct-reacting bilirubin (conjugated) and bile acids
- Urobilinogen

patients with resolved biliary obstructions may have persistently elevated direct bilirubin fractions due to delta bilirubin.

DIAGNOSIS AND MANAGEMENT

The differential hinges on whether the patient has predominantly indirect or direct hyperbilirubinemia.

A patient with predominantly **indirect hyperbilirubinemia** likely has hemolysis, drug-related inhibition of bilirubin uptake or conjugation, or Gilbert syndrome.

Hemolysis or **dyserythropoiesis** is the likely diagnosis in an anemic patient without other evidence of hepatic dysfunction (e.g., normal aminotransferases, alkaline phosphatase, albumin). Patients with hemolysis often have an elevated lactate dehydrogenase and low serum haptoglobin. Check a blood smear, which helps clarify the underlying cause. Since bilirubin metabolism is normal, the direct fraction may also be elevated. Of note, however, the total bilirubin rarely exceeds 4 mg/dL unless there is concurrent hepatic dysfunction that impairs the capacity to conjugate and excrete bilirubin.

Increased bilirubin production
(hemolysis, dyserythropoiesis)

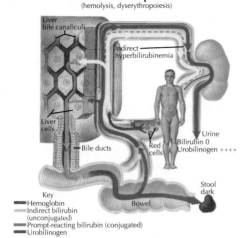

Decreased bilirubin uptake
(rifampin, right heart failure)

Decreased hepatic conjugation
(Gilbert syndrome, atazanavir, indinavir, chloramphenicol)

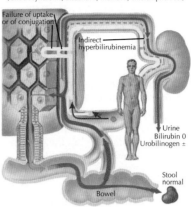

Decreased bilirubin excretion

Extrahepatic obstruction
(choledocholithiasis, pancreatic malignancy, biliary malignancy, primary sclerosing cholangitis, liver flukes, AIDS cholangiopathy, pancreatitis)

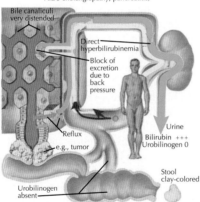

Intrahepatic cholestasis
(pregnancy, medications, infiltrative liver disease, primary biliary cirrhosis)

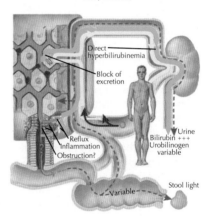

Hepatocellular injury
Defective canalicular excretion
(Dubin-Johnson syndrome, Rotor syndrome)

FIG. 9.2 **Differential Diagnosis for Jaundice.**

Gilbert syndrome is a condition in which patients have a mutated promoter in the *UGT1A1* gene, which encodes a UDP-glucuronosyltransferase that conjugates bilirubin to glucuronic acid. The protein is not absent but is less than half as active as normal. Patients experience intermittent, mild jaundice associated with physiological stresses (such as fasting, fever, or intense physical exertion), probably through a decrease in enteric motility and consequent increase in enterohepatic recirculation. Obtain a blood smear to rule out hemolysis or dyserythropoiesis. No specific treatment is required. The related **Crigler-Najjar syndrome** also results from *UGT1A1* mutations, but the protein is either completely absent or severely impaired; consequently, patients become jaundiced during infancy or childhood and require lifelong therapy.

A patient with predominantly **direct hyperbilirubinemia** likely has biliary obstruction, intrahepatic cholestasis, acute or chronic hepatocellular injury, or a genetic defect in bilirubin excretion.

Direct hyperbilirubinemia associated with elevated alkaline phosphatase levels and normal to moderately elevated aminotransferase levels suggests biliary obstruction or intrahepatic cholestasis.

Biliary obstruction should be ruled out first, especially if the patient has right upper quadrant pain. Obtain an abdominal ultrasound to assess for masses and infiltration of the liver as well as obstruction and/or dilation of the extrahepatic biliary system. The combination of biliary obstruction, fever, and an elevated white blood cell is consistent with acute cholangitis or infection of the biliary system (see Chapter 118 for more details). If obstruction is confirmed or strongly suspected, endoscopic retrograde cholangiopancreatography (ERCP) can provide further information and help restore normal biliary flow. Magnetic resonance cholangiopancreatography (MRCP) offers an alternative, noninvasive means of assessing the intrahepatic and extrahepatic biliary system if ERCP is not readily available.

Once obstruction has been ruled out, **intrahepatic cholestasis** becomes the likely diagnosis. Review all medications or supplements against an online database of drug-induced liver injury, such as LiverTox (maintained by the National Institutes of Health). Order a test for serum antimitochondrial antibodies, which are elevated in primary biliary cirrhosis. Order a pregnancy test in women of childbearing age. If no explanation for cholestasis can be identified, a liver biopsy may be required.

Hyperbilirubinemia associated with markedly (and disproportionately) elevated aminotransferase levels suggests **hepatocellular injury** (see Chapter 35 for more details). In cases of jaundice associated with cirrhosis, or end-stage liver disease, aminotransferases may be only mildly elevated, but there should be other evidence of severe hepatic dysfunction (e.g., physical exam findings, low albumin, prolonged prothrombin time), and a hepatitis workup is indicated.

Finally, direct hyperbilirubinemia with normal alkaline phosphatase and aminotransferase levels suggests a genetic defect in bilirubin excretion.

Dubin-Johnson syndrome occurs when there is a genetic mutation in the *ABCC2* gene, which encodes a protein responsible for exporting bilirubin from the hepatocyte into the bile canaliculus. As in Gilbert syndrome, patients often have mild icterus, especially in the setting of physiological stressors, but only rarely experience more significant hyperbilirubinemia. No specific treatment is required.

Rotor syndrome reflects a genetic mutation affecting hepatic bilirubin reuptake. Normally the hepatocytes nearest the portal tract efficiently take up and conjugate bilirubin, but excretion across the canalicular membrane is a rate-limiting process. Therefore these hepatocytes pump conjugated bilirubin back into the sinusoids for reuptake and excretion by hepatocytes nearer the hepatic vein. In Rotor syndrome, there is a mutation in one of the genes (*SLCO1B1* and *SLCO1B3*) encoding the transporters (OATP1B1 and OATP1B3) responsible for the reuptake process. In addition to causing mild direct hyperbilirubinemia, which manifests as occasional jaundice, these mutations can also affect the metabolism of many medications. Increased urine coproporphyrin levels, reflecting decreased biliary and increased renal coproporphyrin excretion, distinguish Rotor syndrome from Dubin-Johnson syndrome. No specific treatment is required.

CHAPTER 10

Abdominal Pain

CHRISTOPHER R. KELLY

INTRODUCTION

Abdominal pain is a very common symptom that can be either acute, reaching its maximum intensity within hours to days, or chronic, lasting weeks or even months. Pain typically results from mechanical obstruction of the gastrointestinal system or inflammation of the abdominal viscera due to infection, autoimmune disease, or ischemia. This chapter will focus on the approach to acute abdominal pain, the numerous causes of which are shown in Figs. 10.1 and 10.2.

EVALUATION

Establish the time course and tempo of the pain (e.g., progressive or abrupt, colicky or constant) along with its location and quality (e.g., sharp, aching). Clarify if the patient has had similar pain before and what workup may already have been done. Inquire broadly about associated symptoms (e.g., fevers, anorexia, nausea/vomiting, diarrhea, constipation, hematochezia, melena, jaundice, dysuria, hematuria, dyspnea, chest pain). Ask women about vaginal bleeding or discharge. Note any medical comorbidities, medications, and prior surgeries. Inquire about alcohol intake and illicit drug use (e.g., cocaine).

Measure vital signs and perform a focused physical examination. Assess for inflammation of the peritoneum (peritonitis) by gently bumping or moving the stretcher; patients with peritonitis experience pain with even slight movement. Inspect the abdomen for hernias and surgical scars, both risk factors for bowel obstruction. Auscultate the abdomen to determine bowel sounds, which may be hyperactive or high pitched in the presence of bowel obstruction. Palpate the abdomen with the patient's knees flexed (to relax the abdominal muscles) to determine the location of greatest tenderness. Patients with peritonitis involuntarily contract their abdominal musculature (guarding) to reduce movement of viscera against the peritoneum. They also experience pain with the release of deep palpation (rebound tenderness).

Unless the pain is clearly nongastrointestinal, perform a rectal exam to check for masses and/or blood. If a female patient has pain in the lower abdomen or pelvis, perform a pelvic examination.

Obtain a comprehensive metabolic panel, complete blood count, lipase/amylase levels, and urinalysis. Check a pregnancy test in all premenopausal women. If the patient has multiple coronary artery disease (CAD) risk factors, obtain a 12-lead electrocardiogram and measure a serum troponin concentration.

If the patient has severe pain or is hemodynamically unstable, obtain an upright x-ray of the abdomen to assess for bowel obstruction or perforation (which releases free air into the peritoneum that is visible under the diaphragm). If severe pain persists but the x-ray is normal, obtain a contrast-enhanced CT scan. If the patient is overtly jaundiced or has right upper quadrant (RUQ) pain, obtain a RUQ sonogram. If a woman reports predominantly pelvic pain or has an abnormal pelvic examination, obtain a pelvic sonogram.

DIFFERENTIAL DIAGNOSIS AND MANAGEMENT

Patients with **severe, nonfocal abdominal pain** may have life-threatening conditions such as bowel obstruction or acute mesenteric ischemia.

Small or **large bowel obstruction** causes severe, generalized abdominal pain associated with nausea, vomiting, and constipation or obstipation (inability to pass stool or flatus, respectively). The major causes include adhesions (from prior abdominal surgery or bowel inflammation), neoplasms, and hernias. As the bowel becomes increasingly distended, perfusion becomes compromised, and necrosis/perforation may occur. An abdominal x-ray reveals dilated loops of bowel with air-fluid levels. An abdominal CT scan provides detailed anatomical information and can rule out related conditions such as **ileus** and **pseudo-obstruction,** which feature bowel distension without obstruction. Patients with obstruction require emergent surgical consultation. In the meanwhile, resuscitate the patient with intravenous fluid and place a nasogastric tube to relieve distension and reduce pain.

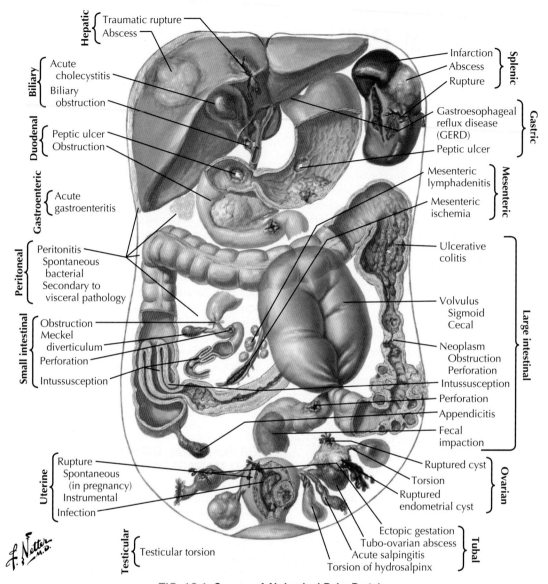

FIG. 10.1 Causes of Abdominal Pain: Part 1.

Acute mesenteric ischemia, resulting from hypoperfusion of the superior or inferior mesenteric arteries, causes severe, nonfocal abdominal pain. Some patients also report bloody diarrhea. About half of cases result from arterial thromboembolism (e.g., from atrial fibrillation, mechanical heart valves, recent endovascular procedures). Less often ischemia results from mesenteric arterial vasoconstriction (e.g., from cocaine use, vasopressor administration), mesenteric venous thrombosis (e.g., from a hypercoagulable disorder), or hypoperfusion without obstruction (e.g., from severe heart failure). A serum D-dimer level is highly sensitive (~95%) but not specific. A venous lactate level is also sensitive but less so in early ischemia. If there is concern for ischemia and another explanation for pain is not apparent, perform an emergent CT angiogram. Surgical intervention is required to restore perfusion and resect infarcted bowel.

Patients with severe pain that progresses from the umbilicus to the right lower quadrant (RLQ) may have **appendicitis.** Most patients also report anorexia and

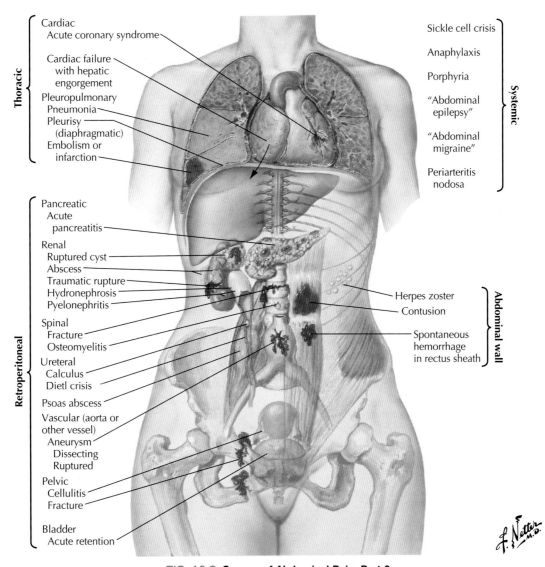

FIG. 10.2 **Causes of Abdominal Pain: Part 2.**

nausea. The inciting event is appendiceal obstruction, usually from lymphoid hyperplasia (in younger patients), fecalith impaction, or tumor. The obstructed appendix initially causes visceral, periumbilical pain, but as distension progresses the peritoneum may become involved and cause RLQ pain. If the appendix is predominantly retrocecal rather than anterior, maximal pain may occur not with abdominal palpation but with extension of the right hip, which compresses the appendix against the psoas muscle (psoas sign). The diagnosis is usually established with contrast-enhanced abdominal CT,

which reveals an enlarged, thickened appendix that does not fill with contrast and has adjacent fat stranding. Administer fluid and empirical antibiotics, and consult a surgeon.

Older patients (>50–60 years old) with lower left or right quadrant pain may have **diverticulitis.** Diverticulitis should be distinguished from **diverticulosis,** the presence of colonic diverticula (saclike mucosal outpouchings that form due to high intraluminal pressures). Diverticulitis occurs when a diverticulum becomes obstructed and inflamed. As with acute appendicitis, the pain may progress from generalized to localized. The diagnosis is established with contrast-enhanced abdominal CT scan. A first episode of uncomplicated diverticulitis (i.e., no evidence of perforation, abscess, or obstruction) can be treated with diet restriction and antibiotics. Patients who fail to improve, have recurrent episodes, or experience complications (e.g., fistulas, abscesses) may require surgery.

Patients with RUQ pain may have cholecystitis or biliary obstruction, the latter being likelier if jaundice is present.

Acute cholecystitis occurs when an impacted gallstone in the cystic duct causes inflammation and in some cases infection of the gallbladder. Jaundice does not occur unless the common bile duct is also obstructed (e.g., Mirizzi syndrome). Most patients have prior episodes of **biliary colic,** in which postprandial gallbladder contractions temporarily propel gallstones into the cystic duct, causing pain and obstruction. Unlike biliary colic, acute cholecystitis causes prolonged pain (>6 hours) and is associated with fever and leukocytosis. The classic physical examination finding is Murphy sign, in which the examiner deeply palpates the RUQ while asking the patient to take a breath. As the patient's diaphragm contracts, the gallbladder becomes compressed against the examiner's hand, causing pain and an abrupt cessation of breathing. The diagnosis is confirmed with ultrasonography, which reveals a sonographic Murphy sign (similar to the exam maneuver), gallbladder wall thickening, and pericholecystic fluid. If the sonogram is

equivocal, a hepatobiliary iminodiacetic acid (HIDA) scan can be performed. Once the diagnosis appears probable, consult a general surgeon.

Common biliary duct obstruction is the most likely diagnosis in a patient with acute RUQ pain and jaundice. The most common cause is gallstones (i.e., choledocholithiasis). Superimposed infection **(cholangitis)** is common. Laboratory assessment typically reveals elevation of aminotransferase levels alongside (and sometimes preceding) an elevation in direct bilirubin concentration (see Chapter 130 for more details). Of note, **acute hepatitis** (e.g., hepatitis A infection) may cause similar symptoms, though the abdominal pain is typically less severe and the onset more subacute.

Patients with episodic gnawing or burning epigastric pain that is either worsened or relieved by food intake may have **peptic ulcer disease** (see Chapter 129 for more details). Finally, patients with epigastric pain that radiates to the back may have **acute pancreatitis,** which is confirmed when serum lipase and/or amylase levels are elevated to >3 times the upper limit of normal (see Chapter 131 for more details).

Patients with mild to moderate, acute or subacute abdominal pain associated with nausea, vomiting, and/or diarrhea may have **infectious gastroenteritis.** A basic laboratory workup may reveal evidence of mild dehydration (e.g., azotemia, metabolic alkalosis) and inflammation (e.g., elevated white blood cell count) but should otherwise be normal (see Chapter 117 for more details).

CHAPTER 11

Gastrointestinal Bleeding

CHRISTOPHER R. KELLY

INTRODUCTION

Gastrointestinal bleeding (GIB) can be abrupt and life threatening or chronic and insidious. The various causes are classified as **upper** or **lower** depending on whether they affect the gastrointestinal (GI) tract proximal or distal to the ligament of Treitz, which marks the transition from duodenum to jejunum. The many different causes are shown in Fig. 11.1.

EVALUATION

The main symptom of GIB is a change in the appearance of stool. **Hematochezia** refers to the passage of fresh, bright-red blood from the anus, either alone (known as bright-red blood per rectum [BRBPR]) or mixed with fecal material. In contrast, **melena** refers to dark, tarry-black stools containing partially digested blood.

Hematochezia is generally secondary to lower GIB, but it can also reflect upper GIB if the rate of bleeding is so great that blood passes undigested through the bowel. Patients with hematochezia due to an upper GIB generally exhibit other symptoms of severe bleeding, such as orthostatic or supine hypotension.

Melena, in contrast, usually reflects upper GIB. Less often, it can result from swallowed blood originating from the mouth, posterior nasopharynx, or respiratory tract. About 50 to 100 cc of blood must be digested to produce melena.

Finally, frank **hematemesis** may occur in patients with rapid upper GIB (e.g., from esophageal varices) due to rapid filling and irritation of the stomach.

The symptoms also depend on the rate of bleeding. A patient with acute, rapid bleeding generally presents with overt melena or hematochezia associated with symptoms of orthostatic or supine hypotension (lightheadedness, syncope). In contrast, a patient with chronic, slow bleeding may be found incidentally to have iron-deficiency anemia without any gross change in the appearance of stool.

If a patient has signs or symptoms consistent with GIB, measure vital signs (including both supine and standing blood pressure) and obtain a focused history.

Determine the time course of symptoms. Ask about the appearance of stool—its consistency, frequency, and color—and any associated abdominal pain and vomiting. Obtain a complete medical history, asking specifically about prior GIB, prior endoscopies, liver disease, and bleeding disorders. Note all outpatient medications, and ask specifically about NSAID use, a major risk factor for peptic ulcer disease, as well as antiplatelet agent and anticoagulant use, which may potentiate bleeding.

Examine the patient's oropharynx for any evidence of oral or nasopharyngeal bleeding. Palpate the abdomen to assess for any regional tenderness. Examine the skin for evidence of cirrhosis and portal hypertension, such as palmar erythema, spider angioma, gynecomastia, caput medusae (dilated periumbilical veins), and ascites (see Chapter 139 for more details). Examine the stool, if any has been collected. Inspect the anus for lesions and perform a rectal examination to check for blood and masses.

Obtain a comprehensive metabolic panel, complete blood count, blood type/antibody screen, and coagulation studies. The blood count can reveal the degree of anemia in subacute and chronic bleeds; however, it may remain normal in the setting of acute bleeding, since the remaining hemoglobin does not become diluted until volume resuscitation occurs or extravascular fluid is redistributed back into the vascular space. An elevated blood urea nitrogen level may be a general sign of volume depletion; however, high levels may also reflect the digestion of blood from upper GIB.

If there is incongruence between the rectal examination and the clinical presentation, card-based **guaiac testing** for fecal blood can be helpful (Fig. 11.2). For example, a patient may present with black or bright-red stool but normal hemodynamics and hematocrit; in this case, it is helpful to confirm that the abnormal color comes from blood rather than food ingestion. (Note, however, that some foods, such as beets, can cause both red stools and false-positive guaiac tests.) Likewise, a patient may have new-onset anemia but normal serum iron levels and normal-appearing stools; guaiac testing offers a rapid means of screening for GIB and may help

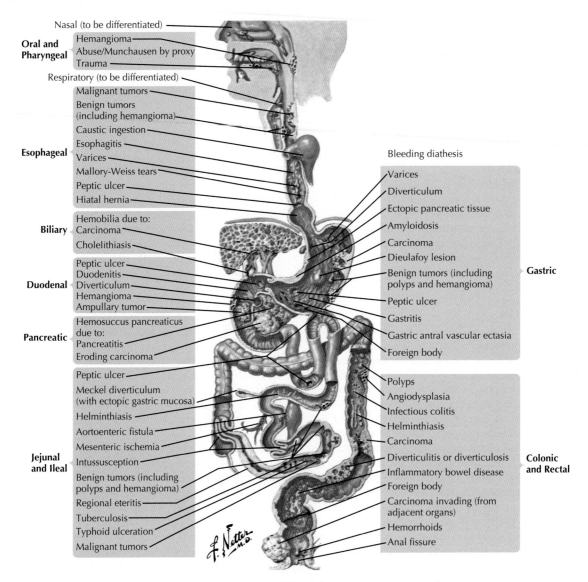

Oral and Pharyngeal
- Nasal (to be differentiated)
- Hemangioma
- Abuse/Munchausen by proxy
- Trauma

Respiratory (to be differentiated)

Esophageal
- Malignant tumors
- Benign tumors (including hemangioma)
- Caustic ingestion
- Esophagitis
- Varices
- Mallory-Weiss tears
- Peptic ulcer
- Hiatal hernia

Biliary
- Hemobilia due to:
  - Carcinoma
  - Cholelithiasis

Duodenal
- Peptic ulcer
- Duodenitis
- Diverticulum
- Hemangioma
- Ampullary tumor

Pancreatic
- Hemosuccus pancreaticus due to:
  - Pancreatitis
  - Eroding carcinoma

Jejunal and Ileal
- Peptic ulcer
- Meckel diverticulum (with ectopic gastric mucosa)
- Helminthiasis
- Aortoenteric fistula
- Mesenteric ischemia
- Intussusception
- Benign tumors (including polyps and hemangioma)
- Regional eteritis
- Tuberculosis
- Typhoid ulceration
- Malignant tumors

Bleeding diathesis

Gastric
- Varices
- Diverticulum
- Ectopic pancreatic tissue
- Amyloidosis
- Carcinoma
- Dieulafoy lesion
- Benign tumors (including polyps and hemangioma)
- Peptic ulcer
- Gastritis
- Gastric antral vascular ectasia
- Foreign body

Colonic and Rectal
- Polyps
- Angiodysplasia
- Infectious colitis
- Helminthiasis
- Carcinoma
- Diverticulitis or diverticulosis
- Inflammatory bowel disease
- Foreign body
- Carcinoma invading (from adjacent organs)
- Hemorrhoids
- Anal fissure

f. Netter m.d.

FIG. 11.1 Causes of Gastrointestinal Bleeding.

focus the anemia workup (though a negative guaiac test does not rule out GIB, especially if no other cause of bleeding is found).

In the guaiac test, stool is applied to guaiac paper, and hydrogen peroxide is applied using a dropper. If the stool contains blood, the hemoglobin acts as a peroxidase that catalyzes a reaction between guaiaconic acid, found in the paper, and hydrogen peroxide. The product, a quinone, turns the paper blue. Several substances can interfere with the guaiac test. False positives can occur if patients eat meat, which contains exogenous hemoglobin, or vegetables with high levels of plant peroxidases (e.g., broccoli, radishes, turnips), which catalyze the reaction in lieu of hemoglobin. Some textbooks state that NSAIDs and anticoagulants cause false-positive guaiac tests by causing bleeding from normal GI mucosa; however, this result is still a true positive, though perhaps of uncertain significance. Meanwhile, false-negative tests can occur if patients consume foods high in vitamin C (e.g., citrus fruits), which interferes with the peroxidation reaction. Oral iron does not interfere with the guaiac test, though it may cause stool to appear dark (though not tarry).

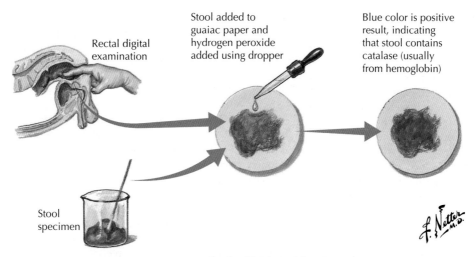

Rectal digital examination

Stool added to guaiac paper and hydrogen peroxide added using dropper

Blue color is positive result, indicating that stool contains catalase (usually from hemoglobin)

Stool specimen

FIG. 11.2 **Guaiac Testing of Stool.**

TABLE 11.1 Glasgow-Blatchford Score									
Blood Urea Nitrogen (mg/dL)		**Hemoglobin (g/dL) for Men**		**Hemoglobin (g/dL) for Women**		**Systolic Blood Pressure (mm Hg)**		**Other Criteria**	
<18.2	0	>13	0	>12	0	≥110	0	Pulse ≥100/min	+1
18.2–22.3	+2	12–13	+1	10–12	+1	100–109	+1	Melena present	+1
22.4–28	+3	10–12	+3	<10	+6	90–99	+2	Presentation with syncope	+2
28–70	+4	<10	+6			<90	+3	Liver disease history	+2
>70	+6							Heart failure history	+2

Reused with permission from Blatchford O, Murray WR, Blatchford M: A risk score to predict need for treatment for uppergastrointestinal haemorrhage, *Lancet* 356(9238):1318–1321, 2000.

MANAGEMENT

Patients with upper GIB may be risk stratified using tools such as the Glasgow-Blatchford score (Table 11.1); those with a score of 0 may be eligible for outpatient care, including urgent referral to a gastroenterologist. Patients with lower GIB who are hemodynamically stable, not anemic, and consistently have only a small amount of hematochezia (e.g., one or two drops of blood at the end of defecation) can also be managed on an outpatient basis.

All other patients with GIB, however, require inpatient care. If a patient exhibits tachycardia, orthostatic hypotension, or supine hypotension, promptly begin aggressive resuscitation with crystalloid solution (e.g., rapid infusion of 1–2 L normal saline). If the patient is hemodynamically unstable and large-volume hematemesis or hematochezia is witnessed, empirically transfuse

two units of blood. If the patient is more stable and the hemoglobin concentration is known, transfuse to achieve a hemoglobin goal of >7 g/dL. If the patient has significant coronary or cerebrovascular disease, a goal of >8 g/dL may be more appropriate.

Transfuse plasma products or platelets as needed to address coagulopathy or thrombocytopenia. If the patient has strong indications for the ongoing use of antiplatelet or anticoagulation agents (e.g., recently implanted drug-eluting stent, mechanical heart valve), early consultation with an appropriate specialist is advisable.

Upper Gastrointestinal Bleeding

If upper GIB is suspected, administer an intravenous bolus of a proton-pump inhibitor (e.g., omeprazole) to deacidify the stomach, as otherwise the low pH will inhibit platelet aggregation and coagulation.

If the patient has or may have cirrhosis, begin an octreotide infusion to constrict the mesenteric arterioles and reduce variceal pressure, in case this is the source of bleeding. Also administer prophylactic antibiotics that provide coverage of gram-negative and anaerobe organisms (e.g., ceftriaxone, piperacillin/tazobactam) to reduce the risk of bacterial translocation.

The definitive therapy for upper GIB is prompt esophagogastroduodenoscopy (EGD) within the first 24 hours of presentation, which can identify and often treat the source of bleeding (see Chapter 45 for more details). If bleeding cannot be controlled endoscopically, surgery or percutaneous arterial embolization may be required.

Lower Gastrointestinal Bleeding

If lower GIB is suspected, the patient should be stabilized and then prepared for colonoscopy (see Chapter 45 for more details) to identify and ideally treat the source. If the patient is unable to tolerate oral intake, the preparation solution may be administered through a nasogastric tube. If adequate bowel preparation does not occur, it is difficult to visualize the source of bleeding.

If significant bleeding is present or the patient is hemodynamically unstable, EGD should be performed alongside colonoscopy to rule out a more proximal source. If the luminal evaluation is negative but the bleeding continues, invasive angiography can localize the source of bleeding as long as the rate exceeds 0.5 mL/min. If necessary, the patient can undergo superselective arterial embolization or surgical resection of the affected bowel segment.

Obscure Gastrointestinal Bleeding or Suspected Small Bowel Bleeding

If bleeding is slow or intermittent and EGD and colonoscopy fail to identify a source, several additional diagnostic tests may be helpful. If the patient has melena, repeating an EGD or performing push enteroscopy permits direct examination of the upper GI tract and/or proximal jejunum. If this is normal, capsule endoscopy can visualize most of the small bowel to help localize the source. If these tests are negative but intermittent brisk bleeding continues, the patient can undergo a CT angiogram or be infused with radiolabeled red blood cells and scanned at regular intervals to locate the source of bleeding; however, this nuclear scan requires a minimum 0.1 mL/min bleeding rate and provides only a general approximation of the source. If the bleeding is more subacute, CT enterography is recommended. Depending on the findings the patient may require deep enteroscopy, interventional angiography, or surgery.

CHAPTER 12

Constipation

YING L. LIU

INTRODUCTION

Constipation is defined as having fewer than three unassisted bowel movements per week, along with any of the following symptoms during 25% or more of defecations: straining, lumpy/hard stools, the sensation of incomplete evacuation, anorectal obstruction or blockage, and reliance on manual maneuvers to promote defecation. The prevalence of constipation is high, estimated to be 16% in adults overall, and may be as high as 30% in certain groups such as the elderly, women, and those with lower socioeconomic status.

Chronic constipation can be primary idiopathic or secondary to other medical processes (Fig. 12.1). Primary idiopathic constipation can be divided into three categories: normal-transit constipation, isolated slow-transit constipation, and defecatory disorders. Some types of slow-transit constipation can be caused by colonic motor disturbances such as reduced propulsion or uncoordinated motor activity. Defecatory disorders include inactive rectal propulsion, incomplete relaxation of the pelvic floor/external anal sphincters, or structure disturbances (including rectoceles and intussusception) (Fig. 12.2). Constipation-dominant **irritable bowel syndrome** should also be considered.

Causes of secondary constipation include medications (frequently opioids), metabolic disturbances, neurological disorders (spinal cord lesions, Parkinson disease), and diseases of the colon (strictures/fissures, cancer, and proctitis).

EVALUATION AND DIAGNOSIS

Evaluation for constipation should begin with a detailed history, including an assessment of symptoms, current regimen and bowel patterns, and a detailed review of all prescription and over-the-counter (OTC) medications. Physical exam should include an external exam of the perineum and a digital rectal exam to assess for rectal tone. Further diagnostic testing should be reserved for patients who do not respond to first-line management or in those with alarm symptoms (weight loss, hematochezia, anemia). Further testing includes colonoscopy, anorectal manometry, rectal balloon expulsion test, and barium or MRI defecography as needed. The American Gastroenterological Association has a detailed algorithm for further testing.

TREATMENT (Table 12.1)

First-line management of constipation includes discontinuation of any offending medications, along with an increase in dietary fiber or fiber supplements. Increasing dietary fiber supplementation has been shown to allow discontinuation of laxatives in 59% to 80% of elderly patients with chronic idiopathic constipation while also improving symptoms. A systematic review of six randomized controlled trials assessing the efficacy of fiber supplementation compared with placebo found that fiber resulted in significant improvements in global symptoms and stools per week. Other types of commonly used fiber supplementations with less evidence include psyllium and docusate, which is a sodium salt that serves to soften stool.

However, 60% to 80% of patients will not respond to first-line fiber supplementation; thus second-line treatment of chronic constipation consists of stimulant **laxatives** such as bisacodyl, milk of magnesia, and senna. The efficacy and safety of bisacodyl treatment in patients with chronic constipation were established in a large, randomized, placebo-controlled multicenter trial in the United Kingdom that demonstrated increased bowel movements as compared to placebo. These agents are well tolerated and considered safe in patients with chronic constipation; however, long-term effects have not been well studied.

Osmotic laxatives, including polyethylene glycol (available OTC) and lactulose (available by prescription), retain water in the colon to soften stool. A recent Cochrane review of 10 randomized, controlled trials evaluated the efficacy of lactulose versus polyethylene glycol in treating chronic constipation and concluded that polyethylene glycol was superior.

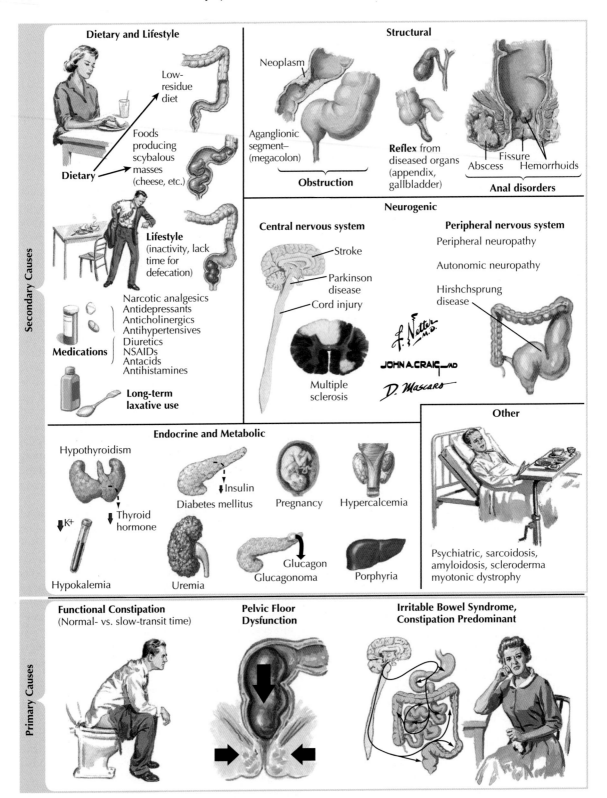

Secondary Causes

Dietary and Lifestyle

Low-residue diet

Foods producing scybalous masses (cheese, etc.)

Dietary

Lifestyle (inactivity, lack time for defecation)

Narcotic analgesics
Antidepressants
Anticholinergics
Antihypertensives
Diuretics
NSAIDs
Antacids
Antihistamines

Medications

Long-term laxative use

Structural

Neoplasm

Aganglionic segment– (megacolon)

Obstruction

Reflex from diseased organs (appendix, gallbladder)

Fissure
Abscess   Hemorrhoids

Anal disorders

Neurogenic

Central nervous system

Stroke

Parkinson disease

Cord injury

Multiple sclerosis

Peripheral nervous system

Peripheral neuropathy

Autonomic neuropathy

Hirshchsprung disease

Endocrine and Metabolic

Hypothyroidism

↓K+

↓ Thyroid hormone

Hypokalemia

↓Insulin

Diabetes mellitus

Uremia

Glucagon
Glucagonoma

Pregnancy

Hypercalcemia

Porphyria

Other

Psychiatric, sarcoidosis, amyloidosis, scleroderma myotonic dystrophy

Primary Causes

Functional Constipation (Normal- vs. slow-transit time)

Pelvic Floor Dysfunction

Irritable Bowel Syndrome, Constipation Predominant

FIG. 12.1 **Etiologies of Constipation.**

Normal pelvis

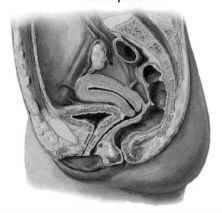

Rectocele

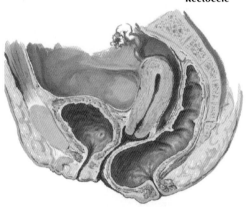
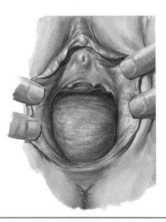

Dyssynergic defecation and fecal impaction

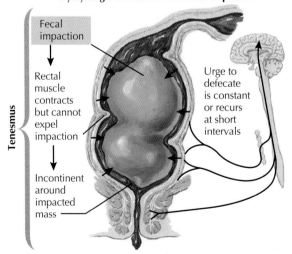

Fecal impaction

Rectal muscle contracts but cannot expel impaction

Tenesmus

Incontinent around impacted mass

Urge to defecate is constant or recurs at short intervals

Fecal impaction, or a large amount of hard stool in the distal rectum obstructing the anal outlet. The presence of a fecal impaction can lead to encopresis as more proximal fecal matter seeps around the impacted fecal mass.

Pelvic floor dysfunction syndrome

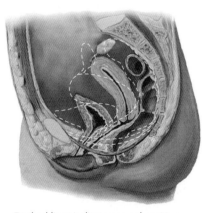

Dashed lines indicate normal position

FIG. 12.2 **Examples of Defecatory Disorders.**

TABLE 12.1
Stepwise Management of Constipation

Line of Treatment	Therapy	Example
1st	Diet and lifestyle changes	Increase fiber, fluids, and exercise
2nd	Stool softeners	Docusate, up to three times a day
3rd	Mild laxatives	Senna up to twice a day
4th	Stronger laxatives	Polyethylene glycol, bisacodyl as needed
5th	Rectal manipulation	Glycerin suppositories, tap water or soap suds enemas; mechanical disimpaction

Several newer agents are now in use to treat chronic constipation. Lubiprostone is an intestinal type 2 chloride channel activator that increases intestinal fluid secretion and improves small intestinal transit and stool passage. It is currently approved for chronic idiopathic constipation, opioid-induced constipation, and irritable bowel syndrome with predominantly constipation in women. Linaclotide, a guanylate cyclase-C agonist, is a small peptide approved for chronic idiopathic constipation and irritable bowel syndrome with constipation. Methylnaltrexone is a peripheral μ-opioid receptor antagonist used in the treatment of opioid-induced constipation when conventional laxative therapy has failed.

Patients with continued constipation despite medical management, particularly those with a defecatory disorder, may benefit from pelvic floor retraining and biofeedback therapy rather than laxatives. These patients may also benefit more from suppositories and **enemas** than oral laxatives alone. Hypertonic sodium phosphate enemas (e.g., Fleet) should be used with caution given reports of severe metabolic derangements, renal abnormalities, and even death. In general, tap water or soap suds enemas are preferred. In rare cases, patients may require manual disimpaction. Patients with refractory constipation, particularly those with slow-transit constipation, may require total colectomy with ileorectal anastomosis, but they first require evaluation by a colorectal surgeon.

CHAPTER 13

Diarrhea

PAUL B. MARTIN

INTRODUCTION

Diarrhea is traditionally defined as either stool volume >300 mL or more than three (typically loose or liquid) bowel movements in a 24-hour period. This definition, however, is more general guidance than a sharp diagnostic tool, as symptoms can vary significantly over time and among cases. Diarrheal illnesses are divided broadly into two categories: **acute** and **chronic.** These categories tend to have divergent underlying diseases, making them useful for diagnostic inquiry. Most acute diarrhea is rapid in onset, brief in duration (commonly <1 week) and resolves without specific intervention. Chronic diarrhea tends to be more insidious in onset, less severe, and lasts at least 4 weeks or sometimes up to many months if diagnosis is delayed.

ACUTE DIARRHEA

Most cases of acute diarrhea are due to infections and resolve without specific treatment. Supportive treatment with oral rehydration and the addition of an antimotility agent (e.g., loperamide) when clinically warranted usually suffices. Major causes include:

- Viruses (e.g., norovirus, rotavirus, and adenovirus)
- Bacteria (e.g., *Salmonella, Shigella, Campylobacter, Escherichia coli*, and **Clostridioides [formerly *Clostridium*] *difficile*)**
- Protozoa (e.g., *Cryptosporidium, Giardia, Cyclospora, Entamoeba*)

Of these, viral causes make up the majority of acute infectious diarrhea. Acute diarrhea with prominent vomiting is usually due to viral enteritis or acute food poisoning. If diarrhea persists, noninfectious causes tend to become more likely.

The two important decisions for clinicians facing a patient with acute diarrhea are whether to perform any specific testing to elucidate the etiology of acute diarrhea and whether any targeted treatment, besides supportive care, is required.

ACUTE DIARRHEA: EVALUATION

No specific testing is required if the diarrhea is watery, mild in severity (i.e., no or minimal change in activities, no fevers, no dehydration), and nonbloody. Patients who present with **dysentery** (diarrhea with visible blood or mucus), or those who manifest moderate-to-severe illness, including fevers, dehydration, or restriction in physical activity, may require microbiologic evaluation with directed antimicrobial treatment based on results. In cases of grossly bloody dysentery, or in cases of **traveler's diarrhea,** empiric treatment with antimicrobials is indicated. Table 13.1 contains information on indications for microbiologic testing.

Stool Cultures

Stool cultures identifying the most common pathogens, such as *Salmonella, Shigella,* and *Campylobacter,* are routinely the first step in testing; more specific tests can be performed as needed and/or suggested by history. For example, in patients with predominantly bloody diarrhea, specific testing for Shiga toxin–producing *E. coli* (looking for *Shiga* toxin) and *Entamoeba* should be considered. Patients with current or recent exposure to antibiotics, or health care facilities within the past 3 months, should be evaluated for *C. difficile.* If diarrhea is persistent and no diagnosis is apparent on initial evaluation, testing for ova and parasites, as well as noninfectious causes, has increasing yield and should be considered. Stool cultures for ova and parasites are also indicated upfront for immunocompromised patients, such as those with advanced HIV/AIDS with CD4 counts <200 or posttransplant patients.

Multipathogen Molecular Panels

If available, novel multipathogen panels have advantages over traditional cultures, including increased diagnostic yield and more rapid diagnosis, which may allow clinicians to withhold or tailor antibiotic therapy. Unfortunately, these methods are so sensitive that they

TABLE 13.1
Features of Acute Diarrhea to Warrant Microbiological Testing

Clinically Severe Illness	Symptoms of Inflammatory Diarrhea	High-Risk Host Features
Profuse diarrhea	Bloody diarrhea	Age >70 years
Persistent diarrhea	Frequent small-volume stools with blood and mucus	High-risk comorbidities[a]
Possible hypovolemia	Fever >38.4°C	Immunocompromised[b]
Severe abdominal pain		Inflammatory bowel disease
Hospitalization required		Pregnancy

[a]Major cardiac/cardiovascular, pulmonary disease.
[b]For example, advanced HIV, transplant recipient.

may detect possible pathogens at subpathogenic levels and have shown increased rates of mixed infections, which can confound the clinical picture.

ACUTE DIARRHEA: TREATMENT

All patients should be treated with oral rehydration; specific diets are usually not indicated, but the avoidance of foods with high fat content may be symptomatically beneficial. Patients with mild, predominantly watery diarrhea should be offered antimotility treatment with loperamide. Unless the diarrhea is severe, antibiotics are not routinely indicated even if a treatable causative agent is identified. Antibiotics may reduce the duration of symptoms but can increase the risk of gastrointestinal side effects or potentially *C. difficile*. Empiric antibiotic therapy is indicated in cases of severe illness, dysentery, or a host susceptible of significant complications (elderly, immunocompromised). Additionally, antibiotic treatment is generally recommended in traveler's diarrhea.

Antibiotics

First-line empiric treatment for acute diarrhea is azithromycin, with a fluoroquinolone (e.g., ciprofloxacin, levofloxacin) as second-line treatment. If patients are at high risk for *C. difficile* based on criteria outlined earlier, especially in severe diarrhea, empiric treatment for *C. difficile* is reasonable while awaiting further testing (see Chapter 119 for further information).

CHRONIC DIARRHEA

Chronic diarrhea, generally defined as diarrheal symptoms lasting >4 weeks, is a challenging diagnostic process, with a wide variety of possible diagnoses ranging from functional **irritable bowel syndrome (IBS)** to inflammatory, malabsorptive, and infectious causes (Fig. 13.1). A first major step in tailoring the diagnostic process is to use the history and exam to categorize the diarrhea as functional or organic. If it is not functional (i.e., an organic process, characterized by profuse watery diarrhea or stool containing fat/blood/mucus), subsequent tailored testing can narrow the diagnosis significantly.

Functional Diarrhea

Functional diarrhea due to IBS is quite common; thus it is often an initial consideration in patients with chronic diarrhea. Patients with IBS can present with a broad range of symptoms, both gastrointestinal and extraintestinal. The hallmark symptoms are chronic lower abdominal pain paired with altered bowel habits without weight loss. Pain tends to be crampy and often is relieved by defecation. Bowel habits can be variable, including constipation and diarrhea alternating, with frequent small-volume stools preceded by extreme urgency that are sometimes described as mucoid. IBS usually presents in young adults and has a female predominance. Weight loss, bloody or greasy stools, large-volume stools, or nocturnal diarrhea are not associated with IBS and warrant further evaluation for organic causes.

Watery Diarrhea

Watery diarrhea can be divided in secretory or osmotic. **Secretory diarrhea** is independent of fasting, occurs day and night, and produces large-volume stools. **Osmotic diarrhea,** on the other hand, is due to high concentrations of solutes within the colon that draw in water, so fasting improves or resolves the symptoms. If the history is not highly suggestive, calculating the **stool osmolar gap,** equal to stool osmolality − [2 × (stool Na + stool K)], can be helpful in differentiating between osmotic and secretory diarrhea. An elevated gap and improvement with fasting suggest dietary **malabsorption,** such as lactose intolerance, which may be supported by hydrogen breath testing, or inadvertent ingestion (e.g., sorbitol). A low stool osmolar gap suggests secretory

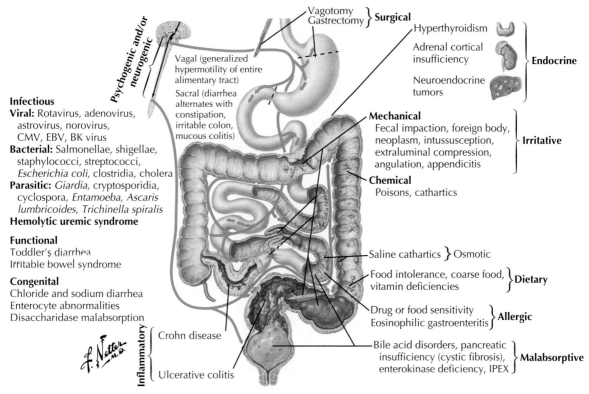

Infectious
Viral: Rotavirus, adenovirus, astrovirus, norovirus, CMV, EBV, BK virus
Bacterial: Salmonellae, shigellae, staphylococci, streptococci, *Escherichia coli*, clostridia, cholera
Parasitic: *Giardia*, cryptosporidia, cyclospora, *Entamoeba*, *Ascaris lumbricoides*, *Trichinella spiralis*
Hemolytic uremic syndrome

Functional
Toddler's diarrhea
Irritable bowel syndrome

Congenital
Chloride and sodium diarrhea
Enterocyte abnormalities
Disaccharidase malabsorption

Inflammatory { Crohn disease
Ulcerative colitis

Psychogenic and/or neurogenic

Vagotomy } **Surgical**
Gastrectomy

Vagal (generalized hypermotility of entire alimentary tract)
Sacral (diarrhea alternates with constipation, irritable colon, mucous colitis)

Hyperthyroidism
Adrenal cortical insufficiency } **Endocrine**
Neuroendocrine tumors

Mechanical
Fecal impaction, foreign body, neoplasm, intussusception, extraluminal compression, angulation, appendicitis } **Irritative**
Chemical
Poisons, cathartics

Saline cathartics } Osmotic
Food intolerance, coarse food, vitamin deficiencies } **Dietary**
Drug or food sensitivity
Eosinophilic gastroenteritis } **Allergic**
Bile acid disorders, pancreatic insufficiency (cystic fibrosis), enterokinase deficiency, IPEX } **Malabsorptive**

FIG. 13.1 **Potential Causes of Diarrhea.** *CMV*, Cytomegalovirus; *EBV*, Epstein-Barr virus; *IPEX*, immunodysregulation, polyendocrinopathy, enteropathy, X linked (syndrome).

diarrhea; possible etiologies include chronic infection, structural anatomical defect, or a systemic process such as thyroid dysfunction, hormone-secreting tumors (e.g., VIPoma), or pheochromocytoma.

Fatty Diarrhea

Fatty diarrhea, or **steatorrhea,** typically presents with stools described as greasy and malodorous and is commonly caused by malabsorption. Malabsorption, in turn, can arise from chronic pancreatitis, bacterial overgrowth of small intestine, and celiac disease (gluten-sensitive enteropathy; see Chapter 133 for details) (Fig. 13.2).

Manifestations of malabsorption can be highly variable, from mild, barely noticeable symptoms to voluminous, foul-smelling diarrhea and significant weight loss despite adequate food intake. Steatorrhea also may result from anatomical defects, which should be evaluated with radiography and/or colonoscopy.

Inflammatory Diarrhea

The most common causes for chronic inflammatory diarrhea are **inflammatory bowel diseases (IBDs)** (including Crohn disease and ulcerative colitis—see Chapter 134 for further information); less common

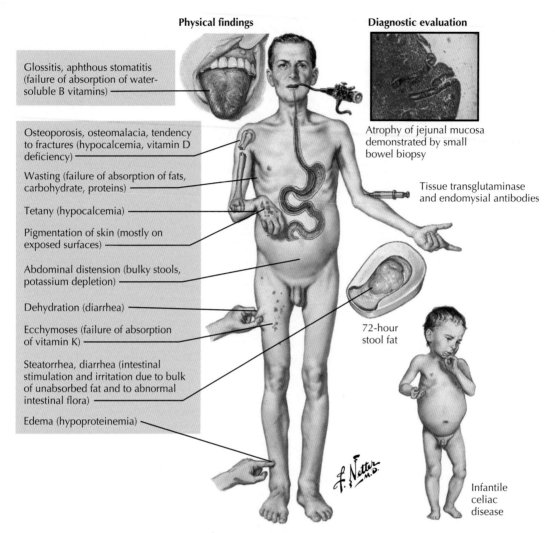

Physical findings

Glossitis, aphthous stomatitis (failure of absorption of water-soluble B vitamins)

Osteoporosis, osteomalacia, tendency to fractures (hypocalcemia, vitamin D deficiency)

Wasting (failure of absorption of fats, carbohydrate, proteins)

Tetany (hypocalcemia)

Pigmentation of skin (mostly on exposed surfaces)

Abdominal distension (bulky stools, potassium depletion)

Dehydration (diarrhea)

Ecchymoses (failure of absorption of vitamin K)

Steatorrhea, diarrhea (intestinal stimulation and irritation due to bulk of unabsorbed fat and to abnormal intestinal flora)

Edema (hypoproteinemia)

Diagnostic evaluation

Atrophy of jejunal mucosa demonstrated by small bowel biopsy

Tissue transglutaminase and endomysial antibodies

72-hour stool fat

Infantile celiac disease

FIG. 13.2 **Celiac Disease and Malabsorption.**

etiologies are microscopic colitis and opportunistic infections such as tuberculosis. Opportunistic infections become more prevalent in resource-poor settings and in patients with immune deficiencies such as advanced HIV. History can be highly suggestive in cases of IBD, and inflammatory markers such as C-reactive protein are usually elevated. Notably, while **fecal leukocytes** are not a good test for inflammatory diarrhea, **fecal calprotectin** is often elevated in IBD and is increasingly utilized. Diagnosis requires endoscopic visualization (usually via colonoscopy) and biopsy.

CHAPTER 14

Hematuria

BALAKUMAR KRISHNARASA • ABHIRAMI VIVEKANANDARAJAH

INTRODUCTION

Hematuria is defined as red blood cells (RBCs) in urine and is categorized into two distinct categories. **Gross hematuria** is visible blood in the urine; the urine itself may be red or brown, but the color change does not necessarily reflect the degree of blood loss, since as little as 1 mL of blood per liter of urine can induce color change.

Microscopic hematuria is detectable only via examination of urine sediment, specifically defined as two to five RBCs found on a urinalysis (UA) on high-power field (HPF) in a spun urine sediment. While point-of-care urine **dipsticks** can detect one to two RBCs/HPF, they can be confounded when semen, myoglobin, or hemoglobin is present; with urine pH >9; or if oxidizing agents are utilized to clean the perineum. A positive urine dipstick therefore must always be confirmed with microscopic examination of the urine.

ETIOLOGY

Hematuria can originate from anywhere in the urinary tract from the kidneys to the urethra (Fig. 14.1). Potential etiologies include:
- Nephrolithiasis
- Infections (including pyelonephritis, cystitis, prostatitis, or urethritis); infection sources include bacterial, viral, fungal parasitic, or mycobacterial
- Traumatic, postprocedural, or postradiation bleeding
- Benign (angiomyolipoma) and malignant (renal cell carcinoma) kidney masses
- Nonrenal malignancies, such as bladder or prostate cancer
- Glomerulonephritis (see Chapter 95 for further details)
- Structural renal disease, such as medullary sponge kidney or autosomal dominant polycystic kidney disease (see Chapter 98 for further information)
- Structural abnormalities (including urethral diverticulum or stricture)
- Vascular injury, such as renal vein thrombus or renal artery embolism that precipitates papillary necrosis

Vigorous exercise can cause hematuria in the absence of underlying urinary tract pathology. It has no known long-term morbidity but remains a diagnosis of exclusion.

EVALUATION AND DIAGNOSIS

Patients with a urine dipstick positive for hematuria should receive a formal UA with microscopic analysis to confirm. Patients who are actively menstruating may have false positives, requiring repeat UA once menstruation has ceased. Patients with hematuria in the setting of vigorous exercise should have repeat testing in 4 to 6 weeks during a period of no exercise. Patients with acute trauma should have a confirmatory UA after 6 weeks.

Historical clues can guide the management of hematuria. Dysuria, increased frequency, and pyuria usually indicate a urinary tract infection but may also occur with bladder malignancy. Unilateral flank pain is common with nephrolithiasis or pyelonephritis but can be seen in malignancy or IgA nephropathy. Patients with a recent upper respiratory infection may suffer from postinfectious glomerulonephritis. Family history of hematuria or renal disease suggests hereditary nephritis, anatomical abnormalities, or sickle cell disease, which can result in vascular complications or papillary necrosis (Fig. 14.2). Older males with hematuria and lower urinary tract symptoms (including hesitancy, difficult stream/dribbling, or nocturia), or with known benign prostatic hyperplasia, should be evaluated for malignancy. Travel history is crucial for assessment of exposure to endemic infections, including *Schistosoma haematobium* and tuberculosis. A thorough medication history can suggest medication-related interstitial nephritis. Hematuria in an anticoagulated patient should be evaluated in the same fashion as in other patients and not be assumed as due to anticoagulation alone, but care must be exercised prior to any invasive procedures or workup.

Patients with hematuria and the following risk factors are at higher risk of urological malignancy:
- Male gender
- Age >40 years

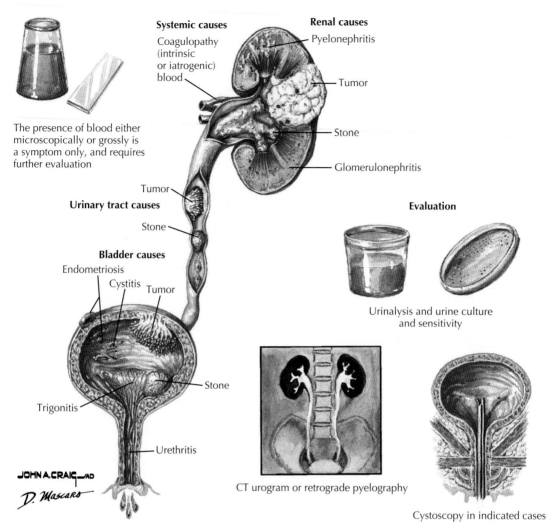

The presence of blood either microscopically or grossly is a symptom only, and requires further evaluation

Systemic causes

Coagulopathy (intrinsic or iatrogenic) blood

Renal causes

Pyelonephritis

Tumor

Stone

Glomerulonephritis

Tumor

Urinary tract causes

Stone

Bladder causes

Endometriosis

Cystitis

Tumor

Trigonitis

Stone

Urethritis

Evaluation

Urinalysis and urine culture and sensitivity

CT urogram or retrograde pyelography

Cystoscopy in indicated cases

JOHN A. CRAIG—MD
D. Mascaro

FIG. 14.1 **Potential Causes and Workup of Hematuria.**

- Past or current smoking history
- Past history of gross hematuria
- History of irritative voiding symptoms
- History of chronic urinary tract infection
- History of pelvic irradiation
- History of a chronic indwelling foreign body
- History of analgesic abuse
- Exposure to chemicals, dyes (benzenes or aromatic amines) in printers, painters, and chemical plant workers
- Exposure to cyclophosphamide

Gross examination of the urine can give several clues. Dark-colored urine is seen in glomerular hematuria, while pink or red urine is typical of nonglomerular hematuria. Visible clots in the urine are due to nonglomerular bleeding. Grossly bloody urine with clots in the absence of recent instrumentation of the urinary tract should trigger an evaluation for a nonglomerular source even if proteinuria is present. Patients with new or worsening hypertension and edema should be evaluated for glomerular disease.

The appearance of RBCs on a centrifuged urine sediment can help localize the source of the bleeding, thus guiding subsequent evaluation. Dysmorphic RBCs, RBC casts, or cola-colored urine suggests a glomerular source of bleeding, but an absence does not necessarily rule out a glomerular source. **Acanthocytes** are defined as ring-shaped RBCs with vesicle-shaped protrusions

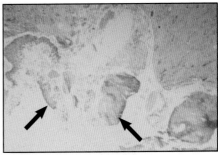

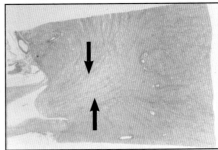

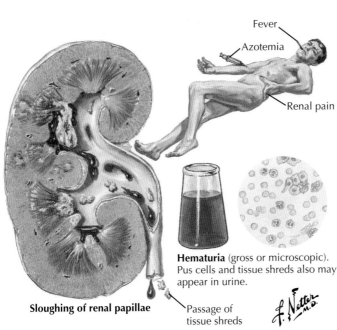

Fever

Azotemia

Renal pain

Papillary necrosis with sloughing. Leaving a concave inner border of the medulla. Detached dead fragments can be found in the urine.

Hematuria (gross or microscopic). Pus cells and tissue shreds also may appear in urine.

Sloughing of renal papillae   Passage of tissue shreds

Papillary necrosis without inflammatory reaction. Believed by some to be characteristic of analgesic papillary necrosis.

FIG. 14.2 **Papillary Necrosis.**

best seen on phase-contrast microscopy; they are the dysmorphic RBCs most predictive of glomerular disease. Nonglomerular bleeding typically produces uniform, round RBCs because they have not been forced through the glomerular filtration apparatus. Proteinuria is more prevalent and severe in patients with glomerular hematuria than in patients with nonglomerular hematuria, but both can have mild to moderate proteinuria. Albuminuria is consistent with glomerular hematuria.

Laboratory testing is directed toward the suspected underlying pathology. A basic metabolic panel is essential to evaluate renal function, and a complete blood count is needed for evaluation of gross hematuria. Urine culture can detect bacterial infections, though serology or specific testing may be needed depending on the suspected pathogen. Urine cytology is no longer recommended due to variable sensitivity and specificity.

Patients with nonglomerular hematuria should receive imaging of the urinary tract. CT of the abdomen/pelvis with and without intravenous contrast, or **CT urography (CTU),** is recommended in patients with otherwise unexplained hematuria. Exceptions include pregnant women, who should instead undergo ultrasound of the kidneys/

bladder to avoid ionizing radiation, and patients with chronic kidney disease (estimated glomerular filtration rate [eGFR] <30), who should not receive contrast for fear of worsening renal function. Fortunately, CTU without contrast is still quite sensitive for detecting nephrolithiasis. MR urography is more sensitive for detecting renal and urothelial tumors but is not as effective at detecting nephrolithiasis. Retrograde pyelography should be considered as an adjunct to **cystoscopy** to evaluate for ureteral abnormalities.

Cystoscopy

Cystoscopy can directly visualize the urethra, prostate, and bladder and may identify the source of the bleeding among patients with gross hematuria. All patients with nonglomerular and noninfectious gross hematuria are recommended to undergo cystoscopy. Cystoscopy is also recommended in patients with microscopic hematuria with no evidence of glomerular or infectious cause, and who have an increased risk of urinary tract malignancy. Cystoscopy can be both diagnostic (identifying the source of bleeding) and therapeutic (direct intervention for bleeding or underlying cause).

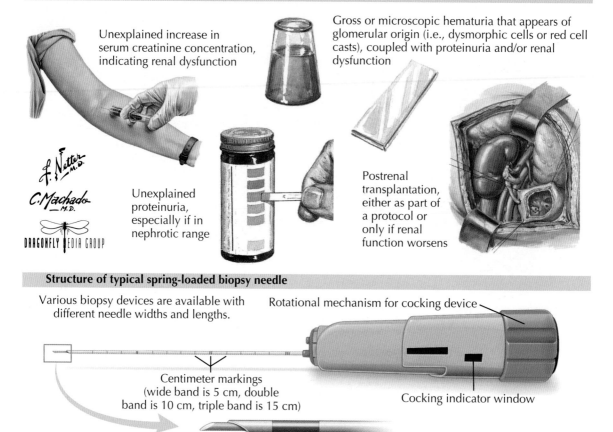

Common indications

Unexplained increase in serum creatinine concentration, indicating renal dysfunction

Gross or microscopic hematuria that appears of glomerular origin (i.e., dysmorphic cells or red cell casts), coupled with proteinuria and/or renal dysfunction

Unexplained proteinuria, especially if in nephrotic range

Postrenal transplantation, either as part of a protocol or only if renal function worsens

Structure of typical spring-loaded biopsy needle

Various biopsy devices are available with different needle widths and lengths.

Rotational mechanism for cocking device

Centimeter markings (wide band is 5 cm, double band is 10 cm, triple band is 15 cm)

Cocking indicator window

Stylet   Cannula

Cannula withdrawn and stylet exposed

FIG. 14.3 **Renal Biopsy: Indications and Structure of Typical Spring-Loaded Needle.**

Kidney Biopsy

Patients with glomerular hematuria, proteinuria, and acute kidney injury should undergo a **kidney biopsy.** Biopsy is also recommended in nondiabetic patients with glomerular hematuria with a persistent urine albumin excretion >30 mg/day (Fig. 14.3).

Kidney biopsy is not usually performed for isolated glomerular and nonglomerular hematuria with no signs of glomerular disease. If kidney biopsy is not performed in a patient with isolated glomerular hematuria, they

should receive periodic monitoring of renal function, urine protein excretion, and UA to detect early signs of progressive disease.

If no diagnosis is apparent from the history, UA, imaging exams, or cystoscopy, then the most likely causes of persistent isolated hematuria are a mild glomerulopathy or nephrolithiasis, particularly in young and middle-aged patients. Current guidelines do not recommend routine screening for hematuria in asymptomatic individuals.

CHAPTER 15

Joint Pain

BRYAN C. LEPPERT

INTRODUCTION

Joint pain is a common presenting complaint with a vast array of underlying causes, including trauma, degenerative joint disease, infection, and inflammation. Treatment goals are to reduce pain, reverse/slow underlying disease, and preserve joint function.

EVALUATION

The history is critical for establishing and focusing the broad differential of joint pain. Several disease characteristics can narrow the differential diagnosis of joint pain, including:

- Location, including how many joints (monoarticular vs polyarticular) and which joints are involved. For example, **rheumatoid arthritis (RA)** classically involves the metacarpophalangeal (MCP) and proximal interphalangeal (PIP) joints, while **osteoarthritis** affects the PIP and distal interphalangeal (DIP) joints.
- Quality of pain, chiefly to distinguish between inflammatory and noninflammatory causes (Table 15.1)
- Timing of onset of pain. Acute pain is more concerning for traumatic or infectious causes. Chronic pain is more often associated with inflammatory or degenerative disease.
- Aggravating/alleviating factors. Elicit any changes in range of motion as a result of pain, or changes in pain with use of the joint. For example, RA usually presents with morning stiffness that improves with movement, while osteoarthritis typically worsens throughout the day with repeated use of the joint.
- Associated symptoms. Extraarticular symptoms such as fatigue, rash, oral ulcers, and dry eyes/mouth are seen in patients with rheumatological diseases. Constitutional symptoms, including fevers, weight loss, and night sweats, suggest an infectious or reactive arthropathy.

Troubling historical symptoms include nocturnal or unremitting pain, systemic symptoms as outlined earlier, and pain that results in significant disability. A history of traumatic injury must be elicited. Family history can reveal patterns of rheumatological disease, including RA and **systemic lupus erythematosus (SLE).** The patient's medication list can reveal predisposing drugs, such as hydrochlorothiazide leading to hyperuricemia and increasing the chance of gout. A detailed travel and infectious history are necessary to rule out infectious causes of arthritis, while sexual history can screen for possible gonococcal or chlamydia-related arthritis.

Physical exam can further refine the differential diagnosis. For a given affected joint, the nonaffected equivalent joint should be examined to provide a normal baseline for comparison in that particular patient. Visual inspection can confirm the affected joints as elicited from history and evaluate for signs of overt trauma (bleeding, foreign body, ecchymoses), joint abnormalities, or erythema (Fig. 15.1). Palpation can reveal signs of **synovitis,** including joint effusion, warmth, and swelling (which may be visually apparent, depending on body habitus), as well as underlying crepitus.

Range-of-motion testing can separate periarticular from articular complaints. In periarticular disease, including bursitis, tendinitis, or other muscle injury, passive range of motion—that is, ability for the examiner to mobilize the joint without any assistance from the patient—is preserved. Active range of motion, in which patients themselves must mobilize the joint unassisted, is reduced in periarticular disease. Decrease in both active and passive range of motion suggests an articular etiology. Specific maneuvers for a given joint or pathology may further clarify the diagnosis; for example, the anterior drawer test assesses for anterior translocation of the tibia characteristic of an anterior cruciate ligament tear.

The remainder of the physical exam can assess for extraarticular symptoms indicative of an underlying systemic disease. Fever is consistent with an inflammatory or infectious arthritis. A malar or discoid rash, alopecia, and oral/nasal ulcers may indicate SLE (see Chapter 106 for further details), while aphthous oral and genital ulcers suggest Behçet disease. Osler nodes, Janeway lesions, and splinter hemorrhages suggest infective endocarditis, which can lead to septic arthritis through

Chronic Heberden nodes.
Fourth and fifth proximal interphalangeal
joints also involved in degenerative process.

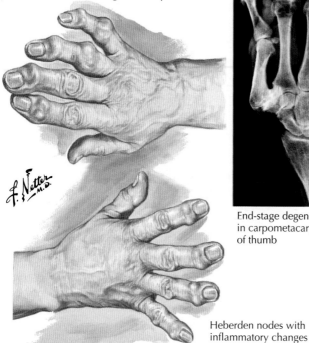

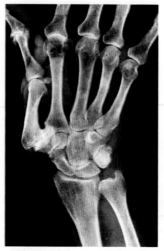

End-stage degenerative changes
in carpometacarpal articulation
of thumb

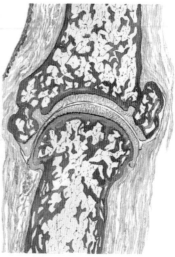

Section through distal interphalangeal
joint shows irregular, hyperplastic bony
nodules (Heberden nodes) at articular
margins of distal phalanx.

Heberden nodes with
inflammatory changes

FIG. 15.1 **Hand Involvement in Osteoarthritis.**

TABLE 15.1
Inflammatory Versus Noninflammatory Pain

Feature	Inflammatory	Noninflammatory
Morning stiffness	>60 minutes	<30 minutes
Activity	Typically worse in the morning and with immobility	Typically worse in the evening and after use
Joint erythema	Sometimes	No
Joint swelling	Yes	Rarely
Joint warmth	Typically yes	Rarely
Constitutional symptoms	Fevers, fatigue, malaise	Absent
Synovial fluid	WBC >2000, mostly neutrophils	WBC <2000, mostly monocytes
Lab work	Elevated ESR, CRP; anemia of chronic disease	Inflammatory markers normal, but could be abnormal from other causes

CRP, C-reactive protein; *ESR,* erythrocyte sedimentation rate; *WBC,* white blood cell.

embolization of infective material. A lacy, reticulated rash or facial exanthem similar to slapped cheeks may signify parvovirus B19 infection.

Laboratory testing in joint pain derives from the history and physical exam. In patients without systemic symptoms or notable physical exam findings, serial evaluation may be acceptable over generalized laboratory testing. The **erythrocyte sedimentation rate (ESR)** and **C-reactive protein (CRP)** are nonspecific markers of inflammation, which can be elevated in patients with symptoms suggestive of an underlying inflammatory condition. While these tests can be followed serially if elevated, care must be taken in their interpretation, as other pathologies (e.g., malignancy, diabetes, infection) can lead to abnormal results.

Basic renal and liver chemistries, as well as a complete blood count, can identify systemic diseases. Notably, leukocytosis may suggest infection but is nonspecific, and the absence of leukocytosis does not rule out infection such as septic arthritis. Hypothyroidism can lead to polyarticular pain without localized tenderness and can be confirmed with an elevated thyroid-stimulating hormone (TSH). Uric acid levels are commonly checked in patients with suspected gout but are nondiagnostic in the acute setting; a below-normal uric acid level makes gout less likely. If viral arthritis is suspected, testing for hepatitis B, C, and parvovirus should be considered. If history and travel are concerning for Lyme disease, appropriate antibodies should be tested. Depending on sexual history elicited, screening for sexually transmitted infections (STIs) may be warranted.

Antibody testing can clarify the diagnosis in patients suspected of having an underlying rheumatological disease. The antinuclear antibody (ANA) is sensitive but not specific for SLE and must be interpreted in the context of other diagnostic criteria for SLE. Rheumatoid factor (RF) and, more specifically, anticyclic citrullinated peptide (anti-CCP), are useful for evaluation of suspected RA (see Chapters 102 and 106 for further details).

Arthrocentesis is the aspiration of synovial fluid in an affected joint and, depending on the clinical circumstance, the injection of medication. Arthrocentesis should be attempted for patients with accessible effusions and for those with signs of inflammatory arthritis, especially septic arthritis and gout. Gross appearance of the fluid can suggest an underlying cause, such as bloody fluid indicative of hemarthrosis or purulent fluid concerning for infection. Typical studies of synovial fluid include:

- Gram stain/culture, useful for isolating a bacterial pathogen in suspected **septic arthritis.**
- Cell count with differential. Normal synovial fluid is largely acellular, and neutrophils account for a small fraction of total white blood cells (WBCs). In inflammatory conditions, the number of WBCs and neutrophils increases dramatically; for example, septic arthritis typically produces >50,000 cells/µL, though this is not an absolute cutoff (see Chapter 103 for further details).
- Crystal analysis to identify crystalline arthropathies. Uric acid crystals in gout are needle shaped with negative birefringence on polarized light microscopy. Crystals in calcium pyrophosphate deposition (CPPD, formerly pseudogout) disease are rectangular or rhomboid shaped and exhibit positive birefringence (see Chapter 104 for further details).

Patients with a history of significant trauma or bony point tenderness on exam should receive plain radiographs to rule out fracture, tumor, or osteonecrosis. Plain radiographs can demonstrate joint effusions that may be amenable to arthrocentesis, with ultrasound useful for real-time guidance. Plain radiographs may be taken with different patient positioning to accentuate pathology, such as weight-bearing films to highlight joint narrowing in osteoarthritis. CT can rule out fracture in patients with demineralized bone from osteoporosis. MRI evaluates the joint itself and surrounding tendons, ligaments, and muscles in suspected periarticular or soft tissue injury.

GENERAL MANAGEMENT

Specific management of joint pain depends on the underlying cause, but some therapeutic options are common across multiple etiologies. Fractures should be immobilized to prevent displacement and any further soft tissue injury; patients with open fractures, in which bone communicates with the environment, or significantly displaced fractures require operative fixation. Braces and supportive devices allow patients to participate in physical therapy and maintain functioning in their activities of daily living. The acronym RICE (rest, ice, compression, elevation) can relieve soft tissue swelling and associated pain.

Pharmacological management of joint pain involves topical, local, and systemic therapies. Topical options are available as patches, gels, or ointments: Common medications include lidocaine and capsaicin, a topical anesthetic derived from chili peppers, while topical **NSAIDs** are finding use in patients who cannot tolerate systemic side effects of NSAIDs (see later discussion). Intraarticular glucocorticoids such as methylprednisolone and triamcinolone can decrease inflammation and reduce pain, but their use is contraindicated in patients with septic arthritis or overlying infection (as the needle could introduce pathogens into the joint space), periarticular

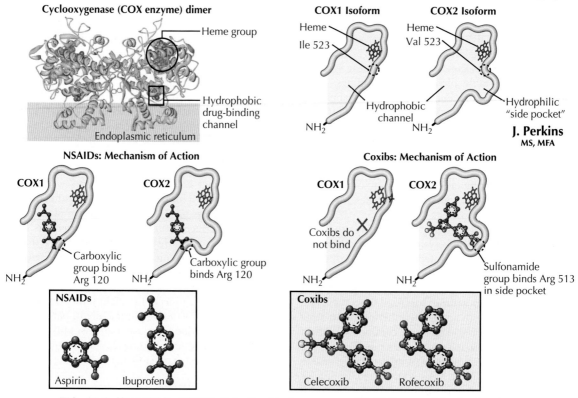

FIG. 15.2 **Nonopioids: NSAIDs, Selective Cyclooxygenase-2 Inhibitors, and Acetaminophen.**

fractures (in which glucocorticoids would inhibit bone healing), and osteoporosis adjacent to the joint (as glucocorticoids would worsen bone density). Systemic glucocorticoids may be utilized in polyarticular joint pain, although care should be exercised to minimize their duration of use given the side effects of glucocorticoids.

Acetaminophen is the most widely used over-the-counter analgesic in the United States and is often a first-line therapy for mild to moderate pain. It possesses both analgesic and antipyretic properties and, owing to its safe side effect profile at recommended doses, has been formulated in combination with numerous other medications. However, acetaminophen overdose can lead to devastating liver damage (see Chapter 135 for further details).

NSAIDs act by inhibiting cyclooxygenase isoenzymes (COX1 and/or COX2), decreasing the synthesis of prostaglandins, which promote inflammation (Fig. 15.2). Common side effects of NSAIDs include decreased prostaglandin-mucosal protection, leading to dyspepsia and predisposing to ulcer formation, which can trigger gastrointestinal (GI) hemorrhage; acute kidney injury through renal vasoconstriction; and increased risk of cardiac events (including myocardial infarction and stroke, especially in patients with established cardiovascular disease and recent cardiovascular events). NSAIDs may be nonselective (e.g., ibuprofen, naproxen, and ketorolac) or COX2 selective (celecoxib), which has a better GI side effect profile. In general, the lowest dose of NSAID for the shortest duration is preferred.

Opioid pain medications are effective at mitigating acute pain, but their use in chronic joint pain is not recommended due to the risk of opioid dependence and respiratory depression.

CHAPTER 16

Altered Mental Status

CHINDHURI SELVADURAI

INTRODUCTION

Altered mental status (AMS) is a general term for a disruption in normal cognitive function. AMS encompasses a multitude of pathological processes, and multiple metrics can help narrow a differential diagnosis:

- Severity, from mild errors in cognition, restricted attention, or changes in behavior to profound confusion and unresponsiveness/coma
- Duration, with presentations ranging from acute (minutes–days), to subacute (days–weeks), to chronic (weeks–months)
- Affected cognitive domains, including language, attention, memory, processing speed, visuospatial function, and reasoning
- Lateralizing or localizing features, particularly in the context of stroke and seizure

Treatment hinges on prompt recognition of the underlying cause, as many conditions can have lasting effects, including death, if not diagnosed readily. One of the most serious etiologies of AMS encountered in the hospital is **delirium,** an acute confusional state with restricted attention, typically characterized by waxing and waning behaviors. Delirium is associated with a very high morbidity and mortality, particularly when it is not diagnosed and reversed promptly.

AMS can be broadly categorized into acute and chronic changes in mental status; this chapter will focus on acute AMS. Briefly, chronic, acquired changes in mental status have a vast array of causes, depending on patient characteristics, and include dementia due to neurodegenerative disease, depression, tumor, poststroke sequelae, and many other chronic brain disorders that may present with a spectrum of cognitive deficits. All patients with chronic changes in mental status are at increased risk for acute disorders of AMS.

INITIAL EVALUATION

Evaluation of patients presenting emergently with acute AMS should focus on searching for potentially reversible causes. Broadly speaking, these include:

- Vascular, including stroke and myocardial infarction
- Primary neurological disease, especially seizures
- Infection, including meningitis, encephalitis, urinary tract infection (UTI), and pneumonia
- Ingestion, including medication/drug overdose or **alcohol withdrawal** (Fig. 16.1)
- Metabolic/endocrine diseases, such as hyponatremia/hypernatremia, hepatic encephalopathy, and uremia

A comprehensive history and physical exam are critical to elucidate the etiology of AMS. Pertinent historical questions include the timing, onset, and duration of AMS, as well as the mental status trajectory (improving or declining). Any recent travel, infectious symptoms, new medications, and trauma history are also important. When possible, clarify the patient's baseline mental status from collateral or chart information, as some patients may have underlying cognitive issues related to dementia. A complete medication history may reveal potential causative agents, including psychiatric medications (antipsychotics resulting in neuroleptic malignant syndrome, or antidepressants leading to serotonin syndrome), opioid pain medications, antihyperglycemics (both oral medications and injectable insulin), and anticholinergic medications, an important cause of AMS in the elderly.

The physical exam can suggest a focal neurological issue, a psychiatric disorder, or potential systemic pathologies. Having cold extremities suggests peripheral vascular disease or hypoperfusion. Fever alongside nuchal rigidity, positive Kernig or Brudzinski sign, pulmonary rales, or suprapubic tenderness suggests underlying infection.

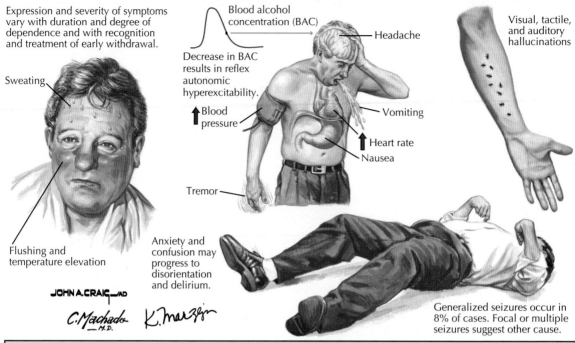

Expression and severity of symptoms vary with duration and degree of dependence and with recognition and treatment of early withdrawal.

Sweating

Flushing and temperature elevation

Blood alcohol concentration (BAC)

Decrease in BAC results in reflex autonomic hyperexcitability.

↑Blood pressure

Anxiety and confusion may progress to disorientation and delirium.

Headache

Vomiting

Heart rate

Nausea

Tremor

Visual, tactile, and auditory hallucinations

Generalized seizures occur in 8% of cases. Focal or multiple seizures suggest other cause.

JOHN A. CRAIG—MD

C. Machado —M.D.

K. marzin

Stages of Alcohol Withdrawal			
	Stage 1	**Stage 2**	**Stage 3**
Hours after alcohol consumption	24 36 (peak) 48	(48–72)	(72–105)
Symptoms	Mild-to-moderate anxiety, tremor, nausea, vomiting, sweating, elevation of heart rate and blood pressure, sleep disturbance, hallucinations, illusions, seizures	Aggravated forms of stage 1 symptoms with severe tremors, agitation, and hallucinations	Acute organic psychosis (delirium), confusion, and disorientation with severe autonomic symptoms delirium tremens

Stage 1 withdrawal usually self-limited. Only small percentage of cases progress to stages 2 and 3. Progression prevented by prompt and adequate treatment.

FIG. 16.1 **Alcohol Withdrawal.**

Patients with suspected drug overdose or intoxication should be examined for track marks from repeated injection or evidence of skin popping. Patients with abdominal ascites may have underlying cirrhosis or have asterixis (inability to maintain wrist extension, causing a flaplike movement), signifying hepatic encephalopathy. The thyroid exam can uncover goiter or tenderness suggesting thyroiditis. Volume depletion may suggest an underlying infection, neglect, or failure to thrive in the chronically ill.

The neurological exam is crucial for the evaluation of the altered patient. While not reviewed in depth here, a comprehensive neurological exam includes assessment of the overall mental status, as well as examination of

cranial nerves, motor and sensory pathways, coordination, reflexes, and gait; various resources, including the American Academy of Neurology, have detailed discussions regarding the comprehensive neurological exam. In patients suspected of having a stroke, the **National Institutes of Health (NIH) Stroke Scale (NIHSS)** quantifies stroke severity and is an essential component of the physical exam.

A mental status exam tests several domains:
- Level of consciousness/responsiveness **(Glasgow coma score [GCS])**
- Orientation (knowledge of place, time, age)
- Attention (e.g., performing multistep tasks, spelling the word world backwards)

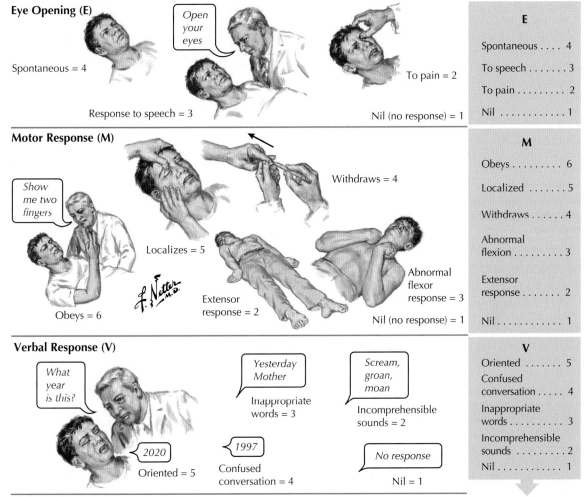

Eye Opening (E)

Spontaneous = 4

Open your eyes

Response to speech = 3

To pain = 2

Nil (no response) = 1

E	
Spontaneous	4
To speech	3
To pain	2
Nil	1

Motor Response (M)

Show me two fingers

Withdraws = 4

Localizes = 5

Obeys = 6

Extensor response = 2

Abnormal flexor response = 3

Nil (no response) = 1

M	
Obeys	6
Localized	5
Withdraws	4
Abnormal flexion	3
Extensor response	2
Nil	1

Verbal Response (V)

What year is this?

2020
Oriented = 5

1997
Confused conversation = 4

Yesterday Mother
Inappropriate words = 3

Scream, groan, moan
Incomprehensible sounds = 2

No response
Nil = 1

V	
Oriented	5
Confused conversation	4
Inappropriate words	3
Incomprehensible sounds	2
Nil	1

Coma score (E + M + V) = 3 to 15

FIG. 16.2 **Glasgow Coma Scale.**

- Memory (providing several common nouns to be recalled after several minutes)
- Language (including object naming, reading, writing, and repetition)
- Calculation (serial 7s or simple currency math, such as "How much money do I have with 7 quarters?")
- Executive functioning, including judgment and insight, obtained during both history and during formal assessment
- Mood and behavior

All patients presenting emergently with AMS require an initial assessment of circulation, breathing, airway patency, and vital signs. The GCS is a scoring system that assesses a patient's level of consciousness on three different metrics: eye opening (4 points), verbal response (5 points), and motor response to pain (6 points) (Fig. 16.2).

All cranial nerves should be examined and can provide information on potential etiologies, though the exam may be limited by a patient's level of consciousness. However, even patients with minimal GCS and suspicion of impending herniation or brain death should undergo testing of extraocular movements and corneal, gag, and cough reflexes. The pupillary exam can reveal pinpoint pupils suggestive of opiate intoxication, or fixed and dilated pupils that suggest herniation or severe anoxic brain injury. Unilateral pupillary defects also raise concern for intracranial pathology. A midposition and fixed pupil is indicative of a lesion in the midbrain. Doll's eyes maneuver is normal if eyes move in opposite direction of head movement. An exhaustive list of findings is beyond the scope of this chapter.

The motor exam in the unresponsive patient involves assessing for flexor or extensor posturing of arms and legs, either with or without stimulation. Otherwise, if the patient is conscious, strength testing may be useful for localizing the neurological lesions seen in stroke. The sensory exam also varies with patient responsiveness, but even the minimally responsive patient may exhibit purposeful movement or reflexive posturing to painful stimuli. Reflexes, including deep tendon reflexes and Babinski, are essential and can localize lesions in addition to distinguishing between upper or lower motor neuron pathology.

DIAGNOSIS AND TREATMENT

As AMS has a broad differential, a systematic approach allows for the best chance to quickly uncover the cause (Table 16.1). Patients who present with coma/profound stupor or concern for airway compromise should be considered for intubation; traditionally in trauma situations, a GCS ≤8 leads to intubation. Patients who do not require intubation should be assessed for acute neurological deficit, which if present should lead to evaluation for stroke, as faster time to intervention directly correlates with long-term prognosis. Patients who do not fall under this category should be evaluated for alternate causes of AMS based around available history and physical exam. Physicians must obtain intravenous (IV) access and, in cases of trauma, immobilize the cervical spine until a fracture has been ruled out.

Initial blood testing in AMS must include a fingerstick glucose, as hypoglycemia is readily reversible and can have significant morbidity if unrecognized. As always, the history and physical exam guide testing, but virtually all patients should receive a basic metabolic panel (BMP), complete blood count (CBC), liver function tests (LFTs), and thyroid-stimulating hormone (TSH). These tests will screen for a variety of AMS causes, including:
- BMP: hyponatremia/hypernatremia, uremia, hypercalcemia
- CBC: leukocytosis, which may indicate infection
- LFT: hyperbilirubinemia and transaminitis, which suggest hepatic disease
- TSH: hypothyroidism or hyperthyroidism

Additionally, alcohol level and urine toxicology can demonstrate intoxicants; due to widespread abuse of heroin and prescription opioids, empirical intranasal naloxone may simultaneously confirm and treat the

TABLE 16.1
Selected Reversible Causes of Altered Mental Status and Associated Treatments

Cause	Approach to Treatment
VASCULAR	
Stroke (ischemic or hemorrhagic)	Activate stroke team; thrombolytics if ischemic BP control
Myocardial infarction	Cardiac catheterization
Subdural hematoma	Neurosurgical intervention
Epidural hematoma	Neurosurgical intervention
Hypertensive encephalopathy	BP control
PRIMARY NEURO	
Seizure/status epilepticus	EEG, anticonvulsant
INFECTION	
Sepsis	Cultures, IV fluids, antimicrobials
Urinary tract infection	Cultures, antimicrobials
Pneumonia	Cultures, antimicrobials
Meningitis/encephalitis	Lumbar puncture with cultures, antimicrobials
INGESTION (CONSIDER ACTIVATED CHARCOAL)	
Opioids	Naloxone
Alcohol	Benzodiazepines; thiamine to prevent Wernicke encephalopathy
Acetaminophen	N-acetylcysteine
METABOLIC/ENDOCRINE	
Thyroid disorder, typically hypothyroidism	Hormone replacement
Hyponatremia/hypernatremia	Evaluate underlying cause (see Chapter 27)
Hypercalcemia	IV fluids, bisphosphonates
Hypoglycemia	Dextrose
Uremia	Dialysis
Wernicke encephalopathy	Thiamine
Hepatic encephalopathy	Lactulose, rifaximin
OTHER	
Hypoxia or hypercarbia	Oxygen and ventilatory support

BP, Blood pressure; *EEG*, electroencephalogram; *IV*, intravenous.

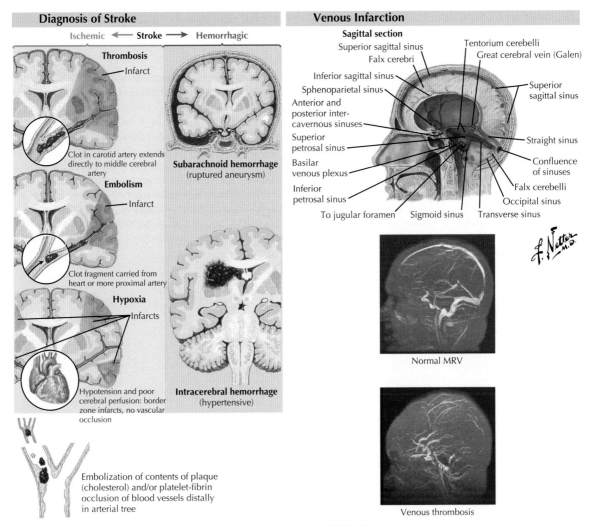

FIG. 16.3 **Diagnosis of Stroke.** *MRV*, MR venography.

AMS. Notably, newer synthetic cannabinoids are not detected on most urine toxicology screens and require specific testing if clinical suspicion is high. Blood and urine cultures can assess for infection; straight bladder catheterization may be required to obtain urine samples and can itself reveal urinary retention, another cause of AMS in the elderly.

Further blood testing should be directly informed by the clinical situation. Elevated prothrombin time (PT) and partial thromboplastin time (PTT) signify coagulopathy and higher risk of intracranial hemorrhage; they may also be elevated in liver failure. While not diagnostic, an elevated ammonia level suggests hepatic encephalopathy and underlying hepatic dysfunction. Patients with known

chronic obstructive pulmonary disease (COPD) or other pulmonary diseases should receive an arterial blood gas with lactate to investigate hypoxia and hypercapnia, either of which can drive AMS. Troponin and concomitant electrocardiogram (ECG) are prudent for patients with suspected myocardial ischemia. Further infectious testing, such as lumbar puncture, may be indicated based on the clinical scenario; examples include patients with fevers and nuchal rigidity, or in patients in whom no clear cause for AMS has been discovered. Blood tests to measure medication levels vary by institution and should be guided by the medication history.

As with blood tests, imaging should be directed by the history and physical exam. Basic chest radiography can uncover pneumonia or pulmonary edema suggestive of heart failure, both of which can lead to hypoxia and resultant AMS. While initial head imaging is often noncontrast CT head, MRI is more sensitive for evaluation of brain parenchyma.

Two common, serious neurological disorders that may present with acute AMS include **stroke** and **seizure.** Stroke is suggested by new, focal neurological deficit, including facial droop, limb weakness, or abnormal speech. Patients with focal neurological signs on exam or suspicion for stroke must receive an emergent noncontrast CT scan of the head to evaluate for intracranial pathology while a stroke team/expert consultant is notified. Strokes are broadly classified into ischemic and hemorrhagic stroke, and while a head CT scan is less sensitive than MRI for ischemic stroke, it is remarkably sensitive for hemorrhagic stroke. Intracranial hemorrhage, including subdural, epidural, or intraparenchymal hemorrhage, are all contraindications to thrombolytics, the treatment of choice in acute ischemic stroke (see Chapter 41 for details) (Fig. 16.3).

Several symptoms suggest seizures, including prodromal aura, loss of bowel/bladder control, tongue biting, and postictal confusion. Actively seizing patients should receive anticonvulsants; options include levetiracetam, phenytoin, lorazepam, and diazepam. Following intracranial imaging, electroencephalography (EEG) can help localize seizure activity. EEG can also provide information suggestive of toxic/metabolic causes for AMS or reveal **status epilepticus,** a neurological emergency. Generalized convulsive status epilepticus is defined as patients having one seizure for >5 minutes or two or more seizures without interval reattainment of neurological function.

CHAPTER 17

Fever

CECILY J. GALLUP

INTRODUCTION

Fever is an elevation in core body temperature and represents an important presenting symptom of myriad disease processes. Although fever technically refers to body temperature above 37°C (98.6°F), a person is usually not considered to have a significant fever until the temperature rises above 38°C (100.4°F). **Hyperpyrexia** refers to excessively high fevers of >41.5°C (106.7°F). In **hyperthermia,** which can be triggered by exogenous heat exposure (e.g., heat stroke) or endogenous heat production (e.g., metabolic processes or pharmacological agents), the hypothalamic setpoint remains unchanged, while body temperature increases uncontrollably.

PATHOPHYSIOLOGY

Body temperature is regulated by the thermoregulatory center in the anterior **hypothalamus,** which tends to maintain a temperature between 37°C (98.6°F) and 38°C (100.4°F). Daily core body temperature fluctuates as we balance metabolic heat production with peripheral heat loss. Older adults have a baseline lower temperature and diminished ability to mount a fever when compared to younger adults and children.

Fever results when the hypothalamic setpoint is raised. Pyrogens are substances that produce fever and can be either endogenous or exogenous. Exogenous pyrogens are usually microbes or their products, including the lipopolysaccharide endotoxin of gram-negative bacteria and the exotoxins of *Staphylococcus aureus*. These exogenous pyrogens trigger the release of endogenous pyrogens, such as **interleukin-1 (IL1)**, **tumor necrosis factor-α (TNFα)**, IL6, and other cytokines; they can also directly trigger Toll-like receptor (TLR) agonists. These cytokines and TLR agonists induce the synthesis of prostaglandin E2 (PGE2) in the hypothalamus, which raises the thermostatic setpoint to febrile levels. This incites the vasomotor center to send signals for heat conservation (vasoconstriction) and heat production (shivering). Heat production occurs within fat or muscle via uncoupling of mitochondrial proteins, which leads to the release of adenosine triphosphate (ATP) and heat. These processes continue until the temperature of the blood that is bathing the hypothalamus reaches the new setpoint.

ETIOLOGIES

The three broad disease processes in which fever can be a presenting symptom are infectious, neoplastic, and inflammatory. Less commonly, fever can result from drug or vaccine side effects, endocrine disorders, or vascular events (Fig. 17.1).

Common sites of infection include the upper and lower respiratory tracts, the gastrointestinal tract, the urinary tract, and the skin. Other infectious processes include meningitis, osteomyelitis, endocarditis, and abscesses. Hospitalized patients may develop fever from intravenous (IV) catheter infections, urinary tract infections associated with indwelling catheters, pneumonias, surgical site infections, decubitus ulcer infections, enteric infection (e.g., *Clostridium [Clostridioides] difficile*), venous thromboembolism, drugs, hematomas, and transfusion reactions. Travelers may be at risk for viral, fungal, parasitic, and atypical bacterial infections, based on the location to which they traveled. Arthropods, including ticks and mosquitoes, can serve as vectors for illnesses, including rickettsiosis, ehrlichiosis, Lyme disease, malaria, and viral encephalitides. Wild animals are vectors for bacterial (including tularemia), viral (including rabies, hantavirus, and Ebola), and fungal infections (including histoplasmosis and cryptococcosis). Diseases from domestic animals include psittacosis from birds; brucellosis, toxoplasmosis, and Q fever from cats; *Salmonella* from reptiles; and *Bartonella*, *Capnocytophaga*, and anaerobic infections from dogs. For further information on infectious causes of fever, refer to Section 10 of this textbook.

Immunocompromised patients, including transplant recipients, patients receiving chemotherapy, and HIV-infected individuals, are susceptible to a wide range of infectious diseases beyond those commonly encountered

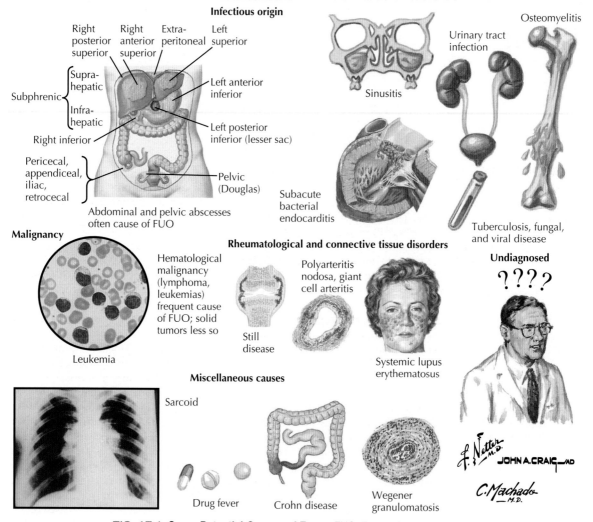

Infectious origin

Right posterior superior   Right anterior superior   Extra-peritoneal   Left superior

Subphrenic { Supra-hepatic / Infra-hepatic }

Left anterior inferior

Left posterior inferior (lesser sac)

Right inferior

Periceceal, appendiceal, iliac, retrocecal

Pelvic (Douglas)

Abdominal and pelvic abscesses often cause of FUO

Sinusitis

Urinary tract infection

Osteomyelitis

Subacute bacterial endocarditis

Tuberculosis, fungal, and viral disease

Malignancy

Hematological malignancy (lymphoma, leukemias) frequent cause of FUO; solid tumors less so

Leukemia

Rheumatological and connective tissue disorders

Still disease

Polyarteritis nodosa, giant cell arteritis

Systemic lupus erythematosus

Undiagnosed

????

Miscellaneous causes

Sarcoid

Drug fever   Crohn disease   Wegener granulomatosis

JOHN A. CRAIG—MD

C. Machado —M.D.

FIG. 17.1 **Some Potential Causes of Fever.** *FUO,* Fever of unknown origin.

in immunocompetent individuals. Invasive viruses (including varicella zoster virus and cytomegalovirus), mycobacteria, fungi (including *Candida, Cryptococcus, Aspergillus, Histoplasma, Coccidioides,* and *Pneumocystis*), and parasites (including *Toxoplasma, Strongyloides, Cryptosporidium, Microsporidia,* and *Cystoisospora belli*) are all of particular concern. Acute HIV infection can also cause fevers.

Fever in patients with malignancy is sepsis related in the majority of cases. However, there are certain neoplastic processes where fever is an associated symptom, such as lymphoma and renal cell carcinoma. Connective tissue diseases, inflammatory bowel disease, and vasculitides such as giant cell arteritis, polymyalgia

rheumatica, or polyarteritis nodosa can all cause fevers. Endocrine disorders such as hyperthyroidism, subacute thyroiditis, and adrenal insufficiency can elevate body temperature. Vascular disorders causing fever include venous thromboembolism (VTE), thrombophlebitis, and hematomas.

Amphetamines, cocaine, MDMA, antipsychotics, and anesthetics can all increase heat production. Certain drugs, including β-lactam antibiotics, sulfa drugs, phenytoin, carbamazepine, procainamide, quinidine, amphotericin B, and interferons, can also trigger fevers. Finally, factitious fever can occur in individuals who manipulate thermometers or inject foreign material through IVs.

EVALUATION

Temperature can be measured peripherally or centrally. The former includes tympanic membrane, temporal artery, axillary, and oral thermometers, whereas the latter includes pulmonary artery catheter, urinary bladder, esophageal, and rectal thermometers. Rectal and tympanic temperatures are 0.3°C to 0.6°C (0.5°F–1°F) higher than oral temperatures. Axillary and temporal temperatures are usually 0.3°C to 0.6°C (0.5°F–1°F) lower than oral temperatures.

Fever characteristics (magnitude, duration, pattern), method of measurement, and last use of an antipyretic are important aspects of the history. Given the broad differential diagnosis for fever, multiple patient factors should be explored. These include:

- Age
- Comorbidities (e.g., HIV infection, rheumatologic disorders, hyperthyroidism, diabetes, cancer, organ transplantation, sickle cell disease, valvular heart disorders)
- Medications (e.g., immunosuppressants, anticonvulsants)
- Immunization status (e.g., hepatitis A and B, meningococcal, pneumococcal, influenza)
- Recent hospitalization or invasive procedures (including dental work)
- Presence of IV or urinary catheters
- Use of mechanical ventilation
- Family history
- Exposure history (e.g., occupation, alcohol or illicit drug use, travel, sexual contacts)

The physical examination should include serial vital signs to confirm the presence of fever. Relative bradycardia is seen in certain infections (e.g., typhoid fever, brucellosis, leptospirosis, some drug-induced fevers) as well as factitious fevers. If there are no localizing symptoms, a thorough physical exam is particularly important. Special attention should be paid to areas of pain and discomfort as well as common sites of infection: the head and neck (in case of suspected meningitis), nasopharynx, lungs, abdomen, genitals, and skin. In hospitalized patients, the sites of peripheral or central IVs, surgical sites, and decubitus ulcers should be carefully examined. Physical exam findings for various infectious etiologies of fever are discussed in separate chapters.

DIAGNOSIS

As noted, history and physical exam should guide the initial evaluation of fever. In an otherwise healthy individual where serious illness is not suspected (e.g., viral upper respiratory tract infection or acute gastroenteritis), simple observation without testing may be appropriate. If more serious infection is suspected, laboratory testing should include a complete blood count with differential. Although white blood cell (WBC) count is often elevated in infection, a low WBC count may represent viral infection or overwhelming bacterial infection. The WBC differential may provide additional information: Neutrophils or immature band forms may be seen in bacterial infection, elevated lymphocytes may be seen in viral or fungal infection, and blasts may be seen in malignancies such as leukemia.

Liver function tests should be obtained if hepatitis or a biliary process is suspected; if abnormal, viral hepatitis serologies can be drawn. Urinalysis and culture can investigate urinary tract infection, and chest radiography and sputum cultures aid in diagnosing pulmonary infection. Stool studies (cultures, microscopy, and multiplex polymerase chain reaction [PCR] panels) may be useful in patients with severe diarrhea to direct treatment. Blood cultures (two sets from different sites) should be drawn before antibiotics are given for suspected systemic infection. Febrile injection drug users with heart murmurs should also receive blood cultures (ideally three sets from different sites) and echocardiography to evaluate for infective endocarditis.

If the initial workup returns unremarkable and fevers persist, physicians can search for less common disease processes. Erythrocyte sedimentation rate (ESR), C-reactive protein (CRP), and lactate dehydrogenase (LDH) provide estimates of the body's inflammatory state and can be trended to normalization if a cause is later found. Further testing includes tuberculin skin test or interferon-γ release assay for tuberculosis (TB), HIV antibody/viral load testing, antinuclear antibodies and rheumatoid factor in suspected rheumatologic disease, or lumbar puncture if there are central nervous system symptoms. Fungal serologies/antigens and thick/thin smears for parasitic infection may be appropriate based on risk factors. If osteomyelitis is suspected, MRI is the gold standard. Further radiological studies (ultrasound, cross-sectional imaging, or functional imaging) may also be useful in the evaluation of fever.

MANAGEMENT

There is considerable debate as to whether fever itself should be treated, and the decision is made largely based on the diagnostic benefit of allowing fever to continue, patient discomfort, and whether the fever is dangerously high. Fevers are generally well tolerated by healthy adults, but extreme temperature elevation (typically >41°C

[105.8°F]), seen with severe sepsis, hyperthermia, illicit drug use, anesthetics, or antipsychotic drugs, can be damaging; complications include organ failure and disseminated intravascular coagulation (DIC). Since fever increases oxygen demand, it can stress adults with preexisting cardiac or pulmonary insufficiency. Fever in healthy children can cause febrile seizures.

Generally, the underlying cause of the fever should be treated in conjunction with antipyretics. Antipyretics decrease the setpoint of the hypothalamus via vasodilation and sweating. As noted, PGE2 plays a key role in fever, and its synthesis is dependent on the enzyme cyclooxygenase. Inhibitors of cyclooxygenases (COX1 or COX2), like aspirin and NSAIDs, are antipyretics. Although acetaminophen does not inhibit cyclooxygenase, its oxidized form does. Corticosteroids are also antipyretics, reducing PGE2 synthesis by inhibiting the activity of phospholipase A2 (which releases arachidonic acid from the membrane to make PGE2) and blocking the transcription of messenger RNA (mRNA) for pyrogenic cytokines. If the patient's temperature is ≥41°C (105.8°F), other cooling measures (e.g., evaporative cooling with tepid water mist, cooling blankets) should also be started. In hyperthermia, because the setting of the thermoregulatory center remains unchanged while body temperature increases and overrides the ability to lose heat, antipyretics are ineffective. Treatment of the underlying pathophysiological process (either infectious, inflammatory, or oncological) is obviously of paramount importance, as outlined in other chapters.

CHAPTER 18

Shock

HANNAH ROEDER

INTRODUCTION

Shock is a clinical state defined by inadequate tissue perfusion to meet metabolic demands. This life-threatening situation leads to the deterioration of cellular function, progressing to multiple organ system dysfunction and death.

In a state of shock, oxygen consumption exceeds oxygen delivery. Apart from a steady oxygen concentration in the environment, adequate oxygen delivery to tissues relies on hemoglobin concentration, **cardiac output (CO)**, and **systemic vascular resistance (SVR)**. Patients with severely low hemoglobin will be unable to carry enough oxygen to meet metabolic demands. To receive oxygen, vital tissues require adequate perfusion by the circulatory system, which depends on CO and SVR. CO is a product of heart rate and stroke volume, which itself relies on preload, myocardial contractility, and afterload. SVR is influenced by vessel diameter, vessel length, and blood viscosity; vessel diameter changes substantially in certain shock states (see Chapter 56 for further details). Perturbations in any of these may contribute to shock.

PATHOPHYSIOLOGY AND EVALUATION

Key to a successful outcome for patients who develop shock is early recognition. Tachycardia can be the earliest warning sign of impending shock and develops prior to hypotension, especially in younger patients. Hypotension is common in, but not synonymous with, shock. For example, an individual who is hypertensive at baseline may have relative hypotension, rather than absolute hypotension, which may be overlooked if baseline blood pressure is unknown. Special attention should be paid to the patient's volume status, as this can give clues to the particular etiology of shock.

Physical exam signs to evaluate volume status include jugular venous distension, presence of axillary sweat and moist versus dry mucous membranes, skin tenting, extremity temperature/pulses, and the presence/absence of edema. A passive straight leg raise or orthostatic vital signs should be checked if clinically feasible, as improved vitals following a passive leg raise or the presence of orthostasis suggests a volume-depleted, and potentially volume-responsive, patient. Delirium, particularly impairments in attention span, may signal cerebral hypoperfusion and be an early indicator of shock. Declining urine output can indicate declining renal perfusion and the onset of acute kidney injury. Skin changes, including mottling and cyanosis, can also occur in shock. Initial lab abnormalities that suggest shock include elevated creatinine and metabolic acidosis from elevated lactate as a result of anaerobic respiration from impaired oxygen delivery.

Etiologies of shock can broadly be delineated as **hypovolemic, distributive, cardiogenic,** and **obstructive.** Many patients manifest a mixed shock presentation. For example, an infection may lead to septic shock, but the patient may also develop cardiogenic shock via **sepsis**-related myocardial impairment. As alluded to earlier, hemodynamic values of CO, SVR, and preload (as measured by the pulmonary capillary wedge pressure [PCWP]) can be used to distinguish between broad categories of shock (Table 18.1).

Hypovolemic Shock

Hypovolemic shock results from inadequate blood or plasma volume. In this clinical state, decreased preload leads to decreased contractility; heart rate subsequently increases to maintain CO, but continued volume loss eventually leads to decreased CO. SVR increases to maintain perfusion despite low circulating blood volume. Causes of hypovolemic shock include severe hemorrhage, severe vomiting and diarrhea, large insensible losses as in heat stroke, severe burns covering significant body area, and so-called third spacing when fluid shifts from the intravascular to interstitial spaces. Third spacing may occur in pancreatitis, cirrhosis, or postoperatively.

In general, the physical exam of a patient with hypovolemic shock is notable for a narrow pulse pressure, cool and clammy extremities, poor capillary refill, and flat neck veins. Patients may also have dry skin, axillae, and mucous membranes. Hemorrhagic shock may be obvious

TABLE 18.1
Hemodynamic Values in Shock

Type of Shock	Preload (PCWP)	CO	SVR
Hypovolemic	↓	Early: Normal to slight ↑ Late: ↓	↑
Distributive	↓	Early: ↑ Late: ↓	↓
Cardiogenic	↑	↓	↑
Obstructive: tamponade	↑	↓	↑
Obstructive: other	Early: Normal Late: ↓	Early: Normal Late: ↓	↑

CO, Cardiac output; *PCWP,* pulmonary capillary wedge pressure; *SVR,* systemic vascular resistance.

on exam, as in the case of large-volume hematemesis, or may require a higher level of clinical suspicion, such as with retroperitoneal bleeding following a femoral artery catheterization, or with internal hemorrhage into the pelvis and lower extremity following trauma.

Distributive Shock

Distributive shock is defined by loss of vascular tone leading to a significantly decreased SVR. Preload falls, but tachycardia can somewhat compensate to maintain CO; patients with late distributive shock can develop decreased CO. Sepsis is the prototype of distributive shock. Other causes of distributive shock include **anaphylaxis,** neurogenic (including acute spinal cord injury and anesthesia-related shock), drug and transfusion reactions, acute adrenal crisis (Addisonian crisis), decompensated hypothyroidism (myxedema coma), and toxic shock syndrome.

In general, patients with distributive shock will manifest a wide pulse pressure, low diastolic blood pressure, and warm extremities. Patients may have flushed, hyperemic skin in early distributive shock, and capillary refill may be normal. In assessing vitals, recall that fever or hypothermia may be present in sepsis. Clinicians can calculate the quick SOFA or complete SOFA score to help determine the severity of sepsis and assess the risk of a poor outcome (see Chapter 111 for further details). Patients with neurogenic shock may manifest bradycardia in the absence of sympathetic tone, and patients with anaphylactic shock often demonstrate signs and symptoms of anaphylaxis, including hives, urticaria, stridor, and airway compromise (Fig. 18.1).

Cardiogenic Shock

Cardiogenic shock most commonly results from decreased myocardial contractility. Cardiogenic shock

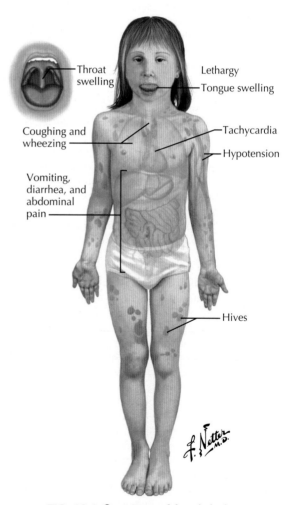

Throat swelling

Lethargy

Tongue swelling

Coughing and wheezing

Tachycardia

Hypotension

Vomiting, diarrhea, and abdominal pain

Hives

FIG. 18.1 Symptoms of Anaphylaxis.

may arise following acute myocardial infarction, viral or drug-induced cardiomyopathy, or decompensated congestive heart failure. Cardiogenic shock can also result from acute or end-stage valvular dysfunction or with dysrhythmia by decreasing filling time.

In cardiogenic shock, there is increased preload but decreased CO, and SVR increases in an attempt to compensate. As a result, physical exam is notable for cool, clammy extremities, poor capillary refill, and a narrow pulse pressure. The proportional pulse pressure (the difference between systolic and diastolic pressure divided by the systolic pressure) is generally <25% in cardiogenic shock, as a result of increased sympathetic activation. Other physical exam findings that may be seen with cardiogenic shock include elevated jugular venous pressure, positive hepatojugular reflex, S3 gallop or new murmur, and pulmonary rales.

Obstructive Shock

Increased afterload can lead to obstructive shock, in which an underlying extracardiac pathology impairs the movement of blood through the cardiopulmonary circuit. These underlying pathologies include acute pulmonary embolus, tension pneumothorax, severe pulmonary hypertension, cardiac tamponade, and constrictive pericarditis.

In obstructive shock, exam reveals cool, clammy extremities, poor capillary refill, and a narrow pulse pressure. An elevated jugular venous pressure may be prominent. In tension pneumothorax, exam will be notable for absent breath sounds over one lung. In cardiac tamponade, Beck triad (distant heart sounds,

hypotension, and jugular venous distension) and Kussmaul sign (distention of jugular veins increasing with inspiration) may be present. Pulsus paradoxus, which is a decrease in systolic blood pressure >10 mm Hg with inspiration, is classically associated with tamponade and constrictive pericarditis but may be seen with other etiologies of shock, including pulmonary embolism, valvular disease, and hypovolemia. Tamponade and cardiogenic shock share similar hemodynamics but can be distinguished by the equalization of pressures seen in tamponade and by the presence of a large pericardial effusion on echocardiography (see Chapter 61 for further details).

DIAGNOSIS AND TREATMENT

Initial management should commence while the diagnosis and etiology of shock are being established. If brief history and physical do not highlight a likely etiology of the patient's shock, a fluid challenge should be considered, typically normal saline or lactated Ringer. The patient's response should be evaluated in real time with the clinician noting effects on heart rate, blood pressure, skin exam, extremity perfusion, and urine output change. A bedside echocardiogram can help differentiate shock etiology, although hypovolemic and septic shock may look similar.

Securing adequate vascular access is key for rapid fluid resuscitation and may involve central venous catheterization. It should be noted that, for emergent fluid resuscitation, triple lumen central lines are not ideal due to lumen diameter and length; shorter, large-bore

TABLE 18.2
Receptor Activities of Common Vasoactive Agents

Medication	α_1	β_1	β_2	Dopamine	V_1	Physiological Effects	Classification
Norepinephrine	++++	++	+			↑↑SVR, ↑CO	Inopressor
Epinephrine	++++	++++	+++			↑↑SVR, ↑↑CO	Inopressor
Phenylephrine	+++					↑↑SVR	Vasopressor
Dobutamine	+	++++	++			↓SVR, ↑↑CO	Inotrope
Dopamine	+ (low dose) +++ (high dose)	+ (low) ++ (high)		++++ (low) ++ (high)		↑CO (low) ↑↑SVR, ↑CO (high)	Inopressor (conc. dependent)
Vasopressin					+++	↑↑SVR	Vasopressor

Action of vasoactive medications depends on the receptors affected; listed are cardiovascular sequelae of receptor activation.
α_1 = Vasoconstriction; β_1 = increased chronotropy, inotropy; β_2 = vasodilation, bronchodilation; dopamine = vasodilation of renal/splanchnic circulation; V_1 (vasopressin) = vasoconstriction.
CO, Cardiac output; SVR, systemic vascular resistance.

IVs or introducer catheters (e.g., Cordis) are preferable. Central venous catheterization provides a safe route for vasoactive medications, as well as for measurement of central venous pressure and central venous oxygen saturation ($ScVO_2$) for ongoing monitoring.

$ScVO_2$ can be helpful in differentiating septic from hemorrhagic and cardiogenic shock, as it reflects the balance between oxygen delivery and oxygen consumption. A normal $ScVO_2$ is roughly 70%. In a state of poor tissue oxygenation, either from pump failure or decreased hemoglobin, oxygen extraction by peripheral tissues is higher, thus an $ScVO_2$ value <65% suggests cardiogenic or hemorrhagic shock. Conversely, in septic shock, vasodilation effectively leads to shunting of arterial blood, and the systemic inflammatory response to sepsis impairs the ability of peripheral tissues to absorb oxygen. This leads to an elevated $ScVO_2$, often over 80%.

Addressing the underlying cause for shock is a cornerstone treatment in all causes (e.g., prompt, broad-spectrum antibiotics for septic shock, needle decompression and chest tube for tension pneumothorax). In the event the patient remains in shock despite resuscitation efforts, vasoactive medications may be required. Vasoactive medications have different activity for α-adrenergic and β-adrenergic, dopaminergic, and vasopressin receptors, and these activities dictate the kinds of shock for which they are used (Table 18.2). Norepinephrine is the first-line agent for septic shock, while patients in cardiogenic shock should receive an inotrope such as dobutamine. Vasoactive medications are titrated to a prescribed effect (e.g., mean arterial pressure >65) and may be combined in severely decompensated patients.

CHAPTER 19

Hypertensive Crisis

LEILA HAGHIGHAT • DAVID J. ENGEL

INTRODUCTION

Hypertensive crisis refers to severely elevated blood pressure (BP) and comprises two separate entities: **hypertensive emergency** and **hypertensive urgency.** According to the Joint National Committee (JNC 7) report, hypertensive urgency is defined as either a systolic blood pressure (SBP) >180 mm Hg or diastolic blood pressure (DBP) >120 mm Hg. About 75% of hypertensive crises are hypertensive urgencies. Hypertensive emergencies meet the aforementioned BP criteria and involve **end-organ damage.** Notably, these cutoffs are not absolute, as a rapid BP increase in a normotensive patient may also result in a hypertensive crisis.

PATHOPHYSIOLOGY

Hypertensive crises arise from a series of vascular injuries, although the pathophysiology is not completely understood. It is triggered by the release of hormones such as norepinephrine and angiotensin II that cause a rise in systemic vascular resistance. As a result, stress is applied against the vascular wall, and the endothelium incurs mechanical damage. Platelet activation and initiation of the coagulation cascade result in a prothrombotic milieu of fibrin deposition, oxidative stress, and inflammation, leading to organ hypoperfusion. This process then leads to a vicious cycle, whereby inadequate perfusion activates the renin-angiotensin system, further exacerbating vascular resistance and endothelial dysfunction.

Box 19.1 outlines etiologies for hypertensive crises. Nonadherence to antihypertensive medications is the most common cause in the United States. Between 1% and 2% of the nation's 50 million people with hypertension will develop a hypertensive crisis. The prevalence is higher among the elderly, black, and male populations.

EVALUATION AND DIAGNOSIS

History taking and a physical exam should focus on identifying the risk factors for developing a hypertensive crisis, the etiology of the current episode, and if there is evidence of end-organ damage. Patients should be asked about cardiovascular, renal, and endocrine diseases. Among patients with known hypertension, it is important to clarify how well controlled the BP has been, medications taken, timing of last dose, and medication adherence. Recent alcohol, food, and drug intake should also be noted. Female patients must be assessed for pregnancy. Table 19.1 lists signs and symptoms of end-organ damage in hypertensive emergency. Even in the absence of end-organ damage, patients may present with severe headache, shortness of breath, epistaxis, and severe anxiety. The most common initial complaint is chest pain. On physical exam, BP should be measured in both arms; discrepancies of >20 mm Hg between upper limbs necessitates checking pressure in the lower limbs to evaluate for aortic dissection. Fundoscopic, cardiac, pulmonary, and abdominal exams should be performed as well.

Patients in hypertensive crisis should receive basic laboratory tests, including basic chemistries to evaluate for renal impairment, urinalysis to identify proteinuria or hematuria, a pregnancy test, and urine toxicology. Anemia and thrombocytopenia on a complete blood count (CBC) may indicate microangiopathic anemia, which can be confirmed with coagulation studies and a blood smear. Endocrine testing, such as free thyroxine (T_4)/thyroid-stimulating hormone (TSH), plasma renin activity, aldosterone, and catecholamines, may be sent to evaluate for other secondary causes of hypertension. Imaging should be ordered as guided by the history. Electrocardiogram (ECG) and chest x-ray can demonstrate myocardial ischemia or pulmonary edema, respectively. The presence of neurological signs should be further evaluated with a head CT, and concern for aortic dissection should prompt CT angiography of the chest/abdomen.

MANAGEMENT

The general principle guiding the management of hypertensive crisis is to provide reduction in BP that is balanced

---

BOX 19.1
Causes of Hypertensive Emergency

- Essential hypertension: poorly controlled blood pressure, antihypertensive drug withdrawal (clonidine, β-blocker)
- Renal parenchymal disease: acute glomerulonephritis, vasculitis, TTP-HUS
- Renovascular disease: renal artery stenosis, fibromuscular dysplasia
- Endocrine disease: pheochromocytoma, renin-secreting tumors, mineralocorticoid hypertension, glucocorticoid excess
- Drugs: cocaine, sympathomimetics, erythropoietin, cyclosporine, interactions with monoamine oxidase inhibitors, amphetamines, oral contraceptive pills, PCP, linezolid, NSAIDs, alcohol
- Autonomic hyperactivity: Guillain-Barré syndrome, acute intermittent porphyria
- CNS disorders: head injury, stroke, brain tumor
- Eclampsia
- Surgery

CNS, Central nervous system; *HUS,* hemolytic-uremic syndrome; *NSAIDs,* nonsteroidal antiinflammatory drugs; *PCP,* phencyclidine, *TTP,* thrombotic thrombocytopenic purpura.

by the harm associated with drastic decline. Hypertension causes a rightward shift in the autoregulatory curve of the vasculature, such that to maintain a certain blood flow, higher pressure is required. Consequently, among patients with hypertension, especially those for whom it is a chronic condition, what is usually considered normotension may in fact result in hypoperfusion. Treatment should be initiated as early as possible, even before the laboratory workup results return.

In hypertensive urgency, the goal for BP reduction is less than 160/110 mm Hg, with no more than a 25% reduction within 1 hour. Normalization of BP to less than 140/90 mm Hg should be achieved within 1 to 2 days. Intravenous antihypertensive medications can be considered initially, but patients will require oral agents for longer term BP control, so treatment with oral medications alone can be considered. The antihypertensive selected must balance a patient's history and current status with side effects (i.e., avoiding ACE inhibitors in patients with acute kidney injury). Medications to consider include labetalol, captopril, clonidine, and furosemide. Sublingual nifedipine is contraindicated, as it produces an unpredictable and potentially unsafe drop in BP. Once the BP is acutely controlled, patients may be started on a long-term oral therapy commensurate with JNC 7 guidelines. The patient should also be scheduled for follow-up with a primary care physician within 1 to 2 weeks.

TABLE 19.1
Symptoms of Hypertensive Crisis

Organ	Symptoms	Signs	Damage
Eyes	Blurry vision	Arteriolar narrowing, AV nicking, cotton wool spots, hemorrhages, hard exudates, papilledema	Hypertensive retinopathy
Kidneys	Hematuria, decreased urine output	New proteinuria, microscopic hematuria, renal bruits, abdominal mass	Acute kidney injury, hypertensive nephropathy
Brain	Nausea, vomiting, confusion, seizures, loss of consciousness	Focal neurological deficits	Stroke (ischemic or hemorrhagic), hypertensive encephalopathy
Lungs	Dyspnea	Rales	Pulmonary edema
Heart	Chest pain, dyspnea	New murmurs, gallops, peripheral edema	Congestive heart failure, acute coronary syndrome
Vascular	Chest, abdominal, or back pain	Blood pressure difference >20 mm Hg between arms, weak pulses, new diastolic murmur	Aortic dissection, ruptured abdominal aortic aneurysm

AV, Arteriovenous.

Hypertensive emergency is treated more aggressively. In general, BP should be reduced by 10% to 20% in the first hour and by a total of ~35% over the first day, but these goals vary with the emergency. Patients should be admitted to the intensive care unit (ICU) for arterial BP monitoring with administration of short-acting intravenous agents that allow for careful titration. Parenteral agents to consider include nicardipine, labetalol, and nitroprusside. While different agents have different side effects and contraindications, systematic reviews have concluded that no single agent is better than the rest. Once adequate BP control is achieved, the patient may be switched to oral therapy with close physician follow-up.

Among patients with **acute ischemic stroke,** hypertension is usually transient and resolves after 24 hours. Patients who are not candidates for fibrinolytic agents should only be treated for BP that is >220/110 mm Hg, with a goal of reducing BP by 15% within 24 hours. For patients receiving fibrinolytic therapy, BP prior to administration should be <185/110 mm Hg to prevent intraparenchymal hemorrhage. In the 24 hours following fibrinolytic administration, BP should be closely monitored and remain <180/105 mm Hg.

Among patients with **hemorrhagic stroke,** a lower threshold for BP control is used to minimize further bleeding. BP >200/150 mm Hg merits aggressive BP reduction. Patients with SBP over 180 mm Hg, together with increased intracranial pressure, should have continuous intracranial pressure monitoring and intervention to maintain cerebral perfusion pressure between 60 and 80 mm Hg. Clonidine should be avoided because centrally acting agents may confound evaluation of mental status. Among patients with subarachnoid hemorrhage, SBP should be maintained under 160 mm Hg.

In **aortic dissection,** the goal is to decrease shear stress to prevent progression of the intimal dissection. This is accomplished by rapidly reducing SBP below 120 mm Hg and heart rate below 60 beats per minute (bpm)—β-blockers such as esmolol are ideal. Caution should be used with vasodilatory agents such as sodium nitroprusside, as vasodilation may result in reflex tachycardia that worsens shearing force on the aortic wall.

In **acute coronary syndromes,** the goal is to decrease myocardial oxygen demand. Appropriate agents to consider include nitrates (decrease preload), β-blockers (decrease chronotropy and inotropy), and nondihydropyridine calcium channel blockers. Dihydropyridine calcium channel blockers should be avoided because of their propensity to cause reflex tachycardia and thereby increase cardiac work. Patients with evidence of left ventricular failure, including those with pulmonary edema, should have reduction in afterload to maximize forward flow resulting from impaired cardiac contractility. Such agents include nitrates, diuretics, and ACE inhibitors.

CHAPTER 20

Tachycardia

GOVIND M. KRISHNAN • DAVID J. ENGEL

INTRODUCTION

The normal adult heart rate (HR) is between 60 and 100 beats per minute (bpm), and any HR faster than this is classified as tachycardia. The rate at which the heart contracts is determined by a complex interplay of the sympathetic and parasympathetic systems, often with increased sympathetic tone or, less often, decreased parasympathetic tone leading to an increased HR. The HR is also largely dependent on the intrinsic electrical conduction system of the heart, with various locations in the heart able to trigger contractile impulses at different rates.

ETIOLOGIES

Essential to evaluating any tachycardia is determining whether the tachycardia originates from the natural pacemaker of the heart (sinoatrial [SA] node) in the right atrium (sinus tachycardia), a different focus above the ventricles other than the SA node (supraventricular tachycardia), or a focus in the ventricle(s) (ventricular tachycardia) (see Chapter 55). This distinction is usually made via a 12-lead electrocardiogram (ECG) or other telemetry device, which can show the presence or absence and morphology of P waves, and whether the patient has a narrow complex tachycardia (QRS complex <120 milliseconds [ms]) or a wide complex tachycardia (QRS complex >120 ms) in the absence of intraventricular conduction abnormalities such as bundle branch block.

Sinus Tachycardia

Normal sinus rhythm is the characteristic regular rhythm of the heart originating from the SA node. Sinus tachycardia therefore is the triggering of impulses over 100 bpm but in sinus rhythm. On an ECG, the P wave has a normal morphology, and a normal sinus P wave always precedes a QRS complex.

The differential for sinus tachycardia is very broad since such a presentation is often a symptom of, or a compensatory response to, an underlying disorder that may be suggested by other signs or symptoms. For example, sinus tachycardia can simply be a normal physiologic response to exercise. Other considerations on this broad differential include fever, pain, anxiety, anemia, hyperthyroidism, hypoxemia, drug use, pheochromocytoma, alcohol withdrawal, or many other such etiologies. Any evaluation and/or treatment of sinus tachycardia must take into account the underlying cause.

Supraventricular Tachycardia

Supraventricular tachycardias (SVT) are a group of arrhythmias that arise in atrial tissue or the atrioventricular (AV) node. The distinguishing feature is that since the impulses are generated at or above the AV node, these impulses are then conducted through the AV node normally, resulting in a normal and narrow QRS complex (<120 ms) on ECG. Exceptions to this exist in patients with abnormal ventricular conduction pathways, such as bundle branch blocks. Common causes of SVTs include ischemic heart disease, heart failure, pulmonary embolism, endocrinopathies, alcohol withdrawal, and stimulants, but SVTs may arise spontaneously in the absence of any of these conditions.

In general, SVT results from either enhanced automaticity or reentry. Enhanced automaticity is the increased generation of action potentials from locations in the atria, either from the SA node (sinus tachycardia [see earlier]) or other foci (atrial tachycardia). Reentry is the continuous excitation of myocardium by an electrical loop, usually involving two interconnected conduction pathways. One pathway is recently depolarized and refractory to conduction, but a second pathway is capable of conducting an impulse. This conduction down the second pathway is slow enough that the first pathway recovers and is able to conduct back the impulse that was initially conducted by the second pathway. In this way, a reentrant loop forms, and the circuit completes when the backwards conduction along the first pathway restimulates the alternative pathway. This creates a repeating loop that conducts impulses at a faster rate than normal, causing tachycardia. Reentrant tachycardia can be further distinguished into **atrioventricular nodal**

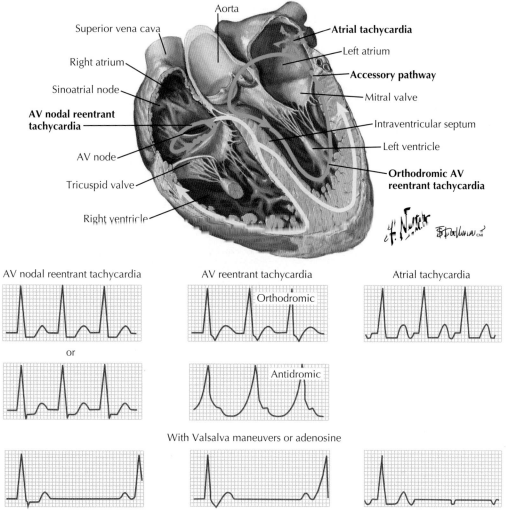

Aorta

Superior vena cava

Right atrium

Sinoatrial node

AV nodal reentrant tachycardia

AV node

Tricuspid valve

Right ventricle

Atrial tachycardia

Left atrium

Accessory pathway

Mitral valve

Intraventricular septum

Left ventricle

Orthodromic AV reentrant tachycardia

AV nodal reentrant tachycardia

or

AV reentrant tachycardia

Orthodromic

Antidromic

Atrial tachycardia

With Valsalva maneuvers or adenosine

FIG. 20.1 **Anatomy and Electrocardiogram of Common Supraventricular Tachycardias.** *AV,* Atrioventricular.

reentrant tachycardia (AVNRT), in which the reentrant circuit exists within the AV node, or **atrioventricular reentrant tachycardia** (AVRT), in which the reentrant circuit may involve the AV node but is not necessarily contained within the node itself (see Fig. 20.1).

A further crucial feature on the ECG or telemetry strip is whether the narrow-complex tachycardia is in regular rhythm or irregular rhythm. The abovementioned diagnoses of sinus tachycardia, atrial tachycardia, AVNRT, and AVRT are all narrow-complex tachycardias that have regular rhythm. However, irregular atrial depolarizations can lead to narrow-complex irregular tachycardias. The most common of these are **atrial fibrillation** and **atrial flutter,** discussed separately in Chapter 60.

Another supraventricular tachycardia of note is **multifocal atrial tachycardia** (MAT). MAT results from multiple areas of increased automaticity or triggered activity within the atria and is diagnosed by the presence of three or more morphologically distinct P waves and an HR between 100 and 140 bpm. It is usually secondary to pulmonary disease and/or hypoxemia, including severe chronic obstructive pulmonary disease (COPD), pulmonary embolism, and congestive heart failure (CHF).

Ventricular Tachycardia

Ventricular arrhythmias, and specifically **ventricular tachycardia** (VT), are an important cause of sudden cardiac death. VT is a potentially life-threatening

QRS >100 ms (continued)
   No P waves (ventricular impulse origin)
      Rate <40/minute: idioventricular rhythm

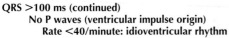

Rate 40 to 120/minute: accelerated idioventricular rhythm (AIVR)

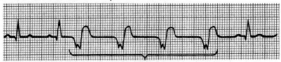
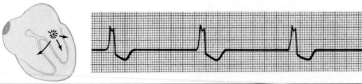

Short bursts (usually <20 seconds) of AIVR, often a few days after myocardial infarction.
Usually asymptomatic with no progression to ventricular tachycardia or ventricular fibrillation

Rate >120/minute: ventricular tachycardia

Infarct
Slowed conduction in margin of
ischemic area permits circular
course of impulse and reentry
with rapid repetitive
depolarization

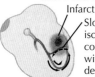
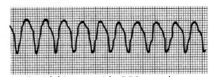

Rapid, bizarre, wide QRS complexes

Ventricular fibrillation

Chaotic
ventricular
depolarization

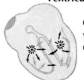
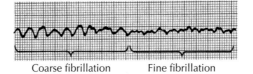

Coarse fibrillation   Fine fibrillation

Pacer rhythm

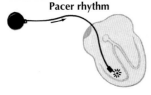

Transvenous pacemaker
produces beat in right
ventricle. Not supraventricular,
and therefore wide QRS

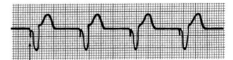

Pacemaker spike (may be small; sometimes missed)

FIG. 20.2 Ventricular Rhythms.

arrhythmia caused by rapid depolarizing impulses that originate in the His-Purkinje system, the ventricular myocardium, or both (Fig. 20.2). VT is most commonly associated with structural and ischemic heart; other triggers include electrolyte abnormalities (hypokalemia, hypomagnesemia), drug toxicity, cardiomyopathy, or long QT syndrome. VT can be either sustained (>30 seconds or featuring hemodynamic collapse) or nonsustained (<30 seconds). It also is characterized by the morphology of the QRS complexes as either monomorphic (similar QRS morphology) or polymorphic (variable QRS morphologies). VT can often degenerate into **ventricular fibrillation** (VF), which reflects a lack of organized ventricular activity; VF is fatal unless terminated within minutes of onset.

EVALUATION, DIAGNOSIS, AND TREATMENT

As evidenced by the varying forms mentioned earlier, tachycardia can present in many different forms with widely variable symptoms and risks. Therefore when presented with a tachycardic patient it is imperative to assess his or her hemodynamic stability, which will be the primary determinant of both treatment urgency and choice. While obtaining a 12-lead ECG, patients must concomitantly be assessed for signs of hemodynamic compromise, including shortness of breath, hypotension, chest pain, shock, or decreased level of consciousness. If these signs are present and the patient is not in sinus tachycardia, immediate **electrical cardioversion** is recommended. Patients with sinus tachycardia and the abovementioned signs must have the underlying cause for sinus tachycardia addressed. In addition, if the tachycardia itself is leading to significant cardiac ischemia, β-blockers may be indicated. If the patient is hemodynamically stable, a nonemergent approach is appropriate. As mentioned, sinus tachycardia can be secondary to a multitude of factors, so a careful review of systems inquiring about fever, causes of pain, symptoms of hyperthyroidism, history of substance abuse, and other common causes of sinus tachycardia is required.

In the case of hemodynamically stable patients with SVT, **vagal maneuvers** may be useful; these maneuvers include **Valsalva,** unilateral carotid massage, and cold calorics. Intravenous adenosine with continuous ECG is recommended if vagal maneuvers fail. Of note, adenosine can be useful to both diagnose and treat unknown narrow-complex tachycardias. It is administered sequentially in 6-mg doses, followed by 12-mg doses if unsuccessful.

In the case of wide-complex tachycardias, the safe approach is to assume that all represent ventricular tachycardia unless proven otherwise. An unresponsive or pulseless patient would fall into standard Advanced Cardiac Life Support (ACLS) algorithm–based treatments. In an unstable but conscious patient, the first step should be to attempt synchronized electrical cardioversion, with conscious sedation if possible. Stable patients should receive a focused diagnostic evaluation to determine the etiology, but often the first step is to attempt synchronized cardioversion with conscious sedation to prevent degeneration into VF. If the patient's tachycardia is recurring or refractory, a class I or III antiarrhythmic is utilized, such as amiodarone, lidocaine, or procainamide. In rare cases, patients known to have VT syndromes in the setting of a structurally normal heart can be treated with calcium channel blockers or β-blockers; however, the decision to do so frequently involves consultation with an electrophysiologist.

CHAPTER 21

Bradycardia

MARGARET INFELD • DAVID J. ENGEL

INTRODUCTION

Bradycardia is defined as a heart rate (HR) less than 60 beats per minute (bpm). Bradyarrhythmias have a wide spectrum of clinical presentations, from physiologic sinus bradycardia in trained athletes to life-threatening complete heart block and bradycardic cardiac arrest. Bradyarrhythmias may be transient due to alterations in vagal tone or may be caused by reversible extrinsic triggers. Evaluation and management of bradycardia is determined by patient symptoms, investigation of and correction of reversible causes, and the location of the defect in the conduction system.

PATHOPHYSIOLOGY

Bradyarrhythmias can result from dysfunction virtually anywhere in the conduction system. In general, the more distal the block, the more serious it is because of a greater potential to degenerate into complete heart block. Distal blocks also usually signify a more diffusely diseased conduction system.

Reviewing the autonomic innervation of the heart is important in the discussion of bradyarrhythmias because both the SA node, the natural pacemaker of the heart, and the AV node, the sole electrical connection between the atria and ventricles in the normal heart, are heavily innervated by both the sympathetic nervous system (SNS) and parasympathetic nervous system (PSNS). Parasympathetic tone decreases SA nodal pacing (and thus HR), conduction speed through the AV node, myocardial inotropy, and the irritability of ectopic foci. The SNS has the opposite actions. Therefore drugs used to treat symptomatic bradyarrhythmias augment the SNS or inhibit PSNS input. Increased vagal tone, as can be seen in athletes or during sleep, can cause relative bradycardia. Noxious stimuli or vagal stimuli such as coughing, gagging, and vomiting (Table 21.1) can cause transient sinus slowing and even heart block in otherwise healthy individuals (Fig. 21.1).

Bradyarrhythmias can arise from extrinsic causes, such as drug effects, and intrinsic causes, such as age-related conduction system fibrosis (see Table 21.1). As the mechanical and electrical systems of the heart are intimately connected, disruption in one can lead to problems in the other. For example, an occlusion in the proximal right coronary artery (RCA) or proximal left circumflex artery (LCX), depending on individual anatomy, can disrupt blood flow through the sinoatrial branch that supplies the SA node. Occlusion in the posterior descending artery (PDA), arising from either the RCA or LCX, can disrupt blood flow through the AV nodal branch and harm the AV node. In the current era of early revascularization in acute myocardial infarction (MI), sinus bradycardia and varying degrees of AV block are seen most commonly with inferior MI and are due to vagal and neurologic reflex mechanisms (e.g., Bezold-Jarisch reflex). Permanent conduction system damage is less common in the current era but can be seen in anterior MI causing extensive damage to the myocardium and conduction system. Rarely, chronic ischemia to the AV node can also result in heart block.

PRESENTATION, EVALUATION, AND DIAGNOSIS

The immediate evaluation and management of bradycardia is determined by hemodynamic stability and severity of symptoms. Vital signs should be checked to ensure hemodynamic stability, as unstable patients require more urgent management. Symptoms arise as a result of decreased cardiac output or chronotropic incompetence. Chronotropic incompetence is the inability to augment heart rate according to a patient's needs during times of increased demand. Symptomatic bradycardia can manifest as lightheadedness, weakness, decreased exercise tolerance, presyncope or, in more severe cases, syncope, symptoms of congestive heart failure, altered mental status and other signs of decreased perfusion. An immediate check of vital signs is required to ensure hemodynamic stability, as unstable patients require more urgent management. Accurate medication reconciliation can reveal medications that cause or exacerbate bradycardia (see Table 21.1). Basic chemistries can reveal reversible causes such as electrolyte disorders, and thyroid function tests should be considered if clinically appropriate.

TABLE 21.1
Bradycardia Causes

Categories	Examples (Not Exhaustive)
Medications	β-adrenergic blockers, nondihydropyridine calcium channel blockers, antiarrhythmic drugs, digoxin
Vagal-mediated	Well-trained athletes can have higher vagal tone; transient sinus slowing and transient AV block can occur with noxious stimuli, carotid sinus massage, or vagal stimuli such as coughing, swallowing, micturition, or defecation
Metabolic/systemic derangements	Hypothyroidism, hyperkalemia, hypoxia, acidosis, hypothermia
Infectious/inflammatory	Acute viral myocarditis, Lyme carditis, Chagas disease, infective endocarditis involving the AV conduction system
Iatrogenic/postprocedural	Following valve surgery, cardiac ablation, or alcohol septal ablation in patients with hypertrophic cardiomyopathy
Ischemia/infarction	Bezold-Jarisch reflex; an extensive infarction can cause permanent high degree AV block; rarely, chronic ischemia of the AV node can cause AV block
Infiltrative processes	Cardiac amyloidosis, hemochromatosis, Fabry disease, glycogen storage diseases, lymphoma
Autoimmune disorders	Cardiac sarcoid, rheumatoid arthritis, systemic lupus erythematosus
Neuromuscular disorders	Muscular dystrophy, Kearns-Sayre syndrome, Charcot-Marie-Tooth disease
Age-related fibrosis of conduction system	Sick sinus syndrome: primary degenerative disease of the conduction system
Familial	Early-onset progressive cardiac conduction disease in patients with structurally normal hearts and a family history of pacemakers or sudden death; may be due to genetic mutations

AV, Atrioventricular.

As with any cardiac condition, a 12-lead electrocardiogram (ECG) is crucial in evaluating bradyarrhythmias. The following are common etiologies of bradycardia based on the ECG.

Sinus Bradycardia

In **sinus bradycardia**, the rhythm originates in the SA node and the rate is less than 60 bpm. Asymptomatic sinus bradycardia often is a normal physiological finding that does not require an evaluation or treatment. However, if symptoms related to the bradycardia are present or if there is evidence of chronotropic incompetence, then further evaluation and cardiac pacing should be considered.

Sick Sinus Syndrome

Sick sinus syndrome (SSS) is typically the result of age-related fibrosis of the conduction system and occurs in patients of advanced age. SSS can present with sinus bradycardia, pauses, or paroxysmal/persistent sinus arrest with replacement by escape rhythms. Other clinical features of SSS may include chronotropic incompetence or the tachycardia-bradycardia syndrome,

an oscillation between paroxysmal atrial fibrillation and sinus bradyarrhythmia.

AV Node Dysfunction

AV node dysfunction similarly can be attributed to the causes listed in Table 21.1. The seriousness of the AV block and whether it needs to be treated is determined by whether the patient is symptomatic and the location of the block within the conduction system. Electrical disease above the His bundle is rarely life-threatening, but conduction block below the His bundle is an indication for permanent pacing, provided that reversible causes have been ruled out or corrected (Fig. 21.2).

First-degree AV block is defined by a PR interval >200 milliseconds (ms) with a preserved 1:1 conduction between the atria and ventricles. It is caused by slowed conduction from the sinus node through the atrium, atrioventricular node, and the His-Purkinje system prior to ventricular depolarization.

Second-degree AV block is separated into two entities:
- **Mobitz I** (also known as **Wenckebach** block) is characterized by a progressively prolonged PR interval leading to a dropped QRS interval. Mobitz Type I is

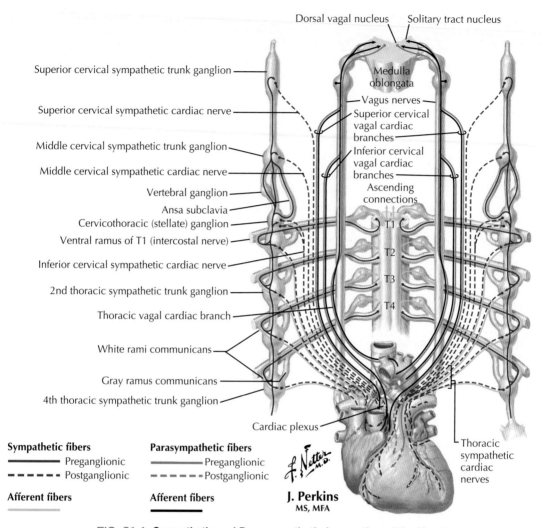

Dorsal vagal nucleus   Solitary tract nucleus

Medulla oblongata

Vagus nerves

Superior cervical vagal cardiac branches

Inferior cervical vagal cardiac branches

Ascending connections

Superior cervical sympathetic trunk ganglion

Superior cervical sympathetic cardiac nerve

Middle cervical sympathetic trunk ganglion

Middle cervical sympathetic cardiac nerve

Vertebral ganglion

Ansa subclavia

Cervicothoracic (stellate) ganglion

Ventral ramus of T1 (intercostal nerve)

Inferior cervical sympathetic cardiac nerve

2nd thoracic sympathetic trunk ganglion

Thoracic vagal cardiac branch

White rami communicans

Gray ramus communicans

4th thoracic sympathetic trunk ganglion

T1
T2
T3
T4

Cardiac plexus

Thoracic sympathetic cardiac nerves

Sympathetic fibers
——— Preganglionic
‐ ‐ ‐ ‐ ‐ Postganglionic

Afferent fibers
———

Parasympathetic fibers
——— Preganglionic
‐ ‐ ‐ ‐ ‐ Postganglionic

Afferent fibers
———

J. Perkins
MS, MFA

FIG. 21.1 **Sympathetic and Parasympathetic Innervation of the Heart.**

typically located in the AV node and does not need to be treated unless the patient is symptomatic.

• **Mobitz II** is characterized by a constant PR interval prior to a dropped QRS interval. Mobitz Type II is typically located below the AV node within the His bundle. Because of its infranodal location, it is a less stable rhythm, and progression to third-degree heart block is common and usually sudden. Because of this, if a reversible cause for Mobitz II is not found, a pacemaker is typically warranted even if the patient is asymptomatic.

Patients who present with 2:1 AV block (two P waves for every QRS complex) on ECG, the distinction between Mobitz I and II is often difficult. The QRS interval duration can be suggestive but is not confirmatory: If the QRS is narrow, it is more likely localized to the AV node and due to Type I Mobitz, while a prolonged QRS is more likely located below the AV node and due to Type II Mobitz.

Pharmacological and physical exam maneuvers can help distinguish between Mobitz I and II in the setting of 2:1 block. Because Mobitz I is usually located at the level of the AV node, it is affected by sympathetic and parasympathetic input. If conduction improves with atropine or exercise, or worsens with carotid sinus massage, the block is in the AV node. For example, if a 2:1 block improves to a 4:3 block (4 p-waves for every 3 QRS complexes) with atropine and unmasks a prolonging PR interval prior to a nonconducted p-wave, then the 2:1 block was due to Mobitz I. If

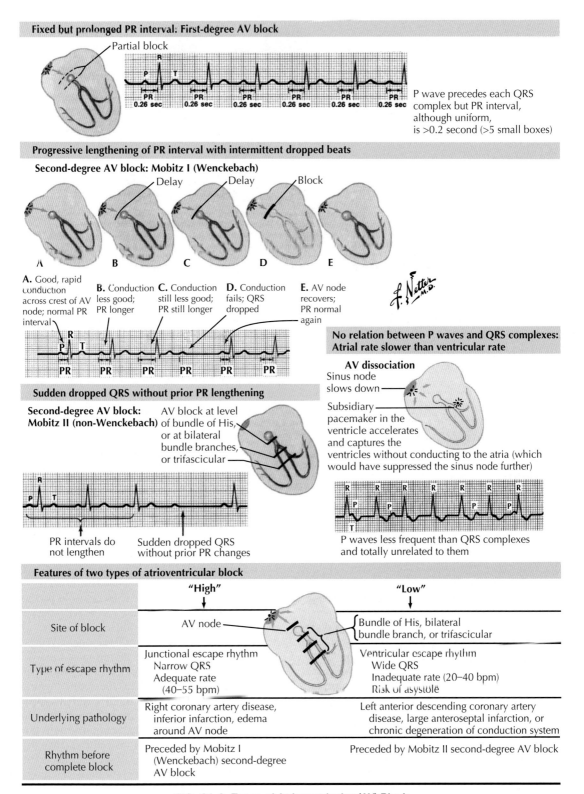

Fixed but prolonged PR interval: First-degree AV block

Partial block

P wave precedes each QRS complex but PR interval, although uniform, is >0.2 second (>5 small boxes)

Progressive lengthening of PR interval with intermittent dropped beats

Second-degree AV block: Mobitz I (Wenckebach)

Delay   Delay   Block

A   B   C   D   E

A. Good, rapid conduction across crest of AV node; normal PR interval

B. Conduction less good; PR longer

C. Conduction still less good; PR still longer

D. Conduction fails; QRS dropped

E. AV node recovers; PR normal again

Sudden dropped QRS without prior PR lengthening

Second-degree AV block: Mobitz II (non-Wenckebach)

AV block at level of bundle of His, or at bilateral bundle branches, or trifascicular

PR intervals do not lengthen

Sudden dropped QRS without prior PR changes

No relation between P waves and QRS complexes: Atrial rate slower than ventricular rate

AV dissociation

Sinus node slows down

Subsidiary pacemaker in the ventricle accelerates and captures the ventricles without conducting to the atria (which would have suppressed the sinus node further)

P waves less frequent than QRS complexes and totally unrelated to them

Features of two types of atrioventricular block

	"High"	"Low"
Site of block	AV node	Bundle of His, bilateral bundle branch, or trifascicular
Type of escape rhythm	Junctional escape rhythm Narrow QRS Adequate rate (40–55 bpm)	Ventricular escape rhythm Wide QRS Inadequate rate (20–40 bpm) Risk of asystole
Underlying pathology	Right coronary artery disease, inferior infarction, edema around AV node	Left anterior descending coronary artery disease, large anteroseptal infarction, or chronic degeneration of conduction system
Rhythm before complete block	Preceded by Mobitz I (Wenckebach) second-degree AV block	Preceded by Mobitz II second-degree AV block

FIG. 21.2 **Types of Atrioventricular** *(AV)* **Block.**

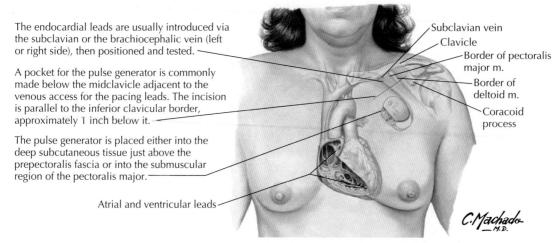

The endocardial leads are usually introduced via the subclavian or the brachiocephalic vein (left or right side), then positioned and tested.

A pocket for the pulse generator is commonly made below the midclavicle adjacent to the venous access for the pacing leads. The incision is parallel to the inferior clavicular border, approximately 1 inch below it.

The pulse generator is placed either into the deep subcutaneous tissue just above the prepectoralis fascia or into the submuscular region of the pectoralis major.

Atrial and ventricular leads

Subclavian vein
Clavicle
Border of pectoralis major m.
Border of deltoid m.
Coracoid process

C. Machado
_M.D.

FIG. 21.3 Implantable (Permanent) Dual-Chamber Cardiac Pacemaker. *m*, Muscle.

the conduction "worsens" in terms of the p-wave: QRS ratio with atropine or exercise (a 2:1 block becomes a 4:1 block), or improves with carotid sinus massage, the block is infranodal and likely Mobitz II.

Third-degree AV block, or **complete heart block,** is characterized by a complete dissociation of electrical activity between the atria and the ventricles. The block can be located at the level of the AV node, at the level of the bundle of His, or below the His bundle. Regardless of symptoms, patients with complete heart block will require a permanent pacemaker.

TREATMENT

Treatment of bradycardia depends on symptoms, location of conduction block, and overall hemodynamic stability. Clear inciting factors leading to bradycardia, particularly myocardial infarction, should be treated urgently.

Asymptomatic patients presenting with sinus bradycardia, first-degree AV block, or Mobitz Type I do not need intervention unless they become symptomatic. If the patient is unable to tolerate required drug therapies because of symptomatic bradycardia (i.e., β-adrenergic blockers for atrial fibrillation with fast rates) or has symptomatic chronotropic incompetence, then a permanent pacemaker is likely indicated. Patients with Mobitz Type II and third-degree heart block without reversible causes should be evaluated by a cardiologist for insertion of a permanent **pacemaker** (Fig. 21.3).

Cardiac pacing is the main treatment for symptomatic or distal conduction system block (Mobitz II or complete heart block). Atropine or sympathomimetic medications like isoproterenol, epinephrine, or dopamine can increase heart rate and cardiac inotropy in the case of hemodynamic instability due to bradycardia in conjunction with transcutaneous or temporary transvenous pacing. Atropine acts to inhibit PSNS input, allowing the SNS to dominate to increase HR, increase AV nodal conduction, and increase heart contraction. Isoproterenol, dopamine, and epinephrine act on β-adrenergic receptors in the heart to augment sympathetic input, resulting in similar effects.

Atropine and sympathomimetic drugs are unlikely to reverse the conduction block in permanent Mobitz II or complete heart block since the block is below the level of the AV node. However, they can reverse transient distal blocks due to increased vagal tone. If β-blocker overdose is suspected, glucagon or calcium gluconate can be administered.

If the patient has symptoms of inadequate perfusion, **transcutaneous pacing** should be started as a temporizing measure pending expert consultation and temporary transvenous pacing. Ideally, pads should be placed anteriorly to the left of the sternum at the point of maximal impulse and posteriorly to the left of the spine just below the left scapula. If the patient is awake, analgesia and light sedation, as tolerated by blood pressure, should be administered as the transcutaneous pacing can cause pain. Cardiac defibrillators can be set to the pacing mode, where goal HR and milliamps delivered can be adjusted to see capture on a cardiac monitor. Ventricular capture will be evident by a pacing spike followed by a wide QRS at the set pacing rate. The patient's pulse should be palpated to ensure that the electrical ventricular capture on the monitor corresponds with an adequate hemodynamic response in the patient. A less painful option for patients is placement of **transvenous pacing** wires through a central venous catheter, though this requires trained personnel to place. Permanent pacemaker placement remains the end therapeutic goal if reversible causes of bradycardia are not found.

CHAPTER 22

Cardiac Murmurs

GEORGE S. A. YANKEY, JR.

INTRODUCTION

Cardiac murmurs are heart sounds caused by turbulent blood flow. Murmurs are generated due to a variety of mechanisms, including blood flow through an obstruction, increased blood flow through normal structures, rapid emptying in a dilated structure, regurgitation of blood flow, and shunting of blood from one area of the heart to another.

PATHOPHYSIOLOGY

To understand and evaluate cardiac murmurs, it is important to review the phases of the cardiac cycle. Systole refers to ventricular depolarization and contraction; it occurs after S1 but before S2. Diastole, on the other hand, refers to ventricular repolarization and filling; it occurs after S2 but before S1. S1 is caused by the closure of the mitral and tricuspid valves following isovolumetric contraction of the left ventricle (LV) and right ventricle (RV). Once the pressure in the ventricles is higher than that of the atria, the valves close, but the higher pressure of the left side allows the mitral valve to close slightly earlier. S2 is caused by closure of the aortic and pulmonic valves. This occurs at the time of isovolumetric relaxation of the LV/RV. Once the pressure in the ventricles is lower than that of the pulmonic artery and aorta, the valves close.

There is a physiological spilt of S2 caused by a slight difference in the timing of closure of the aortic and pulmonary valves (A2 and P2) during inspiration. As the intrathoracic pressure rises during inspiration there is increased blood return delivered to the right side of the heart. This in turn leads to increased flow across the pulmonic valve during systole and, subsequently, delayed P2 closure. There can also be paradoxical splitting, which results from pathology causing prolonged/delayed LV systole, as well as persistent splitting, which results from pathology causing prolonged/delayed RV systole or shortened LV systole.

EVALUATION

The most common descriptive characteristics of murmurs are intensity, pitch, quality, form, location, and phase. **Intensity** of a murmur, reported as a grade, refers to the loudness of a murmur on auscultation. It is influenced by body habitus, velocity of turbulent flow, severity of disease process, and location of auscultation. Systolic murmurs are graded on a scale of 1 to 6, and diastolic murmurs are graded on a scale of 1 to 4. For systolic murmurs, grade 1 is barely audible (not appreciated by many listeners), 2 is quiet (can be appreciated by most listeners), and 3 is easily audible (audible to all listeners). Grades 4 to 6 are associated with a palpable thrill; grade 4 is loud but still requires a stethoscope, grade 5 is audible with the stethoscope partially on the patient, and grade 6 is audible without a stethoscope. For diastolic murmurs, the grading system is the same as for systolic grades 1 to 3, with grade 4 representing a very loud murmur.

Pitch refers to whether a murmur is high or low frequency. High-pitched murmurs tend to be associated with high-pressure gradients, whereas low-pitched murmurs are associated with low-pressure gradients. Low-pitched murmurs are best heard with the bell of the stethoscope.

Quality of a murmur further describes the sound (e.g., harsh, rumbling, squeaky). **Form** describes the magnitude of the murmur throughout auscultation and can be described using the terms crescendo, decrescendo, crescendo-decrescendo, and constant. Crescendo increases in magnitude throughout duration, decrescendo decreases in magnitude throughout duration, crescendo-decrescendo increases in magnitude then decreases before the murmur is complete, and constant has the same magnitude throughout.

Location describes where the murmur can be best heard and if there is associated radiation. Locations correspond to the standard anatomical locations of cardiac auscultation: the aortic (second right intercostal space), pulmonic (second left intercostal space), tricuspid

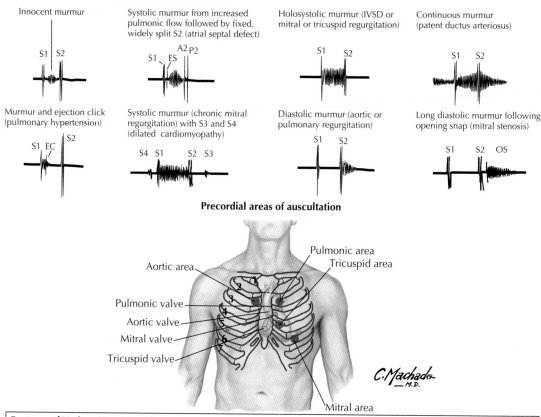

Innocent murmur

S1 S2

Systolic murmur from increased pulmonic flow followed by fixed, widely split S2 (atrial septal defect)

A2 P2
S1 ES

Holosystolic murmur (IVSD or mitral or tricuspid regurgitation)

S1 S2

Continuous murmur (patent ductus arteriosus)

S1 S2

Murmur and ejection click (pulmonary hypertension)

S1 EC S2

Systolic murmur (chronic mitral regurgitation) with S3 and S4 (dilated cardiomyopathy)

S4 S1 S2 S3

Diastolic murmur (aortic or pulmonary regurgitation)

S1 S2

Long diastolic murmur following opening snap (mitral stenosis)

S1 S2 OS

Precordial areas of auscultation

Aortic area
Pulmonic area
Tricuspid area
Pulmonic valve
Aortic valve
Mitral valve
Tricuspid valve

C. Machado
— M.D.

Mitral area

Features of Various Heart Sounds	
Area	**Comment**
Aortic	Upper right sternal border; aortic stenosis
Pulmonary	Upper left sternal border to below left clavicle; second heart sound, pulmonary valve murmurs, VSD murmur, continuous murmur of PDA
Tricuspid	Left fourth intercostal space; tricuspid and aortic regurgitation
Mitral	Left fifth intercostal space, apex; first heart sound, murmurs of mitral or aortic valves, third and fourth heart sounds

FIG. 22.1 **Cardiac Auscultation: Precordial Areas of Auscultation.** *EC,* Ejection click; *ES,* ejection sound; *IVSD,* intraventricular septal defect; *OS,* opening snap; *PDA,* patent ductus arteriosus; *VSD,* ventricular septal defect.

(fourth left intercostal space), and mitral areas (fifth left intercostal space along the midclavicular line) (Fig. 22.1).

Phase identifies when during the cardiac cycle a murmur occurs (systolic, diastolic, or continuous).

Additionally, physicians can take advantage of normal physiology and various exam maneuvers to help better differentiate murmurs. Positioning is key in the cardiac exam, as heart sounds are best heard with patients sitting up and slightly leaning forward because this brings the heart closer to the chest wall. Placing patients in the left lateral decubitus position can be beneficial for mitral murmurs by bringing the LV much closer to the chest

wall. **Inspiration** increases venous return to the right side of the heart leading to increased intensity of right-sided murmurs, both pulmonic and tricuspid.

For most murmurs, increased blood flow across a valve/opening leads to increased intensity. Murmurs due to **hypertrophic cardiomyopathy** (HCM) and **mitral valve prolapse** (MVP), however, increase in intensity when there is less blood flow across the affected area. Standing decreases ventricular filling and leads to decreased intensity of murmurs except for HCM and MVP. Increases in peripheral resistance via squatting leads to an increase in afterload, decreasing the HCM

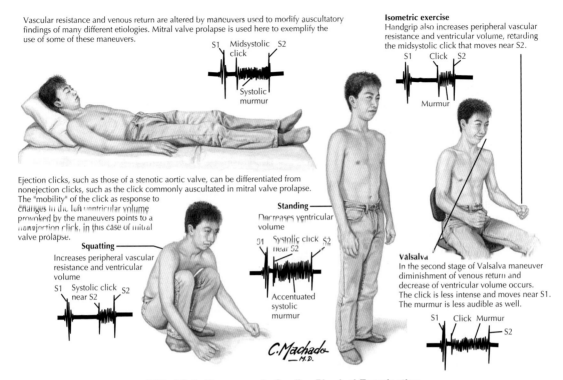

FIG. 22.2 **Maneuvers in Cardiac Physical Examination.**

Vascular resistance and venous return are altered by maneuvers used to modify auscultatory findings of many different etiologies. Mitral valve prolapse is used here to exemplify the use of some of these maneuvers.

S1 Midsystolic S2
click

Systolic
murmur

Isometric exercise
Handgrip also increases peripheral vascular resistance and ventricular volume, retarding the midsystolic click that moves near S2.

S1 Click S2

Murmur

Ejection clicks, such as those of a stenotic aortic valve, can be differentiated from nonejection clicks, such as the click commonly auscultated in mitral valve prolapse. The "mobility" of the click as response to changes in the left ventricular volume provoked by the maneuvers points to a nonejection click, in this case of mitral valve prolapse.

Squatting
Increases peripheral vascular resistance and ventricular volume

S1 Systolic click S2
near S2

Standing
Decreases ventricular volume

S1 Systolic click S2
near S2

Accentuated
systolic
murmur

Valsalva
In the second stage of Valsalva maneuver diminishment of venous return and decrease of ventricular volume occurs. The click is less intense and moves near S1. The murmur is less audible as well.

S1 Click Murmur
S2

C. Machado
M.D.

murmur but increasing **aortic regurgitation, mitral regurgitation** (MR), and **ventricular septal defect** (VSD) murmurs. Handgrip also increases peripheral resistance and afterload, and it can be used as an excluding test. Diastolic murmurs that decrease with handgrip rule out aortic regurgitation and mitral stenosis; for systolic murmurs, increased intensity with handgrip rules out aortic stenosis and HCM, while decreased intensity rules out mitral regurgitation and VSD murmurs.

The Valsalva maneuver can be useful for systolic murmurs and is divided into two phases, strain and release. With strain, there is decreased venous return to the heart as well as decreased peripheral vascular tone, making the murmurs of MVP and HCM louder. In release, the opposite is true making the murmur of aortic stenosis louder (Fig. 22.2).

DIAGNOSIS
Systolic Murmurs
Holosystolic murmurs begin at S1 and continue throughout systole, obscuring S1 and S2. Other systolic murmurs can be separated by their timing within the cardiac cycle. Early systolic murmurs begin at S1 and end

in the middle of systole. In general, both holosystolic and early systolic murmurs are caused by blood flowing from one chamber of higher pressure across a valve and into a chamber of lower pressure. Either can occur in MR, **tricuspid regurgitation** (TR), and VSDs. Chronic TR/MR are more associated with holosystolic murmurs, while acute TR/MR are associated with early systolic murmurs. VSD murmurs without significant shunting tend to present as early systolic murmurs.

Midsystolic ejection murmurs occur in the setting of turbulent flow across the aortic or pulmonic outflow tracts. They tend to be crescendo-decrescendo murmurs starting briefly after S1 and ending before S2. Midsystolic murmurs are heard with **aortic stenosis**/sclerosis, **pulmonic stenosis,** and dilation of the aortic root or pulmonary artery.

Late systolic murmurs are high-pitched, crescendo murmurs occurring after S1 and may obscure either A2 or P2. They result from prolapse of the atrioventricular valves or papillary muscle displacement, and there generally is a click preceding the murmur as the increase in LV pressure pushes back on the valve, causing flow in the regurgitant direction. They occur in **tricuspid valve prolapse,** MVP, and ischemic mitral regurgitation.

Diastolic Murmurs

Early diastolic murmurs are high-pitched, decrescendo, blowing murmurs that initiate at S2 and end during diastole. These murmurs signify regurgitant flow across the semilunar valves as seen in aortic and **pulmonic regurgitation.** When patients progress to severe aortic regurgitation, they can develop an **Austin Flint murmur,** which is a middiastolic murmur thought to be due to the functional mitral stenosis caused by the regurgitant flow from the aortic valve.

Middiastolic murmurs are low-pitched, rumbling murmurs that initiate with an opening snap after S2 and end before an accentuated S1. The opening snap is a result of the fully stenotic valve opening. The timing of the opening snap can give a sense of disease severity, as opening snaps shortly after S2 represent more severe disease due to higher pressure gradient needed to cause earlier opening. S1 is accentuated due to closure of the stenotic valve. Middiastolic murmurs are a result of turbulent flow across the atrioventricular valves and are usually due to **mitral stenosis** and **tricuspid stenosis.**

Late diastolic (presystolic) murmurs are low-pitched, crescendo murmurs that initiate late in diastole and usually end on S1. Similar to middiastolic murmurs, they are a result of turbulent flow across the atrioventricular valves and so can be seen in mitral stenosis and tricuspid stenosis.

Miscellaneous Murmurs

Continuous murmurs start during systole, peak around S2, and continue through diastole. These murmurs are due to flow across high-pressure to low-pressure shunts and thus are not due to valvular disease. Examples of shunts include **patent ductus arteriosus** (classically a machinelike murmur), aortopulmonary window, or arteriovenous fistulas. Murmurs can occur that do not represent a primary cardiac process but instead result from increased blood flow across a normal valve. These are known as **innocent/flow murmurs** and are a diagnosis of exclusion, as they can only be named in absence of other cardiac abnormalities.

TREATMENT

Apart from physical exam, echocardiography is the primary imaging modality used to further characterize the murmur and potential underlying disease process. Transthoracic echocardiography can usually adequately visualize valve structure and function, but a transesophageal approach can provide finer detail (see Chapter 48 for further details). Cardiac CT or MRI can be also used, and cardiac catheterization can more accurately measure valve areas, pressure gradients and resistances, and blood flow across the valves. Murmurs that cause significant symptoms may require intervention, either via catheterization or a surgical approach.

CHAPTER 23

Hypoxemia

PIERRE ELIAS • TALAL DAHHAN

INTRODUCTION

Hypoxemia refers to an abnormally low level of oxygen in the arterial blood. While there are competing definitions, it is generally agreed upon that patients are hypoxemic if they meet one of three criteria:

1. An arterial partial pressure of oxygen (PaO_2) <80 mm Hg
2. A peripheral oxygen saturation (SaO_2) <92% in the absence of structural pulmonary disease
3. A decrease in peripheral oxygen saturation of >5% during physical activity

It is important to recognize the difference between hypoxemia and hypoxia. Hypoxemia refers to oxygen tension within the blood, while **hypoxia** refers to an inadequate oxygenation of a specific organ or the entire body. As such, hypoxemia is often (but not always) a precursor to hypoxia.

EVALUATION

As noted, physicians can evaluate hypoxemia by measuring either the SaO_2 or the PaO_2. An arterial blood gas is required to measure PaO_2, which may be painful for patients and can be technically difficult. While it is more accurate than SaO_2, as the oxygen tension in blood is being directly measured, it only represents a single point in time.

SaO_2, on the other hand, can be measured by **pulse oximetry,** a noninvasive technology that emits light in red and infrared wavelengths and measures how much is absorbed by blood flowing underneath the skin (most commonly, a finger). Pulse oximetry is noninvasive, relatively easy to acquire, and dynamic from second to second. Pulse oximetry, however, has important limitations to consider. Pulse oximetry creates a signal graph, called a plethysmograph, with waves that correspond to pulsatile flow of arterial blood. For accurate pulse oximetry, the waveform must be stable, consistent, and with significant enough amplitude to clearly differentiate peaks from baseline.

Two other physiological points must be considered. The **oxygen-hemoglobin dissociation curve** is sigmoid shaped, approaching an asymptote of 100% SaO_2 despite increases in PaO_2. As a result, large changes in PaO_2 from clinical pathology (e.g., a PaO_2 drop from 140 mm Hg to 100 mm Hg due to pneumonia and impending sepsis) may have minimal effects on SaO_2. In fact, some studies have found that hypoxemia is not present until SaO_2 approaches 85% (Fig. 23.1). Second, pulse oximetry is representative of oxygenation specifically between the emitter and photodetector. Using the fingertips in patients with severe vasoconstriction (such as Raynaud) or abnormal vasculature (such as an arteriovenous fistula) can generate false readings.

Hypoxemia may be suggested by physical exam findings. As can be expected in patients lacking adequate oxygen to meet metabolic demand, hypoxemic patients can present with tachypnea, tachycardia, diaphoresis, and altered mental status. **Cyanosis** is more suggestive of hypoxemia, and it is characterized by the bluish discoloration that occurs from the increased ratio of reduced/oxidized hemoglobin in the peripheral vasculature. The transition from pink to white to ultimately blue predominance in the skin is often a sign of significant hypoxemia. It is more easily detected in people with lightly pigmented skin and is often found at nailbeds, fingertips, and lips.

Patients with chronic hypoxemia may also present with **clubbing.** Digital clubbing presents as enlargement of the terminal segments of digits, often painless and bilateral. This exam finding is sometimes seen in patients with significant pulmonary shunting. While it has been described for centuries, studies have found that there is poor interrater reliability in determining who actually has clubbing, as well as the yield of the diagnostic finding. Available evidence recommends that clubbing is more likely in patients with a distal phalangeal finger depth (DPD) to interphalangeal finger depth (IPD) ratio of >1.0 and a positive Schamroth sign (Fig. 23.2).

DIAGNOSIS AND TREATMENT

Hypoxemia can be separated into five separate mechanisms, which can be evaluated by following the path of

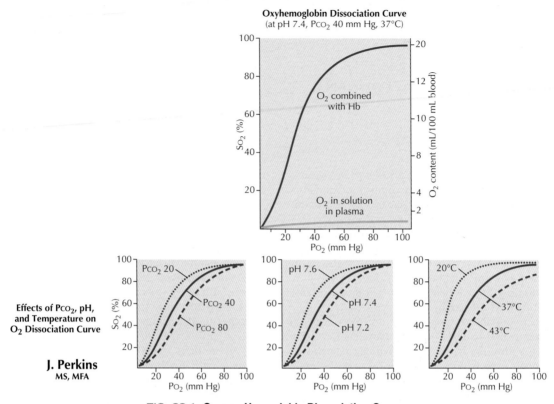

Oxyhemoglobin Dissociation Curve
(at pH 7.4, P_{CO_2} 40 mm Hg, 37°C)

O_2 combined with Hb

O_2 in solution in plasma

S_{O_2} (%)

O_2 content (mL/100 mL blood)

P_{O_2} (mm Hg)

Effects of P_{CO_2}, pH, and Temperature on O_2 Dissociation Curve

P_{CO_2} 20
P_{CO_2} 40
P_{CO_2} 80

pH 7.6
pH 7.4
pH 7.2

20°C
37°C
43°C

S_{O_2} (%)

P_{O_2} (mm Hg)

J. Perkins
MS, MFA

FIG. 23.1 **Oxygen-Hemoglobin Dissociation Curves.**

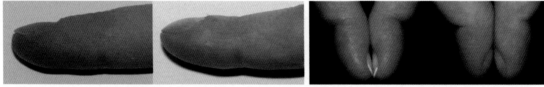

A. The angle between the nailbed and the nailfold (lovibond angle) should normally be ≤165 *(as in the left-hand figure)*. Note the loss of this normal angle in the individual with clubbing *(right-hand image)*.

B. Schramroth sign demonstrated. The diamond-shaped space created by both lovibond angles during apposition of right and left index fingers *(as seen in the left-hand figure)* is lost in the individual with clubbing.

FIG. 23.2 **Digital Clubbing.** (Reused with permission from Florin T, Ludwig S: *Netter's pediatrics,* Philadelphia, 2009, Elsevier, p. 248.)

air from inspiration to the alveolus to the pulmonary circulation. Effective evaluation of hypoxemia requires an arterial blood gas that, along with the patient's clinical presentation, is crucial to determine the cause and severity of hypoxemia. In discussing causes of hypoxemia and abnormal respiration, it is helpful to think of pathology as it relates to ventilation and perfusion. Ventilation can be estimated by the partial pressure of arterial CO_2 ($PaCO_2$), and patients with elevated $PaCO_2$ are deemed unable to breathe off CO_2 created during metabolism. Perfusion, on the other hand, looks at how much blood passes by the alveoli. The adequate removal of CO_2 and delivery of O_2 requires both ventilation (V) and perfusion (Q), and different zones of the lung have different ratios of ventilation and perfusion (V/Q) based on anatomy and positioning; the overall so-called normal average of V/Q ratios in the healthy lung is 0.8 (see Chapter 83).

Calculation of the **alveolar-arterial (A-a) gradient** can reveal defects in gas exchange. The capital **A** represents the partial pressure of oxygen in the alveoli; the lowercase **a** represents the partial pressure in the artery. Alveoli are composed of airspace surrounded by a thin membrane, as the partial pressure of oxygen is at its highest here. Damage to alveoli impairs diffusion of oxygen from alveolar space to pulmonary circulation. The calculated A-a gradient is compared to an age-adjusted normal calculated by ([Age/4] + 4) after age 50; an elevated A-a gradient narrows the differential for hypoxemia.

Patients with an elevated $PaCO_2$ on arterial blood gas have, by definition, a problem of hypoventilation. An elevated $PaCO_2$ and a normal A-a gradient indicate minimal gas exchange and instead pure hypoventilation; an example is a patient presenting with opiate overdose, or patients with Guillain-Barré syndrome who have impaired neural function and respiratory muscle weakness. Patients with elevated $PaCO_2$ and elevated A-a gradient have both hypoventilation and another process. Patients with normal $PaCO_2$ and a normal A-a gradient who nonetheless show hypoxemia are not able to inspire enough oxygen in their environment. The percentage of oxygen in inspired air is called FiO_2. At sea level, FiO_2 is assumed to be 0.21, or 21% oxygen. Decreased FiO_2 is most commonly seen at high altitudes.

Patients with normal $PaCO_2$ and elevated A-a gradient should have supplemental oxygen applied, such as through a nasal cannula or face mask, to determine if the hypoxemia is correctable. Patients whose SaO_2 (easily measured continuously) corrects with oxygen have worsened **V/Q mismatch.** Causes of worsened V/Q mismatch include vascular problems (such as pulmonary hypertension or pulmonary emboli), obstructive airway diseases (such as asthma, chronic obstructive pulmonary disease [COPD], and bronchiectasis), and diffuse interstitial lung disease.

Patients with elevated A-a gradients whose SaO_2 does not correct with oxygen have **shunting,** a form of severe V/Q mismatch. An extreme shunt is described as perfusion without ventilation; mathematically, V is zero, making the V/Q ratio equal to zero. For example, blood in an extreme shunt may travel through the pulmonary circulation but not come into contact with alveolar gas, as in alveolar collapse from pneumothorax or atelectasis. Another example of extreme shunt can be due to complete avoidance of the pulmonary circulation/capillary bed via patent foramen ovale (PFO) or pulmonary arteriovenous malformations (AVMs). Incomplete shunting can be seen in diseases characterized by alveolar filling, such as pneumonia and pulmonary edema, and diffuse alveolar infiltrates such as acute respiratory distress syndrome (ARDS). It is important to remember that, although one process may predominate, multiple causes of hypoxemia can exist at once.

CHAPTER 24

Adventitial Lung Sounds

ZAID I. ALMARZOOQ • TALAL DAHHAN

INTRODUCTION

Auscultation is a cardinal portion of the pulmonary exam, giving the clinician the ability to evaluate airflow within the lungs. The physician primarily uses the diaphragm of the stethoscope to auscultate the posterior, lateral, and anterior chest walls during both inspiration and expiration, although the bell can be used when listening over the apices. Clinicians should evaluate for the quality and intensity of the breath sounds and compare a region with the equivalent region on the opposite lung.

Normal lung sounds are separated into **bronchial** and **vesicular** sounds based on their normal anatomical locations; the presence of either apart from their normal location may indicate a pulmonary pathology. Bronchial and tracheal breath sounds are produced by turbulent airflow in the large airways, whereby a gap occurs between normal, inspiratory lung sounds and louder, expiratory lung sounds. They are normally heard over the trachea and manubrium, corresponding with the anatomical location of the trachea and bronchi. The presence of bronchial breath sounds over the lung parenchyma may be a sign of lung consolidation.

Vesicular lung sounds are produced by airflow conducted through the smaller airways and lung parenchyma, whereby the predominant inspiratory lung sound is followed by the expiratory lung sound without a gap in between. Lung sound intensities can be normal or reduced. Reduced lung sounds occur in chronic obstructive pulmonary disease (COPD) and atelectasis due to decreased airflow, and pleural effusions decrease conduction from parenchyma to the stethoscope, deadening normal lung sounds. Adventitial lung sounds are abnormal, or extra, lung sounds as a result of pulmonary pathology. Several types are detailed in the chapter (Table 24.1).

EXAMINATION FINDINGS
Wheezes

Wheezes are adventitial lung sounds characterized by a high-pitched, musical-like quality. They arise from significant airway narrowing resulting in the continuous oscillation of opposing airway walls that lead to wheezes. Wheezes can occur during inspiration, expiration, or both; airways usually dilate during inspiration and narrow during expiration; thus wheezing is often first heard during the expiratory phase, when airways normally narrow. More severe narrowing, however, can lead to inspiratory wheezing. Despite this, the timing of wheezing is an inaccurate guide to the severity of airflow obstruction—as in very severe airway obstruction, the velocity of airflow is reduced below the level required to produce sound, leading to absent wheezes signifying emergent respiratory compromise. Wheezes also differ in quality; those produced from narrowing of the smaller bronchi result in high-pitched wheezes with whistling quality, while those produced from narrowing of larger bronchi lead to low-pitched wheezes, which are sometimes referred to as **rhonchi.**

Differential diagnosis

The differential diagnosis of wheezes includes asthma, COPD, bronchial spasm, mucosal edema (pulmonary edema), and excessive secretions (pneumonia, bronchiectasis). When wheezes are localized and monophasic, consider a fixed bronchial obstruction, as in carcinoma of the lung. It is important not to confuse wheezes with stridor (reviewed later), given their similarities.

Crackles

Crackles are staccato, interrupted sounds that are thought to result from the opening and closing of small airways. During expiration, peripheral airways collapse; then with inspiration, air enters rapidly into the distal airways leading to a sudden opening of alveoli and small bronchi. Areas that are more compliant open first, followed by less-compliant areas, leading to crackles. Crackles sound akin to the popping noise heard in rice cereals or rubbing strands of hair together next to an ear. Crackles can be separated into higher pitched, fine crackles heard primarily during inspiration and lower pitched, coarse crackles that can be heard in both late inspiration and

TABLE 24.1
Summary of Adventitious Lung Sounds

Adventitial Lung Sound	Description	Differential Diagnosis
Wheezes	Continuous sound secondary to air passing through narrowed airway	Asthma COPD Bronchial spasm Mucosal edema (pulmonary edema) Excessive secretions (pneumonia, bronchiectasis) Lung carcinoma (monophasic)

Crackles	Interrupted, staccato sounds secondary to opening and closing of small airways and alveoli with altered compliance	Early inspiratory crackles
		   COPD
		Late or pan-inspiratory crackles
		   ILD (fine; Velcro-like)
		   Pulmonary edema (medium)
		   Bronchiectasis (coarse)

Stridor	High-pitched, continuous sound secondary to narrowing of the upper respiratory tract	Anaphylaxis Tracheal stenosis or edema Epiglottitis Presence of a foreign body
Pleural friction rub	Continuous or intermittent sound secondary to rubbing of thickened pleura	Pulmonary infarction Pneumonia Pleural malignancy Spontaneous pneumothorax

COPD, Chronic obstructive pulmonary disease; *ILD*, interstitial lung disease.

expiration. It is therefore important to describe their timing, quality (fine, medium, and course), and pitch (low, high).

Differential diagnosis

Crackles have a broad differential diagnosis encompassing many cardiopulmonary pathologies.

Of note, physicians should ask patients to cough when crackles are heard, as they may disappear. Timing crackles can narrow the differential; early inspiratory crackles, which end before mid-inspiration, are associated with small airway disease, especially COPD. Late or pan-inspiratory crackles are related to an alveolar disease. Interstitial lung disease (ILD) is associated with fine, Velcro-like crackles across affected lung fields. Medium crackles are usually due to pulmonary edema, whereby fluid in the alveoli alters the alveoli's resistance due to disruption of the function of surfactant. Coarse crackles are usually due to retained secretions. They are seen in bronchiectasis and any other diseases that lead to retention of secretions.

Pleural Friction Rub

A **pleural friction rub** is a harsh, grating sound, either continuous or intermittent, that occurs when inflamed or thickened pleural surfaces rub together during the respiratory phases. It is often best heard at the axilla or lung bases. The differential diagnosis of pulmonary friction rub includes pulmonary infarction, pneumonia, or (less commonly) spontaneous pneumothorax or pleural malignancy.

Stridor

Stridor is a high-pitched, continuous sound best auscultated over the anterior neck. It is caused by narrowing/obstruction of the upper respiratory tract, which distinguishes it from wheezes, which primarily involve the lower respiratory tract. Indeed, true wheezes are faint, if at all present, over the neck. The differential diagnosis for stridor includes anaphylaxis, tracheal stenosis or edema, epiglottitis, or the presence of a foreign body.

EVALUATION OF ADVENTITIAL LUNG SOUNDS

As with any patient, a thorough history remains a cornerstone in evaluating any complaint. The physical exam should include vital signs, including respiratory rate and oxygen saturation (SpO$_2$); it is key to assess the patient's SpO$_2$ off oxygen, as well as how much supplemental oxygen is needed for an adequate SpO_2. Elements of the respiratory status, including accessory muscle (intercostal, scalene, and sternocleidomastoid) use or tripod posture, are also readily visible prior to the lung exam. Patients may appear cachectic in COPD, congestive heart failure, ILD, or malignancy. Digital clubbing may be present in ILD, empyema, bronchiectasis, asbestosis, and lung malignancy. Examine for signs of congestive heart failure, including cardiac murmurs, elevated jugular venous pressure, ascites, and lower extremity edema.

In addition to basic auscultation, several maneuvers are available to narrow the differential diagnosis for abnormal lung sounds. Physicians test for **egophony** by asking the patient to say "EE" while auscultating over the chest wall. In normal lung, physicians will hear the "EE," but in the presence of underlying consolidation "EE" will become "AY" instead. **Whispered pectoriloquy** involves asking the patient to whisper "ninety-nine"; patients with normal lungs will have only faint transmission through the stethoscope, while consolidation will make the whispers louder. Finally, **tactile fremitus** can be elicited by placing the ulnar surface of the hands at symmetric posterior intercostal spaces and asking a patient to say "ninety-nine." Decreased unilateral fremitus can signify pleural effusion, pneumothorax, or malignancy, while increased unilateral fremitus is seen in consolidation.

CHAPTER 25

Ascites

AHMAD NAJDAT BAZARBASHI

INTRODUCTION

Ascites (from the Greek *askos*, which means "to resemble a sack or winebag") is defined as the pathological accumulation of fluid within the peritoneal cavity resulting in abdominal swelling. An alternate definition is the accumulation of >25 mL of serous fluid within the intraabdominal cavity. Ascites can occur as a consequence of various medical illnesses, though it most commonly occurs as a consequence of decompensated cirrhosis in end-stage liver disease. It is associated with multiple complications as well as significant morbidity and mortality. A series of pathophysiological events leads to ascites, and management usually revolves around symptomatic relief of abdominal distension and reversal of the underlying cause of ascites.

PATHOPHYSIOLOGY

The pathophysiology of ascites involves an intricate network of mediators and a cascade of events that lead to the accumulation of fluid. The specific pathophysiology of ascites varies depending on the underlying cause.

In **cirrhosis,** the most common cause, three key mediators result in ascites. First is **portal hypertension,** which leads to elevated hydrostatic pressure within the hepatic sinusoids resulting in transudation and accumulation of fluid within the peritoneal cavity. Second is splanchnic arteriolar vasodilation caused by local vasodilators, such as nitric oxide, released in portal hypertension. Significant splanchnic vasodilation can decrease arterial blood volume markedly causing arterial pressure to fall, resulting in homeostatic activation of vasoconstrictor and antinatriuretic factors, resulting in sodium and fluid retention. Finally, fall in arterial pressure leads to activation of the sympathetic nervous system, resulting in further sodium and fluid retention.

It is important to note that portal hypertension can occur from causes other than cirrhosis, including portal vein or hepatic vein thrombosis, congestive heart failure, and constrictive pericarditis. Physiological steps in the formation of ascites in noncirrhotic patients involve fluid accumulation from hypoalbuminemia (seen in nephrotic syndrome and protein-losing enteropathy) and peritoneal disease leading to ascitic fluid accumulation (peritoneal carcinomatosis, peritoneal infections, and peritoneal dialysis).

ETIOLOGIES

Cirrhosis is the most common cause of ascites in the United States and accounts for up to 85% of all causes of ascites (Fig. 25.1). The most common underlying cause of cirrhosis is chronic alcohol use, followed by infectious hepatitis (see Chapter 139 for further details). Ascites is the most common complication of decompensated cirrhosis occurring in up to 50% of patients after 10 years of diagnosis. Cirrhotic ascites confers a poor prognosis, with 50% of cirrhotic patients dying within 2 years of developing ascites. Cancer is the second most common cause of ascites in the United States. Various malignancies with or without peritoneal metastases can give rise to malignant ascites. Diagnosis is usually obtained by sending a sample of fluid for cytology to reveal malignant cells. Right-sided congestive heart failure can lead to fluid backup and accumulation in the abdomen (in the form of ascites) and lower extremities. Other potential causes of ascites include tuberculosis (TB) or fungal peritonitis, pancreatic disease, dialysis, or uncommon causes such as ventriculoperitoneal (VP) shunts, endometriosis, hematological malignancies, nephrotic syndrome, and myxedema.

EVALUATION/DIAGNOSIS

When examining a patient with ascites, general inspection from the side of the bed can provide a lot of valuable information. When a patient is supine, look for these signs:

1. Bulging flanks: This results from accumulation of fluid (usually at least 1500 mL) in the paracolic gutters (space between the large bowel and the lateral abdominal wall). This area can also be percussed to

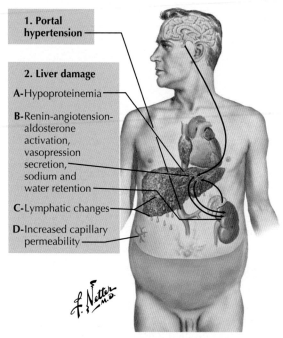

1. Portal hypertension

2. Liver damage

A-Hypoproteinemia

B-Renin-angiotension-aldosterone activation, vasopression secretion, sodium and water retention

C-Lymphatic changes

D-Increased capillary permeability

FIG. 25.1 **Pathogenesis of Ascites in Cirrhosis.**

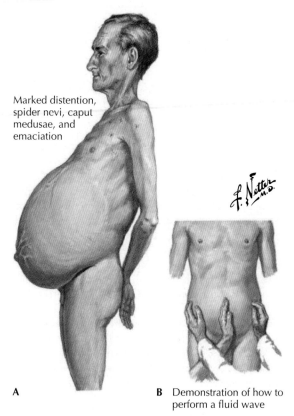

Marked distention, spider nevi, caput medusae, and emaciation

A

B Demonstration of how to perform a fluid wave

FIG. 25.2 **Physical Findings and Assessing for a Fluid Wave in Patients With Ascites.**

reveal dullness, which fades as you percuss toward the midline of the abdomen.

2. **Shifting dullness:** This describes flank dullness that changes locations when a patient rolls from a supine position to a lateral decubitus position. In one study, this test had 83% sensitivity and 56% specificity in detecting ascites.

3. **Fluid wave** or fluid thrill: Have the patient's or an assistant's hand placed in the midline of the abdomen. Place your hand on one flank and tap the other flank. The test is positive if you can feel a "thrill or wave" caused by transmission of the tap across the fluid-filled abdomen. The patient's or an assistant's hand is necessary to halt waves transmitted through the subcutaneous tissue rather than the fluid-filled abdomen (Fig. 25.2).

Ultrasound

Moderate to large ascites can usually be detected on thorough physical examination; however, radiological confirmation is occasionally necessary. Ultrasound is a cost-effective, radiation-free modality that can be utilized to confirm the presence of ascites and is usually the first imaging modality of choice in the diagnosis of ascites. Ultrasound of the abdomen can also comment

on the appearance of the liver, vascular abnormalities that could cause ascites, and intraabdominal malignancy. Other modalities that may be diagnostic for ascites are abdominal CT and MRI scans.

Paracentesis

In the majority of patients, it is imperative to sample ascitic fluid to elucidate the cause of their ascites and rule out malignant disease or possible superimposed infection (bacterial peritonitis). This procedure is called a **paracentesis** and can be performed for diagnostic and/or therapeutic purposes (see Chapter 53 for further details). While paracentesis previously relied on physical examination to determine a suitable pocket of fluid, most paracenteses now occur under the guidance of an imaging modality, usually ultrasound. Samples obtained should be sent to the lab for cell count, Gram stain and culture (to rule out infection), cytology (to rule out malignancy), and protein and glucose levels. To meet criteria for spontaneous bacterial peritonitis (SBP), which is a feared complication in any patient with ascites, the neutrophil count in ascites fluids needs to exceed 250 cells/mm^3 in the absence of other causes of elevated neutrophil counts. Amylase can be sent for concern for ascites secondary to pancreatitis, and acid-fast bacilli stain and culture can be sent if there is concern for TB-associated ascites.

One of the most helpful tests to send on ascitic fluid is the albumin level. The **serum-ascites albumin gradient** (SAAG) is the difference between the serum albumin and the ascites fluid albumin and helps to differentiate portal hypertension–related ascites from peritoneal, nonportal hypertensive causes (Box 25.1). A SAAG of ≥1.1 g/dL indicates portal hypertension or a nonperitoneal cause of ascites, while a SAAG <1.1 g/dL indicates a peritoneal pathology. The SAAG is similar to identifying pleural effusions as transudative or exudative; transudative fluid results from hydrostatic forces moving primarily fluid

---

BOX 25.1
Serum-Ascites Albumin Gradient (SAAG) and the Cause of Ascites

SAAG ≥1.1 g/dL
- Cirrhosis and portal hypertension
- Portal vein thrombosis
- Hepatic vein thrombosis (Budd-Chiari syndrome)
- Heart failure
- Constrictive pericarditis

SAAG <1.1 g/dL
- Peritoneal carcinomatosis
- Peritoneal tuberculosis
- Pancreatitis

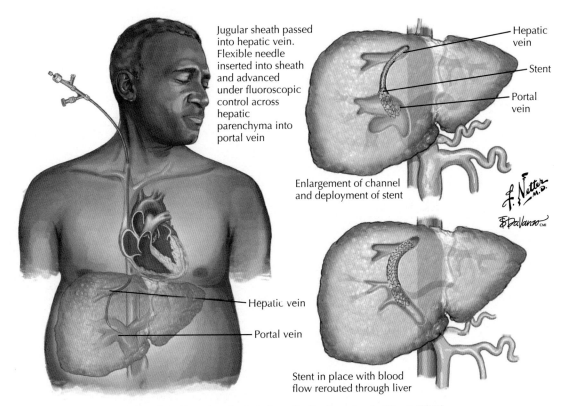

Jugular sheath passed into hepatic vein. Flexible needle inserted into sheath and advanced under fluoroscopic control across hepatic parenchyma into portal vein

Hepatic vein

Stent

Portal vein

Enlargement of channel and deployment of stent

Hepatic vein

Portal vein

Stent in place with blood flow rerouted through liver

FIG. 25.3 **Transjugular Intrahepatic Portosystemic Shunt (TIPS).**

across a membrane and leading to a low fluid protein (or albumin) level, while exudative processes exude both fluid and protein, leading to a high fluid protein (albumin) level. Complications of paracentesis include bleeding, infection, and visceral or blood vessel injury (mainly the inferior epigastric artery).

Note that both congestive heart failure and cirrhosis with portal hypertension can lead to a SAAG ≥1.1 g/dL. One way to distinguish between these two conditions is by looking at the total ascitic fluid protein level. In cirrhosis and portal hypertension, the total ascitic fluid protein level is usually <2.5 g/dL, while in congestive heart failure it is >2.5 g/dL.

DIFFERENTIAL DIAGNOSIS

The differential diagnosis of ascites includes other causes of abdominal distention:
1. Obesity
2. Large ovarian cysts
3. Small bowel obstruction
4. Other causes of abdominal masses, including tumors

MANAGEMENT

Management of ascites revolves around symptomatic relief from abdominal distention while treating the underlying cause of ascites. In patients with volume-related ascites (heart failure) or ascites secondary to cirrhosis/portal hypertension, sodium restriction and the use of diuretics may be beneficial. In cases where patients are resistant to diuresis, large-volume paracentesis can provide significant relief. In refractory cases, a **transjugular intrahepatic portosystemic shunt (TIPS)** may be necessary to relieve portal hypertension as a driver of ascites (Fig. 25.3). Intravenous colloid infusions, such as albumin, which has been the most studied, should be used after large-volume paracentesis to avoid fluid shifts that could lead to circulatory dysfunction. In patients with ascites from peritoneal carcinomatosis, treating the underlying malignancy is the treatment of choice. In select cases with rapidly accumulating malignant ascites, an indwelling Tenckhoff catheter can be useful. Patients with peritoneal infections causing ascites need source control and antibiotics.

CHAPTER 26

Lower Extremity Edema

G. TITUS K. NGENO

INTRODUCTION

Lower extremity edema is a common clinical finding characterized by presence of a palpable lower extremity swelling. It results from increased accumulation of interstitial fluid in the intercellular space and is further classified by whether it is pitting (i.e., if a skin indentation forms upon application of pressure) or nonpitting. It is also described according to laterality of the affected limbs as either unilateral or bilateral and the height to which the edema extends.

The most common cause of acute lower extremity edema is **deep venous thrombosis** (DVT). Other acute causes of swelling include cellulitis, compartment syndrome, ruptured Baker cysts, and rupture of the medial head of the gastrocnemius. The most common cause of chronic edema is **chronic venous insufficiency,** characterized by edema and characteristic skin changes—causes of chronic venous insufficiency include recurrent/untreated DVT, heart failure, renal insufficiency, hepatic dysfunction, and malignancy. Pulmonary hypertension and obstructive sleep apnea have been associated with chronic venous edema, and certain medications can also lead to lower extremity edema; these include calcium channel blockers, NSAIDs, thiazolidinediones (including pioglitazone and rosiglitazone), hormonal therapies, certain chemotherapeutics, dopaminergic agents (such as pramipexole), and antidepressants (such as trazodone).

PATHOPHYSIOLOGY

Increased fluid in the interstitial space results from an imbalance in the distribution of fluid at the capillary level and a disruption in the Starling equation, which governs the exchange of fluid between intravascular and extravascular space. Typically, protein-poor fluid is termed **venous edema,** whereas protein-rich interstitial fluid is called **lymphedema. Lipedema** does not involve changes in interstitial fluid, but is a maldistribution of fat adipocytes often with more proximal involvement and sparring of the feet.

The Starling equation determines the movement of fluid across a membrane separating intravascular and extravascular spaces. The equation takes into account two opposing pressures: **hydrostatic pressure** arising from fluid within a space and **oncotic pressure,** an opposing pressure arising from proteins in fluid, most commonly albumin, that acts to draw water into a space. These pressures interact over a membrane surface area with certain permeability, and changes to these factors will alter the position of fluid within each space.

A decline in intravascular oncotic pressure results in reduced fluid resorption to the intravascular space, thus leading to interstitial edema. Decreased oncotic pressure can be seen in proteinuria (nephrotic syndrome), decreased protein synthesis in hepatic dysfunction, or nutritional inadequacy. On the other hand, increased intravascular hydrostatic pressure also will force fluid into the interstitial space. This can be seen during dysregulation of the renin-angiotensin system seen in heart failure and cirrhosis, venous outflow obstruction as with DVT, or primary increased circulatory volume as with pregnancy.

Increased capillary permeability can arise from systemic venous hypertension seen in right heart failure and pulmonary hypertension. Inflammatory states, such as infection and allergic reactions, result in the release of inflammatory cytokines, which can lead to pericapillary leak and edema. Patients with hypothyroidism have increased deposition of hydrophilic-rich molecules, such as glycosaminoglycans and mucopolysaccharides, in the tissue matrix of connective tissue protein, resulting in **myxedema.** Idiopathic edema has also been described to occur in menstruating women as well as in cases of diuretic abuse, obesity, and depression.

Untreated edema presents several complications, most notably lower extremity deformations and overall debilitation. Chronic edema interrupts the protective skin barrier, leading to dermatitis and skin tears. Unaddressed, these can progress to **venous ulcers** and cellulitis (Fig. 26.1). Patients who are unable to walk due to untreated

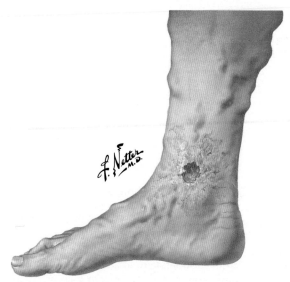

FIG. 26.1 Ulceration and Varicose Veins in Chronic Venous Insufficiency.

edema suffer complications of immobility, including DVTs, which can exacerbate lower extremity edema.

Lymphedema results from occlusion of lymphatic drainage systems. Occlusion often arises from inflammation and fibrotic changes that result from chronic insults, such as venous stasis, radiation, and sometimes infection by filarial worms. Obstruction by mass effect is also common, especially from direct mass effect of neoplastic disease or enlarged lymph nodes in the pelvis (Fig. 26.2).

EVALUATION

A detailed past medical history is important to characterize potential causes as well as to elicit subtle presentations of swelling. Early, acute-stage presentations may be described by patients as a feeling of increased heaviness, fullness, or induration. Chronic presentations tend to be overt and easily recognizable on visual inspection. Clinical symptoms such as improvement overnight and recurrence during the day are associated with venous edema and are due to positional changes and gravity effects; lymphedema tends to be persistent throughout the day.

On examination, venous edema is characteristically pitting with loss of skin creases in the early stages. Progressive deposition of hemosiderin results in typical dark brown skin discoloration and, in later stages, skin ulceration. Dependent edema is associated with atypical atrophic skin resulting from defective vascular innervation in immobilized patients.

Lymphedema, on the other hand, is classically described as nonpitting. Sharp skinfolds are present, and cysts tend to be more prominent. However, the distinction between chronic pitting edema and nonpitting edema is not always clear. For example, chronic pitting venous edema due to venous insufficiency results in persistent inflammation and fibrosis, leading to impaired lymphatic flow and resultant nonpitting lymphedema.

Diagnostic imaging is useful to evaluate local causes of edema. Duplex ultrasonography is the preferred imaging modality, able to evaluate DVT and chronic venous insufficiency. Where suspicion is high with no alternate explanation of the cause, MRI may be warranted to rule out pelvic vein thrombosis and pelvic masses. Lymphatic scintigraphy allows for evaluation of lymphatic flow obstruction as a cause of lymphedema.

Diagnostic testing for systemic causes of edema includes evaluation of synthetic function with serum albumin and coagulation studies, thyroid function tests, urine dipstick assays for proteinuria, and assessment of renal function. Patients with suspected infectious causes of edema should receive a complete blood count. The D-dimer assay, while not specific for DVT, is extremely sensitive and can rule out thrombosis. Screening tests for heart failure such as pro–B-type natriuretic peptide (pro-BNP), alongside echocardiographic evaluation for ventricular dysfunction and pulmonary hypertension, are warranted based on clinical presentation.

DIAGNOSIS AND TREATMENT

Treatment for lower extremity edema is primarily targeted at the cause alongside adjunctive supportive therapy. In chronic edema, the goal is often not curative but rather minimization of deformation, prevention, and treatment of infection as well as return to functionality. Prior to initiation of treatment for edema, the **ankle-brachial index** (ABI) should be measured to rule out arterial insufficiency, as **compression stockings,** the mainstay of therapy for edema from a nonsystemic cause, may be contraindicated depending on the degree of peripheral vascular disease as measured by the ABI (Fig. 26.3).

If possible, patients should have underlying causes of edema treated before chronic changes develop. DVT is treated by initiation of anticoagulant therapy. Early recognition mitigates against complications, such as postthrombotic syndrome and chronic venous insufficiency. In addition, adjunctive use of compression stockings significantly reduces the risk of postthrombotic syndrome. Patients with venous hypertension from volume overload, such as heart failure, nephrotic syndrome, or cirrhosis, should be treated with **diuretics** to avoid development

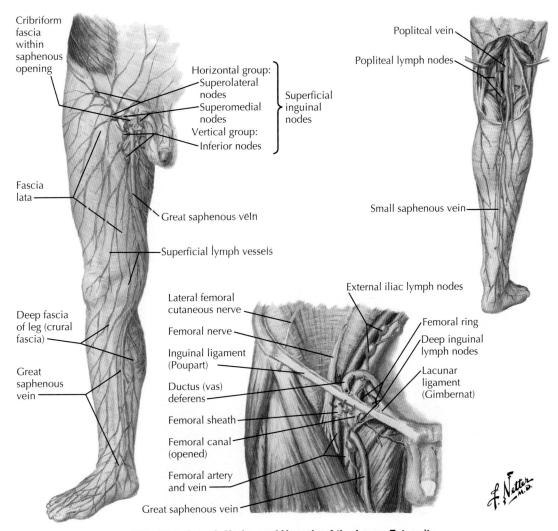

Cribriform fascia within saphenous opening

Horizontal group:
Superolateral nodes
Superomedial nodes
Vertical group:
Inferior nodes

Superficial inguinal nodes

Fascia lata

Great saphenous vein

Superficial lymph vessels

Deep fascia of leg (crural fascia)

Great saphenous vein

Popliteal vein
Popliteal lymph nodes

Small saphenous vein

External iliac lymph nodes

Lateral femoral cutaneous nerve

Femoral nerve

Inguinal ligament (Poupart)

Ductus (vas) deferens

Femoral sheath

Femoral canal (opened)

Femoral artery and vein

Great saphenous vein

Femoral ring

Deep inguinal lymph nodes

Lacunar ligament (Gimbernat)

FIG. 26.2 Lymph Nodes and Vessels of the Lower Extremity.

of chronic venous insufficiency. Care must be paid to side effects, including hypovolemia from overdiuresis and metabolic derangements. However, it is key to understand that diuretics offer no benefit in lymphedema.

For patients with chronic edema leading to chronic venous insufficiency, the main therapeutic approach is application of compression dressings and limb elevation. Compression stockings are applied in a graduated manner from the most distal portion of the foot where pressure is highest. The pressure applied by the garment (measured in mm Hg) is adjusted depending on severity of the edema. In patients with arterial insufficiency, intermittent pneumatic compression devices have shown some benefit, as has oral horse chestnut seed extract. Skin

changes are treated by using emollients and intermittent application of topical steroids to prevent onset of cellulitis and dermatitis.

Treatment for severe lymphedema is initiated with a combination of deep tissue massage and pneumatic compression dressings. Subsequently, nonelastic dressings are applied before transition to graduated compression stockings. A thicker, knit material and layering is used in lymphedema to prevent uneven compression, especially along skin crevices. Other supportive treatment strategies include limb elevation, early treatment of tinea pedis, and prophylactic antibiotics for recurrent cellulitis. Surgical debulking and bypass procedures are limited to refractory cases.

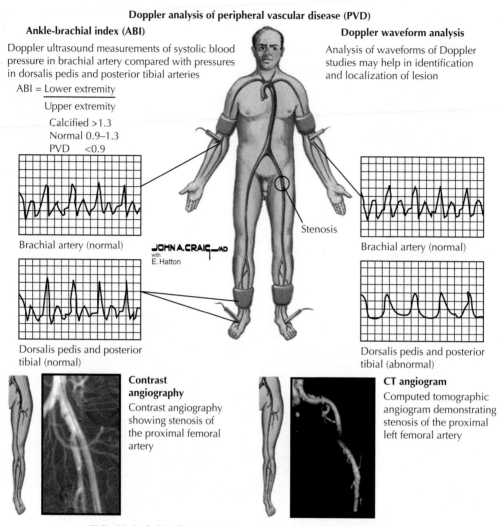

Doppler analysis of peripheral vascular disease (PVD)

Ankle-brachial index (ABI)

Doppler ultrasound measurements of systolic blood pressure in brachial artery compared with pressures in dorsalis pedis and posterior tibial arteries

ABI = Lower extremity
Upper extremity

Calcified >1.3
Normal 0.9–1.3
PVD   <0.9

Brachial artery (normal)

JOHN A. CRAIG___AD
with
E. Hatton

Dorsalis pedis and posterior tibial (normal)

Doppler waveform analysis

Analysis of waveforms of Doppler studies may help in identification and localization of lesion

Brachial artery (normal)

Stenosis

Dorsalis pedis and posterior tibial (abnormal)

Contrast angiography

Contrast angiography showing stenosis of the proximal femoral artery

CT angiogram

Computed tomographic angiogram demonstrating stenosis of the proximal left femoral artery

FIG. 26.3 **Ankle-Brachial Index and Peripheral Vascular Disease.**

CHAPTER 27

Hyponatremia and Hypernatremia

DANIEL EDMONSTON • RUEDIGER W. LEHRICH

HYPONATREMIA

Pathophysiology

Hyponatremia and serum osmolality

The serum sodium concentration is the main determinant of the serum osmolality, with smaller contributions from other endogenous (e.g., blood urea nitrogen [BUN], glucose) and exogenous (e.g., alcohols) osmoles. The equation for osmolality is generally given as:

$$2 * sodium + \frac{BUN}{2.8} + \frac{glucose}{18} + \frac{ethanol}{4.6} \qquad \textbf{EQ. 27.1}$$

Hyponatremia, defined as a serum sodium concentration of <135 mEq/L, usually occurs because of a relative excess of free water to serum osmoles. This phenomenon is known as hypo-osmolar (or dilutional) hyponatremia.

Less often, hyponatremia occurs because of an excess of other osmoles (i.e., hyperglycemia, mannitol administration, high BUN secondary to renal failure, alcohol intoxication), which draws water out of cells and dilutes the serum sodium. This phenomenon is known as hyperosmolar (or translocational) hyponatremia.

In rare cases, apparent hyponatremia occurs in the setting of normal serum osmolality and very high serum lipid concentrations. In such cases, the serum sodium concentration is normal, but the increase in the nonaqueous fraction of serum introduces errors when the sodium concentration is measured using dilution-based methods (i.e., flame photometry, indirect ion-specific electrodes). This phenomenon is known as pseudohyponatremia.

Causes of hypo-osmolar hyponatremia

Hypo-osmolar (dilutional) hyponatremia, the focus of this chapter, occurs either because of an imbalance in free water and solute intake or because of a failure to appropriately dilute urine.

The average Western diet consists of 600 to 900 mOsm of solute per day, and a normal kidney can dilute urine to a concentration of 50 mOsm/L. Thus given a typical osmolar load, one can ingest approximately 12 L free water per day before the kidneys are unable to excrete enough free water despite maximal urine dilution (600 mOsm/day divided by 50 mOsm/L is 12 L/day). If solute intake is low, even a typical volume of water intake may result in hyponatremia (e.g., a diet of 150 mOsm/day will result in hyponatremia if water intake exceeds 3 L/day). The threshold for a positive water balance becomes even lower if the tubules cannot maximally dilute urine (e.g., in advanced chronic kidney disease).

Urine concentration is under the control of **antidiuretic hormone** (ADH, also known as **vasopressin**), which binds to vasopressin 2 (V2) receptors in the cortical collecting ducts, and thereby promotes aquaporin-2 channel expression and insertion in the luminal membrane (Fig. 27.1). Water is transported through these channels from the urine to the peritubular capillaries. Thus higher ADH concentrations are associated with free water retention and concentrated urine, while low concentrations are associated with free water excretion and diluted urine.

The primary stimulus of ADH release is an increase in serum osmolality. A secondary stimulus for ADH release is intravascular volume depletion, either from true hypovolemia or third spacing of fluids (e.g., heart failure, cirrhosis, nephrotic syndrome). Once engaged, the secondary stimulus assumes primacy, such that patients with intravascular volume depletion retain free water regardless of serum osmolality.

The increased level of ADH in response to hyperosmolality and hypovolemia is physiologically appropriate, in that it addresses the underlying stimulus. Additional stimuli for ADH release that are not appropriate include nausea, pain, pulmonary inflammation and/or infection, various intracranial processes, medications, and (rarely) ADH-secreting tumors. The ADH release/resulting

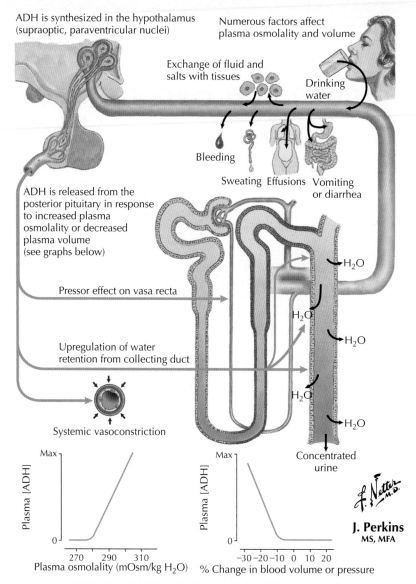

ADH is synthesized in the hypothalamus
(supraoptic, paraventricular nuclei)

Numerous factors affect
plasma osmolality and volume

Exchange of fluid and
salts with tissues

Drinking
water

Bleeding

Sweating Effusions Vomiting
or diarrhea

ADH is released from the
posterior pituitary in response
to increased plasma
osmolality or decreased
plasma volume
(see graphs below)

H_2O

Pressor effect on vasa recta

H_2O

H_2O

Upregulation of water
retention from collecting duct

H_2O

H_2O

Systemic vasoconstriction

Concentrated
urine

Max

Plasma [ADH]

0

270   290   310
Plasma osmolality (mOsm/kg H_2O)

Max

Plasma [ADH]

0

−30 −20 −10 0 10 20
% Change in blood volume or pressure

J. Perkins
MS, MFA

FIG. 27.1 Antidiuretic Hormone *(ADH)* (Vasopressin).

hyponatremia associated with these stimuli is termed the syndrome of inappropriate ADH (SIADH).

Diagnostic Approach

A diagnostic approach to hypo-osmolar hyponatremia should start with a comprehensive history and the measurement of serum osmolality, urine osmolality, and urine sodium (Fig. 27.2).

In some cases, the history will reveal a profound ingestion of free water or a very small amount of solute

intake. A urine osmolality of <100 mOsm/L confirms that ADH levels are appropriately low but that free water intake (relative to solute intake) exceeds the kidney's capacity to produce sufficient dilute urine. The diagnosis is primary polydipsia (excessive free water intake in the setting of a normal solute load) or a tea and toast diet (normal free water intake in the setting of a very low solute load). Beer potomania, a phenomenon similar to the tea and toast diet, occurs when patients consume large quantities of beer—a low-solute, high-calorie,

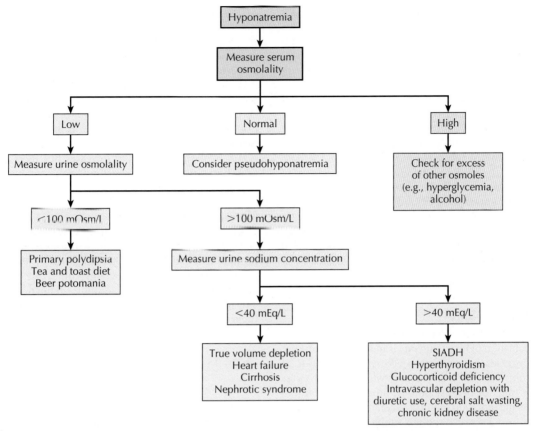

FIG. 27.2 **Approach to Hyponatremia.** *SIADH,* Syndrome of inappropriate antidiuretic hormone.

alcohol-containing beverage—but not other solute-containing foods.

All other causes of hypo-osmolar hyponatremia are ADH mediated (i.e., the kidneys are retaining free water, and the urine osmolality is >100 mOsm/L). An analysis of the urine sodium concentration provides additional insights. If the urine sodium concentration is low (<20 mEq/L), the renin-angiotensin-aldosterone system has been engaged in response to either true hypovolemia (ADH release is appropriate since volume needs to be retained) or third spacing of fluids (ADH release is maladaptive since overall volume is high).

If the urine sodium concentration is elevated (>40 mEq/L), the patient is euvolemic and may have SIADH. It is important, however, to first rule out hypothyroidism and glucocorticoid deficiency, since these can also cause elevated ADH levels and hyponatremia through uncertain mechanisms. In addition, patients may have high sodium excretion despite decreased effective arterial volume (and appropriate ADH release) in the

setting of diuretic use, advanced chronic kidney disease, and cerebral salt-wasting syndrome.

Management

The treatment of hyponatremia depends on the time course and presence or absence of symptoms. A rapid decrease in the serum sodium concentration can cause cerebral edema and associated symptoms, such as seizures and coma. Therefore patients with symptoms of hyponatremia, or patients known to have acute (<24 hours) hyponatremia (e.g., hospitalized patients with regular laboratory monitoring, patients reporting a single large water ingestion), generally require rapid correction with hypertonic saline.

In contrast, patients with chronic, asymptomatic hyponatremia should be corrected more slowly (<8 mEq/24 hours), since the brain has already compensated for the change in osmolality by reducing intracellular osmoles, and rapid overcorrection can cause osmotic demyelination. The specific treatment depends on the underlying cause. Patients with polydipsia or volume overload, for example, should be placed on fluid restriction. Patients with true volume depletion should receive a slow infusion of normal saline, anticipating that ADH secretion will cease with restoration of intravascular volume, and serum sodium may rapidly rise in response.

Meanwhile, patients with SIADH should be fluid restricted and placed on a high osmole diet as the underlying cause is addressed. If this proves inadequate, a combination of salt (or urea) tabs and loop diuretics may be attempted next. Loop diuretics are helpful because they block the ability of the medullary countercurrent transport system to maintain an osmotic gradient between the tubular lumen and peritubular space, thereby limiting the ability to concentrate urine regardless of ADH levels. ADH receptor antagonists may be useful in limited situations, such as in patients with SIADH who fail to improve despite the abovementioned measures or in patients with severe heart failure.

HYPERNATREMIA

Pathophysiology and Diagnostic Approach

The evaluation of hypernatremia is more straightforward. In most cases, hypernatremia occurs either because of hypotonic fluid losses in a patient with impaired access to free water or because of a hypothalamic lesion that impairs the sensation of thirst. Very rarely, hypernatremia results from excessive sodium supplementation.

The most common causes of large-volume hypotonic fluid losses are urinary (diabetes insipidus, osmotic diuresis, postobstructive diuresis), gastrointestinal (vomiting, excessive drainage from gastric tubes, osmotic diarrhea), and sweating.

Even a slight rise in plasma osmolality results in a profound increase in thirst. Thus patients usually ingest enough free water to offset hypotonic losses. If the sensation of thirst occurs but the patient is unable to access free water (e.g., due to debilitation), hypernatremia will occur. If plasma osmolality increases but there is no sensation of thirst, then by definition the patient has a hypothalamic lesion.

Management

The free water deficit (FWD) represents the amount of free water necessary to correct the serum sodium back to normal. It is equal to the total body water (50%–60% of the body weight in kilograms) times the fraction above the normal serum sodium (defined here as 140 mEq/L, though this can be altered if the target is higher or lower):

$$FWD = 0.5 \times \text{weight (kg)} \times \frac{\text{serum sodium}\left(\frac{mEq}{L}\right) - 140\ mEq/L}{140\ mEq/L}$$

EQ. 27.2

As with hyponatremia, it is important not to correct the FWD too rapidly, as cerebral edema may occur.

CHAPTER 28

Hyperkalemia and Hypokalemia

ANTHONY VALERI

INTRODUCTION

Potassium is primarily an intracellular cation and, with sodium, creates the membrane potential necessary for muscle and nerve function. Potassium is freely filtered at the glomerulus and reabsorbed throughout the proximal convoluted tubules and the loop of Henle, such that nearly all of the filtered potassium has been reabsorbed by the time the urine reaches the distal convoluted tubules. At this point, potassium handling is determined by the rate of sodium delivery and fluid flow along the distal nephron and by the activity of **aldosterone.**

Aldosterone is produced by the zona glomerulosa of the adrenal gland and acts on mineralocorticoid receptors to control the expression of the **epithelial sodium channels (eNaC),** which allow for sodium uptake in the distal tubules and collecting ducts. Sodium uptake here creates a lumen-negative electrical gradient that, along with upregulation of sodium-potassium pumps (the Na-K ATPase) on the basolateral surface (opposite the lumen), facilitates potassium excretion into the lumen through renal outer medullary potassium channels (ROMK). The **renin-angiotensin-aldosterone system (RAAS)** regulates distal tubular potassium excretion, allowing for potassium homeostasis.

Hyperkalemia and hypokalemia result from perturbations to normal homeostatic mechanisms. These can be at the level of kidney, such as excessive loss of potassium (hypokalemia) or failure to excrete excess potassium (hyperkalemia), or throughout the body due to transcellular potassium shift, which leaves total body potassium unchanged.

HYPERKALEMIA (Table 28.1)

Hyperkalemia is defined as a potassium level above the testing reference range, usually >5 mEq/L. Symptoms of hyperkalemia include muscle weakness, but higher levels can lead to muscle/nerve conduction dysfunction manifesting as paralysis and cardiac arrhythmias. Evaluation of hyperkalemia should focus on three possible etiologies:

1. **Pseudohyperkalemia**
2. Causes of transcellular shifts from intracellular to extracellular stores
3. Causes of impaired potassium excretory ability by the kidney, either due to acute or advanced chronic renal disease or due to an absolute or relative aldosterone deficiency (Fig. 28.1)

Hyperkalemia is unlikely due to increased potassium ingestion (unless acute), as the kidneys are efficient at excreting excess potassium in the absence of impaired function.

Pseudohyperkalemia results from release of potassium from cells in the test tube after phlebotomy. Blood may undergo hemolysis due to shear stress while being drawn (often if drawn through an intravenous catheter). Pseudohyperkalemia also can occur in the setting of marked leukocytosis (white blood cell [WBC] count >100,000/cm^3) or thrombocytosis (platelet count >1,000,000/cm^3).

Potassium may shift from the intracellular to the extracellular space in the setting of metabolic acidosis, as H+/K+ pumps shift hydrogen ions intracellularly and potassium extracellularly to buffer blood pH against the underlying acidosis. Insulin is a major driver of intracellular potassium shift, so patients with insulin deficiency, either relative or absolute (as in type 1 diabetes), may have hyperkalemia. Potassium may also be released from intracellular stores in the setting of cellular lysis. Common causes include rhabdomyolysis (confirmed by elevated creatine kinase levels); hemolysis (confirmed with schistocytes on blood smear and very reduced/absent haptoglobin and elevated lactate dehydrogenase); or tumor lysis, leading to hyperkalemia, hyperphosphatemia, and hyperuricemia. Patients with rapidly proliferating tumors that are drug sensitive, especially leukemia and lymphoma, are at the highest risk for tumor lysis. **Hyperkalemic periodic paralysis** is due to an inherited autosomal dominant mutation of the muscle sodium channel causing intermittent acute, transcellular potassium shifts often precipitated by extremes of heat or cold.

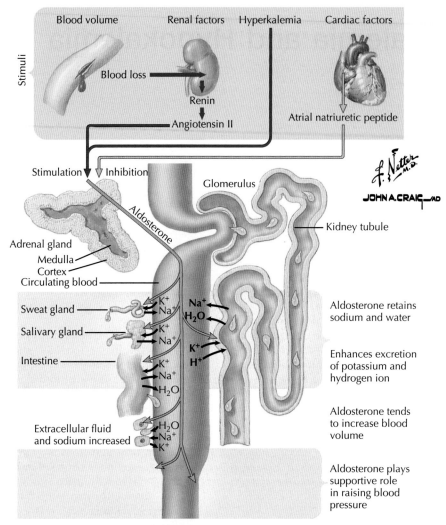

FIG. 28.1 **Actions of Aldosterone.**

TABLE 28.1
Hyperkalemia With Metabolic Acidosis

		PLASMA RENIN ACTIVITY (PRA)	
		Elevated	**Suppressed**
ALDOSTERONE	Elevated	Mineralocorticoid receptor antagonists eNaC inhibitors (amiloride, triamterene, trimethoprim) PHA, type 1 (low-normal BP)	
	Suppressed	Addison disease ACE inhibitors ARBs	Direct renin inhibitors NSAIDs Diabetic nephropathy PHA, type 2 (Gordon syndrome) Calcineurin inhibitors

ARBs, Angiotensin-2 receptor blockers; *BP,* blood pressure; *eNaC,* epithelial sodium channels; *PHA,* pseudohypoaldosteronism.

Decreased urinary potassium excretion is a major underlying cause of hyperkalemia, most commonly patients with low glomerular filtration rate (GFR) <10 mL/min, including those with chronic kidney disease or acute kidney injury. Patients with shock have impaired sodium/water delivery to the distal nephron, leading to impaired potassium secretion.

Impaired aldosterone function can be divided into conditions of aldosterone deficiency and aldosterone resistance. Impaired aldosterone function can lead to the development of a **type 4 renal tubular acidosis (RTA)**, characterized by hyperkalemia. Hyperkalemia inhibits ammoniagenesis in the proximal convoluted tubule, thus limiting net acid excretory capacity by the kidney and inducing a mild, nonanion gap metabolic acidosis.

Patients with aldosterone deficiency can be separated by renin level, or **plasma renin activity (PRA)**. Addison disease, or primary adrenal insufficiency, leads to a hyperreninemic hypoaldosterone state; renin is upregulated to drive aldosterone secretion, which is impaired by the underlying disorder. ACE inhibitors and angiotensin-2 receptor blockers (ARBs) also lead to hyperreninemic hypoaldosteronism. Hyporeninemic hypoaldosteronism can result from diabetic nephropathy, NSAID use (via suppression of renal prostaglandin E formation), and direct renin inhibitors, such as aliskiren.

Aldosterone resistance can directly result from loss of function mutations in the mineralocorticoid receptor or, more commonly, from medications that inhibit the receptor (e.g., spironolactone, eplerenone). Drugs that inhibit eNaC also lead to hyperkalemia and include amiloride, triamterene, and high-dose trimethoprim. Resistance to aldosterone can also be seen in conditions causing chronic tubulointerstitial disease, including sickle cell nephropathy, chronic obstructive uropathy, and medullary cystic kidney disease.

Pseudohypoaldosteronism is divided into two types: Type 1 is a rare genetic disorder characterized by resistance to aldosterone action, due to a mutation in the mineralocorticoid receptor. Patients are generally normotensive and have elevated (though ineffective) aldosterone levels. Type 2 is known as **Gordon syndrome**, characterized by a gain-of-function mutation in the sodium-chloride cotransporter (NCC) leading to competitive inhibition of eNaC; patients present hypertensive. Calcineurin inhibitors activate the NCC as well, which produces the same syndrome.

Patients with hyperkalemia should first receive an electrocardiogram (ECG), as hyperkalemia raises the potential for life-threatening arrhythmias. Characteristic findings first include peaked T waves and a shortened QT interval; with time, the PR interval prolongs, followed by loss of P waves, a widened QRS, and finally a sine wave pattern that portends imminent cardiac arrest (Fig. 28.2). Emergent management centers on shifting potassium intracellularly, which is much faster than

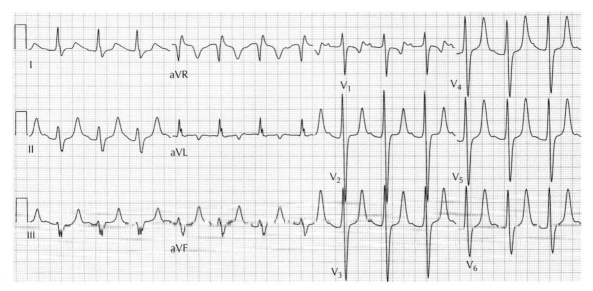

Example of the ECG changes associated with hyperkalemia. It is recorded from a 29-year-old woman with chronic renal disease. The P wave is broad and difficult to identify in some leads. The QRS is diffusely widened (0.188 sec), and the T wave is peaked and symmetrical. These changes are characteristic of severe hyperkalemia, and in this patient, the serum potassium concentration was 8.2 mM.

FIG. 28.2 **Early Electrocardiogram *(ECG)* Changes in Hyperkalemia.**

TABLE 28.2
Hypokalemia With Metabolic Alkalosis

| | | PLASMA RENIN ACTIVITY (PRA) | |
		Elevated	Suppressed
ALDOSTERONE	Elevated	Nasogastric suction Bartter syndrome Gitelman syndrome	Cushing syndrome Conn syndrome
	Suppressed		Liddle syndrome (high BP)

BP, Blood pressure.

eliminating potassium from the body. Patients with ECG changes should receive intravenous calcium (gluconate peripherally, or chloride with central venous access) to stabilize the cardiac membrane. Options for intracellular shifting include:

- Inhaled β-agonists, such as albuterol (although the fastest acting, its duration of effect is short)
- Intravenous insulin (5–10 units) with intravenous dextrose to counteract hypoglycemia
- Intravenous sodium bicarbonate, which activates H+/K+ pumps to shift hydrogen extracellularly and potassium intracellularly

Removing potassium from the body can be achieved with loop diuretics, though their use may be limited by blood pressure or volume status. Loop diuretics with or without sodium bicarbonate (to deliver sodium with a poorly reabsorbed anion to the distal nephron to enhance potassium excretion) can be used long term in patients with chronic kidney disease and hyperkalemia. Sodium polystyrene sulfate absorbs potassium from the gut but takes hours to work; patients with bowel obstruction should not receive sodium polystyrene sulfate due to risk of bowel necrosis. Patiromer is another large nonabsorbed polymer that will exchange sodium for potassium in the intestines. Finally, hemodialysis can directly filter potassium from the blood. Fludrocortisone (a mineralocorticoid) may be useful chronically in patients with aldosterone deficiency, although it is often limited due to increased sodium resorption in the kidney and worsening hypertension and volume overload.

Further evaluation should focus on medication history and assessment of comorbidities while attempting to correct any underlying renal dysfunction. Renin and aldosterone levels, if ordered, must be interpreted with caution and in the context of the patient's volume status and other medications. Of note, the transtubular potassium gradient has questionable utility.

HYPOKALEMIA (Table 28.2)

Patients with hypokalemia have a potassium level <3.5 mEq/L. Symptoms of hypokalemia include generalized weakness and malaise, progressing to muscle dysfunction, paralysis, and cardiac arrhythmias as severity worsens. Potential etiologies for hypokalemia include inadequate dietary intake (uncommon), transcellular potassium shifts, or excessive loss of potassium through the gastrointestinal tract or kidney.

Patients with metabolic alkalosis will develop hypokalemia as the body shifts hydrogen ions extracellularly (and potassium intracellularly) through H+/K+ pumps to buffer the pH change. The serum potassium will fall 0.4 mEq/L for every 0.1 rise in arterial pH. Medications that induce potassium shifts include insulin, sympathomimetics, including albuterol and epinephrine, and phosphodiesterase inhibitors such as caffeine. **Hypokalemic periodic paralysis** is a rate inherited disorder of the muscle sodium, potassium, or calcium channel causing intermittent acute transcellular potassium shifts, often precipitated by large carbohydrate meals (insulin release) or exercise (catecholamine release) and often in patients with associated hyperthyroidism, and is more prevalent in Asian patients.

The most common etiology for hypokalemia is excessive potassium loss. A 24-hour urine potassium is the most accurate quantification of urinary potassium excretion, but by definition takes 1 day. Quicker testing includes spot urine potassium and the fractional excretion of potassium (FE_K), calculated as:

$$(U_K/P_K)/(U_{creat}/P_{creat}) \qquad \textbf{EQ. 28.1}$$

A U_K <40 mEq/L, U_K/U_{creat} <13 mEq/g creatinine, and FE_K <6.5% suggests extrarenal potassium loss, such as through diarrhea (seen often with a nonanion gap metabolic acidosis). This is conceptualized as the kidney working to reabsorb any filtered potassium due to losses beyond its control.

A U_K >40 mEq/L, U_K/U_{creat} >13 mEq/g creatinine, and FE_K >9.5% suggests renal dysfunction as a cause of excessive potassium loss. Patients with a concomitant nonanion gap metabolic acidosis may have an RTA. **Type 1 (distal RTA)** typically produces inappropriately alkalotic urine (pH >5.5), while **type 2 (proximal RTA)** has appropriately acidic urine (pH <5.5).

If the patient has a concomitant metabolic alkalosis, then either primary or secondary hyperaldosteronism may be to blame. Patients with primary hyperaldosteronism have low PRA with elevated aldosterone resulting from **Conn** or **Cushing syndrome.** Secondary hyperaldosteronism, on the other hand, has both elevated PRA and aldosterone levels. Patients with secondary hyperaldosteronism with elevated blood pressure may have accelerated or malignant hypertension, **renal artery stenosis,** reninoma, or be in a scleroderma renal crisis.

Secondary hyperaldosteronism patients with low/normal blood pressure should be evaluated for **Bartter and Gitelman syndromes.** Bartter syndrome is a loss-of-function mutation in either the sodium-potassium-2 chloride transporter (NKCC), chloride-bicarbonate exchanger, or ROMK, and produces a urinary phenotype similar to patients on a loop diuretic (i.e., hypercalciuria). Gitelman syndrome is a loss-of-function mutation of the NCC in the distal nephron, producing a urinary phenotype similar to patients on a thiazide diuretic (i.e., hypocalciuria). Gitelman syndrome is more often associated with hypomagnesemia compared to Bartter syndrome, which often may be used to clinically distinguish between the two syndromes prior to genetic testing. Finally, patients with both low renin and aldosterone levels should be tested for Liddle syndrome, a gain-of-function mutation in eNaC resulting in hypokalemia, hypertension, and metabolic alkalosis.

While determining the underlying etiology for hypokalemia, patients can receive oral and intravenous potassium supplementation. Intravenous potassium may be limited, as potassium is a vesicant (destructive to veins) and requires a central line for vigorous supplementation. In general, every 10 mEq of supplementation raises the serum potassium by 0.1 mEq/L.

CHAPTER 29

Hypercalcemia and Hypocalcemia

TARA HOLDER

INTRODUCTION

Calcium exists in blood in three forms: ionized, protein bound, and complexed. About half of the total calcium is ionized and metabolically active. Forty percent is bound to proteins, primarily albumin. Ten percent is chelated to sulfate, citrate, and phosphorus.

In clinical practice, it is common to measure the total calcium and **ionized calcium** concentrations. The total calcium assay measures all three forms and is thus sensitive to changes in protein-bound calcium, even when ionized calcium is normal. Thus it must be corrected to account for albumin. At a normal pH of 7.4, 1 g/dL of albumin binds to about 0.2 mmol/L (0.8 mg/dL) of calcium; therefore

$$\text{Corrected [Ca] (mg/dL)} = \text{Measured total [Ca] (mg/dL)}$$
$$+ [0.8 \times (4 - \text{patient's albumin [mg/dL])}]$$

EQ. 29.1

The ionized calcium assay, in contrast, measures only the active form of calcium and is thus a more clinically relevant test. Unfortunately, ionized calcium is not routinely used due to cost and the lack of standardized measurements. The total serum calcium typically ranges between 8.5 mg/dL and 10.2 mg/dL (2.19–2.76 mmol/L), while the ionized calcium ranges between 4.5 and 5.5 mg/dL (1.01–1.26 mmol/L); notably there is mild variability of these ranges between laboratories.

Corrected calcium is relevant as hypoalbuminemia causes **pseudohypocalcemia**, in which total calcium is low but the more clinically relevant, ionized (active) calcium is normal. Causes of hypoalbuminemia include (but are not limited to) malnutrition, chronic illness, sepsis, nephrosis, burns, volume overload, and cirrhosis.

PATHOPHYSIOLOGY

An average, healthy adult body weighing 70 kg contains approximately 1 to 1.3 kg of calcium, 99% of which is contained in the skeleton in hydroxyapatite. The remaining 1% is in extracellular fluid (ECF) and soft tissue. The ECF calcium concentration is tightly regulated by homeostatic fluxes between the ECF, kidney, bone, and gut. The three primary regulatory hormones are **parathyroid hormone (PTH), calcitonin,** and **1,25-dihydroxyvitamin D (calcitriol).**

Calcium homeostasis is regulated primarily by calcitriol and PTH, which is released from the parathyroid glands in response to hypocalcemia, hyperphosphatemia, or reduced calcitriol levels. PTH and calcitriol both increase serum calcium concentrations by stimulating osteoclasts and promoting bone resorption. PTH also stimulates hydroxylation of 25-hydroxyvitamin D $(25[\text{OH}]D_3)$ to the active $1,25\text{-}(\text{OH})_2D_3$ (calcitriol) form (primarily in the kidney) and, furthermore, promotes calcium reabsorption and phosphate excretion by the kidney. Calcitriol also increases the intestinal absorption of calcium and phosphate. Calcitonin, which appears to be primarily regulated by the concentration of ionized calcium, reduces serum calcium by inhibiting osteoclastic bone resorption and reabsorption from urine. Its effects appear to be short term, however, and its overall significance in humans is unclear (Fig. 29.1).

HYPERCALCEMIA
Presentation and Differential Diagnosis

Hypercalcemia is defined as a serum level of total calcium >10.2 mg/dL (2.76 mmol/L). Hypercalcemia causes nonspecific symptoms such as fatigue, depression, constipation, and anorexia (typified by the mnemonic "bones, stones, groans, and moans"), as well as abnormal electrocardiogram (ECG) findings. The extent of these symptoms depends on the severity and duration of hypercalcemia. Abnormal ECG findings include QT shortening, prolonged PR, widened QRS, and atrioventricular (AV) block.

The two most common causes of hypercalcemia, accounting for 80% to 90% of all cases, are primary hyperparathyroidism (PHPT) and malignancy. PHPT is the abnormal overproduction of PTH, altering calcium homeostasis and causing hypercalcemia (see Chapter 74 for further information). Risk factors include postmenopausal state and family history of HPT or multiple endocrine neoplasia.

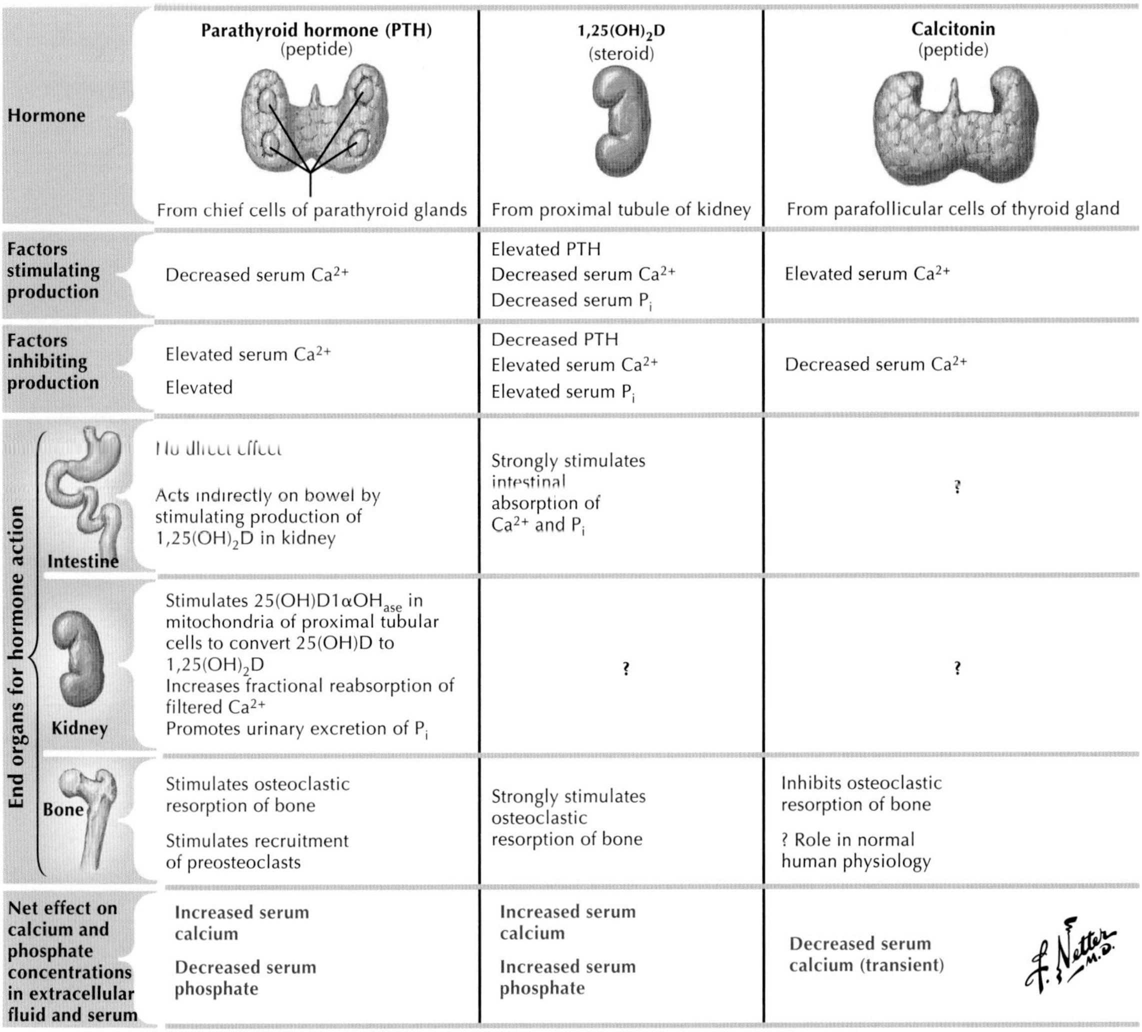

	Parathyroid hormone (PTH) (peptide)	1,25(OH)₂D (steroid)	Calcitonin (peptide)
Hormone	 From chief cells of parathyroid glands	 From proximal tubule of kidney	 From parafollicular cells of thyroid gland
Factors stimulating production	Decreased serum Ca^{2+}	Elevated PTH Decreased serum Ca^{2+} Decreased serum P_i	Elevated serum Ca^{2+}
Factors inhibiting production	Elevated serum Ca^{2+} Elevated	Decreased PTH Elevated serum Ca^{2+} Elevated serum P_i	Decreased serum Ca^{2+}
End organs for hormone action — Intestine	No direct effect Acts indirectly on bowel by stimulating production of 1,25(OH)₂D in kidney	Strongly stimulates intestinal absorption of Ca^{2+} and P_i	?
End organs for hormone action — Kidney	Stimulates 25(OH)D1αOH_ase in mitochondria of proximal tubular cells to convert 25(OH)D to 1,25(OH)₂D Increases fractional reabsorption of filtered Ca^{2+} Promotes urinary excretion of P_i	?	?
End organs for hormone action — Bone	Stimulates osteoclastic resorption of bone Stimulates recruitment of preosteoclasts	Strongly stimulates osteoclastic resorption of bone	Inhibits osteoclastic resorption of bone ? Role in normal human physiology
Net effect on calcium and phosphate concentrations in extracellular fluid and serum	Increased serum calcium Decreased serum phosphate	Increased serum calcium Increased serum phosphate	Decreased serum calcium (transient)

FIG. 29.1 **Regulation of Calcium and Phosphate Metabolism.**

Malignancy causes hypercalcemia by various mechanisms, most notable of which is **humoral hypercalcemia of malignancy** (HHM), where tumors secrete **parathyroid hormone-related protein** (PTHrP). Squamous cell carcinomas account for ~50% of HHM cases, in addition to breast cancer and renal cell carcinoma. In lymphoproliferative (e.g., Hodgkin and non-Hodgkin lymphomas) or granulomatous disorders (e.g., sarcoidosis), 1,25(OH)₂D₃ (calcitriol) is typically elevated. In both lymphoproliferative and granulomatous diseases, the primary abnormality responsible for hypercalcemia is increased intestinal calcitriol absorption, though there may also be some contribution from calcitriol-induced bone resorption. Plasma cell dyscrasias, such as multiple myeloma, and malignancies with a tendency to be metastatic to the bone, such as prostate cancer, can also induce hypercalcemia through lytic lesions.

In the ambulatory setting, the majority of hypercalcemic patients have PHPT, while in the hospitalized population, underlying malignancy is more common. Patients with PHPT generally have chronic, stable mild hypercalcemia. In contrast, patients with hypercalcemia of malignancy generally have a more acute presentation, with higher serum calcium concentration.

The third most common cause of hypercalcemia is **milk-alkali syndrome,** which is reported to be as high as 12% of cases. Milk-alkali is due to the ingestion of large amounts of calcium-containing supplements,

Condition	Serum Ca²⁺	Serum P$_i$	Serum PTH	Serum 25(OH)D	Serum 1,25(OH)₂D	Associated findings
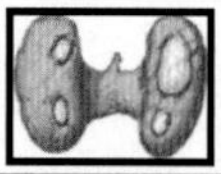 Primary hyperparathyroidism	↑	N or ↓	High N or ↑	N	N or ↑	80% Asymptomatic Nephrolithiasis Osteoporosis Hypercalcemic symptoms
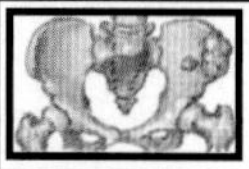 Cancer with extensive bone metastases	↑	N or ↑	↓	N	↓ or N	History of primary tumor, destructive lesions on radiograph, bone scan
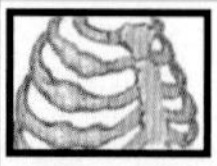 Multiple myeloma and lymphoma	↑	N or ↑	↓	N	↓ or N	Abnormal serum or urine protein electrophoresis, abnormal bone radiographs
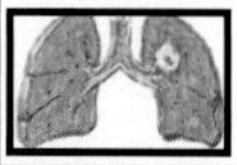 Humoral hypercalcemia of malignancy	↑	N or ↓	↓	N	↓ or N	↑PTHrP Solid malignancy usually evident
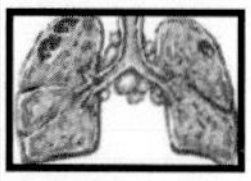 Sarcoidosis and other granulomatous diseases	↑	N or ↑	↓	N	↑	Hilar adenopathy, interstitial lung disease, elevated angiotensin-converting enzyme
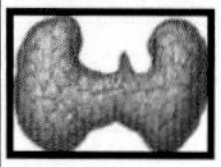 Hyperthyroidism	↑	N	↓	N	N	Symptoms of hyperthyroidism, elevated serum thyroxine
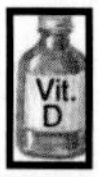 Vitamin D intoxication	↑	N or ↑	↓	Very ↑	N or ↑	History of excessive vitamin D intake
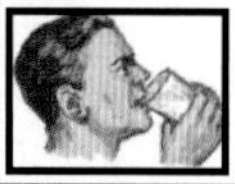 Milk-alkali syndrome	↑	N or ↑	↓	N	N or ↓	History of excessive calcium and alkali ingestion, heavy use of over-the-counter calcium-containing antacids
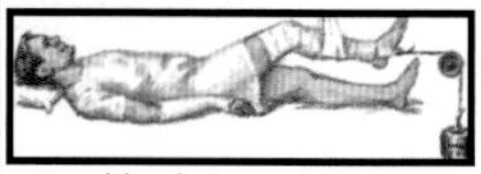 Total body immobilization	↑	N or ↑	↓	N	↓ or N	Multiple fractures, paralysis (children, adolescents, patients with Paget disease of bone)

FIG. 29.2 Differential Diagnosis of Hypercalcemic States. *PTH*, Parathyroid hormone; *PTHrP*, parathyroid hormone-related protein.

particularly over-the-counter (OTC) antacids, such as calcium carbonate, used for the treatment of dyspepsia. The typical presenting features include hypercalcemia, metabolic alkalosis, and acute kidney injury. A review of OTC medications is important in this assessment.

Diagnostic Approach (Fig. 29.2)

The majority of hypercalcemia will be ionized (active) calcium. Initial steps in evaluation include rechecking calcium values to ensure accuracy, correcting for serum albumin, and reviewing previous values for serum calcium. Long-standing asymptomatic hypercalcemia is suggestive of PHPT. PTH should be the initial laboratory test in differentiating the cause of hypercalcemia. A PTH level distinguishes between PTH-mediated hypercalcemia, which includes PHPT and the rare disorder familial hypocalciuric hypercalcemia (FHH),

and non–PTH-mediated hypercalcemia, which includes malignancy and milk-alkali syndrome.

If the serum PTH level is suppressed, follow-up laboratory studies should include PTHrP, 25(OH)D₃, and 1,25(OH)₂D₃ (calcitriol). Elevated PTHrP suggests HHM. If 1,25(OH)₂D₃ is elevated, consider lymphoproliferative or granulomatous disorders. Elevated 25(OH)D₃ alone is suggestive of excess oral vitamin D intake. If none of these initial tests are diagnostic, consider laboratory studies of serum protein electrophoresis (SPEP), urine protein electrophoresis (UPEP), and serum free light-chain assay for multiple myeloma and reassess the patient history for excess calcium intake to suggest milk-alkali syndrome.

Treatment

Hypercalcemia causes reversible kidney injury resulting in the inability to concentrate urine and polyuria. The

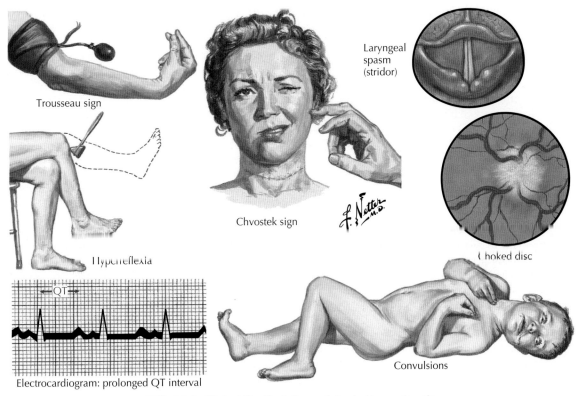

Laryngeal
spasm
(stridor)

Trousseau sign

Chvostek sign

Hyperreflexia

Choked disc

Convulsions

Electrocardiogram: prolonged QT interval

FIG. 29.3 **Clinical Manifestations of Acute Hypocalcemia.**

goals of hypercalcemia treatment are to correct dehydration and acute kidney injury, enhance renal excretion of calcium, reduce bone resorption, and treat the underlying disorder. Asymptomatic patients with mild hypercalcemia (<12 mg/dL) do not require immediate treatment and can be further evaluated and treated in the outpatient setting. Symptomatic patients, or patients with moderate (12–14 mg/dL) to severe (>14 mg/dL) hypercalcemia, should receive intravenous isotonic saline at a rate of 2.5 to 4 L daily along with a loop diuretic (only once they are volume resuscitated) to promote urinary excretion of calcium. Although these interventions can help reduce the serum calcium concentration, they do not affect the underlying mechanism, which is usually excessive mobilization of calcium from bone (with the exception of milk-alkali syndrome). Only in milk-alkali syndrome will the removal of the offending oral agent (isotonic saline) and loop diuretic completely resolve the hypercalcemia without rebound elevated calcium as there is no underlying stimulus when compared to PHPT or malignancy.

Bisphosphonates are indicated in patients with severe hypercalcemia and those who continue to be

symptomatic after administration of saline and loop diuretics. Intramuscular calcitonin (nasal spray not efficacious) can also be considered when acutely treating severe hypercalcemia, but its effect is only transient. Finally, the underlying disorder must be treated.

HYPOCALCEMIA
Differential Diagnosis

Hypocalcemia, defined as a serum total calcium concentration of <8.5 mg/dL (2.12 mmol/L), is a common abnormality. When it is severe, patients can experience seizures, arrhythmias, and muscular irritability such as tetany, **Chvostek sign,** and **Trousseau sign** (Fig. 29.3). Abnormal ECG findings include QTc prolongation, T-wave inversion, complete heart block, and torsades de pointes. In adults, after calcium is corrected for albumin and pseudohypocalcemia is excluded, the main causes of hypocalcemia include **hypoparathyroidism,** hypomagnesemia, hyperphosphatemia, alkalemia, and vitamin D deficiency.

Primary causes of hypoparathyroidism include postsurgical (thyroidectomy or parathyroidectomy) or autoimmune (autoimmune postglandular syndrome) processes. Hypomagnesemia causes decreased PTH secretion and PTH resistance in bone. Low PTH decreases serum calcium that is derived from bone or reabsorbed by the kidneys; it also results in increased serum phosphate, which can then bind and precipitate out calcium, contributing to acute hypocalcemia. Alkalemia contributes to increased binding of calcium to albumin, therefore decreasing active calcium. Vitamin D deficiency is seen with decreased sun exposure, poor nutritional intake, chronic kidney disease, chronic liver disease, and malabsorptive disease (e.g., celiac sprue). The most common cause of hypocalcemia in the primary care setting is vitamin D deficiency.

Diagnostic Approach

It is important to first rule out pseudohypercalcemia. Once true hypocalcemia is confirmed, initial studies should include PTH, $1,25(OH)_2D_3$, and a complete metabolic panel, which are sufficient to distinguish between the various causes listed earlier.

Treatment

The treatment of hypocalcemia depends on the cause, severity, acuity, and symptomatology. Symptomatic patients (seizures, tetany, ECG changes) and asymptomatic patients with acute decreases in serum corrected calcium concentration to <7.6 mg/dL (1.9 mmol/L) should be treated preferably with intravenous calcium gluconate, though calcium chloride can be used with central venous access. All patients should have continuous ECG monitoring as arrhythmias can occur with rapid correction and serum calcium measurements every 4 to 6 hours. Mildly symptomatic (paresthesias) and asymptomatic patients with serum corrected calcium concentration >7.6 mg/dL (1.9 mmol/L) can be treated with oral calcium carbonate or calcium citrate supplementation. If mild symptoms do not improve with oral supplementation, intravenous calcium is recommended.

If patients have concurrent hypomagnesemia <2 g (16 mEq), magnesium sulfate should also be infused. In hypocalcemia with concurrent vitamin D deficiency, supplementation with **vitamin D_2 (ergocalciferol)** or **vitamin D_3 (cholecalciferol)** is required. In patients with hypoparathyroidism, lifelong calcium and calcitriol supplementation is needed, as patients are no longer able to maintain calcium homeostasis or calcitriol production. Long-term treatment of hypoalbuminemia, electrolyte and PTH abnormalities, and vitamin D deficiency depends on the underlying disease.

CHAPTER 30

Acute Kidney Injury

CHIDIEBUBE C. EGWIM

INTRODUCTION

Acute kidney injury (AKI) is defined as a rapid decrease in glomerular filtration rate (GFR) over the course of hours to days. The term AKI encompasses a spectrum of renal injury and impairment, ranging from asymptomatic changes in laboratory values to the need for renal replacement therapy. Because even minor changes in renal function have been associated with increased mortality among hospitalized patients, the term AKI is more sensitive and relevant than the previously used term acute renal failure.

CRITERIA

AKI is defined and staged according to changes in serum creatinine concentration and urine output, which are both surrogates of GFR. According to the widely used criteria established by the Kidney Disease: Improving Global Outcomes (KDIGO) AKI Work Group, AKI is defined as any of the following:
1. An increase in serum creatinine by ≥0.3 mg/dL within 48 hours
2. An increase in serum creatinine to ≥1.5 times baseline over the course of 7 days
3. Urine output <0.5 mL/kg/hour for 6 hours

AKI is further subclassified into stages based on the degree of the abnormalities (Table 30.1).

ETIOLOGY

The etiology of AKI is customarily divided into prerenal, intrarenal (or intrinsic renal), and postrenal causes (Fig. 30.1). Prerenal AKI refers to physiological, reversible decreases in filtration that result from renal hypoperfusion. Intrarenal AKI refers to renal dysfunction resulting from direct structural injuries to the renal vasculature, glomeruli, tubules, and/or interstitium. Postrenal AKI refers to obstruction of the urine collecting system, which raises pressures in nephrons and thereby interferes with effective glomerular filtration. (Of note, patients can have obstructions sufficient to cause AKI without becoming anuric.)

Prerenal Acute Kidney Injury

The compensatory response to a reduction in blood pressure is activation of the sympathetic nervous system (SNS), which increases systemic vascular resistance. In the kidneys, the SNS causes vasoconstriction of afferent arterioles, which reduces both renal blood flow and GFR. If the effect on GFR is sustained, the patient experiences prerenal AKI. (Of note, when hypotension is severe enough to cause renal ischemia, acute tubular necrosis [ATN] may occur, as described later.)

The major causes of prerenal AKI include true volume depletion, intraarterial volume depletion (i.e., heart failure, cirrhosis), sepsis, and medication use (e.g., NSAIDs, angiotensin receptor inhibitors).

True volume depletion can result from vomiting, diarrhea, hemorrhage, diuretic use, cutaneous losses (e.g., fevers, burns), and poor oral intake.

Effective intraarterial volume depletion results from heart failure or abnormal third spacing of plasma fluid, as seen in cirrhosis. In heart failure, low cardiac output causes chronic activation of the SNS, resulting in renal hypoperfusion. High right atrial pressures are also transmitted to the renal veins, which reduces renal perfusion pressure. In cirrhosis, high portal pressures and low serum albumin levels lead to pooling of blood in the splanchnic system and translocation of fluid into the peritoneum, reducing overall blood pressure. The effective depletion of volume causes chronic activation of the SNS, further impairing renal perfusion.

In sepsis, generalized vasodilation causes hypotension and renal hypoperfusion. In addition, severe inflammation can be directly cytotoxic to the kidneys resulting in ATN.

Some medications also cause physiological changes that can cause or worsen prerenal AKI. Prostaglandins, for example, promote afferent arteriolar vasodilation, but the use of NSAIDs inhibits their synthesis and may worsen renal perfusion in patients with chronic SNS overactivation (e.g., secondary to heart failure). Likewise, angiotensin II is produced in response to renal hypoperfusion and constricts efferent arterioles, thereby increasing glomerular pressure and filtration. The use of

TABLE 30.1
Acute Kidney Injury: Staging

AKI Stage	Serum Creatinine	Urine Output
Stage 1	Increase in serum creatinine by ≥0.3 mg/dL **or** an increase to 1.5–1.9 from baseline	Urine output <0.5 mL/kg/h for 6 12 h
Stage 2	Increase in serum creatinine to 2.0–2.9 times from baseline	Urine output <0.5 mL/kg/h for ≥12 h
Stage 3	Increase in serum creatinine to 3.0 times the baseline **or** increase in serum creatinine to ≥4.0 mg/dL **or** need for RRT **or** in patients <18, decrease in GFR to <35 mL/min per 1.73 m²	Urine output <0.3 mL/kg/h for ≥24 hours **or** anuria for ≥12 h

Reused with permission from KDIGO AKIWG: Kidney Disease: Improving Global Outcomes (KDIGO) clinical practice guideline for acute kidney injury, *Kidney Int* 2(Suppl 2012):S1–S138, 1–141, 2012.
GFR, Glomerular filtration rate; *RRT*, renal replacement therapy.

ACE inhibitors or angiotensin receptor blockers, however, blocks this compensatory mechanism and causes GFR to fall.

Intrarenal Acute Kidney Injury

Intrarenal AKI results from damage to the tubules, glomeruli, interstitium, and/or renal vasculature.

Tubular disease

ATN is the most common cause of renal tubular disease and may result from either severe ischemia, exposure to nephrotoxins, or profound inflammatory states. Common exogenous nephrotoxins include antibiotics (e.g., aminoglycosides), iodinated contrast, acyclovir, and multiple chemotherapies. Common endogenous nephrotoxins include hemoglobin, bilirubin, uric acid, and light chains.

Glomerular disease

Glomerulonephritis occurs when abnormal activation of the immune system results in direct injury to the glomerular capillaries. The major causes are categorized based on the pattern of inflammation into immune complex mediated (e.g., immunoglobulin A [IgA] nephropathy, lupus nephritis, postinfectious glomerulonephritis, cryoglobulinemia), pauci-immune/antineutrophil cytoplasmic antibody (ANCA) associated (i.e., microscopic

polyangiitis, polyangiitis with granulomatosis [Wegener disease]), and antiglomerular basement membrane (anti-GBM) antibody mediated (e.g., Goodpasture disease). See Chapter 95 for further details.

Interstitial disease

Acute interstitial nephritis (AIN) occurs when inflammation of the renal interstitium results in the destruction and obliteration of tubules. The major causes include medications (e.g., β-lactams, NSAIDs, proton-pump inhibitors) and, to a much lesser extent, infections and autoimmune diseases.

Vascular disease

Vascular disease can affect both large and small vessels. A renal artery, for example, may become acutely occluded from aortic dissection or a large thromboembolus; the resulting impact on GFR will depend on the extent of renal injury and, in the case of a large infarct, the capacity of the contralateral kidney to compensate. One or both renal arteries may also become stenotic due to atherosclerotic disease or fibromuscular dysplasia, causing AKI during states of hypoperfusion or with the use of NSAIDs, ACE inhibitors, or angiotensin receptor blockers.

Meanwhile, the microvasculature can become thrombosed and occluded secondary to the thrombotic microangiopathies (TMAs), which include thrombotic thrombocytopenia purpura, hemolytic-uremic syndrome, disseminated intravascular coagulation, malignant hypertension, and scleroderma renal crisis.

Postrenal Acute Kidney Injury

Postrenal AKI results from obstruction to urinary flow, which increases pressures through the tubules and interferes with glomerular filtration. The most common cause is prostatic hypertrophy either due to age or cancer. Ureteral obstruction secondary to metastatic cancer, nephrolithiasis, or retroperitoneal fibrosis can also lead to postrenal AKI if both kidneys are obstructed, a solitary kidney is obstructed, or the unobstructed kidney is already chronically diseased and unable to compensate for the obstructed kidney.

CLINICAL FEATURES

The presentation of AKI depends in part on the etiology. Patients with prerenal AKI may have signs of volume depletion (e.g., tachycardia, dry mucous membranes, hypotension). Patients with intrarenal AKI may experience hematuria or signs of other systemic disease (e.g., fever, rash). Patients with postrenal AKI may have abdominopelvic pain related to the obstruction. The

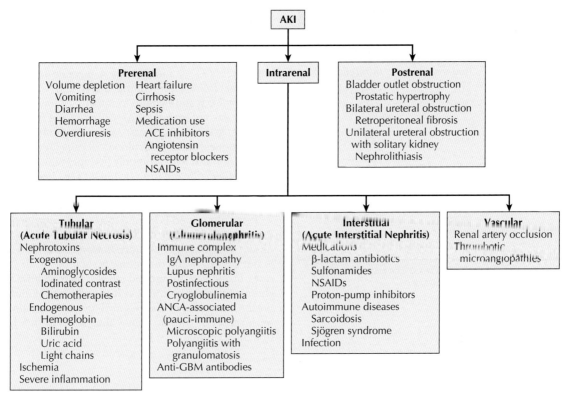

FIG. 30.1 **Causes of Acute Kidney Injury *(AKI)*.** *ANCA,* Antineutrophil cytoplasmic antibody; *GBM,* glomerular basement membrane; *IgA,* immunoglobulin A.

remaining symptoms depend on the severity of the renal injury. Urine output can range from anuria (<50 mL/day) to oliguria (<500 mL/day) to normal. Patients with significant loss of renal function can present with edema, hypertension, and even symptoms of uremia (nausea, confusion, bleeding due to platelet dysfunction).

Workup

All patients should undergo a comprehensive history and physical to assess for the various causes of AKI. The history should identify comorbid illnesses and exposures to possible nephrotoxins, in particular medications (including over-the-counter and herbal medications) and intravenous contrast. The physical examination should assess overall volume status and check for signs of systemic illness.

The most useful laboratory tests include urine osmolality, urine electrolytes, and a basic metabolic panel. The urine electrolytes can be used to calculate the fractional excretion of sodium (FENa), which is equal to the fraction of filtered sodium that is ultimately excreted in the urine. It is necessary to normalize this value using the fraction of serum creatinine present in the urine, to account for changes in urine electrolyte concentration related to the reabsorption of water:

$$\frac{(\text{urine sodium})/(\text{serum sodium})}{(\text{urine creatinine})/(\text{serum creatinine})} \times 100 \qquad \textbf{EQ. 30.1}$$

The FENa can be interpreted along with the urine osmolality, urine sodium concentration, and serum blood urea nitrogen (BUN):creatinine ratio to distinguish prerenal AKI from intrarenal AKI (Table 30.2). In prerenal AKI, high levels of norepinephrine, angiotensin, and aldosterone promote the reabsorption of sodium from the nephron to maintain plasma volume, leading to low urine sodium levels. As urea is passively reabsorbed along with sodium, this also results in elevated serum BUN levels out of proportion to the elevation in creatinine. Of note, however, urine-based sodium assays are inaccurate in the setting of diuretic use. The fractional excretion of urea, which is less sensitive to diuretic use, is more accurate in this setting (<35% indicates prerenal disease).

A urinalysis can further help determine the etiology of AKI, especially when paired with microscopy to

TABLE 30.2
Laboratory Findings That Indicate Prerenal or Intrarenal AKI

	Prerenal	Intrarenal
FENa	<1%	>2%–3%
Urine osmolality (mOsm)	>500	250–300
Urine sodium concentration (mmol/L)	<20	>40
BUN:Cr	>20:1	<20:1
Urinalysis	Bland sediment (possibly hyaline casts), no proteinuria	Active sediment (cells, casts), proteinuria

AKI, Acute kidney injury; *BUN:Cr,* blood urea nitrogen:creatinine ratio; *FENa,* fractional excretion of sodium.

determine the presence of cells and casts (aggregates of cells and proteinaceous material formed in the thick ascending limb). The presence of urine protein (particularly albumin) indicates glomerular dysfunction; high levels (3+ or more) suggest possible nephrotic syndrome (>3.5 g proteinuria daily) and warrant a spot protein:creatinine ratio for quantification. Muddy brown casts are typical of ATN but are not found in all cases. Red blood cell casts are pathognomonic for glomerulonephritis. White blood cell casts may be seen in AIN (or much less commonly pyelonephritis) but are not sensitive. A bland urine sediment (i.e., free of cells or casts), or the presence of only acellular hyaline casts, suggests prerenal AKI (See Chapter 37 for further details).

Renal ultrasound is helpful to assess for obstruction in patients with suggestive findings or pertinent history. Absent such findings or history, however, an ultrasound is not necessary for the initial evaluation of all AKI cases. In addition, ultrasound can also help establish the chronicity of kidney injury if it is unknown. With the notable exceptions of diabetes mellitus and amyloidosis, most causes of chronic kidney disease result in a loss of kidney volume.

CHAPTER 31

Acid-Base Disturbances

MELISSA S. MAKAR • EUGENE C. KOVALIK

INTRODUCTION

The body tightly controls serum acid and base concentrations to maintain equilibrium. Bicarbonate, the body's main extracellular buffer, helps maintain normal pH by neutralizing acids, including those produced from carbon dioxide. The bicarbonate buffering system is based on the principle that carbon dioxide (CO_2) is in equilibrium with carbonic acid (H_2CO_3), which is in equilibrium with bicarbonate (HCO_3^-). This relationship is summarized as:

$$dissolved\ CO_2 + H_2O \longleftrightarrow H_2CO_3 \longleftrightarrow HCO_3^- + H^+ \quad \textbf{EQ. 31.1}$$

The **Henderson-Hasselbalch equation** is derived from this principle and simplifies to $H^+ = 24 \times (PaCO_2 / HCO_3^-)$, where $PaCO_2$ is the partial pressure of CO_2. This equation highlights the key fact that the body can only maintain acid-base equilibrium by either controlling $PaCO_2$ through the respiratory system or by controlling HCO_3^- through the renal system (Fig. 31.1). A disturbance in one of these two systems leads to a partial correction by the other system known as compensation.

TYPES OF ACID-BASE DISORDERS AND COMPENSATION

There are four acid-base processes or disorders: metabolic acidosis, metabolic alkalosis, respiratory acidosis, and respiratory alkalosis (Fig. 31.2). An acidosis is a process that generally leads to a state of acidemia, defined as a pH <7.35. An alkalosis is a process that generally leads to a state of alkalemia, defined as a pH >7.45. It is possible, however, to have multiple concurrent processes, such as both a respiratory alkalosis and metabolic acidosis. In such cases, the overall effect on pH is variable.

A **metabolic acidosis** is a process that increases H^+ or decreases HCO_3^-. In either case, the respiratory system attempts to restore equilibrium by increasing ventilation and thereby reducing CO_2. The increases in respiratory rate and tidal volumes are rapid, starting within minutes to hours. Similarly, the respiratory system responds rapidly in response to **metabolic alkalosis,** a disorder of elevated bicarbonate. Rather than hyperventilation, however, hypoventilation occurs to raise $PaCO_2$.

Respiratory acidosis is the process by which decreased ventilation leads to an accumulation of CO_2. The kidneys compensate by secreting more hydrogen ions in the urine and generating new bicarbonate (via the process of ammoniagenesis), which is reabsorbed into the blood. Renal compensation is slow and can take several days to complete. Early in this process, the respiratory acidosis is termed acute. Later on, when the kidneys are maximally secreting hydrogen ions, the respiratory acidosis is chronic.

Finally, in **respiratory alkalosis,** hyperventilation leads to decreased CO_2 levels. To compensate, the kidneys secrete more bicarbonate and less hydrogen in the urine, both of which decrease the serum bicarbonate concentration. Again, the full renal response is slow, resulting in both acute and chronic forms of respiratory alkalosis.

IDENTIFYING THE ACID-BASE DISORDER

There are several methods for evaluating acid-base disorders. The following abbreviated version requires measurement of the arterial pH and $PaCO_2$ using an arterial blood gas (ABG), along with measurement of HCO_3^- and other electrolytes using a basic metabolic panel (BMP). For accuracy, it is important to draw the ABG and BMP at the same time.

Step 1: Examine the pH. The pH will determine if the combination of all acid-base processes present has led to a state of acidemia or alkalemia.

Step 2: Examine HCO_3^- and $PaCO_2$ levels, which help identify whether the primary issue is a metabolic or respiratory disturbance. If the patient is acidemic, a low HCO_3^- indicates a metabolic acidosis, while a high $PaCO_2$ indicates a respiratory acidosis. If the patient is alkalemic, then a high HCO_3^- indicates a metabolic alkalosis, while a low $PaCO_2$ indicates a respiratory alkalosis.

Step 3: Calculate the anion gap. The BMP reports the major anions in serum (bicarbonate and chloride) as well as the major cation (sodium). Because it is burdensome to measure all the anions (phosphate, sulfate, albumin, organic anions) and cations

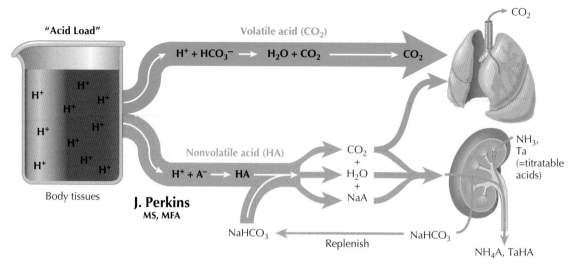

FIG. 31.1 **Role of Lungs and Kidneys in Acid-Base Balance.**

(potassium, calcium, magnesium, some immuno-globulins), these unmeasured ions are accounted for with the anion gap (AG), which is the difference between unmeasured anions and unmeasured cations:

$$Na - (Cl^- + HCO_3^-) \qquad \textbf{EQ. 31.2}$$

The AG for the population at large is typically around 10 mEq/L +/− 3. For a given individual, however, what his or her AG should be depends on the primary unmeasured anion, serum albumin. If there is not an increase in another unmeasured anion, the AG for an individual should be 2.5 times serum albumin, in g/dL. Thus in a patient with an albumin of 2 g/dL, the appropriate calculated AG would be 5. If it were instead found to be 12, this would indicate the presence of a high anion gap acidosis due to an increased unmeasured anion, regardless of the overall pH.

Step 4: Assess for appropriate compensation. In the presence of a metabolic disorder the lungs should respond by altering the $PaCO_2$, while a respiratory disorder should stimulate the kidneys to respond by altering the concentration of HCO_3^-. Several equations exist to predict the expected degree of compensation for a given acid-base disorder and allow assessment of whether alterations in HCO_3^- and $PaCO_2$ are appropriate compensations or are instead evidence of a second concurrent disorder. The most well known is Winters formula for predicting the respiratory response to metabolic acidosis:

$$(1.5 \times HCO_3^-) + 8 +/-2 \qquad \textbf{EQ. 31.3}$$

If the $PaCO_2$ is higher than the value predicted by the formula, then the patient has a respiratory acidosis (in addition to the metabolic acidosis). If the $PaCO_2$ is lower than predicted, the patient has a respiratory alkalosis. The formulas for appropriate compensation are shown in Table 31.1.

COMMON CAUSES OF ACID-BASE DISORDERS

High anion gap metabolic acidosis reflects overproduction or underexcretion of acids. The various causes can be categorized as endogenous (acid production through metabolism) or exogenous (ingestion of acid-generating substances).

The common endogenous causes include diabetic ketoacidosis (DKA), lactic acidosis, and renal failure. In DKA, a lack of insulin results in an overproduction of ketones. Lactic acidosis commonly results from impaired tissue perfusion, such as seen in septic shock. In renal failure, acids from sulfate, phosphate, and urate accumulate because of impaired clearance.

The exogenous causes of high anion gap metabolic acidosis include salicylate, ethylene glycol, methanol, and propylene glycol. Salicylate is commonly found in over-the-counter pain medications (e.g., aspirin) and can lead to a mixed respiratory alkalosis and high anion gap metabolic acidosis. Ethylene glycol is traditionally found in antifreeze, while methanol has a variety of industrial applications. Finally, propylene glycol is used as a solvent for intravenous benzodiazepines and accumulates when patients receive prolonged infusions in the intensive care unit.

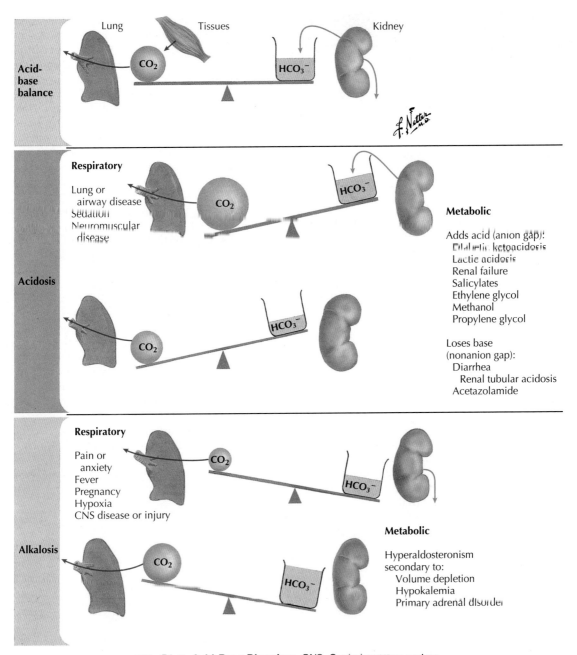

FIG. 31.2 **Acid-Base Disorders.** *CNS,* Central nervous system.

Normal anion gap metabolic acidosis reflects the loss of serum bicarbonate through diarrhea, renal tubular acidosis (RTA), or acetazolamide use. RTAs result from dysfunction in the renal proximal tubules (RTA type II) or distal tubules (RTA types I and IV). The common causes of RTAs include monoclonal gammopathies, heavy metal toxicity, autoimmune disorders (e.g., Sjögren syndrome, systemic lupus erythematosus), diabetes mellitus, and chronic interstitial nephritis. Acetazolamide is a diuretic that reduces renal bicarbonate reabsorption (and hence increases its excretion in urine) by inhibiting carbonic anhydrase in the proximal tubule.

TABLE 31.1
Normal Compensation for Acid-Base Disorders

RESPIRATORY RESPONSES TO METABOLIC DISORDERS

Primary disorder	Expected PaCO$_2$ with appropriate compensation
Metabolic acidosis	$(1.5 \times HCO_3^-) + 8$ +/− 2
Metabolic alkalosis	$40 + 0.7 \times (HCO_3^- - 24)$ +/− 5

METABOLIC RESPONSES TO RESPIRATORY DISORDERS

Primary disorder	Expected HCO$_3^-$ with appropriate compensation
Respiratory acidosis	Acute: $24 + \left(\dfrac{PaCO_2 - 40}{10} * 1 \right)$ Chronic: $24 + \left(\dfrac{PaCO_2 - 40}{10} * 3.5 \right)$
Respiratory alkalosis	Acute: $24 - \left(\dfrac{40 - PaCO_2}{10} * 2 \right)$ Chronic: $24 - \left(\dfrac{40 - PaCO_2}{10} * 5 \right)$

Metabolic alkalosis is most commonly caused by volume depletion, such as from diuretic use or vomiting. Aldosterone is released in response to volume depletion and promotes sodium reabsorption in the distal nephron, which creates an electrical gradient that favors potassium and hydrogen secretion into the urine. The net result is hypokalemia and metabolic alkalosis. A similar phenomenon occurs in patients with Bartter or Gitelman syndrome, in whom impaired sodium reabsorption in more proximal tubular segments results in increased sodium delivery and reabsorption (and thus potassium and hydrogen secretion) in the collecting duct. Finally, primary hyperaldosteronism, or any state that leads to hypokalemia and thus aldosterone secretion, can cause a metabolic alkalosis process in the same manner. In many cases, the treatment of hypokalemia and/or volume depletion will lead to resolution of the alkalosis (see Chapter 28 for further details).

Respiratory acidosis can be categorized as acute and chronic based on the degree of renal compensation, as described earlier. The most common etiology is carbon dioxide retention secondary to chronic obstructive pulmonary disease (COPD). Carbon dioxide can also be retained in patients with obesity, obstructive sleep apnea, and disorders that impair alveolar gas exchange, such as pulmonary edema and pneumonia. Finally, respiratory acidosis can develop due to hypoventilation resulting from an inhibited respiratory center in the brain, such as from opiates, or from dysfunction of the respiratory muscles and chest wall, which can occur acutely in myasthenia gravis, Guillain-Barré syndrome, and severe hypophosphatemia or chronically in amyotrophic lateral sclerosis and multiple sclerosis.

Respiratory alkalosis, which can also be categorized as acute or chronic, reflects hyperventilation that can occur in response to hypoxemia, fever, pain, and other conditions that cause direct stimulation of the respiratory center in the brain (e.g., pregnancy or salicylate intoxication).

CHAPTER 32

Anemia

JIGAR CONTRACTOR

INTRODUCTION

Anemia, one the most common laboratory abnormalities in clinical practice, is defined as a pathological reduction in the number of circulating red blood cells (RBCs) or RBC mass.

Anemia is most commonly assessed by measuring the serum concentration of **hemoglobin,** the primary oxygen-carrying protein. A hemoglobin molecule consists of a tetramer of two α-globin and two β-globin proteins, each of which is bound to a heme molecule with an iron-containing porphyrin ring. Anemia may also be assessed by measuring the **hematocrit,** or packed spun volume of intact RBCs expressed as a percentage of the whole blood volume.

Anemia is defined as a reduction in hemoglobin or hematocrit to less than two standard deviations below the normal ranges for men and women. Although the specific threshold values vary across laboratories, many clinicians define anemia in men as a hemoglobin concentration of <13.5 g/dL (or hematocrit <41%) and in women as a hemoglobin concentration of <12 g/dL (or hematocrit <36%).

Of note, hemoglobin and hematocrit may not accurately reflect RBC mass in certain clinical situations. For example, diarrhea may lead to the loss of plasma volume and relative RBC hemoconcentration, increasing the hemoglobin concentration and hematocrit without affecting RBC mass. In contrast, heart failure may cause plasma expansion and relative RBC hemodilution, lowering the hemoglobin concentration and hematocrit. Meanwhile, the simultaneous loss of both red cells and plasma, as occurs in acute hemorrhage, may not cause any immediate change in hemoglobin concentration or hematocrit despite significant losses of RBCs.

PATHOPHYSIOLOGY

Normal RBCs remain in the circulation for an average of 120 days, after which they are cleared from the circulation by the reticuloendothelial system, primarily in the spleen. Under normal circumstances, the rate of RBC production closely matches the rate of consumption. In anemia, however, this equilibrium becomes disturbed by dysfunctional RBC synthesis (e.g., from iron or other micronutrient deficiency, thalassemia, or other hemoglobinopathies) or accelerated RBC loss (e.g., from bleeding or hemolysis).

The RBC concentration and cardiac output are the main determinants of tissue oxygenation. In response to anemia, several compensatory mechanisms help acutely preserve adequate oxygenation of vital organs; these include an increase in heart rate and cardiac ejection fraction, a selective reduction in the perfusion of skin and other peripheral soft tissues, and an increase in tissue oxygen extraction. More chronically, hypoxia also induces mechanisms to help correct the underlying anemia. Specifically, the increased production of hypoxia-inducible transcription factors promotes the renal synthesis of erythropoietin, which augments RBC production and accelerates the release of reticulocytes (the immediate precursors of RBCs) into the circulation (Fig. 32.1). These mechanisms, however, may have limited effects when the anemia is secondary to dysfunctional RBC production.

DIAGNOSTIC APPROACH

The assessment of anemia requires a systematic approach that considers the overall clinical picture and several key laboratory markers. First, the clinician should consider the possibility that the observed abnormalities in hemoglobin and/or hematocrit may reflect changes in plasma volume, rather than in RBC mass, as described earlier. If anemia is believed to reflect a true reduction in RBC mass, the diagnostic approach can be further refined based on (1) **chronicity** (if known), (2) **mean corpuscular volume** (MCV), and (3) **reticulocyte count** (Fig. 32.2).

Chronicity

Rapid-onset anemia most often reflects blood loss or hemolysis. By contrast, subacute or insidious-onset

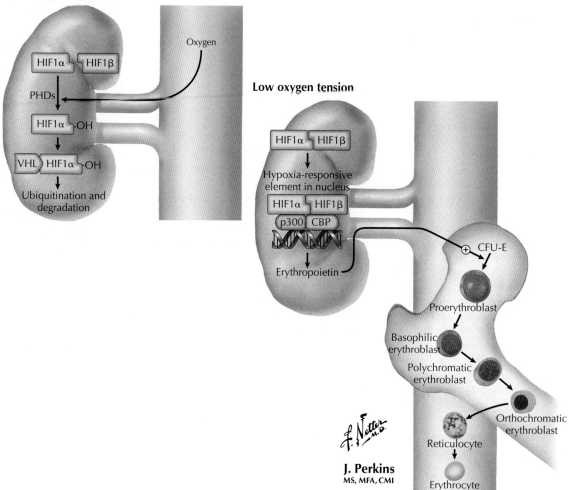

High oxygen tension

Low oxygen tension

FIG. 32.1 **Role of Kidneys in Erythropoiesis.** *CBP*, CREB (cAMP-response element-binding protein)-binding protein; *CFU-E*, colony forming unit-erythroid; *HIF*, hypoxia-inducible factor; *OH*, hydroxide; *PHDs*, prolyl hydroxylases; *VHL*, von Hippel-Lindau.

anemia may reflect a developing micronutrient deficiency or, less commonly, a bone marrow disorder.

Mean Corpuscular Volume

The MCV measures the average RBC size in femtoliters (fL). Anemia is classified as microcytic when the MCV is <80 fL, normocytic when between 80 and 100 fL, and macrocytic when >100 fL.

Microcytic anemia

In **microcytic anemia** (MCV <80 fL), RBCs contain a decreased amount of hemoglobin, typically because of dysfunctional synthesis. The major causes of microcytic

anemia include iron deficiency, thalassemia, anemia of chronic disease, and sideroblastic anemia.

Iron-deficiency anemia (IDA) may be caused by iron loss (e.g., from gastrointestinal or vaginal bleeding), dietary restriction, or gastrointestinal malabsorption (e.g., from gastric bypass or celiac sprue). Several blood tests can help establish the diagnosis of IDA, including the concentration of iron; the total iron binding capacity (TIBC), which reflects levels of transferrin (the major protein responsible for iron transport in the blood); the iron saturation, defined as the ratio of iron to TIBC; and the concentration of ferritin (the major protein responsible for iron storage in tissues). In classic IDA,

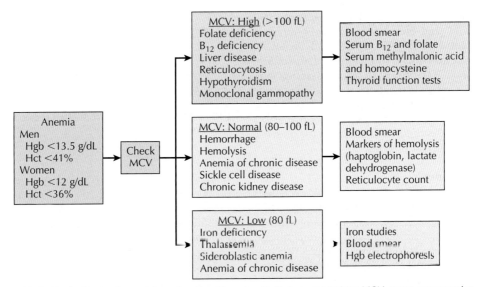

FIG. 32.2 **Basic Evaluation of Anemia.** *Hct*, Hematocrit; *Hgb*, hemoglobin; *MCV*, mean corpuscular volume.

the iron concentration is low; the TIBC is elevated, from increased production of transferrin; the iron saturation is low; and the ferritin concentration, as a measure of total body storage iron, is low. The peripheral blood smear in IDA classically reveals microcytic RBCs with hypochromia (increase in RBC central pallor to greater than one-third of the RBC diameter) and anisopoikilocytosis (broad distribution of RBC sizes and shapes, including pencil-shaped RBCs). It is imperative that the diagnosis of IDA be followed by a thorough investigation of potential causes.

Thalassemias occur when abnormalities in either the α-globin or the β-globin genes cause impaired or absent synthesis. α-Thalassemias result in an accumulation of excess β-globin proteins, while β-thalassemias result in an accumulation of excess α-globin proteins. See Chapter 141 for further details on classification of α- and β-thalassemias.

The hallmark of thalassemia is ineffective erythropoiesis, which in severe cases results in extramedullary hematopoiesis that manifests as splenomegaly and characteristic skeletal and facial abnormalities. Because of ineffective erythropoiesis and constant RBC turnover, thalassemia frequently causes iron overload, partly as a result of chronic blood transfusion therapy and partly from transfusion-independent processes. The peripheral blood smear usually reveals target RBCs, which have an abnormal membrane-to-cytoplasm ratio secondary to defective hemoglobin synthesis. Hemoglobin electrophoresis can diagnose β-thalassemia, while

more specific DNA analysis is required to diagnose α-thalassemia trait.

Iron studies, hemoglobin electrophoresis, blood smear, and family history can help distinguish IDA from the thalassemia. In addition, the red cell distribution width (RDW), which measures the variability in RBC size, is classically high in iron deficiency (due to anisopoikilocytosis) but low in thalassemia. Lastly, the Mentzer index, or ratio of MCV to RBC count, is commonly high in IDA due to a reduction in RBC count, but low in mild forms of thalassemia as the number of RBCs produced is often normal.

Sideroblastic anemia is a rare cause of microcytic anemia that arises from a disruption in the incorporation of iron into heme, resulting in iron accumulation in mitochondria. Acquired sideroblastic anemia may occur with lead poisoning, alcohol use, or deficiencies of copper, zinc, or pyridoxine. Inherited sideroblastic anemia is usually X-linked. The diagnosis of sideroblastic anemia is established on a bone marrow biopsy, which reveals RBCs containing rings of iron-laden mitochondria (known as ringed sideroblasts).

Anemia of chronic disease, also known as anemia of inflammation, is most often associated with normocytosis but can, in about one in five cases, cause microcytosis. Anemia of chronic disease occurs when inflammatory states cause increased production of hepcidin, a regulator of iron homeostasis that suppresses gastrointestinal iron absorption as well as iron utilization. Iron indices have a characteristic pattern, including a low or normal serum iron concentration, low TIBC, low or normal iron saturation, and elevated ferritin concentration. Ferritin concentrations become elevated both because of increased tissue iron storage (from impaired iron utilization) and because ferritin is an acute-phase reactant. Other markers of inflammation, such as erythrocyte sedimentation rate or C-reactive protein, may also be elevated. The characteristic finding on blood smear is rouleaux, aggregates of RBCs that form in the presence of acute-phase reactant proteins.

Normocytic anemia

Normocytic anemia (MCV 80–100 fL) typically reflects acute hemorrhage, hemolysis, or deficient production of erythrocyte precursors. Common causes of deficient erythrocyte production include anemia of chronic disease, as described earlier; chronic renal disease, which is associated with impaired erythropoietin production; and sickle cell disease. Although acute hemorrhage can lead to normocytic anemia in the short term, microcytosis occurs more chronically as iron deficiency occurs.

Macrocytic anemia

Macrocytic anemia (MCV >100 fL) may be classified as either megaloblastic or nonmegaloblastic. Megaloblastic anemia usually results from deficiency of vitamin B_{12} or folic acid. During the process of erythropoiesis, the RBC volume progressively decreases. As vitamin B_{12} and folic acid are essential cofactors in nucleic acid biosynthesis, deficiencies in either micronutrient leads to dyssynchrony of nuclear and cytoplasmic maturation, causing overall enlargement of erythrocyte size and the formation of large, immature nuclei. As a result, peripheral blood smear findings include macro-ovalocytes (large, oval-shaped RBCs) and hypersegmented neutrophils (containing six or more lobes). Biochemically, a deficiency of folic acid may give rise to an elevation in homocysteine, while a deficiency of vitamin B_{12} often causes elevations of

> *Reticulocyte Production Index =*
> *(%reticulocyte × hct/normal hct) / maturation factor*
> Maturation Factors:
> Hct ≥ 35%: 1.0
> 35% > Hct ≥ 25%: 1.5
> 25% > Hct ≥ 20%: 2.0
> 20% > Hct: 2.5

FIG. 32.3 **Reticulocyte Production Index.** *Hct,* Hematocrit.

both homocysteine and methylmalonic acid. Laboratory measurements of vitamin B_{12} do not always reliably reflect physiologic vitamin B_{12} status, so when working up a potential case of vitamin B_{12} deficiency, homocysteine and methylmalonic acid levels should be checked.

The nonmegaloblastic causes of macrocytosis and macrocytic anemia include liver disease and hypothyroidism (from abnormal lipid deposition in the RBC membrane), reticulocytosis (reflecting the enlarged size of a reticulocyte compared to a mature RBC), and monoclonal gammopathies.

Reticulocyte Count

The reticulocyte count measures the percentage of total circulating RBCs represented by reticulocytes. The reticulocyte production index (RPI) helps determine if the bone marrow response is appropriate given the degree of anemia, and thus whether the anemia is likely related to deficient erythropoiesis (RPI <2%) or RBC loss (RPI >2%). The RPI relies on a maturation factor that takes into account the increased life span of reticulocytes in the circulation when released early (Fig. 32.3). Hypoproliferative anemias, characterized by a low RPI, include micronutrient deficiencies, anemia of inflammation, and anemia of renal disease. Hyperproliferative anemia, characterized by a high RPI, may be seen in hemolysis and acute blood loss.

CHAPTER 33

Thrombocytopenia

STEPHANIE J. TANG • ALICE J. TANG • ALFRED LEE

INTRODUCTION

Platelets are produced in the bone marrow by mega-karyocytes. In normal circumstances, the bone marrow produces 35 to 50 × 10³ platelets per day, which survive for an average 8 to 10 days. Thrombocytopenia is defined as a platelet count <150 × 10³/μL. Patients with throm-bocytopenia generally do not experience bleeding until the platelet count is <50 × 10³/μL. Major spontaneous bleeding, such as an intracranial hemorrhage, does not generally occur until the platelet count is <10 × 10³/μL.

PATHOPHYSIOLOGY

Thrombocytopenia can reflect decreased platelet produc-tion, increased platelet destruction, splenic sequestration, and/or dilution.

Decreased platelet production can occur in a variety of settings, including nutritional deficiencies of vitamin B_{12} or folate; infections such as HIV, Epstein-Barr virus, cytomegalovirus, or viral hepatitis; myelodysplastic syn-drome, aplastic anemia, and other primary bone marrow problems; infiltration of the bone marrow by solid tumor malignancies or other processes not native to the bone marrow (a.k.a., myelophthisis); and medications, drugs, and toxins (including alcohol, chemotherapy, and radiation exposure). In addition, liver disease can cause both a hypoproliferative thrombocytopenia due to impaired production of thrombopoietin and a sequestrative thrombocytopenia due to hypersplenism (details to come).

Increased platelet destruction can occur secondary to consumption, mechanical destruction, or immune-mediated processes. Platelet consumption occurs in conditions such as disseminated intravascular coagulation (DIC) and the thrombotic microangiopathies (TMAs). DIC is a state of uncontrolled concurrent systemic coagulation and fibrinolysis that may occur in the setting of sepsis, major trauma, and malignancy. The TMAs cause widespread formation of platelet-rich thrombi in the microvasculature; two major subtypes of TMAs include thrombotic thrombocytopenia purpura and hemolytic-uremic syndrome. (See Chapters 142 and 144 for discussions of microangiopathic hemolytic anemia and DIC, respectively.)

Mechanical platelet destruction most commonly occurs in the setting of mechanical heart valves or extracorporeal circuits (e.g., extracorporeal membrane oxygenation, continuous veno-venous hemofiltration).

The autoimmune diseases most frequently associ-ated with thrombocytopenia include systemic lupus erythematous, **idiopathic thrombocytopenia purpura** (ITP), **heparin-induced thrombocytopenia** (HIT), antiphospholipid syndrome (APS), posttransfusion alloimmune destruction, and drug reactions. Drugs can induce thrombocytopenia via either marrow suppression (detailed earlier) or a drug-induced ITP with development of drug-dependent antiplatelet antibodies. The drugs that most often cause thrombocytopenia are antibiotics (e.g., β-lactams, ceftriaxone, trimethoprim-sulfamethoxazole, vancomycin, linezolid, daptomycin), antiepileptics (phenytoin, carbamazepine, valproic acid), analgesics (naproxen, acetaminophen), furosemide, proton-pump inhibitors, and antihistamines (ranitidine, famotidine).

Splenic sequestration is a normal process, typically retaining one-third of the body's platelets in equilibrium with the circulating pool. In times of stress, the splenic stores are reduced to increase the circulating pool. Condi-tions that increase spleen size (e.g., infiltrative disorders such as sarcoidosis or amyloidosis, or storage disorders such as Gaucher disease) or cause splenic congestion (e.g., chronic liver disease or other causes of portal hypertension, splenic vein thrombosis, or hemolytic conditions such as hemoglobinopathies or red blood cell disorders), however, increase the sequestration of platelets in the spleen, leading to decreased peripheral platelet counts. Unlike other causes of thrombocytopenia, in splenic sequestration the total platelet mass in the body is normal, and platelets sequestered in the spleen remain available for use in hemostatic processes, so splenic sequestration as a sole cause of thrombocytopenia rarely leads to bleeding complications.

Finally, **dilutional thrombocytopenia** can occur when patients receive massive transfusions or certain types of fluid resuscitation (particularly colloids, which remain in the vasculature and do not readily extravasate), but the effect of this on platelet count is somewhat minor due to physiologic splenic sequestration and the ability of platelets to mobilize from the spleen.

PRESENTATION, EVALUATION, AND DIAGNOSIS

Thrombocytopenia is often an incidental finding but should be suspected in any patient with a history of recurrent bleeding (especially from mucosal surfaces, such as the gingiva) and/or a **petechial** rash.

The first step in the evaluation of thrombocytopenia is to repeat the test and rule out laboratory artifact. Some patients produce an antibody that causes in vitro platelet clumping after exposure to ethylenediaminetetraacetic acid (EDTA) additives, which are typically present in the tubes used for complete blood counts, leading to a falsely low measure of platelet count as measured on an automated counter, a phenomenon known as pseudothrombocytopenia. In pseudothrombocytopenia, the peripheral blood smear in a standard EDTA preparation

will show clumps of platelets, and an accurate platelet count can be obtained by submitting a blood sample in a tube containing sodium citrate.

Once the diagnosis of thrombocytopenia is confirmed, a careful history, physical exam, and focused laboratory analysis should be performed. Special attention should be paid to findings that suggest highly morbid disorders, such as acute leukemia, DIC, TMAs, or HIT. Chronicity and potential risk factors such as alcohol use, infectious exposures, or exposures to medications, recreational drugs, supplements, or toxins should be ascertained. A history of hemorrhagic diarrhea should raise concern for *Shiga* toxin–mediated hemolytic-uremic syndrome. Certain diets or prior gastrointestinal surgeries may predispose to nutritional deficiencies. A personal or familial history of recurring bruising or bleeding suggests a congenital or chronic disorder.

Patients should also be assessed for systemic diseases. For example, cirrhosis is a major cause of splenic sequestration and should be considered in patients with alcohol abuse, intravenous drug use, blood transfusions, and high-risk sexual behavior. Likewise, a report of

HELLP Syndrome (Hemolysis, Abnormal Liver Function Tests, Low Platelets)

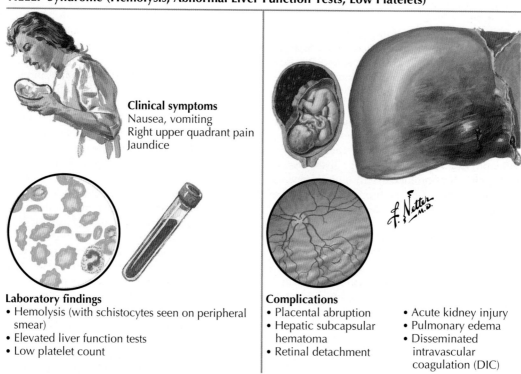

Clinical symptoms
Nausea, vomiting
Right upper quadrant pain
Jaundice

Laboratory findings
- Hemolysis (with schistocytes seen on peripheral smear)
- Elevated liver function tests
- Low platelet count

Complications
- Placental abruption
- Hepatic subcapsular hematoma
- Retinal detachment
- Acute kidney injury
- Pulmonary edema
- Disseminated intravascular coagulation (DIC)

FIG. 33.1 **Clinical and Laboratory Findings in HELLP (*h*emolysis, elevated *l*iver enzymes, *l*ow *p*latelets).**

rashes or arthralgias may raise concern of an underlying autoimmune disorder. In hospitalized patients or those who have been recently hospitalized, the possibility of sepsis and exposure to heparin or extracorporeal circuits should be assessed.

A targeted physical examination is also essential. Thrombocytopenia generally causes petechiae, purpura on the skin or mouth, or ecchymoses; the concomitant presence of hemarthrosis or deep soft tissues, muscle, or body cavity hematoma strongly suggests a concurrent disorder of coagulation, as may occur in DIC. Limb swelling or necrosis may indicate arterial or venous thrombosis, which can occur secondary to HIT or APS. Patients should be evaluated for stigmata of cirrhosis (e.g., splenomegaly, ascites, jaundice, encephalopathy) and rheumatological disorders (serositis, joint swelling, skin rash). Lymphadenopathy or splenomegaly may suggest hematological malignancy or viral infection.

The laboratory examination should begin with a complete blood count to determine if other hematopoietic cell lines are also abnormal. A peripheral smear is imperative to evaluate for immature blasts, which would suggest acute leukemia, and schistocytes, which suggest a TMA. Markers of coagulation and fibrinolysis (prothrombin time, activated partial thromboplastin time, D-dimer level, fibrinogen) should also be assessed; the combination of prolonged clotting times, elevated D-dimer level, hypofibrinogenemia, and thrombocytopenia is diagnostic of DIC. The risk of HIT should be assessed using the 4Ts score, which takes into account timing of thrombocytopenia in relation to heparin exposure, magnitude of thrombocytopenia, presence or absence of thrombosis, and likelihood of other causes of thrombocytopenia other than HIT. For patients with an intermediate or high 4Ts score, a platelet factor 4 antibody test should be checked, which if positive should be followed by a serotonin release assay to confirm the diagnosis of HIT. Premenopausal women should be tested for pregnancy, which can cause **HELLP** (*h*emolysis, *e*levated *l*iver enzymes, *l*ow *p*latelets) (a type of TMA) (Fig. 33.1).

A few clinical pearls are worth keeping in mind:

- In patients with isolated thrombocytopenia (i.e., thrombocytopenia without anemia or leukopenia) and platelet counts <100,000/μL, ITP needs to be considered.
- In patients with severe, isolated thrombocytopenia (i.e., platelet count <10,000–20,000/μL), an immune-mediated cause such as ITP, drug-induced ITP, or alloimmunization should be considered.
- In patients with the combination of thrombocytopenia and thrombosis, HIT and APS should be considered.

The treatment of thrombocytopenia is typically focused on addressing the underlying diagnosis (i.e., discontinuing potentially causative drugs, treating underlying sepsis/infection). In the absence of bleeding, platelet transfusions are generally not indicated until platelet counts are $<10 \times 10^3$ per μL, while in patients with thrombotic thrombocytopenic purpura or HIT, platelet transfusions should generally be avoided.

CHAPTER 34

Abnormal Coagulation Studies

GINA P. JABBOUR

INTRODUCTION

Hemostasis occurs in two distinct phases. **Primary hemostasis** describes the process of platelet activation resulting in platelet plug formation. **Secondary hemostasis** refers to the **coagulation cascade,** which produces a meshwork of cross-linked fibrin on the surfaces of platelet plugs. These processes are illustrated in Figs. 34.1 and 34.2.

In primary hemostasis (see Fig. 34.1), exposure of subendothelial collagen at a site of endothelial injury leads to platelet adhesion, mediated by von Willebrand factor (vWF), which tethers platelets to subendothelial collagen via platelet glycoprotein receptor Ib/IX/V. Platelets become activated, release their granule contents, and bind to each other via platelet glycoprotein receptor IIb/IIIa (integrin $\alpha_{IIb}\beta_3$ or fibrinogen receptor), forming a platelet plug.

Secondary hemostasis (see Fig. 34.2), or the coagulation cascade, consists of **extrinsic, common,** and **intrinsic pathways.** In each of these pathways, the coagulation factors exist as inactive zymogens, which are cleaved into active proteins at specific steps in the coagulation cascade. All coagulation factors are synthesized predominantly in the liver, with the exception of factor VIII, which is produced in both liver and endothelial cells, and vWF, which is produced in megakaryocytes, endothelial cells, and subendothelial collagen.

EXTRINSIC COAGULATION CASCADE

Tissue factor (TF) is a transmembrane receptor expressed by endothelial cells. Under normal circumstances, TF is segregated from circulating factor VII, but when the endothelial surface is disrupted, TF becomes exposed and binds factor VII, converting it to activated VIIa. The TF/VIIa complex, known as the **tenase complex,** converts factor X into activated factor Xa and factor IX into activated factor IXa.

COMMON COAGULATION CASCADE

Factor Xa binds to activated factor Va to form the **prothrombinase complex,** which converts factor II (prothrombin) into activated IIa (thrombin). Thrombin then cleaves fibrinogen into fibrin, factor XIII into activated XIIIa, and factor V into activated Va. The fibrin molecules form strands whose individual molecules become cross-linked via XIIIa, forming an insoluble fibrin meshwork on the surfaces of platelets.

INTRINSIC COAGULATION CASCADE

Upon contact with negatively charged surfaces such as glass or silica, factor XII (Hageman factor) becomes activated into factor XIIa, which then converts factor XI into XIa, which in turn binds to and activates factor IX into IXa. Factor IXa then binds factor VIII (which normally circulates in nonactivated form bound to vWF), resulting in an activated VIIIa/IXa complex, which converts factor X into Xa, propagating the common coagulation pathway. It should be noted that physiologically, factor XII is not thought to play a major role in coagulation in vivo.

CELL-BASED MODEL OF HEMOSTASIS AND COAGULATION

In the last decade, an alternate cell-based model of hemostasis and coagulation has been proposed, consisting of initiation, amplification, and propagation phases. **Initiation,** the start of coagulation, occurs on cells expressing TF and consists of tenase-mediated activation of Xa and IXa, generating a small amount of thrombin. During **amplification,** thrombin activates platelets, factor V, and factor VIII, leading to assembly of multiple coagulation factors on the surfaces of the activated platelets. In **propagation,** the prothrombinase complex generates large amounts of thrombin, which convert fibrinogen to fibrin. The individual mechanisms

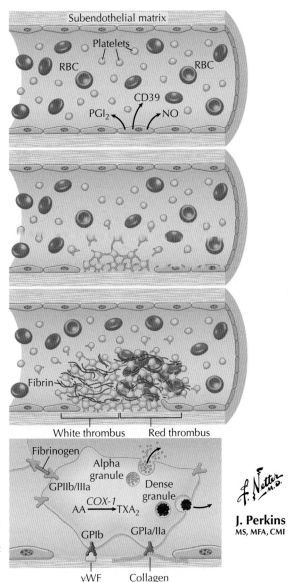

Platelets circulate individually and in an unactivated form. The intact vascular endothelium produces nitric oxide (NO), prostacyclin, and CD39, substances that inhibit platelet activation and aggregation.

If endothelial integrity is interrupted, for example by atherosclerosis or trauma, exposure of subendothelial matrix triggers a hemostatic response with rapid adhesion of platelets to the injured vessel wall. Platelets then release thromboxane A_2 and products of their storage granules that lead to aggregation and recruitment of additional platelets.

As more platelets aggregate, a fibrin network develops and stabilizes the mass into a "white thrombus." If the thrombus develops further, red blood cells become enmeshed in the platelet-fibrin aggregate to form a "red thrombus," which can grow and block the vessel lumen. Either platelet-fibrin aggregates or more fully formed clots may break off, leading to embolization in distal arteries.

Platelets attach to the injured endothelium (adhesion) and to other platelets (aggregation) via specific surface glycoproteins. During platelet activation, cyclooxygenase converts arachidonic acid (AA) into thromboxane A_2 (TXA$_2$), a strong platelet agonist and vasoconstrictor. The content of alpha and dense granules is released, contributing to further growth of the platelet plug.

FIG. 34.1 Role of Platelets in Arterial Thrombosis. *COX-1,* Cyclooxygenase-1; *RBC,* red blood cell; *vWF,* von Willebrand factor.

of coagulation factor activation take place in a manner similar to what is described in the classical model of coagulation, although the ways in which these components interact are more complex.

COAGULATION TESTS

The coagulation cascade is most often assessed by two laboratory tests: the **prothrombin time (PT)** and the **activated partial thromboplastin time (aPTT).**

Prothrombin Time (PT)

PT is a measure of extrinsic coagulation activity. It reflects the time it takes for a fibrin clot to form after a sample of blood is exposed to TF and phospholipids. The usual reference range is 11 to 13 seconds. As the PT can vary depending on the reagent used and particulars of the individual laboratory performing the test, a standardized value known as the **international normalized ratio (INR)** is often used instead of PT. The INR is a ratio of the calculated PT to a control PT, the latter determined

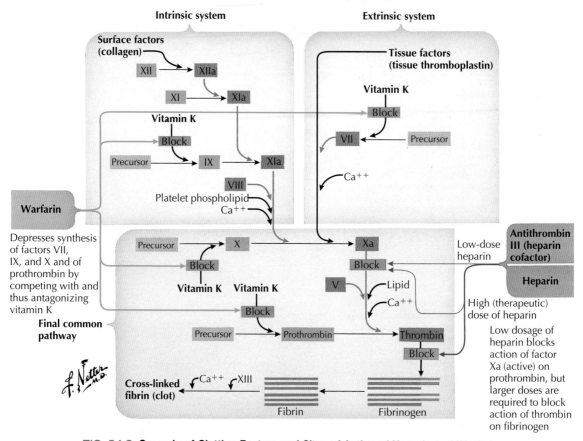

FIG. 34.2 Cascade of Clotting Factors and Sites of Action of Heparin and Warfarin.

using a reference thromboplastic reagent developed by the World Health Organization.

The most common clinical application of the INR is to monitor therapeutic activity of **warfarin,** which inhibits synthesis of the vitamin K–dependent factors II, VII, IX, and X, as well as proteins C and S, which mediate anticoagulation activity in the body. Although these factors comprise all three pathways in the coagulation cascade, the short half-life of factor VII renders the INR a particularly sensitive and accurate measure of warfarin anticoagulant activity.

Activated Partial Thromboplastin Time (aPTT)

aPTT is a measure of intrinsic coagulation activity. It is similar to PT, except that the reaction is performed without TF (hence the term **partial thromboplastin time**) and with addition of a negatively charged substance (e.g., silica), which activates the intrinsic coagulation pathway. The usual reference range is 25 to 35 seconds.

The most common clinical application of the PTT is to monitor **heparin** activity. Heparin binds to and greatly enhances the activity of **antithrombin,** which inactivates multiple coagulation factors in the intrinsic (XIIa, XIa, IXa) and common (Xa, IIa) coagulation pathways.

APPROACH TO A PATIENT WITH PROLONGATION OF THE PT AND/OR aPPT

Since PT measures extrinsic coagulation activity, an isolated prolongation of PT indicates that there is an impairment in factor VII (or VIIa) activity. Because aPTT measures intrinsic coagulation activity, an isolated prolongation of aPTT indicates that there is an impairment in activity of factor(s) XII (or XIIa), XI (or XIa), IX (or IXa), and/or VIII (or VIIIa). Prolongation of both PT and aPTT indicates an impairment of factors in both the extrinsic and intrinsic coagulation pathways, or in the common pathway (i.e., factor[s] X/Xa, V/Va, or fibrinogen/fibrin).

TABLE 34.1
Causes of Abnormal PT and/or aPTT

PT	aPTT	Mixing Study Corrects	Mixing Study Does Not Correct
Normal	High	• Factor VIII deficiency • Factor IX deficiency • Factor XI deficiency • Factor XII deficiency • Von Willebrand disease	• Inhibitor to factors VIII, IX, XI, and/or XII • Heparin • Lupus anticoagulant
High	Normal	• Factor VII deficiency • Warfarin • Vitamin K deficiency • Liver disease	• Inhibitor to factor VII
High	High	• Factor X deficiency • Factor V deficiency • Factor II deficiency • Dysfibrinogenemia or hypofibrinogenemia • Disseminated intravascular coagulation • Vitamin K deficiency (severe) • Warfarin (supratherapeutic)	• Inhibitor to factors X, V, and/or II • Heparin (supratherapeutic)

aPTT, Activated partial thromboplastin time; *PT*, prothrombin time.

The first step in the evaluation of an unexplained prolongation of PT and/or aPTT is to repeat the tests, since improper collection technique can introduce errors. Inadequate mixing of the blood tubes may allow the blood to clot prematurely, invalidating the sample for coagulation testing. Shaking of the collection tubes, or delays in processing the collected samples, can lead to premature activation or degradation of clotting factors. Marked polycythemia will prolong the PT and aPTT as the resultant low plasma volumes lead to a relative excess of citrate in the collection vial. Blood drawn from heparinized indwelling catheters can also prolong coagulation times if the heparin in the tubing is not appropriately removed.

If the coagulation abnormalities persist on repeated testing, the next step is to perform a mixing study to determine whether a coagulation factor inhibitor or a deficiency is responsible for the coagulation impairment. In a mixing study, a patient's plasma is mixed with normal plasma (containing normal amounts of coagulation factors) in a 1:1 mixture. Correction of PT or aPTT after mixing indicates a factor deficiency, while persistent prolongation of PT or aPTT after mixing indicates the presence of a factor inhibitor. Individual coagulation factor activities can then be measured to elucidate the specific coagulation factor impairment(s). Causes of prolonged PT and/or aPTT tests, categorized according to mixing study results, are shown in Table 34.1.

In general, a coagulation factor impairment due to a factor deficiency or inhibitor will lead to an increased risk of bleeding. An exception to this rule is a lupus anticoagulant, which may prolong aPTT, yet is typically associated with an increased risk of clotting due to antiphospholipid syndrome (reviewed in Chapter 145). Lupus anticoagulants are antiphospholipid antibodies that cause thrombosis through a variety of cell-dependent and cell-independent mechanisms. Because such antibodies bind and sequester phospholipids from the aPTT reaction mixture, aPTT times in patients with lupus anticoagulant are often prolonged in vitro. In patients with an isolated prolongation of aPTT, who have no significant bleeding history and in whom a 1:1 aPTT mixing study fails to correct, a lupus anticoagulant should be suspected.

CHAPTER 35

Abnormal Liver Function Tests

RACHEL FEDER

INTRODUCTION

The term **liver function tests** (LFTs) generally refers to a laboratory panel that includes the serum concentrations of albumin, alanine aminotransferase **(ALT)**, aspartate aminotransferase **(AST)**, alkaline phosphatase **(ALP)**, and **bilirubin.** This term is a misnomer, however, as these tests do not measure actual liver synthetic function; the term **liver chemistries** is more appropriate.

AST and ALT are aminotransferases involved in amino acid metabolism. AST converts aspartate and α-ketoglutarate to oxaloacetate and glutamate. ALT converts α-ketoglutarate and alanine to glutamate and pyruvate. AST is present in highest concentrations in the liver, though it is also present in cardiac muscle, skeletal muscle, and the kidneys, and to a much lesser extent in the brain, pancreas, lungs, leukocytes, and erythrocytes. In contrast, ALT is largely liver specific but is also present at low concentrations in the kidney, cardiac muscle, skeletal muscle, and pancreas. During hepatocellular injury and breakdown, AST and ALT in hepatocytes leak into the serum, raising their serum concentrations. For both, the upper limit of normal is 30 U/L in a male and 20 U/L in a female.

ALP is an enzyme that catalyzes dephosphorylation and is mainly produced in the liver, biliary epithelial cells, bone, intestine, and placenta. In the setting of bile duct obstruction, retained bile acids increase ALP production, leading to elevated serum concentrations. A concurrent elevation in the serum concentration of γ-glutamyl transpeptidase (GGT) generally confirms the ALP elevation reflects underlying biliary obstruction. GGT is produced in the canalicular membrane of hepatocytes and biliary epithelial cells, as well as in the kidney, pancreas, and small intestine. Biliary obstruction increases GGT production and elevates serum concentrations.

Bilirubin is a metabolite of heme normally conjugated in the liver and excreted into bile. The liver chemistry panel includes both direct and indirect bilirubin fractions. As detailed in Chapter 9, the direct fraction represents primarily conjugated bilirubin, while the indirect fraction represents unconjugated bilirubin. Indirect hyperbilirubinemia may reflect overproduction (usually from hemolysis) or impaired uptake or conjugation of bilirubin. In contrast, direct hyperbilirubinemia occurs when conjugated bilirubin is not properly excreted into the bile ducts or when hepatocytes are damaged and bilirubin leaks into the serum.

Given the location and function of these enzymes, liver chemistry abnormalities are often categorized into one of four patterns: hepatocellular injury, cholestasis, isolated hyperbilirubinemia, or a mixed pattern (Table 35.1). The hepatocellular injury pattern features elevated AST and ALT concentrations, a variable amount of direct hyperbilirubinemia, and a normal or only mildly elevated ALP. The cholestatic pattern features elevated ALP concentrations, milder AST and ALT abnormalities, and some degree of direct hyperbilirubinemia. In isolated hyperbilirubinemia, direct and/or indirect bilirubin concentrations may be elevated but the other values are normal. A mixed pattern features multiple abnormalities without a clear predominance.

Although the serum concentrations of these enzymes can be used to diagnose and monitor many diseases of the liver and biliary system, they are not markers of hepatic synthetic function and can be normal in patients with advanced liver disease. In contrast, serum albumin concentration and prothrombin time more accurately reflect hepatic synthetic function, since the liver synthesizes albumin and coagulation factors.

EVALUATION AND DIAGNOSIS
Hepatocellular Injury Pattern

The differential diagnosis depends on the degree of abnormality (Box 35.1). If a comprehensive review of medical comorbidities, medications, and supplements does not point to a specific cause, further workup should include an abdominal ultrasound with color Doppler imaging and additional laboratory tests. Of note, if a patient presents with **hepatocellular injury** and also has an elevated prothrombin time and/or encephalopathy, an urgent liver consultation should be undertaken to

TABLE 35.1
Liver Chemistry Abnormality Patterns

	AST/ALT	Alkaline Phosphatase	Bilirubin
Hepatocellular injury	↑↑	↑	↑
Cholestasis	↑	↑↑	↑↑
Isolated hyperbilirubinemia			↑↑

AST/ALT, Aspartate aminotransferase/alanine aminotransferase.

BOX 35.1
Differential Diagnosis for Hepatocellular Injury Pattern

AST AND ALT 2–5× THE UPPER LIMIT OF NORMAL

- Drug-induced hepatitis
- Chronic viral hepatitis
- Nonalcoholic fatty liver disease
- Alcoholic liver disease
- Hemochromatosis
- Autoimmune hepatitis
- Thyroid disease
- Celiac disease
- α1-antitrypsin antibody
- Wilson disease
- Adrenal insufficiency
- Congestive hepatopathy
- Myopathy
- Hepatic infiltration (sarcoidosis, amyloidosis, tuberculosis, malignancy)

AST AND ALT >5–10× THE UPPER LIMIT OF NORMAL

- Acute viral hepatitis
- Alcoholic hepatitis
- Drug-induced hepatitis (especially acetaminophen)
- Ischemic hepatitis ("shock liver")
- Budd-Chiari syndrome
- Autoimmune hepatitis
- Malignant infiltration of liver
- HELLP (hemolysis, elevated liver enzymes, low platelets) syndrome
- Toxin-induced hepatitis (e.g., wild mushroom ingestion)

ALT, Alanine aminotransferase; *AST,* aspartate aminotransferase.

assess for acute liver failure, which would warrant referral to a liver transplant center.

If AST and ALT are two to five times the upper limit of normal, the initial laboratory testing should include tests for chronic viral hepatitis (hepatitis B surface antigen [HBsAg], hepatitis B surface antibody [HBsAb], antibody against hepatitis C virus [anti-HCV]) and hemochromatosis (serum iron panel). If these are unremarkable, the next set should include tests for autoimmune hepatitis (antinuclear antibody, anti–smooth muscle antibody, anti–liver-kidney antibody, quantitative immunoglobulins), thyroid disease (thyroid-stimulating hormone [TSH], free thyroxine [T_4]), and celiac disease (anti–tissue transglutaminase antibodies). If these are also unremarkable, next check for Wilson disease (serum ceruloplasmin, urinary copper level), serum α1-antitrypsin antibody, adrenal insufficiency (morning cortisol/adrenocorticotropic hormone [ACTH], cortisol stimulation test), and myopathies (creatine kinase).

If AST and ALT are >5 to 15 times the upper limit of normal, the initial laboratory testing should include tests for acute viral hepatitis (anti–hepatitis A virus [anti-HAV] IgM, HBsAg, anti–hepatitis B core antigen [anti-HBc] IgM, anti-HCV), hemochromatosis, Wilson disease, acetaminophen overdose (serum level), and autoimmune hepatitis. In women of childbearing age, order a serum human chorionic gonadotropin (hCG) test and consider HELLP (hemolysis, elevated liver enzymes, low platelets) syndrome if anemia and thrombocytopenia are also present.

In those with ALT or AST levels >15 times the upper limit of normal, or a massive elevation ALT (>10,000 IU/L), the most likely diagnosis is either acetaminophen toxicity or ischemic hepatopathy (shock liver).

If AST and ALT concentrations remain persistent and unexplained despite extensive workup, a liver biopsy may be appropriate.

- Choledocholithiasis
- Acute cholangitis
- Malignant obstruction (primary or metastatic)
- Biliary stricture (malignancy, chronic pancreatitis, postinstrumentation)
- Infection (liver fluke, *Ascaris lumbricoides*, hepatic abscess, AIDS cholangiopathy)
- Primary sclerosing cholangitis
- Primary biliary cirrhosis
- Medications (see LiverTox database)
- Pregnancy
- Hepatic infiltration (sarcoidosis, amyloidosis, tuberculosis, malignancy)

Cholestatic Pattern

The differential diagnosis for the **cholestatic pattern** is shown in Box 35.2. If the history and physical examination do not suggest a particular cause, an appropriate initial workup is an abdominal ultrasound. If this is normal, the next step is to test for antimitochondrial antibodies, which are present in primary biliary cirrhosis, and perform a magnetic resonance cholangiopancreatography (MRCP). A liver biopsy may be necessary if ALP remains elevated without an explanation.

Isolated Hyperbilirubinemia

For isolated conjugated hyperbilirubinemia, the differential diagnosis is Dubin-Johnson or Rotor syndrome. For isolated unconjugated hyperbilirubinemia, the differential diagnosis is hemolysis, the use of certain medications (rifampin, probenecid), or Gilbert syndrome (see Chapter 9).

CHAPTER 36

Elevated Troponin

TOI N. SPATES

HISTORY OF DIAGNOSTIC TESTING

While the troponin complex within the cardiomyocyte was identified in the mid-1960s, it was not until the 1990s that technology made it feasible to detect serum troponin levels. Prior to that development, a variety of markers were used to evaluate myocardial injury. Aspartate aminotransferase (AST) was first used in the 1950s, but its ubiquity offered limited specificity for cardiac injury. The 1970s saw the use of creatine kinase (CK) and lactate dehydrogenase (LDH), but although they were more specific for cardiac injury, significant overlap with other pathology remained. The isoenzyme **CK-MB** (creatine kinase-myocardial band, as it was developed using electrophoresis) was more specific for cardiac damage and was in use through the 1990s until the development of radioimmunoassays for troponin. Troponin proved more sensitive and specific, and it became the primary cardiac-specific biomarker in clinical use. In the 2010s, the fifth-generation high-sensitivity troponins were developed to detect much smaller concentrations of troponin as compared to the predecessors, aiding in the ability to efficiently detect those with trends consistent with acute myocardial infarction (AMI).

Each of these biomarkers, although of varying sensitivity and specificity, are detected the following times after myocardial injury: AST 3 to 4 hours, LDH 5 to 10 hours, CK-MB 3 to 8 hours, and troponin I/T 3 to 8 hours. Time to peak for frequently used biomarkers includes CK-MB after 24 hours and troponin I/T after 12 to 24 hours (depending on the infarct size).

BACKGROUND AND PATHOPHYSIOLOGY

The cardiomyocyte contains two key structural components: thick filaments containing **myosin** and thin filaments containing **actin**. Regulatory contractile units derived from troponin protein complexes and tropomyosin control the interaction of myosin and actin (Fig. 36.1). Coordination of these components, along with calcium-triggered adenosine triphosphate (ATP) use, yields muscle contraction. The troponin protein complex is crucial in the initial step of calcium binding and is derived from three distinct subunits: troponin C, T, and I. Thus troponin is a fundamental component of the cardiomyocyte and is typically only present in the serum in pathological states where the myocardium experiences a demand event resulting in injury. Because troponin C is also found on noncardiac skeletal muscle, hospital assays for cardiac-specific troponins detect either troponin T or I. The troponin subunits exist bound to cardiac filaments within the free cytosolic pool.

Myocardial demand is any increased work or stress experienced by the myocardium. Demand increases when the rate of myocardial contraction exceeds the body's ability to supply oxygenated blood to the myocardium during diastolic filling of the coronary arteries. As a result, the myocardium can suffer injury during episodes of increased demand, leading to release of the cytosolic pool and troponin residing there. Prolonged demand causes accumulated myocardial injury, leading to myocardial necrosis, cell death, and further release of troponin. The classic scenario of myocardial demand and injury is that of an acute thrombotic event resulting in myocardial infarction (MI), but the dynamic of myocardial demand and myocardial injury can be seen in a number of clinical scenarios.

DIFFERENTIAL DIAGNOSIS

When a patient has elevated troponin, the most important diagnostic breakpoint is whether the underlying cause is related to myocardial necrosis from acute coronary syndrome (ACS) or is due to nonthrombotic myocardial injury. (Refer to Chapter 58 for further details on the diagnosis and management of ACS.) A discussion of instances of nonthrombotic myocardial injury follows; in each of these scenarios there is effective ischemia from inadequate perfusion without evidence of a thrombotic coronary event and cell necrosis. The progression from ischemia to true MI and cell necrosis can be produced by a continuum of prolonged injury or demand despite the absence of discrete thrombosis.

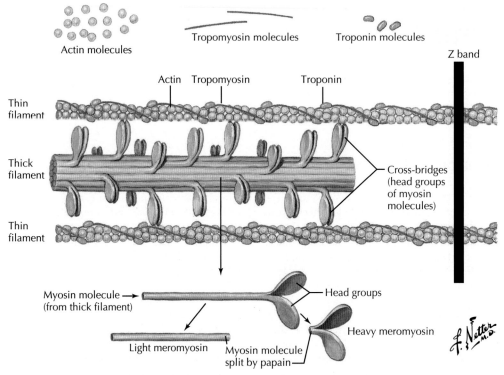

FIG. 36.1 **Composition and Structure of Myofilaments.**

For patients with left ventricular (LV) dysfunction, volume overload, or tachyarrhythmias, troponins are often released in small but detectable amounts secondary to either stretch release of troponins or rate-dependent myocardial injury. These scenarios can be further confounded in patients with chronic kidney disease, because of the cumulative effect of multiple episodes of demand and the limited ability to excrete troponin filtered by the kidney. A baseline troponin level in patients with chronic kidney disease and known cardiovascular disease is useful to evaluate the degree of elevation and the likelihood of a true ACS event.

LV dysfunction can be seen in patients with severe **congestive heart failure,** fulminant **myocarditis,** or cor pulmonale. In patients with congestive heart failure, myocardial oxygen demand is increased during episodes of increased ventricular volume and pressure. Increased volume and pressure lead to increased ventricular wall tension, causing stretch-mediated release of troponins. Ventricular dysfunction in patients with elevated troponin is generally more severe than those patients with no detectable troponin.

Another cause of non-ACS troponin release is **Takotsubo stress cardiomyopathy,** often identified as a diagnosis of exclusion. Takotsubo stress cardiomyopathy can present with both the symptomatology and electrocardiogram (ECG) changes consistent with an AMI but diagnostically shows no evidence of coronary disease on cardiac catheterization. Myocardial injury is related to a direct catecholamine surge seen in patients under stressful situations, causing apical ballooning, dyskinesis, and general LV dysfunction (Fig. 36.2).

Troponin elevation can also be seen in direct trauma to the myocardium in patients with cardiac contusions, recent defibrillation, or ablative procedures. Each of the preceding etiologies results in an elevation of serum troponins in the absence of a thrombotic event characteristic of MI.

Noncardiac causes of elevated troponin include pulmonary embolism, cardiotoxic medications, hypoxic respiratory failure, arrhythmias, severe anemia, hemispheric cerebral infarct, or generalized cardiac inflammation. Patients with sepsis (in particular, septic shock) have elevated troponin through increased myocardial demand, poor myocardial perfusion consistent with shock, and an independent cytokine effect. Tumor necrosis factor-α (TNF-α), interleukin-1 (IL-1), and IL-6 are all released in sepsis, and part of this characteristic dysregulated

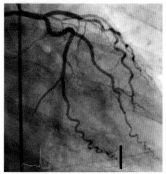

A. Coronary angiogram showing nonobstructive disease of the left coronary artery.

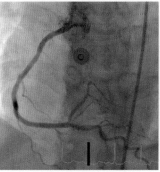

B. Coronary angiogram showing nonobstructive disease of the right coronary artery.

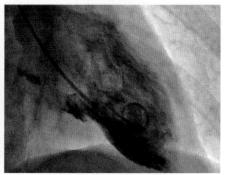

C. Normal end-diastolic left ventriculogram.

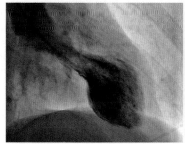

D. End-systolic left ventriculogram showing apical ballooning.

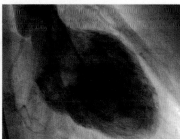

E. Normal end-diastolic left ventriculogram.

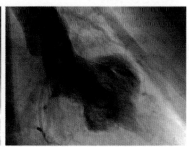

F. End-systolic left ventriculogram showing midventricular ballooning.

FIG. 36.2 **Takotsubo Stress Cardiomyopathy.**

inflammatory response is resultant increased membrane permeability promoting troponin leak. An increase in inflammatory-mediated cytokines and cortisol seen after large strokes also potentiates a small elevation in troponin.

DIAGNOSIS

A thorough history and physical exam helps the clinician delineate potential etiologies of troponin elevation. While a pattern of illness will arise to direct testing, it is always important to rule out true ACS with serial troponin levels and ECGs as guided by the clinical situation.

Basic blood work, including basic metabolic panel and complete blood count, can evaluate for chronic kidney disease that leads to decreased troponin clearance and anemia, which can decrease the heart's ability to respond to increased demand. Other tests to consider include brain natriuretic peptide (BNP) for congestive heart failure, D-dimer and the modified Wells score for pulmonary embolism, and urine toxicology for sympathomimetics such as cocaine.

The ECG is critical for evaluating a patient with elevated troponin (see Chapter 38 for further details). In addition to patterns of MI, the ECG can reveal signs of strain indicative of LV dysfunction. A bedside echocardiogram can elucidate wall motion abnormalities consistent with a particular vascular territory, implying coronary artery disease.

CHAPTER 37

Urinalysis

ANTHONY VALERI

INTRODUCTION

Urinalysis screens for the presence of several substances in the urine, which can indicate underlying pathology. This broad applicability has made it one of the most common screening tests available, enhanced by its availability as a point-of-care test with rapid interpretation. Colloquially, a **urine dipstick** is a simple bedside test that assesses urine by multiple parameters and is discarded once interpreted (Fig. 37.1). More specific testing, including sediment evaluation and microscopy, can be ordered as clinically warranted or if the dipstick is positive for certain findings (e.g., heme-positive urine can be further evaluated to determine the number of red blood cells [RBCs] per high-power field [HPF]).

While not part of the typical dipstick, **urine electrolytes** provide crucial information on the kidney's ability to concentrate urine and handle the metabolism of several electrolytes.

DIPSTICK

Proteinuria results from multiple pathologies and is readily detected on urinalysis. The urinalysis can detect albumin and other large molecular weight proteins, but small molecular weight proteins may not be detected. When positive, the amount should be quantified with a spot urine protein to creatinine ratio (UP:UC) and a spot urine albumin to creatinine ratio (UA:UC) to determine precisely the amount and type of protein; 24-hour urine collections are the most accurate but can be time consuming, and urine protein electrophoresis can quantify the amounts of each protein subtype present.

As small molecular weight proteins may not be detected on routine urinalysis, a significant discrepancy between the dipstick proteinuria and the UP:UC (higher UP:UC out of proportion to the dipstick proteinuria) suggests the presence of an excess of a small molecular weight protein, such as Bence-Jones protein. Bence-Jones proteins are immunoglobulin light chains, which collect in the renal tubules. This should prompt a further investigation for a possible plasma cell dyscrasia, including monoclonal gammopathy of undetermined significance (MGUS) or multiple myeloma (see Chapter 146 for further details).

Protein may be qualified on a urinalysis as trace to 4+, each level of which has an associated approximate quantity. For specific measures, a UA:UC <30 μg of albumin per 1 g creatinine is considered normal. Micro-albuminuria (an early indicator of diabetic nephropathy) is 30 to 299 μg/g, while macroalbuminuria is >300 μg/g.

The UP:UC accounts for all protein in the urine; a UP:UC >3 g protein per 1 g creatinine, or a UA:UC >2000 μg/g, is consistent with nephrotic range proteinuria. The **nephrotic syndrome,** however, requires additional criteria, including serum albumin <3.5 g/dL and peripheral edema (see Chapter 97 for further details). Subnephrotic proteinuria can be found in early/mild forms of glomerular disease, such as diabetic nephropathy, or in tubulointerstitial renal diseases.

The most common cause of elevated glucose in the urine **(glycosuria)** is an elevated serum glucose, frequently from diabetes mellitus. Glycosuria in a nondiabetic patient with normal serum glucose may represent proximal renal tubular injury (renal glycosuria) with consideration of nephrotoxic injury, such as recent chemotherapy (e.g., cisplatin). Light-chain Fanconi syndrome is a proximal tubulopathy arising from excess monoclonal immunoglobulin light-chain accumulation. Other features suggestive of Fanconi syndrome with proximal tubular injury and renal wasting include hypophosphatemia, hypouricemia, and hypomagnesemia (all due to excessive renal excretion of those electrolytes) and a type II renal tubular acidosis (RTA).

The heme parameter on a standard urinalysis detects the presence of globin in the urine. Thus a heme-positive high urine osmolality, free hemoglobin in the blood due to intravascular hemolysis, or free myoglobin due to rhabdomyolysis.

Both **leukocyte esterase** and **nitrites** assess for the presence of a urinary tract infection (UTI). Leukocyte esterase is produced by white blood cells (WBCs), and positivity suggests the presence of WBCs in the urine. Nitrites suggest the presence of *Enterobacteriaceae*, which convert urinary nitrates to nitrites. Notably, the presence of WBCs does not necessarily guarantee a UTI (e.g., chronic interstitial nephritis), and positive nitrites indicate bacteriuria but not necessarily infection (e.g., colonization). Microscopy and sediment analysis can quantify the number of WBCs in the urine (**pyuria** >5 WBCs/HPF), but any test result must be correlated with symptoms before treatment is considered.

The urine specific gravity (SG) can approximate urine osmolality, with a low SG corresponding to dilute urine. However, actual measurement of urine osmolality is crucial for patients with hyponatremia, hypernatremia, acute kidney injury, and polyuria. Urinary ketones can indicate a fasting state or, in a patient with diabetes, diabetic ketoacidosis.

SEDIMENT ANALYSIS AND MICROSCOPY
(Fig. 37.2)

Sediment analysis and microscopy can further refine findings on a dipstick and detect a wide array of substances not tested on a standard dipstick. **Hematuria,** or RBCs in the urine, signifies bleeding anywhere along the urinary tract. This includes glomerular hematuria manifested by dysmorphic RBCs, nephrolithiasis, tumors, or infections in the urinary tract (see Chapter 14 for further details).

Pyuria is usually associated with a UTI or acute interstitial nephritis. Acute interstitial nephritis most often results from medications and is suggested by negative urine culture and/or the presence of peripheral eosinophilia with fever/rash. Eosinophils in the urine support the diagnosis but are not required.

Casts are structures formed within a tubular lumen. They are comprised of embedded cells (including RBCs and WBCs) in a matrix of Tamm-Horsfall protein, which is present in the loop of Henle. RBC casts suggest a proliferative glomerulonephritis, but their absence does not rule it out. WBC casts indicate interstitial inflammation. Granular casts are degenerated cells within the Tamm-Horsfall cast matrix, often appearing in the setting of renal injury; muddy-brown granular casts are seen in acute tubular necrosis. Hyaline casts are common in concentrated urine or in patients taking diuretics.

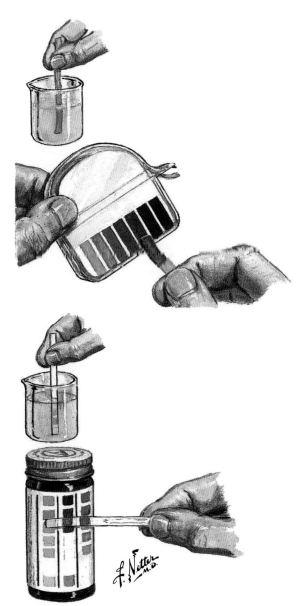

Aside from measuring the urine pH *(top)*, the dipstick combines several tests on the same strip. Color changes for each measurement are compared to the key found on the outside of the testing kit *(bottom)*.

FIG. 37.1 Dipstick Testing.

urinalysis can derive from RBCs, free hemoglobin, or myoglobin in the urine. Microscopic evaluation is key to further evaluate heme-positive urinalysis. If no RBCs are visualized on urine sediment analysis, it suggests either RBC lysis in the urine due to very low or very

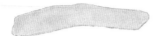

Hyaline casts
- Seen in normal individuals and prerenal state
- Formed by aggregation of Tamm-Horsfall mucoprotein in distal tubule, especially when there is low urine flow

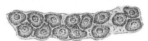

Epithelial cell casts
- Formed by sloughed renal tubular cells and Tamm-Horsfall mucoprotein in distal tubule
- Often (but not always) seen in acute tubular necrosis

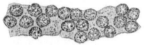

White blood cell casts
- Formed by leukocytes that enter tubules and aggregate with Tamm-Horsfall mucoprotein
- Seen in acute interstitial nephritis, exudative glomerulonephritis, and severe pyelonephritis

Red blood cells
- May reflect glomerular disease, papillary necrosis, pyelonephritis, cystitis, urinary tract malignancy, urolithiasis, and many others

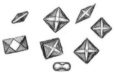

Oxalate crystals
- May be seen with calcium oxalate stones
- Also indicate ethylene glycol ingestion or other hyperoxaluria

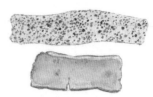

Coarsely granular casts
Waxy casts
- Formed by the breakdown of cellular casts
- Nonspecific indicators of intrarenal disease
- Muddy brown pigmentation of coarsely granular casts may be seen in acute tubular necrosis

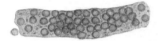

Red blood cell casts
- Formed by red blood cells that enter the tubules at the glomerulus and then aggregate with Tamm-Horsfall mucoprotein
- Indicate glomerular disease

Dysmorphic red blood cells
- Formed as red blood cells pass through pores in damaged glomerular capillaries
- Indicate glomerular disease

White blood cells
- Major causes are cystitis, pyelonephritis, and acute interstitial nephritis

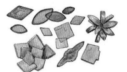

Uric acid crystals
- May be seen with uric acid stones
- May also be seen in tumor lysis syndrome

FIG. 37.2 **Possible Urine Sediment Findings.**

Crystal structures may be visible in the urinary sediment as well and can represent an underlying pathology.

Urine Electrolytes

Urine electrolytes are helpful in the evaluation of several renal-related diseases. Urine sodium can be useful in acute kidney injury by calculation of the **fractional excretion of sodium (FE$_{Na}$)** or in the evaluation of hyponatremia. Patients with acute kidney injury who have received diuretics should have a **FE$_{urea}$** measured, as the urine sodium will be inappropriately high due to

diuretic effect (see Chapters 27 and 30 for further details). The urine potassium, along with the U$_K$:U$_{creat}$ ratio and the FE$_K$, can help distinguish the cause of hypokalemia as extrarenal (e.g., gastrointestinal losses) or intrarenal (e.g., renal potassium wasting) (see Chapter 28).

Urine chloride, along with FE$_{Cl}$, is helpful in distinguishing the cause of a metabolic alkalosis. A U$_{Cl}$ <20 or FE$_{Cl}$ <1% suggests a chloride-deficient metabolic alkalosis (formerly known as a contraction alkalosis) due to volume depletion. A U$_{Cl}$ >40 or FE$_{Cl}$ >3% suggests a chloride-replete metabolic alkalosis, more likely due to a primary or secondary hyperaldosteronism or to an inherited syndrome, such as Bartter, Gitelman, or Liddle syndrome.

The **urinary anion gap** can help determine the cause of a nonanion gap metabolic acidosis. The urinary anion gap is calculated as:

$$(U_{Na} + U_K) - U_{Cl} \qquad \textbf{EQ. 37.1}$$

A negative urinary anion gap suggests the production of NH_3 (ammoniagenesis) in the proximal renal tubules, which in turn suggests a nonrenal cause of metabolic acidosis (diarrhea, etc.) or a type I or II RTA. A positive urinary anion gap indicates impaired ammoniagenesis, often due to hyperkalemia, as seen in a type IV RTA.

CHAPTER 38

Electrocardiogram (ECG)

PAULA ROY-BURMAN

INTRODUCTION

The electrocardiogram (ECG) is a noninvasive and inexpensive diagnostic tool used to assess the structure and function of the heart. It is the cornerstone in the workup of cardiac complaints and diseases, especially chest pain and cardiac arrhythmias. It is also used to evaluate metabolic and pharmacological effects on the heart.

In addition to understanding the waveforms that comprise a normal tracing, accurate interpretation requires a systematic approach. In this chapter we will first describe the elements to obtain a recording (i.e., the ECG grid and leads). After a description of the waveforms and the conduction system, we will discuss a generalized, stepwise method to reading an ECG.

BASIC PRINCIPLES: PAPER AND LEADS

The ECG is a graph of voltage over time recorded on specialized paper incorporating a 1×1-mm grid. Every fifth line of the grid is bolded to create 5×5-mm large boxes. Conventionally, every 10 mm in height is equal to 1 mV, and the paper is run at a speed of 25 mm/s; these measurement parameters are specified in the corner of every ECG but may vary depending on the ECG machine used. In this standard convention, each 1-mm square or small box represents 0.04 s (40 ms), and each 5-mm large box represents 0.20 s (200 ms).

The complete ECG recording captures 10 s in time and portrays 12 electrical views of the heart. A 2.5-s interval is graphed for each lead in the first three rows of the ECG. The last row is called the rhythm strip and is a full 10-s recording from a single, preselected lead (Fig. 38.1).

The 12 leads of the ECG are divided into **limb** and **precordial leads.** The six limb leads are obtained by placing four electrodes—right arm (RA), right leg (RL), left arm (LA), and left leg (LL)—onto their respective appendages. Notably, the RL electrode serves as an electrical ground and does not otherwise contribute to the tracing. The limb leads capture electrical activity

from the frontal plane. They are subdivided into bipolar (I, II, and III) and unipolar augmented (aVR, aVL, and aVF) leads. The bipolar leads record the difference in electrical potential between two given limbs (e.g., lead I is the change in potential from RA to LA). The augmented unipolar leads record the potential between one limb and the average of the remaining limbs (e.g., lead aVR is the change in potential from the combination of LA and LL to RA) (Fig. 38.2).

The remaining six leads are the precordial leads (V_1–V_6). Like the augmented leads, these leads are unipolar, but each lead has its own electrode. The leads are oriented along the horizontal plane with V_1 and V_2 placed at the fourth intercostal space (ICS) on the right and left side of the sternum, respectively. Lead V_4 is placed at the fifth ICS at the left midclavicular line, and V_6 is placed at the left midaxillary line at the level of V_4. The remaining leads, V_3 and V_5, are placed midway between V_2 and V_4, and V_4 and V_6, respectively.

ECG TRACING AND RELATED PHYSIOLOGY OF THE CONDUCTION SYSTEM

The ECG tracing is composed of waves (P, QRS, T, and U), segments (PR, ST, and TP), and intervals (PR, QRS, and QT). These components relay information regarding the propagation of electrical activity through the cardiac conduction system (Fig. 38.3).

The **P wave** represents sequential right then left atrial depolarization. When arising from the sinoatrial node, the deflection is positive (or upright) in all leads except aVR where it is negative (inverted). The wave may be slightly notched in the limb leads and is often biphasic (i.e., first upright then inverted) in leads V_1 and V_2.

The impulse then slows as it travels through the atrioventricular (AV) node and His-Purkinje system. This passage of time is represented by the PR segment, which exists between the end of the P wave and the beginning of the **QRS complex.** The **PR interval,** which combines

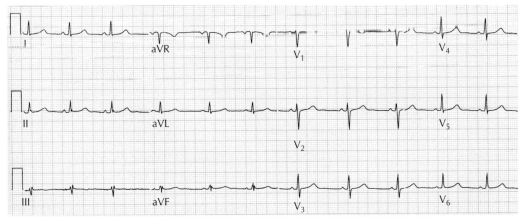

Example of a normal ECG recorded from a 24-year-old woman. Note that the P wave is upright in leads I and II and inverted in aVR. The QRS complex gradually changes from negative in V_1 to positive in V_6. Note that the polarity of the T wave is similar to that of the QRS complex.

FIG. 38.1 **Normal Electrocardiogram *(ECG)***

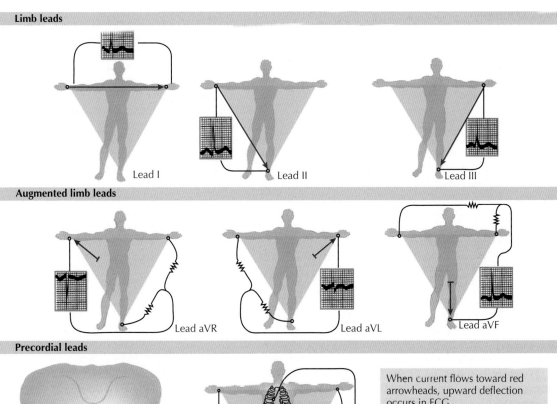

Limb leads

Lead I   Lead II   Lead III

Augmented limb leads

Lead aVR   Lead aVL   Lead aVF

Precordial leads

V_6
V_5
V_1 V_2 V_3 V_4

When current flows toward red arrowheads, upward deflection occurs in ECG

When current flows away from red arrowheads, downward deflection occurs in ECG

When current flows perpendicular to red arrows, no deflection or biphasic deflection occurs

FIG. 38.2 **Limb and Precordial Leads.** *ECG,* Electrocardiogram.

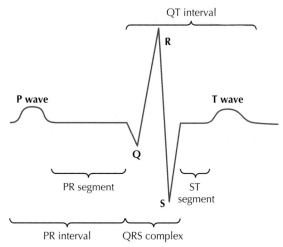

FIG. 38.3 **Basic Components of the Electrocardiogram.**

the P wave and the PR segment, lasts between 120 and 200 ms, or 3 to 5 small boxes.

Next, the impulse travels through the left and right bundle branches to depolarize the ventricles, which corresponds to the QRS complex. By convention, the first positive deflection is the **R wave;** a negative deflection before the R wave is a **Q wave,** while a negative deflection following the R wave is the **S wave.** On occasion, the S wave is followed by a second positive deflection referred to as an **R′ wave**. Moving across the precordial leads, the R-wave amplitude will increase (with a concordant decrease in S-wave amplitude) known as R-wave progression. The normal duration (or width) of the QRS complex, also known as the QRS interval, is 60 to 100 ms, or 1.5 to 2.5 small boxes.

There is a brief period of ventricular recovery **(ST segment)** followed by rapid ventricular repolarization **(T wave).** The ST segment is generally isoelectric, whereas the T wave is an asymmetric, broad, and positive wave (except in aVR and V_1, where it is negative). A general measure of ventricular repolarization is ascertained by the **QT interval,** consisting of the QRS complex, ST segment, and T wave. Normal duration is <440 ms in men and <460 ms in women; however, the measurement is quite sensitive to changes in rate. Thus formulas are used to calculate a **corrected QT (QTc).**

The last elements of the ECG tracing are the TP segment and the U wave. The TP segment represents the period between cardiac cycles in which the myocardial cells are electrically silent. The segment is isoelectric and used as the baseline to determine whether other portions of the ECG are elevated or depressed. The source of the U wave remains unclear. When present, it is a broad and positive wave of small amplitude immediately following the T wave. It is usually associated with an abnormality (e.g., bradycardia or hypokalemia), but it is sometimes seen in the midprecordial leads of a normal ECG.

SYSTEMATIC APPROACH TO INTERPRETING THE ECG

There are multiple approaches to reading the ECG. The six-step method presented here is a broad framework and is by no means comprehensive. We will start by assessing the rate, rhythm, and axis, followed by evaluation of intervals, chamber size, and infarct/ischemia.

The normal ventricular rate is between 60 and 100 beats per minute (bpm). Rates <60 bpm are bradycardic and those >100 bpm are tachycardic. The ventricular rate is calculated by counting the number of QRS complexes across one row (usually the rhythm strip) of the standard ECG and multiplying by six. If the QRS complexes recur in regular intervals, the number of large boxes can be counted between two R waves and divided into 300 (i.e., rate = 300/number of large boxes).

Rhythm is determined by assessing for the presence of P waves, the regularity of QRS complexes, and the association between P waves and QRS complexes. If P waves are absent and QRS complexes are regular, consider a rhythm arising from the AV node or ventricles. If the rhythm is irregular and lacking P waves, consider atrial fibrillation. If P waves do not precede every QRS complex, consider AV nodal block or complete dissociation (Fig. 38.4) (see Chapter 21 for further details).

The rotation of the heart in the frontal plane is known as the axis, which is normally between −30 degrees and +90 degrees (Fig. 38.5).
- **Left axis deviation (LAD)** falls between −30 degrees and −90 degrees.
- **Right axis deviation (RAD)** is between +90 degrees and 180 degrees.
- An axis between −90 degrees and 180 degrees is an **extreme axis** (extreme right or left).

The simplest method to determine the axis involves looking at leads I, aVF, and II. If the vector of the QRS complex is positive (i.e., the sum of forces is directed above the TP baseline) in I and aVF, the axis is normal. If they are both negative, there exists an extreme axis deviation. If I is negative but aVF is positive, there exists RAD. If I is positive but aVF is negative, the axis may be normal (i.e., between 0 degrees and −30 degrees) or leftward. Lead II is used as a tie-breaker. If II is positive, the axis is normal. If negative, there is LAD (Fig. 38.6).

AV Nodal Reentrant Tachycardia

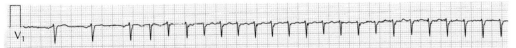

A. Lead V_1 recorded from a patient with abnormal cardiac rhythms. This tracing shows the onset of AV nodal reentrant tachycardia in a 47-year-old man. There are three sinus beats followed by an atrial premature beat, which initiates a run of AV nodal reentrant tachycardia, with a rate of 170 bpm.

Ventricular Tachycardia

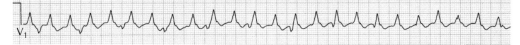

B. Ventricular tachycardia with a rate of 150 bpm from a 56-year-old man. The QRS complex is widened, and there is AV disassociation. The P waves, with an atrial rate of 73 bpm, are marked with an asterisk.

Atrial Fibrillation

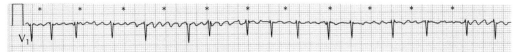

C. Example of atrial fibrillation in a 50-year-old woman. Note the undulating baseline and the irregularly irregular QRS complexes, with a rate of 105 bpm.

Complete AV Block

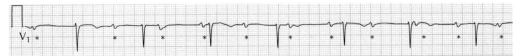

D. Complete AV block from a 78-year-old woman. The atrial rate is 70 bpm, and the ventricular rate is 46 bpm. There is no relation between the P waves *(asterisks)* and the QRS complexes.

FIG. 38.4 **Select Cardiac Arrhythmias.** *AV,* Atrioventricular; *bpm,* beats per minute.

Prolongation of the PR, QRS, or QT interval is pathological. AV nodal blocks are diagnosed in the setting of PR prolongation (i.e., >200 ms). QRS intervals >100 ms can be seen in the setting of aberrant conduction such as **right bundle branch block** (manifesting a QRS >120 ms and rSR′ pattern in V_1–V_2), **left bundle branch block** (QRS >120 ms and broad or notched R wave in I, aVL, and V_5–V_6), and preexcitation syndromes such as **Wolff-Parkinson-White** (Fig. 38.7). A wide QRS also is seen in rhythms originating from the ventricles. QT prolongation has wide-ranging causes, including electrolyte abnormalities (e.g., hypokalemia and hypocalcemia), hypothermia, myocardial infarction, and congenital long

QT syndrome. However, the most frequent causes of QT prolongation are medications, including antiarrhythmics, (e.g., amiodarone), antipsychotics (e.g., haloperidol), antidepressants (e.g., citalopram), antihistamines (e.g., loratadine), and antimicrobials (e.g., erythromycin).

The morphology of the P wave and QRS complex can be evaluated for atrial and ventricular enlargement, respectively. Leads II and V_1 are used to determine atrial enlargement. **Right atrial enlargement** is defined by an exaggerated P-wave height (i.e., >2.5 mm in II, or >1.5 mm in V_1). **Left atrial enlargement** is more subtle, suggested by P-wave duration >110 ms (lead II), interpeak interval >40 ms in a notched P (lead II), or duration >40 ms in the inverted portion of the P wave (lead V_1).

Left ventricular hypertrophy (LVH) is evaluated by multiple criteria; commonly used criteria include:

- R in aVL >11 mm (Sokolow-Lyon)
- S in V_1 + tallest R in V_5 or V_6 >35 mm (Sokolow-Lyon)
- R in aVL + S in V_3 >28 mm (men) and >20 mm (women) (Cornell) (Fig. 38.8)

Right ventricular hypertrophy (RVH) is defined by the presence of RAD, a dominant R wave in V_1 (i.e., >7 mm or R/S ratio >1), and a dominant S wave in either V_5 or V_6 (i.e., >7 mm or R/S ratio >1).

In the last step, we evaluate for ischemia and infarct by reviewing the ST segments, T waves, and QRS complexes. It is important to note that, in the absence of appropriate clinical history or physical exam findings, abnormality of ST segments or T waves is nonspecific. They can either occur as normal variants in healthy patients or represent other metabolic or cardiopulmonary disease.

In the setting of **acute coronary syndrome (ACS)**, elevation or depression of ST segments is seen with concomitant T-wave changes (Fig. 38.9). These must occur in two or more contiguous leads, which follow an anatomical pattern (Table 38.1). ST-segment depression is a downward deviation of ≥0.5 mm from the TP baseline. It is measured 2 mm after the J point (i.e., the junction between the terminus of the QRS complex and the start of the ST segment). ST-segment elevation is measured at the J point and, with the exception of leads V_2 and V_3, is defined as an upward deviation of ≥1 mm. The elevation thresholds in leads V_2 and V_3 are ≥2.5 mm in men <40 years old, ≥2 mm in men ≥40 years old, and ≥1.5 mm in women of any age. While T-wave changes may be seen in normal patients or more benign conditions, new or deep T-wave inversions, especially those that fluctuate on serial ECGs, are concerning for ACS (see Chapter 58 for further details).

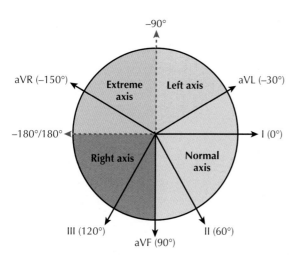

FIG. 38.5 **Axis on the Electrocardiogram.**

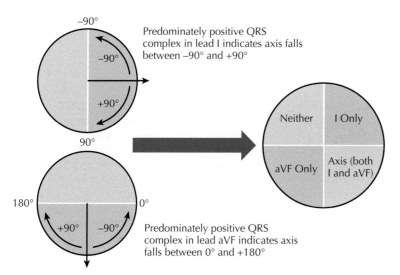

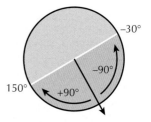

FIG. 38.6 **Identifying Normal Axis.**

Bundle Branch Block

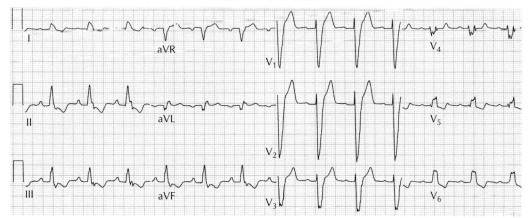

A. ECG showing left bundle branch block. It was recorded from a 73-year old man. Note that the QRS complex is diffusely widened with broad R waves in I, V_5, and V_6 (lateral leads) and notching in V_3–V_6. Note also that the T wave is directed opposite to the QRS complex. This is an example of a secondary T-wave change

Ventricular Preexcitation

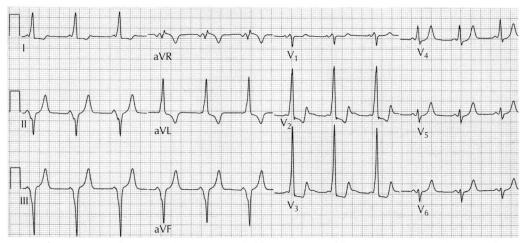

B. ECG showing ventricular preexcitation. It is recorded from a 28-year-old woman. Note the short PR interval (0.9 s) and the widened QRS complex (0.134 s). The initial portion of the QRS complex appears slurred. This is referred to as a delta wave. This combination of short PR interval and widened QRS complex with a delta wave is characteristic of Wolff-Parkinson-White, a specific type of ventricular preexcitation. Note also that the T wave is abnormal, another example of a secondary T-wave change.

FIG. 38.7 **Bundle Branch Block and Ventricular Preexcitation.** *ECG,* Electrocardiogram.

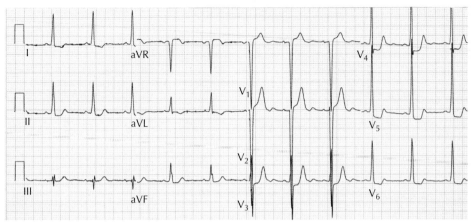

Example of the ECG changes of LVH. It is recorded from an 83-year-old woman with aortic stenosis and insufficiency. Note the increase in QRS amplitude, the slight increase in QRS duration to 100 ms, and the ST-segment and T-wave changes.

FIG. 38.8 **Left Ventricular Hypertrophy *(LVH)* on Electrocardiogram *(ECG)*.**

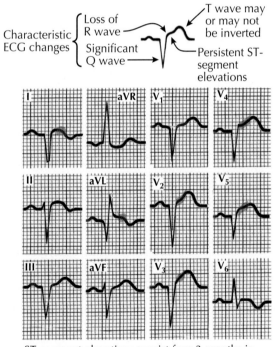

ST-segment elevations persist for >3 months in area of infarct

FIG. 38.9 **ST Elevations.** *ECG*, Electrocardiogram.

TABLE 38.1
Anatomical and Electrocardiographic Correlates

Leads	Wall	Artery
I, aVL, V$_5$, V$_6$	Lateral wall	Left circumflex
II, III, aVF	Inferior wall	Right coronary
V$_1$, V$_2$	Septum	Left anterior descending
V$_3$, V$_4$	Anterior wall	Left anterior descending

The hallmark of an old or evolving infarct is the Q wave. Pathological Q waves occur in two or more contiguous leads and are variably defined (e.g., >1 mm wide, >2 mm deep, or ≥25% of the QRS height). A prior anterior wall infarction may not manifest as Q waves, but instead as poor R-wave progression across the precordium or as QS waves (an entirely negative QRS complex) in leads V$_2$ and V$_3$. An evolving infarct will have Q waves in the presence of ongoing ST-segment and T-wave changes.

CHAPTER 39

Chest Radiography

THEODORE T. PIERCE

INTRODUCTION

The chest radiograph is one of the most commonly performed radiographic exams. Its rapidity, portability, and ability to identify life-threating conditions make it an integral component in diagnostic evaluation. While skilled radiograph interpretation yields remarkable diagnostic information, cross-sectional techniques, such as CT, are useful for providing a more detailed evaluation of thoracic structures and confirming critical findings.

TECHNIQUE

A chest radiograph is obtained by exposing the chest to electromagnetic radiation within the x-ray spectrum. At these energy levels, different tissues attenuate the beam to varying degrees, allowing only some photons to travel through the patient to be measured by a detector. Metal and bone, owing to their density and chemical composition, attenuate x-rays to the greatest degree and will appear whiter (more opaque). Air attenuates the beam to a lesser degree and will appear blacker (more lucent). Water and fat are of intermediate density and will appear grey with fat relatively more lucent. When two structures of differing density are in contact, a crisp line demarcating the structures will be visible when the x-ray beam is tangential to the boundary. Absence of an expected interface is known as the **silhouette sign,** which can localize pathological processes.

High-quality frontal chest radiographs are typically obtained in the upright position, with the patient in full inspiration and the x-ray beam traversing the patient from posterior to anterior (PA—as opposed to anterior posterior [AP]). An accompanying lateral projection can be particularly helpful in identifying lower lobe pneumonia, pleural effusions, and localizing masses. Specialized views can be obtained as needed (e.g., oblique images of the chest wall to assess for rib fracture, decubitus views to diagnose fluid loculation, and expiratory images to identify air trapping).

Given that three-dimensional anatomical delineation can be challenging on a two-dimensional radiograph,

straying from these technical parameters will significantly reduce the sensitivity and specificity of the exam for detecting pathology. Semiupright or supine radiographs can easily obscure the detection of intraperitoneal free air, pleural effusions, or pneumothoraces, and images obtained during shallow inspiration can result in lung opacities that mimic pulmonary edema or pneumonia. AP radiographs result in magnification of the cardiomediastinal silhouette, mimicking a pericardial effusion. Lastly, due to a variety of technical limitations, portable x-ray machines generate inferior images compared to fixed imaging systems. As a result, PA/lateral radiographs should be sought unless the patient's clinical status is so tenuous as to limit patient positioning or prohibit the patient from traveling to the radiology department for an exam.

KEY DIAGNOSES

Pneumonia

At the microscopic level, pneumonia results in replacement of intraalveolar air with bacteria, inflammatory cells, cellular debris, and fluid. This material has a greater density on chest radiograph, appearing as an opacity, which may be confined to part of a lobe, all of a lobe, or multiple lobes (see Chapter 114 for further details). Given that the air is replaced by material, the opacity should be space occupying, with no loss of volume as seen in atelectasis.

The silhouette sign is used to localize pneumonia. Obscuration of the normal diaphragmatic contour suggests lower lobe pneumonia, while loss of the right cardiac border suggests right middle lobe involvement (Fig. 39.1). Upper lobe pneumonia can be difficult to definitively identify on a frontal radiograph alone, given the significant overlap of the upper lobes with the superior segment of the lower lobes, but the lateral radiograph is often definitive in differentiating the two. The lateral radiograph also is helpful for identifying posterior lower lobe pneumonia, which can be obscured on the frontal projection. Under normal conditions, the

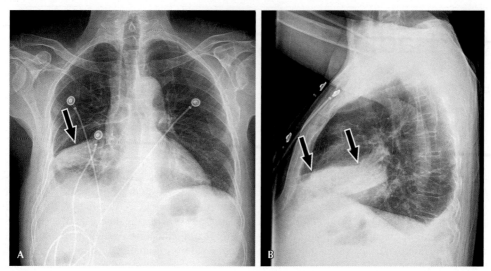

FIG. 39.1 **Right Middle Lobe Pneumonia.** A 57-year-old man presents with chest pain and fever. (A) PA chest radiograph shows a consolidative opacity in the right midlung zone *(arrow)* compatible with pneumonia. Obscuration of the right heart border suggests that the infection affects the middle lobe. (B) Lateral chest radiograph confirms the presence of pneumonia in the right middle lobe *(arrows)*, located anteriorly and beneath the minor fissure. A small pleural effusion is also present.

thoracic vertebral bodies should appear more lucent as one moves inferiorly. Failure of this progression is known as the **spine sign;** it suggests an abnormal opacity, such as pneumonia.

Radiographic findings must be interpreted clinically in the context of symptoms, physical exam findings, and concurrent laboratory values. Certain noninfectious processes can mimic pneumonia radiographically, while certain infectious processes may be radiographically occult. If there is a high suspicion for pneumonia, chest CT and/or empiric therapy should be considered. Furthermore, pneumonia can herald an underlying malignancy, even in young patients, so follow-up imaging to ensure resolution should be considered.

Atelectasis

While the precise pathophysiology of atelectasis is quite complex, the result is reduced aeration of alveoli. The resultant crowding of relatively radiodense vessels and pulmonary parenchyma results in an opacity on chest radiograph. Unlike pneumonia, empty alveoli result in volume loss. Sequela of volume loss include:
- Elevation of the ipsilateral hemidiaphragm
- Ipsilateral mediastinal shift
- Displacement of the minor fissure toward the opacity
- Displacement of the ipsilateral hilum toward the abnormality
- Asymmetrically small ipsilateral hemithorax

Unfortunately, these findings are not universally present, making the distinction between atelectasis and pneumonia difficult. Additionally, radiography is insensitive for the detection of small pneumonic foci within atelectatic lung, although patients who have clear volume loss findings and lack infectious symptoms are more likely to have isolated atelectasis.

Atelectasis can involve small areas of the lung (subsegmental or segmental atelectasis), an entire lobe, or the entire lung. Atelectasis is a common radiographic finding, often resulting from insufficient inspiratory effort, and its clinical consequence varies on the clinical context. However, atelectasis can be a sentinel sign for a more sinister process, such as a malignant mass causing airway obstruction. Persistent atelectasis without a clear etiology should prompt additional diagnostic evaluation—often CT or bronchoscopy. Atelectasis on CT manifests as bright, homogeneous enhancement, while pneumonia will have areas of heterogeneous hypoenhancement.

Pulmonary Edema

Pulmonary edema is excess fluid accumulation within the lung parenchyma and may involve the interstitium or alveoli. Excess interstitial fluid causes blurred and indistinct pulmonary vessel margins. Fluid in the interstitium between the alveolar lobules can result in interlobular septal thickening. When viewed tangentially on radiograph, these thickened septae appear as discrete, long lines (1–2 cm) most apparent along the pleural surface, termed **Kerley B lines.** Since lymphatic fluid clearance is more efficient centrally and inferiorly, pulmonary edema is most apparent in the upper lung zones and peripherally.

Fluid-filled alveoli manifest as a patchy, hazy opacity. Notably, hazy bilateral opacities are not specific for pulmonary edema and can be seen in multifocal pneumonia, diffuse alveolar hemorrhage, aspiration, and/or acute respiratory distress syndrome (ARDS); thus clinical contextualization remains paramount. Pulmonary edema is often bilateral and symmetric, although it can be asymmetric or even unilateral.

Increased intravascular volume, a common cause of pulmonary edema, presents as prominence of the segmental and subsegmental pulmonary veins. Likewise, cardiac enlargement (cardiomediastinal width greater than half of the thoracic diameter) can be seen in patients with dilated cardiomyopathy.

Pulmonary edema can be correctly diagnosed on a high-quality radiograph, but portable AP radiographs with low lung volumes significantly confound the diagnosis. These radiographs may demonstrate vascular indistinctness, patchy opacities (often secondary to atelectasis), widening of the vascular pedicle (space between the superior vena cava and the left subclavian artery), and cardiac magnification, even in healthy normal patients—all findings that would otherwise suggest pulmonary edema. Interlobular septal thickening and pleural effusions are unlikely to be artefactual, even on a low-quality radiograph, but the former is radiographically uncommon, and the latter are nonspecific.

Pleural Effusion

Pleural effusions reflect fluid within the pleural space. Simple pleural effusions appear as a homogeneous, increased density with smooth borders in the dependent periphery of the thoracic cavity (i.e., the costophrenic angle in upright images), often with a meniscus. Lateral radiographs are more sensitive for detecting small pleural effusions, located posteriorly and obscured behind the diaphragm on frontal views. Unless the fluid is loculated (bound in place by thin membranes) the fluid will change appearance based on patient positioning, such as with decubitus views. On a single view, fluid density in a nondependent position or with convex borders suggests loculation. When patients are imaged supine or semierect, simple effusions may layer posteriorly, obscuring the meniscus and making diagnosis difficult. In the absence of secondary findings such as prior surgery, the etiology of pleural effusions cannot be determined radiographically

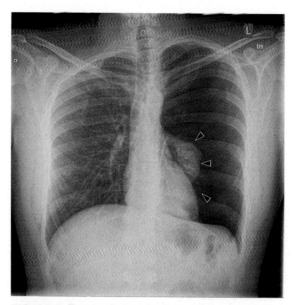

FIG. 39.2 Tension Pneumothorax. A 26-year-old man with acute onset pleuritic chest pain. Fontal chest radiograph shows a unilateral lucent left hemithorax with absent pulmonary vascular markings compatible with pneumothorax. The left hilar opacity reflects the collapsed left lung *(arrowheads)*. Ipsilateral left rib space widening, hemithoracic volume expansion, diaphragmatic inversion, and contralateral mediastinal/tracheal displacement suggest tension pneumothorax.

and must be done clinically (see Chapter 52 for further details).

Pneumothorax

Pneumothorax is a potentially life-threatening condition in which air accumulates within the pleural space. In a tension pneumothorax, increased intrathoracic pressure decreases venous return to the heart, resulting in cardiovascular collapse (Fig. 39.2). The chest radiograph plays a crucial role in the diagnosis of pneumothorax, as early clinical findings, including pain, cough, and shortness of breath, are nonspecific but commonly evaluated by chest radiograph. Careful evaluation for pneumothorax should be performed on every radiograph regardless of the indication.

A pneumothorax will appear as a peripheral, intrathoracic lucency without lung markings, adjacent to a thin, uniformly thick radiopaque line, reflecting the pleura. In upright patients, pleural air often rises cranially, leading to apical pneumothoraces. Air filling the costophrenic angle can produce a **deep sulcus sign,** though this is a rare finding.

Common mimics of pneumothorax include skinfolds, bony margins, and emphysema. A skinfold will appear as an area of relatively increased density bordering an area of relatively decreased density. A key differentiating factor is that the margin of a skinfold may extend beyond the anatomical confines of the chest, unlike a pneumothorax. The radiodense boundaries of the ribs can be mistaken for a pneumothorax. For equivocal findings, repeat chest radiograph may be helpful, while chest CT is often definitive.

Radiographs with pneumothorax should be investigated for findings of tension, although patient clinical status supersedes the radiographic findings. Contralateral tracheal and mediastinal shift may be present but are easily fabricated by rotating the patient. Other findings, such as ipsilateral rib splaying, ipsilateral diaphragmatic flattening or inversion, and ipsilateral increased hemithoracic volume, are more specific for tension.

Thoracic Masses

While CT has largely replaced plain radiography for assessing thoracic masses, the sheer volume of chest radiographs performed leads to a significant number of incidentally discovered masses. Masses appear as focal areas of increased density with convex borders. Localization of the mass to the mediastinum, lung, or beyond the lung (pleura and chest wall) is crucial for forming a reasonable differential diagnosis. The finding of a mass on radiograph rarely leads to a specific diagnosis and often requires additional evaluation with contrast-enhanced CT and, when necessary, tissue sampling.

Mediastinal masses appear as abnormal mediastinal contours. They are classified as anterior, middle, or posterior based on the apparent center of the mass; these designations do not reflect strict anatomical boundaries, but rather help to group structures that may give rise to the mass, aiding in differential diagnosis. Large masses commonly involve multiple mediastinal compartments.

The classic differential diagnosis for anterior mediastinal masses is described by the five T's:
- *Teratoma* (germ cell tumors)
- *Thymic* lesions (thymoma, thymolipoma, thymic carcinoma)
- *Terrible* lymphoma
- *Thyroid* (often related to a goiter, but discontinuous thyroid tissue is possible)
- *Thoracic* aortic aneurysm

While multiple pathologies can lead to middle mediastinal masses, many are uncommon or have nonspecific appearances. Bilateral hilar adenopathy may arise from sarcoidosis, lymphoma, metastasis, and infection.

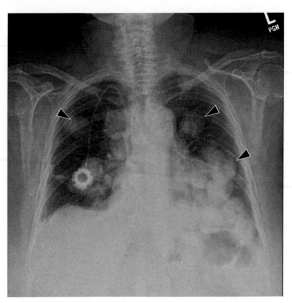

FIG. 39.3 Pulmonary Metastases. A 67-year-old woman with a history of melanoma presents with shortness of breath. Frontal chest radiograph shows multiple bilateral circumscribed round nodules/masses *(arrowheads)* in a basal to apical gradient compatible with metastases. Note the presence of the port overlying the right chest, used for chemotherapy administration.

Unilateral lymphadenopathy is more suspicious for metastasis (especially from a primary lung malignancy) or infection, although there is considerable diversity in the presentation of sarcoidosis and lymphoma. Posterior mediastinal masses most often arise from nerves, bones, or adjacent soft tissues.

Masses within the lung often appear as rounded opacities with a complete border, although large masses or those abutting the pleura may demonstrate an incomplete border. The differential for pulmonary masses is long and includes malignancy, infection, and vascular malformations. Primary lung cancer often presents as a solitary mass and is more common in the upper lobes. Metastatic lesions often present as multiple masses or nodules (masses <3 cm) in a basal to apical gradient (Fig. 39.3). Fungal infection and septic emboli can present as multiple bilateral masses. Bacterial, mycobacterial, and fungal infections can lead to cavitary lesions possessing a central lucency, although certain cancers (particularly squamous cell) or vasculitides have a similar appearance. Masses identified on chest radiography frequently require further evaluation with CT.

CHAPTER 40

Peripheral Blood Smear

HANA I. LIM • ALFRED LEE

INTRODUCTION

The peripheral blood smear is a basic, yet powerful tool utilized for the diagnostic and therapeutic evaluation of a myriad of hematological abnormalities in children and adults. In addition to diagnosis, the peripheral blood smear can be used to monitor disease progression and therapeutic response in patients with established hematological diseases. Although modern automatic hematology analyzers can reliably report blood counts and morphology data, a manual review of the peripheral blood smear can provide clinicians with subtle yet crucial findings in different clinical contexts. Common clinical scenarios in which manual examination of a blood smear is indicated include the evaluations of anemia, thrombocytopenia, leukocytosis, and pancytopenia, where the morphologies of different blood cells can provide the first clues needed to establish accurate and timely diagnoses and develop appropriate treatment plans.

SLIDE PREPARATION

When requested, trained medical laboratory technicians manually prepare the peripheral blood smear. Typically, a drop of blood is placed near one end of a slide, and the back of a second slide (i.e., the spreader slide) held at an angle of 30 to 45 degrees touches the blood drop. Upon contact, the blood spreads along the edge of the spreader slide, which is then pushed rapidly to generate the blood smear. An optimal blood smear consists of a thick area containing a high density of blood cells, gradually transitioning to a thin area containing evenly separated red blood cells (RBCs). The slide is then air-dried and stained with both acidic and basic dyes.

The most commonly used stains for peripheral blood smears are the Wright, Giemsa, and May-Grünwald stains. All three utilize a similar principle consisting of a combination of an acidic **eosin** that stains alkaline cellular components (e.g., hemoglobin or eosinophilic granules) a red-orange color and an alkaline **methylene blue** dye that stains acidic components of cells (e.g., nucleic acids such as deoxyribonucleic acid [DNA]

and ribonucleic acid [RNA], basophilic granules, and nucleoproteins) a blue-purple color.

SLIDE EXAMINATION

Clinicians should interpret their findings on a peripheral blood smear alongside clinical information. Microscopic review of the peripheral blood smear starts with scanning the slide under low power (10× or 20× objective). Low-power examination can be used to determine uniformity and adequacy of staining, and to detect overt abnormalities in cell number, type, and aggregation. While on low power, the lateral and the end (feathered) edges of the smear are first examined. These areas are where white blood cells (WBCs) and larger forms tend to congregate, rendering the lateral and feathered edges particularly well suited to look for abnormal WBC types (including leukemic blasts), platelet clumps, or parasites such as microfilaria. Next, the RBC monolayer is examined, which can be identified as a thin area of the smear in which the RBCs form a single layer, sometimes touching, but rarely overlapping one another. The red cell monolayer is ideally suited to study red cell morphology and overall blood cell counts; it also can be examined for abnormal-appearing WBCs, although, as indicated earlier, the leukocytes tend to cluster in the thicker areas of the smear.

Next, the blood smear should be examined at higher power (50× and 100×), under oil immersion, which allows for an assessment of detailed characteristics of each cell type. RBCs can be evaluated for distribution, shape, size, color, cellular inclusions, and fragmentation. Platelets are evaluated for clumping, satellitism, and granularity. WBCs are assessed for nuclear chromatin pattern, presence or absence of nucleoli, cytoplasmic granules, vacuoles, and inclusions.

RBC EXAMINATION

A healthy individual's RBCs appear as uniform disc shapes with slight central pallor occupying about one-third of the diameter. The size of a normal RBC is similar to the size

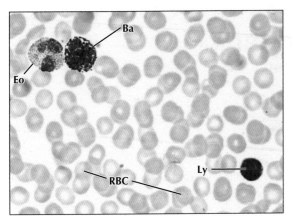

Light micrograph of a blood smear showing typical erythrocytes and leukocytes. Two kinds of granular leukocytes seen are an eosinophil *(Eo)* and a basophil *(Ba)*. They are distinguished by the staining pattern of their granules. A lymphocyte *(Ly)*, an agranular leukocyte, has a densely stained nucleus and lacks cytoplasmic granules. Erythrocytes *(RBC)*, the most numerous formed elements of blood, lack nuclei and have a uniform size: 7–10 μm in diameter and 2 μm wide. They are eosinophilic, with pale centers because of their biconcave disc like shapes. 690×. *Wright.*

FIG. 40.1 **Typical Red Blood Cells (*RBCs*) and White Blood Cells.** (Reused with permission from Ovalle W, Nahirney P: *Netter's essential histology*, ed 2, Philadelphia, 2013, Elsevier.)

of a mature lymphocyte nucleus, about 6 to 8 μm (Fig. 40.1). Microcytic RBCs are smaller than the expected size, while macrocytic RBCs are generally >9 μm; both may be indicative of anemia (see Chapter 32 for further details). A variation in RBC size, or **anisocytosis,** is commonly seen in various kinds of anemia and reflected as a wide red cell distribution width on automated blood counts. Diminished RBC color with increased central pallor is described as **hypochromasia,** which is characteristic of anemia. A number of different RBC morphologies may be seen (Fig. 40.2), with descriptive names often reflecting their appearances; some of the major ones and their associated conditions are:

- *Target cells.* These RBCs contain a central darkened area. They arise as a result of an imbalance in the ratio of RBC membrane and RBC cytoplasm. They may be seen in conditions of anemia, particularly thalassemias, or in liver disease.
- *Spherocytes.* These cells are spherical in shape and have no central pallor. They may be seen in warm autoimmune hemolytic anemia or hereditary spherocytosis (a rare inherited RBC cytoskeletal condition).

- *Schistocytes.* These are fragmented cells containing two pointed edges. They are characteristic of thrombotic microangiopathy (i.e., microangiopathic hemolytic anemia) (see Chapter 142).
- *Degmacytes (bite cells).* These are cells in which part of the membrane and adjacent cytoplasm has been removed, typically via phagocytosis by splenic macrophages. They are characteristic of glucose 6-phosphate dehydrogenase deficiency.
- *Elliptocytes.* These cells are elliptical in shape and may be seen in iron deficiency or in hereditary elliptocytosis (another rare inherited RBC cytoskeletal condition similar to hereditary spherocytosis).
- *Acanthocytes.* These cells contain regularly spaced spiked projections of cell membrane. They are characteristic of liver disease.
- *Echinocytes.* These contain irregularly spaced, smooth undulations of the cell membrane. They are characteristic of renal disease.
- *Tear drops.* Shaped like a tear or a raindrop, these are characteristic of myelofibrosis or myelophthisis (i.e., infiltration of the marrow by nonhematopoietic cells).

A smear containing a variety of different shapes of RBCs is described as demonstrating **poikilocytosis.**

RBCs can also have a number of intracellular inclusions. Some of the major inclusions are:

- *Howell-Jolly bodies.* These are singular remnants of DNA that would ordinarily be removed by splenic macrophages. Their presence is indicative of hyposplenia or asplenia, as may be seen in splenectomized patients.
- *Basophilic stippling.* This is characterized by the presence of numerous basophilic granules in the cytoplasm. These granules contain RNA. They can be seen in many conditions and are classically described in sideroblastic anemia and lead poisoning.
- *Pappenheimer bodies.* These are small, cytoplasmic flecks of basophilic material, consisting of iron. They can be seen in a variety of conditions, including thalassemia, sickle cell disease, sideroblastic anemias, and myelodysplastic syndromes (MDS).
- *Parasites.* Two of the major parasites that have an intracellular RBC phase are malaria (which typically shows ring forms, often with a headphone-like appearance) (Fig. 40.3) and Babesia (which occasionally forms tetrads in a so-called Maltese cross configuration).

PLATELET EXAMINATION

Platelet examination and count estimation can be done on the thin area of the smear where RBC morphology is

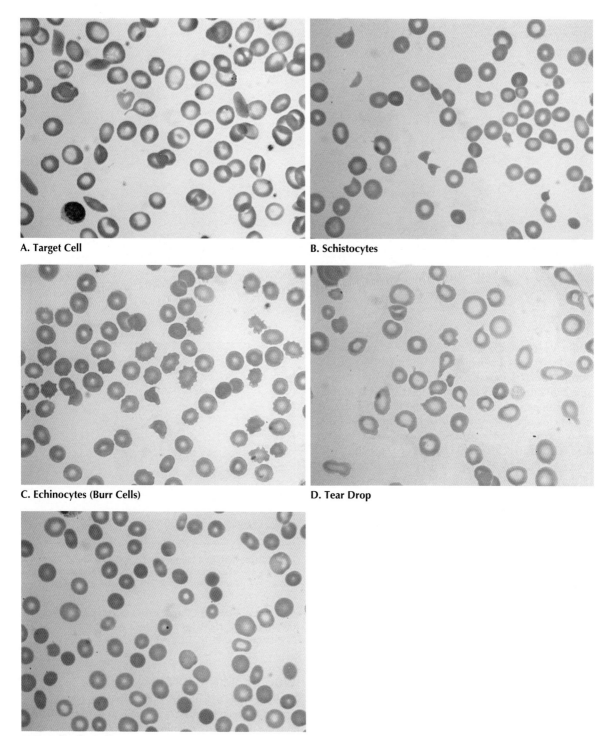

A. Target Cell

B. Schistocytes

C. Echinocytes (Burr Cells)

D. Tear Drop

E. Howell-Jolly Bodies

FIG. 40.2 **Red Blood Cell Morphologies.**

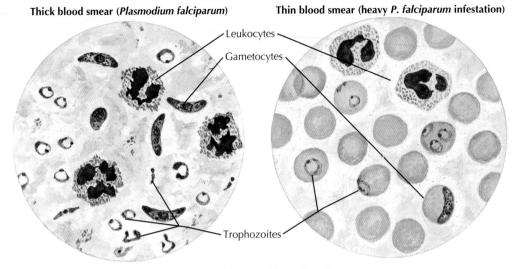

Thick blood smear (*Plasmodium falciparum*)   **Thin blood smear (heavy *P. falciparum* infestation)**

Leukocytes

Gametocytes

Trophozoites

FIG. 40.3 **Malaria on Thick/Thin Smear.**

optimally observed. Platelets are anucleate and typically range from 2 to 4 μm in diameter. Under the microscope, normal platelets appear generally round to oval shaped and contain granules that stain light blue to purple. Approximately 1 platelet per 20 to 30 RBCs is expected in a microscope field. Under oil immersion (100×) field, about 15 to 20 platelets are normally seen in each viewing field; at least 10 fields should be counted, averaged, and then multiplied by 10 for a manual platelet count. Some of the more common platelet morphologies observed include:

- *Platelet clumping* (i.e., pseudothrombocytopenia) (Fig. 40.4). This classically occurs as a result of platelet antibodies that become active in the presence of ethylenediaminetetraacetic acid (EDTA), a calcium-chelating agent that is used in standard complete blood count measurements. The presence of such EDTA-depending platelet clumping leads to an artifactual reduction in the number of platelets that are counted. It is purely an in vitro phenomenon of generally no clinical consequence.
- *Large or giant platelets.* These can sometimes be seen in conditions of increased platelet destruction (e.g., immune thrombocytopenia), certain congenital platelet disorders (e.g., Bernard-Soulier syndrome), or myeloproliferative neoplasms but are generally nonspecific.
- *Agranular platelets.* These are characteristically observed in gray platelet syndrome, a congenital platelet disorder marked by absence of platelet α-granules.

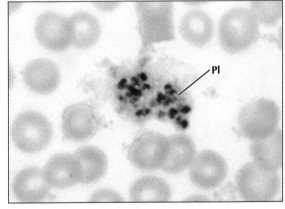

PI

Light micrograph of a clump of platelets in a blood smear. Platelets *(PI)* are round to oval discs containing a dark-staining central granulomere surrounded by a homogeneous, pale hyalomere. 900×. *Wright.*

FIG. 40.4 **Platelet Clump.** (Reused with permission from Ovalle W, Nahirney P: *Netter's essential histology*, ed 2, Philadelphia, 2013, Elsevier.)

WBC EXAMINATION

All three types of leukocytes (granulocytes, lymphocytes, and monocytes) should be examined in both the thick and the thin areas. Overall numbers of leukocytes can be increased, normal, or decreased, and the dominant type of leukocyte should be noted. Granulocytes (neutrophils, eosinophils, and basophils) contain granules in abundant

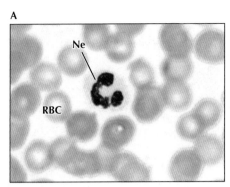

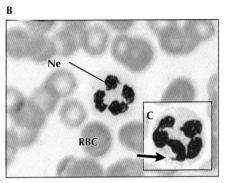

Light micrographs of neutrophils in blood smears. (A) The young neutrophil *(Ne)* has a U-shaped, darkly stained nucleus. (B) The neutrophil is more mature; its nucleus has four lobes connected by fine strands. The cytoplasm of both cells is pale and finely speckled. Their granules are difficult to distinguish. Surrounding erythrocytes *(RBC)* are smaller than neutrophils, which are 9–12 μm in diameter. 1000×. (C) The inset shows a Barr body *(arrow)* on the neutrophil nucleus. It has a drumstick shape and appears to be attached to a lobe of the nucleus by a thin strand of chromatin. Present in females, it is inactive heterochromatin of one of the two X chromosomes. 1500×. *Wright.*

FIG. 40.5 **Neutrophils.** *RBC,* Red blood cell. (Reused with permission from Ovalle W, Nahirney P: *Netter's essential histology*, ed 2, Philadelphia, 2013, Elsevier.)

cytoplasm that stain with various colors that designate their names, as follows:

- *Neutrophils* (Fig. 40.5). These are the most common WBCs and have segmented nuclei with between two and five lobes. Hypersegmentation, defined as six or more lobes of nuclei in neutrophils, is an important diagnostic feature for megaloblastic anemias such as vitamin B_{12} or folic acid deficiency. As granulocytes, neutrophils contain neutral-colored granules, which stain blue-gray to gray-purple; absence of these granules may suggest a primary bone marrow disorder such as MDS. Immature forms of neutrophils, including **bands** (containing a nonlobar, bandlike nucleus), metamyelocytes, and myelocytes can be seen in the peripheral blood due to inflammatory, infectious, or malignant etiology.
- *Lymphocytes* (Fig. 40.6). These cells constitute about 20% to 40% of WBCs. They are small cells with scant blue cytoplasm generally devoid of granules, and round or oval-shaped nuclei typically about the same size as a RBC. During active infections, lymphocytes may acquire a larger cytoplasm and unusual shape, sometimes forming a scalloped edge in contact with adjacent RBCs; such cells are referred to as atypical lymphocytes and are characteristic of viral infections such as Epstein-Barr virus (EBV). In certain autoimmune diseases, a small population of large lymphocyte-containing sparse blue granules, known as large granular lymphocytes, may also be observed.

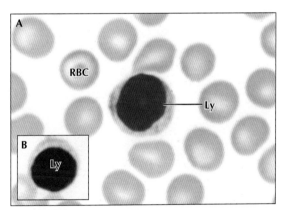

Light micrographs of lymphocytes in a blood smear. (A) A rim of blue-gray cytoplasm caps a darkly stained round nucleus in a large lymphocyte *(Ly)*. Erythrocytes *(RBC)* are also in view. (B) A small lymphocyte at the same magnification is shown for comparison. 1275×. *Wright.*

FIG. 40.6 **Lymphocytes.** *RBC,* Red blood cell. (Reused with permission from Ovalle W, Nahirney P: *Netter's essential histology*, ed 2, Philadelphia, 2013, Elsevier.)

- *Monocytes* (Fig. 40.7). These cells usually represent about 5% to 10% of total circulating WBCs. They are large cells, about four to five times larger than a RBC, with abundant gray-blue cytoplasm and purple, clefted nuclei. Monocytes can be irregularly shaped with cellular projections, or pseudopods. When activated, the cytoplasm may contain a small

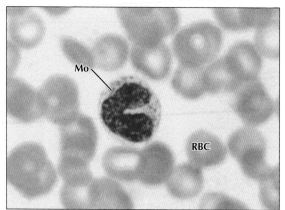

Light micrograph of a monocyte in a blood smear. A monocyte *(Mo)* nucleus is highly indented and less densely stained than that of lymphocytes. Throughout the light blue cytoplasm are many faintly stained granules, so the cytoplasm looks dusty. The monocyte is twice as large as the erythrocytes *(RBC)*. 1350×. *Wright.*

FIG. 40.7 **Monocyte.** *RBC*, Red blood cell. (Reused with permission from Ovalle W, Nahirney P: *Netter's essential histology*, ed 2, Philadelphia, 2013, Elsevier.)

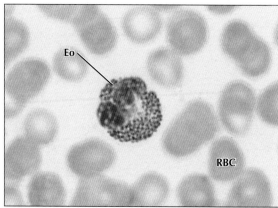

Light micrograph of an eosinophil in a blood smear. The distinctive, closely packed eosinophilic granules fill the cytoplasm of the eosinophil *(Eo)*. The usually bilobed nucleus has an irregular shape. This granular leukocyte has a larger diameter than that of the erythrocytes *(RBC)*. 1350×. *Wright.*

FIG. 40.8 **Eosinophil.** *RBC*, Red blood cell. (Reused with permission from Ovalle W, Nahirney P: *Netter's essential histology*, ed 2, Philadelphia, 2013, Elsevier.)

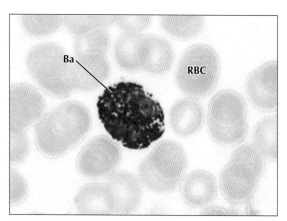

Light micrograph of a basophil in a blood smear. The easily recognized basophil *(Ba)* has many large basophilic specific granules that are blue. The nucleus, being masked by the granules, is less evident. The erythrocytes *(RBC)* are smaller than the basophil. 1200×. *Wright.*

FIG. 40.9 **Basophil.** *RBC*, Red blood cell. (Reused with permission from Ovalle W, Nahirney P: *Netter's essential histology*, ed 2, Philadelphia, 2013, Elsevier.)

number of granules and may have large vacuoles as well.

- *Eosinophils* (Fig. 40.8). These cells usually comprise ≤5% of total circulating WBCs. They have large, intensely orange cytoplasmic granules with a bilobed nucleus. They are seen in increased numbers in allergic and atopic states, including drug reactions and asthma, and also in parasitic infections.
- *Basophils* (Fig. 40.9). These cells comprise ≤1% of total WBCs in the peripheral blood. They contain large, highly basophilic or blue granules. The presence of large numbers of basophils can be associated with myeloproliferative neoplasms, most characteristically chronic myeloid leukemia.

CHAPTER 41

CT Scan of the Head

THEODORE T. PIERCE

INTRODUCTION

CT is one of the great advancements of modern diagnostic medicine, allowing for rapid, noninvasive, and relatively inexpensive three-dimensional evaluation of malignancy, trauma, infection, and other pathology. For radiologists, a thorough reproducible search pattern is crucial to efficiently and accurately interpret CT exams, while clinicians can leverage presenting signs and symptoms for targeted image evaluation. Collaboration between radiologists and clinicians is critical to increase sensitivity for detecting the etiology of a patient's symptoms and optimize the exam's diagnostic yield. CT is not without its issues, however, such as the small, but widely accepted, cancer risk associated with ionizing radiation. Furthermore, advances in technology have revealed ever more subtle abnormalities resulting in debate over the integration of these incidental findings into relevant clinical decisions.

This chapter will provide an overview of CT technique, followed by a discussion of the CT scan of the head. Chapter 42 will discuss the utility of contrast (specifically intravenous [IV]), its side effects, and allergic reactions. Chapter 43 will discuss oral contrast and the effect of radiation.

CT TECHNIQUE

CT images are acquired by rotating an x-ray source and corresponding detector array around a patient to obtain images from multiple directions, or projections (each similar to a single radiograph). Each projection provides a one-dimensional plot of transmitted x-ray intensity. Utilizing a technique called back projection, the different projections are combined to produce a single two-dimensional image. Artifacts resulting from this process can be substantially reduced by applying a predetermined, mathematical function as a filter; this entire process is known as **filtered back-projection (FBP)** and is the cornerstone for CT image reconstruction. Technological and computational advancements have led to the development of novel virtual reconstructed images with unique properties and iterative reconstruction to improve image quality and reduce radiation dose.

FBP combined with iterative reconstruction provides high-quality single axial images, but additional steps must be taken to image a patient (unless only one slice is desired). While the first CT scanners could only complete a single rotation before needing to unwind and step to the next imaging position, today's scanners utilize a slip ring to allow continuous rotation of the x-ray source/detector ring construct. The patient is moved through the scanner in a continuous motion, and with respect to the patient's reference frame, the x-ray source traces a helix, giving rise to the **helical CT.** Mathematical analysis allows the data to be parsed into individual axial slices and analyzed by FBP with iterative reconstruction.

One particular advantage of helical scanning over axial scanning is that helical data sets are inherently volumetric, thereby allowing the data to be cut in any desired plane. This allows the simple creation of coronal and sagittal images or any other plane that can be imagined (including nonlinear planes). This is in contrast with the majority of MRI sequences, which inherently prohibit multiplanar reformats. Another relatively recent advance is the improved temporal resolution of CT, which now permits effective imaging of rapidly moving structures such as the heart.

HEAD CT

CT of the head is often the first-line diagnostic tool in the evaluation of a new neurological deficit or suspected intracranial abnormality. The rapidity of CT scanning is particularly beneficial, as intracranial processes typically require prompt intervention. While MRI offers superior tissue characterization compared with CT, CT is superior in the identification of intracranial abnormalities that necessitate the most prompt treatment (e.g., intracranial hemorrhage). The absence of contrast improves sensitivity of intracranial hemorrhage detection, which can be obscured by contrast-opacified cerebral vessels. Correct patient positioning helps to project artifact (often from dental amalgam) away from the brain. Postcontrast images in an arterial or venous phase can assess the intracranial vessels. The role of postcontrast images

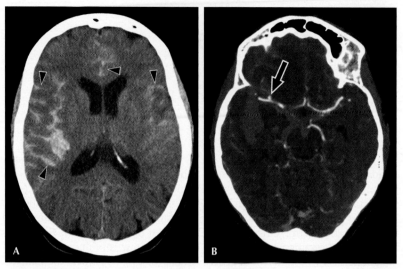

FIG. 41.1 **Subarachnoid Hemorrhage.** A 64-year-old woman with severe headache underwent CT imaging. (A) Axial noncontrast CT head shows extensive hyperdense fluid (blood) interdigitating between the right cerebral gyri and to a lesser extent anteriorly and on the left *(arrowheads)* compatible with subarachnoid hemorrhage. (B) Subsequently performed contrast-enhanced CT angiogram shows a 3-mm focal outpouching *(arrow)* from the right middle cerebral artery consistent with an aneurysm. The combination of findings suggests aneurysm rupture.

for brain parenchymal evaluation has largely been replaced by MRI and is typically only used when MRI is contraindicated.

KEY DIAGNOSES

Hemorrhage

Intracranial hemorrhage occurs in various anatomical spaces; precise localization helps to predict the underlying etiology and to guide management. An **epidural hematoma** is a collection of blood products between the skull and the dura mater, appearing as a hyperdense, lentiform collection that does not cross the sutures. Typically, epidural hematomas result from injury to the middle meningeal artery secondary to an underlying fracture. Skull fractures may be challenging to detect, but the presence of an epidural hematoma prompts detailed interrogation of the adjacent bone. The arterial nature of the bleed can lead to rapid expansion, brain herniation, and death. Heterogeneity of the fluid collection suggests ongoing bleeding.

A **subdural hematoma** occurs beneath the dura mater and appears as hyperdense, crescentic collection conforming to the cerebral convexity but not interdigitating within the sulci. Subdural hematomas are not bound by sutures. These hemorrhages typically result from torn bridging veins in trauma, even when mild. Older patients with

brain parenchymal volume loss may be at greater risk for subdural hematoma development.

Subarachnoid hemorrhage is common in patients with a history of trauma. Blood products beneath the arachnoid mater will appear as hyperdensities interdigitating within the sulci. Common locations include the frontal and anterior temporal sulci, which may be best assessed on sagittal images. Small volume, temporally stable subarachnoid hemorrhages are likely to resolve with conservative management. In the absence of trauma, subarachnoid hemorrhage can signify a ruptured aneurysm (Fig. 41.1). These patients require prompt angiographic evaluation and careful interrogation of each intracranial vessel, especially at arterial bifurcations.

Lastly, **intraparenchymal hemorrhage** can appear as a rounded, hyperdense mass. The differential diagnosis is broad and includes prior trauma, hypertension, vascular malformation, and underlying malignancy (which is better assessed on MRI). Hemorrhage can extend into the ventricles, typically layering in the dependent portions of the lateral ventricles (often the posterior horns, as the patients are imaged supine) or extending into the basal cisterns. These blood products can obstruct cerebrospinal fluid (CSF) resorption at the arachnoid granulations, resulting in rapidly progressing hydrocephalus that may require urgent intervention to prevent parenchymal compression and herniation.

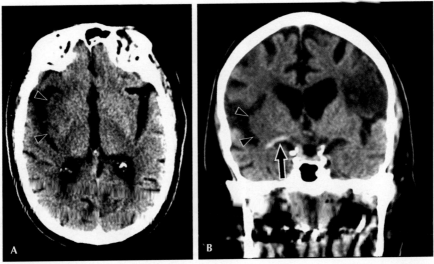

FIG. 41.2 **Right Middle Cerebral Artery Territory Infarct.** A 71-year-old man presents with left-side weakness and left facial droop. (A) Axial noncontrast head CT shows asymmetric edema and loss of gray-white differentiation in the right insular cortex *(arrowheads)*. (B) Coronal oblique reformatted image again shows early signs of insular infarction *(arrowheads)*. The ipsilateral proximal right middle cerebral artery *(arrow)* appears hyperdense to the contralateral vessel compatible with acute thrombus. These findings support the diagnosis of acute right middle cerebral artery territory infarct, which explains the new-onset neurological deficits.

Stroke

Ischemic stroke is a major cause of morbidity; however, prompt diagnosis and treatment can result in substantial clinical improvement. Although imaging plays a key role in stroke management, the most important management aspect is the clinical evaluation, which dictates who requires imaging (based on a history and physical exam suspicious for stroke, along with the National Institutes of Health Stroke Scale [NIHSS]) and who is eligible for treatment (based in part on symptom duration). For treatment-eligible patients, the major role of imaging is to identify or exclude major contraindications for thrombolysis, especially intracranial hemorrhage, for which noncontrast head CT is quite sensitive. Since CT is insensitive to detect small/early infarcts, patients can be treated with thrombolytics empirically on the basis of clinical criteria even in the absence of imaging confirmation of infarct, provided that contraindications are absent. While MRI is more sensitive for the detection of small/early infarcts, the longer exam duration, compared to CT, may unnecessarily delay treatment, although diagnostic strategies (CT vs. MRI) vary by institution.

The CT appearance of infarction varies with time. Early strokes may have no CT manifestations. As the infarct progresses, the gray-white differentiation within a vascular territory will be lost, as the relatively hyperdense outer gray matter will become equal in attenuation to the inner white matter. Evaluation of the insular cortex is of particular utility, as this region is often involved in middle cerebral artery infarcts (Fig. 41.2). Later, the gray and white matter will become increasingly edematous and more hypodense. This edema can have mass effect and result in compression or herniation of key cerebral structures. Ribbonlike hyperdensity may appear along the cortex, reflecting microhemorrhage, a result of cortical laminar necrosis. Larger areas of internal hyperdensity may reflect hemorrhagic conversion. In the chronic phase, the infarcted tissue will atrophy, resulting in asymmetric parenchymal volume loss with previously occupied space replaced with fluid density.

In examining vessels, identification of an asymmetrically hyperdense vessel (noting that certain iterative reconstruction algorithms may make both vessels artefactually hyperdense) may reflect acute thrombus within that vessel and be the p recipitant for symptoms. The length and location of the thrombus have prognostic implications; long thrombi may be more difficult to lyse, while location affects the decision to pursue catheter-directed thrombectomy or intraarterial thrombolysis.

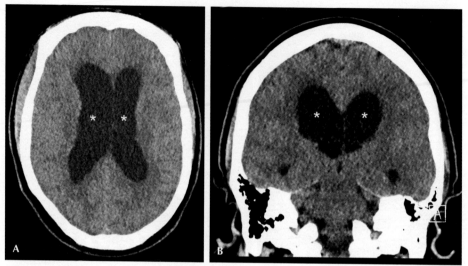

FIG. 41.3 Normal Pressure Hydrocephalus. A 53-year-old man with progressively worsening memory impairment, gait disturbance, and urinary incontinence underwent head CT. (A) Axial noncontrast head CT shows symmetric dilatation of the lateral ventricles *(asterisks)* with preservation of brain parenchymal volume demonstrated by the absence of sulcal prominence. (B) Coronal reformatted image at the level of the posterior commissure again shows dilated lateral ventricles *(asterisks)*, which result in a narrow callosal angle. No obstructing mass is identified. These findings support the clinical diagnosis of normal pressure hydrocephalus.

Vascular imaging of head and neck, often with IV contrast-enhanced CT angiography (CTA), is crucial following identification of a cerebral infarct or transient ischemic attack (TIA). Imaging of the intracranial arteries may demonstrate the abrupt termination of a vessel suggesting an occlusion, which may prompt catheter-directed intraarterial treatment. Also, identification of carotid artery atherosclerotic disease, with the possibility of medical or surgical intervention, is crucial to minimize risk for future stroke. MR angiography (MRA) remains an option for vessel evaluation, especially in patients who cannot tolerate the iodinated contrast used in CTA.

Hydrocephalus

Hydrocephalus is characterized by abnormal ventricular dilatation. This dilatation must be differentiated from ventricular enlargement as a consequence of brain parenchymal volume loss, which is typical in older patients. Diffuse parenchymal volume loss will cause enlargement of *both* ventricles and sulci, while isolated ventricular enlargement in the absence of prominent sulci is suspicious for hydrocephalus. Concomitant hydrocephalus and volume loss can occur and is challenging to identify.

Hydrocephalus can be divided into obstructive and communicating hydrocephalus. **Obstructive hydrocephalus,** or noncommunicating hydrocephalus, results from impeded CSF flow through the ventricles. Key points at risk for obstruction include the foramen of Monroe, the third ventricle, the cerebral aqueduct, and the fourth ventricle. These areas should be carefully evaluated to exclude an underlying mass. Patients with obstructing lesions often require CSF shunting and/or surgical excision of the mass.

In the absence of an obstructing lesion, the hydrocephalus is termed communicating hydrocephalus and can be managed conservatively or with medication, although a shunt catheter may ultimately be needed. Normal pressure hydrocephalus is a subtype of communicating hydrocephalus characterized by the classic triad of dementia, urinary incontinence, and gait disturbance (Fig. 41.3).

CHAPTER 42

CT Scan of the Chest

THEODORE T. PIERCE

IMAGE CONTRAST

As in conventional radiography, CT images can delineate six distinct densities: metal (white/opaque) → bone → soft tissue → water → fat → air (black/lucent). Individual pixel intensities are measured on a standardized scale known as **Hounsfield units,** in which pure water is defined as zero with more dense substances being positive and less dense ones negative. As the range of values along this spectrum is too broad for the human eye to note subtle differences, images are viewed in different windows to optimize evaluation of the organ or pathology of interest (i.e., bone, soft tissue, stroke windows).

Since many disease processes are difficult to distinguish from normal background structures, contrast agents are used to make abnormalities more obvious. The two major groups of CT contrast are intravenous and enteric (intraluminal digestive tract). In addition to improved conspicuity, intravenous contrast provides the important diagnostic role of a surrogate marker of vascularity or lesional blood flow. For a discussion of enteric contrast, refer to Chapter 43.

Intravenous Contrast

Intravenous CT contrasts are iodine-based compounds, which increase the density of structures that have internal vascularity. Intravenous contrast demonstrates unequivocal benefit in many clinical situations and should be considered for the evaluation of vascular structures, intraabdominal solid organs, or soft tissues throughout the body. The radiologist can tailor the timing of image acquisition following contrast administration to create optimal images depending on the structure of interest. This makes communication of the relevant clinical history by the requesting physician a critical element. For example, arterial phase images may be needed to diagnose renal cell carcinoma metastases, although these additional images may not be routinely obtained in the absence of a provided history of known renal cancer.

While intravenous contrast, and to a lesser extent oral contrast, are crucial in many scenarios, there are times when such agents can be omitted for equal or better diagnostic evaluation. For example, intravenous contrast can obscure subdural hemorrhage on a head CT, making a noncontrast exam preferable. Noncontrast exams are often sufficient for most musculoskeletal indications, such as fracture evaluation, or when evaluating solely for nephrolithiasis.

Intravenous Contrast Allergy/Premedication

All patients are at risk for an adverse reaction following the administration of intravenous contrast, even if they have successfully received contrast in the past. Iodinated contrast reactions are uncommon, while reactions to gadolinium-based contrast agents are quite rare. In general, these reactions can be divided into two groups, physiological and allergic, and occur on a spectrum of severity.

Physiological contrast reactions include warmth, nausea, flushing, hypertension, or occasionally hypotension and bradycardia due to increased vagal tone. These reactions are often transient and self-resolving, though persistent symptoms may require symptom-directed treatment; for example, patients with increased vagal tone can receive intravenous fluids for hypotension and, if persistent, atropine for bradycardia. Premedication is generally unhelpful to prevent future physiological reactions. Fortunately, mild physiological contrast reactions do not preclude future contrast-enhanced exams, provided that the patient is willing to tolerate the adverse effects.

Allergic-type contrast reactions can be identified by the presence of hives, sneezing, itching, facial swelling, laryngeal edema, bronchospasm, or anaphylactic shock. Mild reactions can be managed with observation or diphenhydramine. Moderate and severe reactions, characterized by hypotension, tachycardia, and airway compromise, can be life threatening and require prompt treatment with intramuscular epinephrine and intravenous fluids. Antihistamines may be administered as an adjunct.

Patients with prior contrast reactions, regardless of severity, are at increased risk for subsequent severe reactions. Patients with a history of allergic-type contrast reaction should receive premedication prior to contrast administration, typically a combination of steroids and antihistamines (detailed protocols may be institution specific). Breakthrough reactions may still occur, so physicians must exercise great caution before rechallenging a patient who has a known moderate or severe contrast reaction history.

Intravenous Contrast and Renal Dysfunction

Contrast-induced nephropathy (CIN) is an adverse consequence following intravascular iodinated contrast injection resulting in impaired renal function. Although the precise biochemical mechanism is still being investigated, the typical clinical course includes a rising creatinine in the first 24 to 48 hours following contrast, peaking at 3 to 4 days and then falling; patients less commonly progress to oliguria. Initially felt to be common, CIN is now thought to be a real, but rare, entity. Impaired renal function following contrast injection (postcontrast acute kidney injury [PC-AKI]) remains common, but the causative factor is often felt to be coexisting confounding illnesses (e.g., sepsis, decompensated heart failure, severe trauma), which prompt the contrast-enhanced imaging rather than the contrast itself. Indeed, the major risk factor for contrast nephropathy is already impaired renal function, either acutely or chronically (especially creatinine clearance <30 mL/min). Of note, end-stage renal disease (ESRD) patients on hemodialysis without residual renal function are not at risk for contrast nephropathy, as there is no baseline renal function to damage.

Apart from omitting intravenous contrast if diagnostically feasible, no single strategy can fully mitigate the risk of contrast nephropathy. The primary strategy utilized is intravenous hydration with isotonic fluid if tolerated by the patient. Insufficient data exist to support the use of sodium bicarbonate, N-acetylcysteine, or diuretics. Likewise, prompt hemodialysis has shown no significant benefit for renal protection and should only be recommended for ESRD patients in whom there is a concern for volume overload secondary to the administered volume of fluid.

Unlike iodinated contrast for CT, gadolinium-based contrast agents used in MRI have fewer direct nephrotoxic effects. Unfortunately, patients with severe renal dysfunction (ESRD or creatinine clearance <30 mL/min) receiving gadolinium can develop **nephrogenic systemic fibrosis (NSF),** a debilitating disease characterized by multiorgan system fibrosis. In patients with renal dysfunction, the renally excreted contrast remains in the body longer, allowing dissociation of free gadolinium, which incites a fibrotic reaction throughout the body. Newer, more stable contrast agents may reduce the level of free gadolinium in the body, but due to the absence of effective NSF treatments, gadolinium remains contraindicated in these patients. Recent reports also suggest that gadolinium may persist in certain tissues long after intravenous injection (even in patients with normal renal function), the significance of which is not known.

KEY DIAGNOSES
Masses

Masses and masslike lesions are common findings that can occur in any anatomical compartment. While many masses are ultimately benign, the key differential consideration is malignancy (Fig. 42.1). The goal of imaging is to distinguish between masses that are clearly benign, for which additional evaluation may induce undue anxiety or clinical harm; masses that are clearly malignant, which can lead to prompt treatment; and masses that are indeterminate, which often require close imaging follow-up or definitive histopathological diagnosis. While the role of CT varies by malignancy, general uses include assessing tumor extent (both locally and distant metastases), response to therapy, and screening for recurrence.

CT is an optimal technique for evaluating lung masses and nodules (solid lesions <3 cm). The rapid acquisition of CT images can be completed within a single breath hold, minimizing artifact and permitting evaluation of small lesions. Adjacent aerated lung provides excellent intrinsic contrast against nodules and masses, so intravenous contrast is not necessarily required but may be useful to identify potential nodal disease spread within the mediastinum.

In evaluating pulmonary nodules, a helpful diagnostic feature is internal composition; calcification or macroscopic fat is nearly always benign. Spatial distribution (centrilobular, perilymphatic, or random) can help to formulate a differential diagnosis, especially in the setting of diffuse lung disease. Temporal stability in size suggests benignity. Unfortunately, many soft tissue nodules will be indeterminate and require follow-up imaging or biopsy. The **Fleischner criteria,** which apply to patients age >35 years, who are not immunocompromised, and without known/suspected malignancy, provide recommendations on further workup for an incidentally discovered pulmonary nodule based on size, composition, and number of nodules. Finally, CT plays a growing role in the management of lung cancer through CT lung

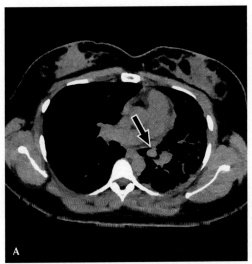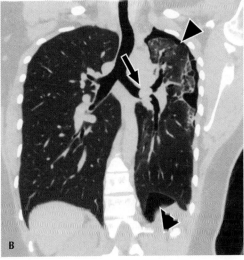

FIG. 42.1 **Endobronchial Mass.** A 25-year-old woman presented for evaluation of left chest wall pain and hemoptysis. (A) Axial noncontrast chest CT in soft tissue windows at the level of the left mainstem bronchus demonstrates a 16-mm endobronchial soft tissue density filling defect *(arrow)*. (B) Coronal oblique reformatted CT image in lung windows again shows the lesion at the bifurcation of the left main bronchus *(arrow)*. A left pneumothorax with the peripheral lung *(arrowheads)* displaced from the chest wall by air is likely the cause of chest pain. Pathology results following transbronchial biopsy and debulking revealed carcinoid tumor, typical for this age group and location.

cancer screening, CT-guided percutaneous biopsy, and CT-guided ablation.

Lymphadenopathy broadly describes abnormal lymph nodes without attributing an etiology. Lymphadenopathy is divided into two general categories: reactive and malignant. Malignant lymph nodes are those in which cancer has spread; these are critical to identify, as they often play a role in biopsy site selection, staging, prognosis, and treatment selection/planning. Reactive lymph nodes are physiologically enlarged secondary to an ongoing nearby infectious or inflammatory process; they typically regress following resolution of the primary insult. Rounded lymph nodes without a fatty hilum measuring >1 cm in short-axis diameter are, in general, considered abnormal. Knowledge of normal lymphatic drainage patterns helps to identify expected locations of disease spread.

Trauma and Thoracic Emergencies

CT, a cornerstone of evaluating patients with acute trauma, is able to quickly and accurately identify life-threatening injuries. The optimal CT should be performed with intravenous contrast to evaluate for vascular and solid organ injury. Oral contrast is often omitted to avoid CT scanning delays and mitigate the aspiration risk in these critically ill patients. Life-threating complications of trauma include pneumothorax, which may be

under tension, pericardial effusion/hemopericardium (raising suspicion for clinical cardiac tamponade), and **hemothorax.** Pulmonary contusions and lacerations can be readily identified by CT. Traumatic aortic injury commonly occurs at specific locations, including the ligamentum arteriosum and the diaphragmatic hiatus. Bone integrity should be assessed by reconstructing additional CT images with a dedicated bone algorithm to increase sensitivity for fracture detection. Identification and characterization of thoracic spine injuries help to guide management to reduce the consequences of spinal cord trauma. While rib fractures may result in underlying lung injury, multiple contiguous fractured ribs broken in at least two places can present as **flail chest,** which may necessitate clinical/surgical intervention.

Pulmonary Embolism (See Chapter 89 for Further Details)

Pulmonary embolism (PE) is the migration of material into the pulmonary arteries, classically a thrombus arising in the deep venous system. As clinical signs of PE are often insensitive and nonspecific, imaging is the cornerstone of PE diagnosis.

The most widely used diagnostic test for identification of PE is the contrast-enhanced CT chest. Since image acquisition parameters are adjusted to optimize the

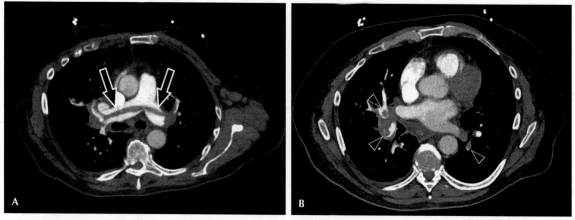

FIG. 42.2 **Saddle Pulmonary Embolus.** A 70-year-old man presented with 1 week of shortness of breath, asymmetric painful right lower extremity swelling, and inguinal/cervical lymphadenopathy. (A) Axial oblique contrast-enhanced pulmonary embolism protocol chest CT image at the level of the main pulmonary artery shows a linear filling defect *(arrows)* straddling the pulmonary artery bifurcation diagnostic of saddle embolus. (B) A second CT image more inferiorly shows additional extension of clot into the right lower lobar, right middle lobar, and left lower lobe segmental pulmonary arteries. The patient was ultimately diagnosed with a right lower extremity deep venous thrombosis and follicular lymphoma, both risk factors for the development of pulmonary embolism.

visualization of potential pulmonary arterial thrombi (which may not be visible on routine chest CT scans), the decision to evaluate for PE must be decided a priori. For example, the timing between contrast injection and image acquisition is changed such that scanning occurs when the contrast is within the pulmonary artery to maximize contrast between thrombus and blood pool. Emboli appear as soft tissue–density filling defects within the pulmonary arteries. A large embolus straddling the pulmonary bifurcation and involving both main pulmonary arteries is termed a **saddle embolus** (Fig. 42.2). Motion artifact can mimic small thrombi, predominantly in the segmental and subsegmental pulmonary arteries. In the event that an embolus is identified, the heart can be evaluated for signs of right heart strain, including right > left ventricular diameter, flattened intraventricular septum, or paradoxical septal bowing into the left ventricle. Dual-energy CT may be helpful to identify areas of reduced pulmonary perfusion or infarction resulting from emboli.

Aortic Dissection (See Chapter 64 for Further Details)

Aortic dissection (Fig. 42.3) results from a defect within the intima layer of the aorta, permitting high-pressure arterial blood to pass longitudinally between the layers of the aortic wall, creating a false lumen. While any imaging modality can identify findings of dissection,

multiphase CT without and with contrast is the most prevalent choice due to high sensitivity and rapid image acquisition.

The first step in dissection imaging is a noncontrast CT to assess for **intramural hematoma**, a dissection equivalent, which presents as a high-density, crescentic thickened aortic wall reflecting clotted intramural blood products. Contrast administration can obscure this high-density hematoma. The noncontrast exam can also identify the overall size of the aorta (often enlarged in the setting of dissection) and displaced intimal calcification. Apart from these findings, the arterial-phase contrast-enhanced CT scan is the crucial acquisition for dissection assessment. This acquisition optimizes opacification of the aorta and increases conspicuity of the intraluminal soft tissue flap (or intimal flap) that is diagnostic of dissection. Following arterial phase images, delayed images are often obtained to increase sensitivity for active extravasation of contrast. Oftentimes there is marked differential flow between the true lumen and false lumen resulting in incomplete contrast opacification of the slower flow lumen. This can mimic thrombosis on arterial phase images, but delayed images can demonstrate delayed luminal enhancement indicative of slow flow rather than thrombosis.

According to the Stanford classification, type A dissections involve any part of the aorta from the aortic valve to the take-off of the left subclavian artery.

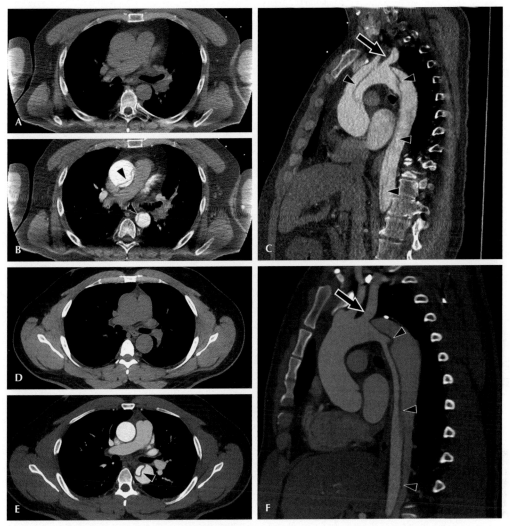

FIG. 42.3 Type A and Type B Aortic Dissection. (A–C) A 42-year-old man with sharp tearing substernal chest pain underwent multiphase CT showing type A thoracic aortic dissection. (A) Axial noncontrast CT at the level of the midascending aorta shows a dilated ascending aorta but is otherwise unrevealing. (B) Axial arterial phase contrast-enhanced CT at the same level shows the presence of an intimal flap in the ascending and descending thoracic aorta *(arrowheads),* diagnostic of type A dissection. (C) Sagittal oblique (candy cane) reformatted image shows the extent of the dissection flap in the ascending aorta, aortic arch, and descending aorta *(arrowheads)* as well as involvement of the left subclavian artery *(arrow).* (D–F) A 39-year-old man with acute onset substernal chest pain radiating to his back underwent multiphase CT showing type B aortic dissection. (D) Axial noncontrast CT at the level of the midascending aorta shows a prominent caliber descending aorta but is otherwise unrevealing. (E) Axial arterial phase contrast-enhanced CT at the same level shows the presence of an intimal flap in the descending thoracic aorta *(arrowhead)* with sparing of the ascending aorta. (F) Sagittal oblique (candy cane) reformatted image shows the dissection flap *(arrowheads)* beginning at the origin of the left subclavian artery *(arrow),* diagnostic of type B aortic dissection.

Extension into the aortic root and pericardium leading to hemopericardium, into the coronary vessels resulting in myocardial infarction, or into the carotid arteries resulting in stroke can all be identified by CT. When the intimal flap is present only within the descending aorta distal to the origin of the left subclavian artery, the dissection is categorized as type B. Major aortic branch vessels should be evaluated for involvement and occlusion, as this can cause organ ischemia and may require procedural intervention.

CHAPTER 40

CT Scan of the Abdomen and Pelvis

THEODORE T. PIERCE

ORAL/ENTERIC CONTRAST

Enteric contrast agents have long been used for evaluation of the digestive tract, possessing an excellent safety profile and minimal risk. The typical contrast appears opaque/white on CT, termed **positive contrast**; examples include barium sulfate or a dilute iodinated contrast. Enteric contrast allows for expanded evaluation of the bowel, including:

- Proximal hollow viscous perforation, as extraluminal contrast is diagnostic of perforation and can provide localizing clues
- **Bowel obstruction,** which can be seen by delayed contrast passage or narrowed lumen
- Abscess, as contrast-opacified bowel can be more easily distinguished from extraluminal fluid collections

Contrast can also be instilled into other anatomical openings, including the rectum, bladder, or an ostomy to evaluate for perforation, strictures, or fistulae.

A second type of oral contrast is **negative contrast,** essentially a large volume of water that is retained within the bowel lumen. This appears as low-density intraluminal fluid, allowing for improved identification of mucosal enhancement that may indicate inflammation. Indeed, the major utility of negative contrast is in assessing inflammatory bowel disease, although a major limitation is the inability to distinguish between loops of bowel and abscess. Hypervascular metastases to bowel (i.e., from melanoma) are more conspicuous with negative oral contrast agents, as positive oral contrast can obscure the enhancing masses.

Despite these benefits and safety profile, oral contrast administration is disliked by many patients, increases cost, and can delay imaging; the urgency of the exam must be balanced with the potential benefit of oral contrast. Utilization of oral contrast varies widely by institution.

RADIATION IN CT

The risks of ionizing radiation have been well covered in both medical and popular literature, and a basic understanding is crucial for all providers to accurately discuss risks with patients and avoid propagating myths. A single high dose of radiation can lead to hair loss, bone marrow suppression, radiation sickness, and death. Patients exposed to these high doses also are predisposed to various malignancies, largely based on studies of Japanese atomic bomb survivors and nuclear accidents. These doses of radiation, however, are orders of magnitude greater than those used for diagnostic imaging exams, and it remains unclear if results can be extrapolated to medical imaging.

Several theoretical models attempt to elucidate the risk of malignancy from repeated diagnostic imaging, but controversy exists regarding each model's assumptions and ability to accurately predict future malignancy. The **linear no-threshold model** is the most widely accepted and conservative model assuming that any amount of radiation is harmful and that radiation risk is proportional to dose. Other, unproven models opt for a specific threshold of radiation exposure at which risk of malignancy increases. Until further data are available, the linear no-threshold model provides the most cautious approach to radiation exposure. It should be noted that a significant lag time (on the order of a decade) is present between ionizing radiation exposure and the development of a radiation-induced malignancy. As a result, patients with limited life expectancy are likely at lower risk for developing radiation-induced malignancy. Nonetheless, all exams exposing patients to ionizing radiation should abide by the ALARA (as low as reasonably achievable) principle to reasonably minimize radiation exposure.

In recent years, there have been significant decreases in radiation dose per exam due to technical advancements (e.g., improved scanner hardware, iterative image reconstruction techniques), tendency away from multiphase CT exams, and a willingness to compromise on image quality. The most important factor in population-wide radiation dose stewardship, however, remains the appropriate utilization of radiological exams, in particular CT.

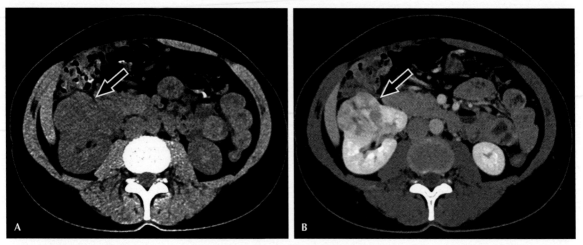

FIG. 43.1 **Renal Mass.** A 45-year-old woman underwent renal mass protocol CT to characterize an incidental right renal lesion detected at ultrasound. (A) Noncontrast axial CT shows lobulated soft tissue *(arrow)* contiguous with and isodense to the right kidney. Other than the contour abnormality, the mass is difficult to identify or distinguish from the background kidney. The absence of intrinsic hyperdensity suggests against a hemorrhagic cyst. (B) Contrast-enhanced axial CT clearly demonstrates a solid right renal mass *(arrow)*, hypoenhancing compared to normal renal parenchyma. Subsequent biopsy reveals to the lesion to be an oncocytoma, a known mimic of renal cell carcinoma.

KEY DIAGNOSES

Masses

Unlike lung lesions, abdominopelvic solid organ masses arise on a background of soft tissue instead of air, dramatically reducing their conspicuity, which necessitates intravenous contrast for their identification and characterization. Routine abdominal evaluation times image acquisition to the portal venous phase to maximize conspicuity of common pathologies, but certain lesions may only be visible on other phases of contrast enhancement. Arterial phase acquisitions allow for identification of hypervascular lesions, such as hepatocellular carcinoma or hypervascular metastases. While multiple different postcontrast phases can be acquired following a single contrast bolus, the trade-off is an increased radiation dose to the patient. As masses can arise in any organ, it is crucial to have a systematic search of each CT exam to identify incidental masses, which can be lifesaving, especially when tumors are identified early.

The most common lesion in the solid organs, such as liver and kidney, is the benign **simple cyst,** which will appear as well-circumscribed and fluid attenuation (~0 Hounsfield units [HU]). Metastases, common in the liver, manifest as numerous, hypodense (but greater density than fluid) hepatic lesions, often in patients with known malignancy, such as colon cancer or lung cancer. The liver metastases from certain cancers (e.g.,

melanoma, thyroid, renal, neuroendocrine) are more typically hypervascular. Primary arterially enhancing liver lesions include both benign (hemangioma, focal nodular hyperplasia, hepatic adenoma) and malignant (hepatocellular carcinoma) etiologies. Many liver lesions may be indeterminant by CT for which liver MRI may be helpful.

For renal masses, the key role of CT is to differentiate benign lesions (simple cysts, angiomyolipoma) from indeterminate or suspicious lesions (enhancing masses, complex cysts), which must be further evaluated for malignancy. On noncontrast CT, renal masses can be difficult to identify from background parenchyma. On a single-phase postcontrast CT, high-density material (hemorrhage or protein) within a simple cyst can mimic enhancement. Definitive diagnosis of an enhancing renal mass may require precontrast and postcontrast CT acquisitions (Fig. 43.1).

The adrenal gland deserves special mention due to the high number of incidentally identified masses, termed **incidentalomas.** Many of these adrenal lesions will ultimately prove to be benign. Small masses (<4 cm) that measure <10 HU on noncontrast CT are almost universally benign adenomas and do not require additional evaluation. Some adenomas do not meet this criterion and may require evaluation of contrast kinetics with multiphasic CT to correctly diagnose. Some benign adenomas are hormonally hyperfunctioning (see Chapter 79 for further details). The most common malignant adrenal mass is metastasis, often from lung cancer. Primary adrenal malignancies are exceedingly rare, especially when the mass is <4 cm. In the absence of definitive benign findings, and in masses >4 cm, resection is frequently required due to increased probability for malignancy.

Masses also arise in the remainder of the abdomino-pelvic organs. Colon cancer appears as circumferential, segmental **bowel wall thickening,** although nondistended bowel and inflammation can mimic this appearance. Pancreatic masses can be quite challenging to identify, even with dedicated imaging acquisitions, although the presence of main pancreatic duct dilatation (>2–3 mm) with abrupt cutoff should raise high suspicion for an occult mass. Pelvic organs such as the bladder, uterus, and ovaries can be difficult to evaluate by CT, but gross abnormalities can be further evaluated by ultrasound or MRI. Osseous metastatic lesions may not present as masses, but instead as focal, rounded areas osteolysis. Certain primary tumors, such as prostate cancer and breast cancer, may result in sclerotic metastases. Many chemotherapy treatments can cause bone metastases to appear more sclerotic; this should not be interpreted as disease progression.

For a discussion of evaluation of lymphadenopathy, refer to Chapter 42.

Trauma and Abdominal Emergencies

Intravenous contrast-enhanced CT is typically used in the setting of trauma to improve sensitivity to detect and grade intraabdominal organ injury. If there is high clinical suspicion or CT evidence of liver, spleen, kidney, bladder, or vascular injury, delayed images should be obtained to increase sensitivity for contrast extravasation, which may alter surgical management. For this reason, it is often helpful to have a radiologist directly monitor the CT examination to make a real-time determination about the need for additional imaging.

Hemorrhage appears as hyperdense fluid, typically >30 HU. Clinically occult life-threatening hemorrhage can accumulate within four compartments: the pleural space, the peritoneum, the retroperitoneum, and either thigh, necessitating evaluation of each. Relatively more dense hemorrhage may be noted near the site of ongoing bleeding **(sentinel clot sign),** which can help to localize bleeding. Over time, the components of hemorrhage can separate, with a predilection for the hyperdense components to deposit in dependent positions, often within the pelvis. This can be a useful sign for identifying the combination of low-density ascites and superimposed hemorrhage.

Due to the intrinsic contrast between air and soft tissue, an abnormal collection of air is typically easy to identify. Extraluminal free intraperitoneal air heralds underlying gastrointestinal perforation, often a surgical emergency (Fig. 43.2). However, air is adept at dissecting through soft tissue and spreads widely, making localizing of such a perforation difficult. Free air may be present following abdominal surgery and does not necessarily indicate pathology in this setting. Tubular air in the liver may be within the biliary system or portal venous system. **Pneumobilia,** which appears as branching, centrally located lucencies, is often an incidental finding following endoscopic retrograde cholangiopancreatography (ERCP) or prior biliary-enteric anastomosis. Portal venous gas, however, is an ominous sign suggesting the presence of **bowel wall pneumatosis** (air within the bowel wall), which has dissected into the portal system and migrated to the liver. Although potentially benign, pneumatosis is worrisome for bowel ischemia. Differentiating pneumatosis from fecal material mixed with air can be challenging. Air within the bladder lumen is typically iatrogenic related to catheterization.

Bowel Wall Thickening and Obstruction

Bowel wall thickening is a common imaging feature of multiple disease processes affecting the bowel and thus is often nonspecific. Focal wall thickening suggests an underlying mass (more common in colon than small bowel), while segmental or diffuse wall thickening can result from infectious, inflammatory, or ischemic processes. **Fat stranding,** a change in the attenuation of fat surrounding an inflamed structure, can highlight adjacent pathology.

Infectious causes of bowel wall thickening are often viral, and in most cases cannot be distinguished from bacterial causes. Marked diffuse colonic wall thickening in a patient recently taking antibiotics should raise concern for *Clostridioides* (formerly *Clostridium*) *difficle* infection, while marked cecal/ascending colonic wall thickening in a neutropenic patient suggests **typhlitis.** Bowel wall thickening adjacent to colonic diverticula, along with pericolonic fat stranding, suggests **diverticulitis.** Terminal ileal wall thickening with adjacent necrotic mesenteric lymph nodes can indicate tuberculous infection, especially in endemic areas. While inflammatory processes can be difficult to distinguish from infectious causes, diffuse continuous colonic involvement may suggest ulcerative colitis, while terminal ileal involvement may suggest Crohn disease.

The etiology of ischemia dictates the imaging phenotype. Bowel wall thickening in watershed areas (e.g., the colonic splenic flexure) can result from systemic hypotension. Mesenteric venous thrombosis presents as

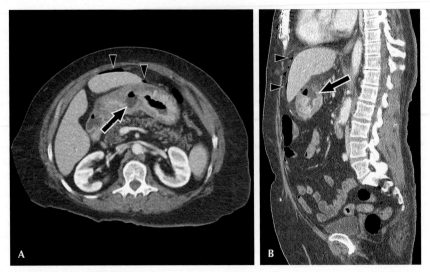

FIG. 43.2 **Gastric Perforation.** A 56-year-old woman presented to the emergency department with hematemesis. (A) Axial contrast-enhanced CT demonstrates antidependent foci of intraperitoneal free air *(arrowheads)*, which herald underlying hollow viscous perforation. Careful inspection reveals an adjacent ulcer in the gastric antrum *(arrow)*, which is more clearly shown on sagittal reformatted images (B); also showing additional foci of gas anterior to the liver *(arrowheads)*. Subsequent surgical resection revealed ulcerated/perforated poorly differentiated signet ring gastric adenocarcinoma.

marked segmental bowel wall thickening with absent superior mesenteric vein/portal vein enhancement. **Mesenteric thromboembolism** appears as a segmental area of bowel wall hypoenhancement distal to an occluded supplying artery; wall thickening may be only modest given reduced blood inflow.

Radiographic identification of a suspected bowel obstruction and its associated findings can influence whether medical or surgical management is appropriate. Bowel obstruction presents as disproportionately dilated loops of proximal bowel (compared with distal bowel) with an abrupt **transition point.** In general, the diameter of normal small bowel is <3 cm. The principal differential consideration is **ileus,** in which the bowel is diffusely dilated without a focal transition point. Obstruction more often affects the small bowel than the large bowel. In the setting of distal large bowel obstruction, the cecum dilates to a greater degree than the transverse colon. Thus cases in which the transverse colon is larger than the cecum invariably represent ileus rather than obstruction (note that the converse is not true). In the setting of bowel obstruction, decreased mural enhancement, pneumatosis, and intraperitoneal free air are concerning for bowel necrosis, which would necessitate surgical intervention. Two transition points identified in close geographic proximity (a variable length of intervening bowel may be present) suggest a closed-loop bowel obstruction, a surgical emergency due to the risk of bowel ischemia.

Cirrhosis

Morphological findings of hepatic cirrhosis include hepatic nodularity, hypertrophy of the caudate and left lateral segments, and right lobe atrophy. Ascites may be present as a result of portal hypertension, appearing as a homogenous low attenuation structure, which molds around adjacent structures. This is in contrast to an abscess, which appears as a fluid collection with a clearly defined enhancing wall. The volume of fluid is typically greater than the trace pelvic fluid present normally in women of reproductive age. Spontaneous bacterial peritonitis is not well diagnosed by imaging. Other sequela of portal hypertension include splenomegaly (size thresholds vary by height) and portosystemic collateral vessel formation. Collateral vessels are identified anatomically as gastroesophageal **varices,** perirectal varices, periumbilical varices secondary to recanalization of the umbilical vein, and retroperitoneal collaterals such as portorenal shunts.

Pancreatitis

The major role of imaging in **pancreatitis** is to detect and localize pancreatitis-associated complications and assist in operative planning. Acute interstitial edematous

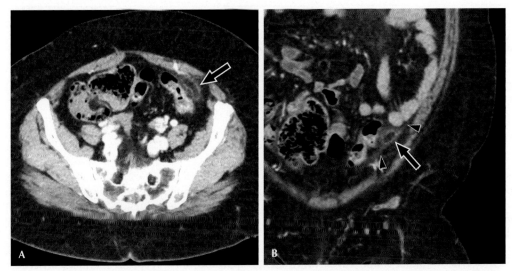

FIG. 43.3 **Epiploic Appendagitis.** A 58-year-old woman underwent contrast-enhanced CT to evaluate 4 days of left lower quadrant abdominal pain. (A) Axial image shows a left lower quadrant pericolonic fat lobule *(arrow)* surrounded by a soft tissue rim with adjacent fat stranding. (B) Coronal reformatted image shows reactive fascial thickening *(arrowheads)* adjacent to the inflamed fat lobule *(arrow)*; typical findings of epiploic appendagitis.

pancreatitis may show only peripancreatic fat stranding with preservation of normal pancreatic parenchymal enhancement. More severe inflammation can organize into acute peripancreatic collections and later evolve into a **pseudocyst.** Necrotizing pancreatitis is identified as an area of absent parenchymal enhancement or an area of peripancreatic fat necrosis. Acute necrotic collections may develop and ultimately form walled-off necrotic collections over time. Percutaneous drainage or surgical debridement may be indicated on the basis of the imaging findings. Inflammation related to pancreatitis can be florid, extending through the abdomen and pelvis along retroperitoneal fascial planes. Gallstones, an important cause of pancreatitis, can be identified on CT but may be occult; MRI and ultrasound are more sensitive for the detection of gallstones. For additional discussion of gallbladder pathology, refer to Chapter 44.

Pyelonephritis

Pyelonephritis is a clinical diagnosis made on the basis of presenting symptoms, physical exam findings, and laboratory evaluation, since imaging findings are insensitive. The CT finding of pyelonephritis, when present, is that of alternating bands of hypoenhancement throughout the renal parenchyma (striated nephrogram). Rather than diagnose pyelonephritis, the role of CT is to identify infectious complications such as renal abscess or an infectious nidus such as **nephrolithiasis,** which appear as focal high-density structures within the renal collection system.

Epiploic Appendagitis

Epiploic appendagitis is an underrecognized cause of acute abdominal pain (Fig. 43.3). The epiploic appendices are small fat lobules hanging from the peripheral margin of the colon, nourished by vasculature embedded within the pedicle (base) of the appendage. This pedicle is prone to torsion, which results in ischemia and death of the epiploic appendage, leading to severe abdominal pain. Imaging demonstrates a small rounded fat density adjacent to the outer margin of the colon with surrounding inflammation, but little to no colonic wall thickening. Unlike many other diagnoses, epiploic appendagitis is self-limiting and does not warrant aggressive therapy, either surgical or medical.

CHAPTER 44

Abdominal Ultrasound

THEODORE T. PIERCE

INTRODUCTION

Ultrasound is a cross-sectional modality that creates images based on differential absorption and reflection of sound waves. Ultrasound probes of differing shape and transmit frequency are used for a diverse array of clinical applications. Within a single transducer, piezoelectric crystals produce sound waves, which are reflected back by underlying structures and received in the same transducer. For a traditional B-mode image, the ultrasound machine displays an image based on the time to receive an echo and the corresponding echo intensity. Additional ultrasound modes, such as M mode, color Doppler, power Doppler, pulse wave Doppler, and elastography, provide numerous tools to noninvasively interrogate intraabdominal organs (Fig. 44.1).

Advantages of ultrasound include dynamic, real-time imaging allowing for functional evaluation, ability to use provocative maneuvers, relatively low cost, widespread availability, and lack of ionizing radiation. Its main limitations include difficulty imaging through air (e.g., bowel gas), bone, and obese patients. Technical artifacts are common on ultrasound, and both pathological and normal findings can be misconstrued. Lastly, ultrasound is operator dependent, with image quality highly dependent on skill and experience.

KEY STRUCTURES

Appendix

Appendicitis is characterized by appendiceal inflammation, often resulting from luminal obstruction by an appendicolith producing right lower quadrant pain, anorexia, and nausea. The normal appendix is a tubular, blind-ending structure with a diameter of ≤6 mm. It can be quite challenging to identify due to the small size and large amount of adjacent bowel, which can mimic the appendix in appearance. Failure to identify the appendix is reassuring but unfortunately does not exclude appendicitis.

On ultrasound, an inflamed appendix will be dilated, fluid filled (anechoic, or homogeneously black), and

thick walled (Fig. 44.2). A small amount of adjacent fluid may result from the inflammation, although a large fluid collection may reflect abscess formation following appendiceal rupture. Echogenic (bright on ultrasound) mesenteric fat, the ultrasound equivalent of fat stranding on CT, can suggest adjacent inflammation. A mineralized appendicolith will appear as a markedly echogenic arc with absent signal posteriorly (**posterior shadowing,** owing to blocked sound waves). An appendicolith is important to identify when present, since it increases the probability of both appendicitis and conservative treatment failure. Lymph nodes, appearing as hypoechoic masses, may be identified within the mesentery of the terminal ileum but are more common in viral enteritis; as such, mesenteric adenopathy makes appendicitis less likely.

When appendicitis is excluded or not identified, other common mimics such as **cholecystitis, nephrolithiasis,** and ovarian pathology can be evaluated during the same ultrasound exam. Indeterminate sonographic exams may require performing CT, on which a normal appendix can be more confidently identified or appendicitis more readily diagnosed. MRI should be utilized in circumstances where ionizing radiation is relatively contraindicated, such as in pregnancy.

Gallbladder

Acute cholecystitis typically results from cystic duct obstruction from impacted gallstones. Patients classically present with fevers and epigastric or right upper quadrant pain. These nonspecific symptoms fail to distinguish cholecystitis from nonsurgical conditions (hepatitis, cholangitis, and pancreatitis), so a high degree of suspicion is required. Ultrasound is particularly adept at evaluating the gallbladder for cholecystitis. CT and MRI may clarify equivocal ultrasound findings, while **cholescintigraphy,** such as a **HIDA scan,** can assess for cystic duct patency.

On ultrasound, the normal gallbladder lies inferior to the liver and appears as a round fluid-filled structure with a thin wall (≤3 mm). Findings of cholecystitis include

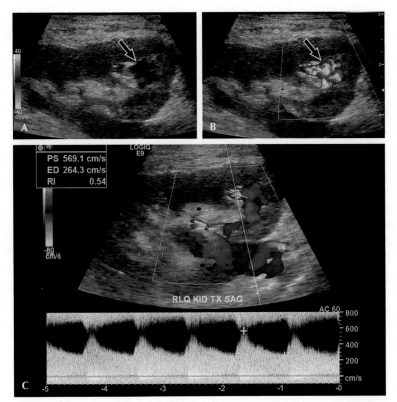

FIG. 44.1 **Renal Transplant Arteriovenous Fistula.** A 57-year-old man with vomiting and shortness of breath underwent sonographic evaluation of his right lower quadrant renal transplant. (A) Sagittal B-mode ultrasound image of the renal allograft shows focal fluid in the lower pole *(arrow)*. (B) The corresponding color Doppler image demonstrates the structure to be vessels *(arrow)* rather than hydronephrosis or a cystic renal lesion. (C) Spectral Doppler interrogation of the vascular structure shows markedly elevated flow in a low resistance pattern compatible with arteriovenous fistula.

gallbladder wall thickening due to edema, pericholecystic fluid, and a positive sonographic **Murphy sign.** Echogenic foci with shadowing are typical findings of cholelithiasis (sludge will appear echogenic without shadowing), which is a risk factor for, but does not confirm, cholecystitis. Sonographers can image patients in both supine and decubitus positions, noting that gallstones should be mobile and change location with patient repositioning, unlike gallbladder polyps, which remain fixed. One notable exception is an impacted gallstone at the gallbladder neck that may not move.

On physical exam, Murphy sign involves applying right upper quadrant pressure during inspiration. As the diaphragm contracts, the gallbladder moves downward and impacts the examiner's fingers; if the gallbladder is inflamed, this causes increased pain and breath-catching. Direct pressure to the gallbladder using an ultrasound transducer has the added benefit of directly localizing the

gallbladder; thus sonographic Murphy sign has a higher positive predictive value than the traditional maneuver.

Ultrasound can also image the hepatic and common bile ducts for evidence of dilation that may represent an obstructing common bile duct stone, termed **choledocholithiasis.** If dilation is present but no stone is identified, **MR cholangiopancreatography (MRCP)** can better evaluate the patency of the biliary tree and assess for any associated obstructing masses.

Kidney

The kidneys are best imaged by placing the transducer on the patient's flank in the intercostal spaces to prevent interference by ribs and bowel gas. Readily identified pathologies include **hydronephrosis,** nephrolithiasis, and mass lesions, though operator ability remains important. For subtle or equivocal findings, CT and MRI can provide more conclusive results.

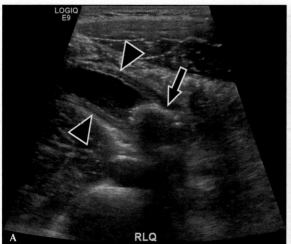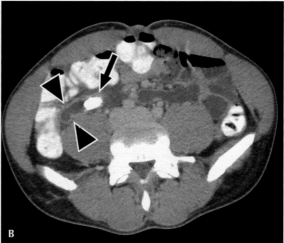

FIG. 44.2 **Appendicitis.** A 32-year-old man presents to the emergency department with 1 week of right lower quadrant abdominal pain. (A) Focused right lower quadrant ultrasound, performed with graded compression, reveals a dilated, 17-mm, noncompressible blind-ending tubular structure *(arrowheads)* compatible with appendicitis. A shadowing echogenic structure *(arrow)* reflects an appendicolith. (B) Axial contrast-enhanced CT confirms the sonographic findings of a dilated appendix *(arrowheads)* and a calcified appendicolith *(arrow)*. Imaging findings were confirmed at the time of surgery.

Hydronephrosis results from the impedance of normal urinary drainage resulting from an obstruction within the urinary tract between the renal collecting system and the urethra. Hydronephrosis is frequently more visible than the underlying obstruction and should prompt close inspection or further evaluation for the obstructive source. On ultrasound, hydronephrosis appears as dilated, fluid-filled calyces and renal pelvis, with blunting of the medullary pyramids in more severe cases. A leading cause of hydronephrosis is nephrolithiasis, which will appear as round, echogenic structures with posterior shadowing. Notably, small stones may not demonstrate clear shadowing, while normal renal sinus fat may also appear as a nonshadowing echogenic focus. Obstructing stones are often found at the ureterovesicular or ureteropelvic junction. When not identified in these locations, stones may be lodged within the midureter, an area difficult to interrogate with ultrasound requiring CT for diagnosis.

While ultrasound can identify the presence of a renal mass, these masses have a variety of appearances and often require cross-sectional imaging for characterization. **Renal cysts,** a common finding, appear as anechoic, round structures with increased **through transmission** (increased signal deep to the lesion; opposite of posterior shadowing as in nephrolithiasis), a barely perceptible wall, and absent internal color flow. While renal cysts are benign and generally do not require treatment, complex cysts are associated with an increased risk of malignancy.

Complex cysts may demonstrate septations, thickened walls, or solid components; these may require additional evaluation with CT or MRI.

Uterus

While low-frequency curvilinear ultrasound probes used in abdominal exams can visualize the uterus, transvaginal imaging allows the probe to be placed much closer to the structure of interest, resulting in vastly superior image quality. **Transvaginal ultrasound** is the cornerstone of ultrasound evaluation of the uterine myometrium, endometrium, and early pregnancy.

Leiomyomas, or **fibroids,** are benign tumors of smooth muscle cells arising from the uterine myometrium and are the most common pelvic tumor in women, often presenting during reproductive age. On ultrasound, fibroids typically are well-circumscribed, hypoechoic intramural myometrial masses, although atypical appearances are common due to the high incidence of fibroids. Fibroids may project into the endometrial canal (submucosal fibroid) or bulge beyond the normal uterine contour (subserosal fibroid). Interestingly, fibroids may arise less commonly from structures other than the uterus, such as the broad ligament or round ligament. Perhaps stranger, fibroids can spread throughout the body, yet remain benign (benign metastasizing leiomyoma). Fibroids, and their malignant counterpart, **leiomyosarcoma,** can be nearly impossible to distinguish from each other by imaging in the absence of overt invasion of adjacent structures. Thankfully, leiomyosarcoma is quite rare.

Adenomyosis occurs when endometrial glands invade the myometrium, leading to abnormal uterine bleeding and painful menses. On ultrasound, adenomyosis may appear as a bulky uterus with diffusely heterogeneous myometrium and, on occasion, myometrial cysts. More focal clusters of endometrial glands within the myometrium can form an adenomyoma, a potential mimic of a fibroid. Adenomyosis can be a challenging sonographic diagnosis in some cases, for which MRI can be useful.

The endometrium is well evaluated by transvaginal ultrasound, appearing as a thin, echogenic strip within the uterus. An abnormal, thickened endometrium may represent **endometrial hyperplasia** or cancer; in postmenopausal women who present with vaginal bleeding, an endometrial thickness of ≥5 mm warrants tissue sampling. Premenopausal women can have thicker endometria on account of ongoing menstruation. Endometrial polyps can be identified as rounded echogenic filling defects within the endometrial canal containing a vascular stalk (seen on Doppler ultrasound). Sonohysterography (ultrasound following instillation of fluid into the endometrial canal) can increase conspicuity of polyps.

Ovary

The ovaries appear as a mass of soft tissue and, in premenopausal women, will demonstrate numerous small cystic structures reflecting follicles, a normal finding.

Transabdominal evaluation should be performed with a full bladder to improve image quality, while transvaginal ultrasound further improves diagnostic ability for ovarian pathology, including torsion, mass, or **ectopic pregnancy**.

Ovarian torsion results when the ovarian pedicle twists, resulting in venolymphatic obstruction, which leads to impaired venous outflow, swelling, and ischemia. Torsed ovaries swell to >4 cm in size, a key sign for torsion. Arterial occlusion is not required for ischemia in the setting of torsion, so the presence of arterial waveforms on Doppler imaging does not exclude torsion. Furthermore, torsion may be intermittent, and Doppler flow may be present during temporary detorsion. Ultimately, imaging findings may be insensitive and nonspecific; experienced expert clinical consultation is invaluable for diagnosing ovarian torsion.

Complex **ovarian cysts** are a common finding; the majority are benign. Hemorrhage within a normal follicular cyst is common and can appear homogeneous with low-level internal echoes and no internal flow on Doppler ultrasound. As clot evolves, it can take on irregular appearances that can mimic malignancy but are best followed with short-term serial ultrasounds to confirm resolution. Multilocular cysts with thick septations, or those with solid components, are more suspicious for malignancy. As a general rule, indeterminate, but presumably benign, sonographic lesions can go to MRI for confirmation and avoidance of surgery, while suspicious lesions should go to CT for staging prior to surgical excisional and histopathological diagnosis. As

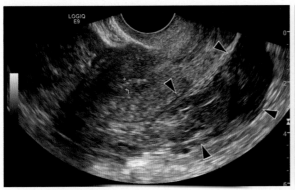

A. Sagittal Uterus

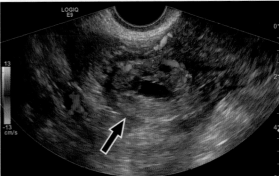

B. Right Adnexa

FIG. 44.3 Ruptured Ectopic Pregnancy. A 39-year-old woman presents to the emergency department with lower abdominal pain and β-human chorionic gonadotropin (βhCG) >10,000 IU/L. (A) Sagittal B-mode ultrasound image through the uterus shows a normal endometrium (calipers) without an intrauterine gestational sac. Large-volume hemoperitoneum is present in the cul-de-sac *(arrowheads)*. (B) Color Doppler image of the right adnexa reveals a complex vascular mass *(arrow)*. This combination of clinical and sonographic findings is highly suspicious for ruptured ectopic pregnancy, which was subsequently confirmed by laparoscopy.

the ovary lacks a capsule to act as a barrier to tumor spread, intraabdominal dissemination can occur shortly after cancer development.

Ectopic pregnancy occurs when the gestating embryo implants somewhere other than the endometrium, most commonly the fallopian tubes (Fig. 44.3). Due to the life-threatening nature of potential rupture, accurate diagnosis is key. In the setting of a positive pregnancy test, the presence of an adnexal mass is worrisome, although the absence of such a finding certainly does not exclude ectopic pregnancy. On the other hand, identifying an intrauterine gestation essentially excludes the possibility of ectopic pregnancy (although heterotopic pregnancy can be seen following assisted reproductive techniques such as in vitro fertilization). In the absence of an intrauterine gestation, the possibility of ectopic pregnancy must be entertained, but early intrauterine pregnancy (below the resolution of imaging) and early pregnancy failure (missed abortion) appear similarly. Close clinical follow-up and repeat ultrasound are often needed.

CHAPTER 45

Endoscopy and Colonoscopy

MARGOT E. COHEN

OVERVIEW

Esophagogastroduodenoscopy (EGD) is a procedure that allows direct visualization of the upper gastrointestinal tract with the ability for direct interventions as indicated. EGD, or upper endoscopy, provides visualization of the oropharynx, esophagus, stomach, and proximal duodenum. This procedure is typically performed by a trained gastroenterologist or surgeon with nurse or physician-guided sedation.

Colonoscopy allows direct visualization of the lower gastrointestinal tract with the ability to provide interventions. Colonoscopy, or lower endoscopy, visualizes the rectum and colon (ascending, transverse, descending, sigmoid) and can access the terminal ileum. A separate procedure must be performed to visualize the remainder of the small bowel (e.g., jejunum, proximal ileum) (see "Related Procedures" later in the chapter). As stated, colonoscopy is generally performed by a gastroenterologist or colorectal surgeon with sedation/anesthesia support.

INDICATIONS

Endoscopy and colonoscopy may be performed for a variety of indications, including diagnostic, surveillance-related, and therapeutic purposes. The decision to perform a biopsy (and the number of samples taken) is determined by the performing physician based on the specific indication and findings of the procedure. Biopsies may be sent for further evaluation, including for *Helicobacter pylori* testing, viral staining if high suspicion for infection, particularly in an immunosuppressed patient, or pathology if highly suspicious for malignancy.

Endoscopy (Fig. 45.1)

A variety of symptoms should prompt consideration of an EGD: dysphagia, odynophagia, early satiety, anorexia, weight loss (particularly if associated with other upper abdominal symptoms), persistent or recurrent reflux symptoms, persistent vomiting of unclear etiology, hematemesis, coffee-ground emesis, melena, or chronic diarrhea with suspicion of small bowel origin (e.g., celiac disease). Any of these symptoms that persist despite a trial of empiric therapy or that present in an individual over 50 years of age should prompt an EGD evaluation.

Alternative reasons to perform an EGD include:

- Confirmation of diagnoses demonstrated radiologically (e.g., suspected malignant lesion, stricture, or obstruction)
- Chronic iron-deficiency anemia after negative colonoscopy evaluation
- Documentation or treatment of esophageal varices in patients with suspected portal hypertension (e.g., cirrhosis)
- Deployment of pH reflux monitor
- Assessment of damage after caustic ingestions
- Malignancy surveillance in patients with Barrett esophagus, gastric intestinal metaplasia, or familial genetic syndromes

Therapeutic interventions include removal of foreign bodies, treatment of acute gastrointestinal bleeding (e.g., clipping, electrocautery, laser photocoagulation, injection therapy, variceal banding), stenting of esophageal or duodenal strictures, placement of feeding or decompressive gastrostomy tube, management of achalasia (e.g., botulinum toxin injection, dilation), and therapy of intestinal metaplasia or stenosing malignant lesions. Endoscopy is contraindicated if a perforated viscus is known or suspected or, as in any nonemergent invasive procedure, informed consent cannot be obtained from the patient or designated proxy.

Colonoscopy

The following symptoms should prompt consideration of a colonoscopy: hematochezia, positive fecal occult blood test, melena if upper gastrointestinal source has been excluded, clinically significant diarrhea of unclear etiology, or weight loss associated with any of these symptoms. Suspicion of inflammatory bowel disease may also prompt colonoscopy for biopsy and confirmation of the suspected diagnosis or to assess the response to therapy in those with a previously confirmed diagnosis.

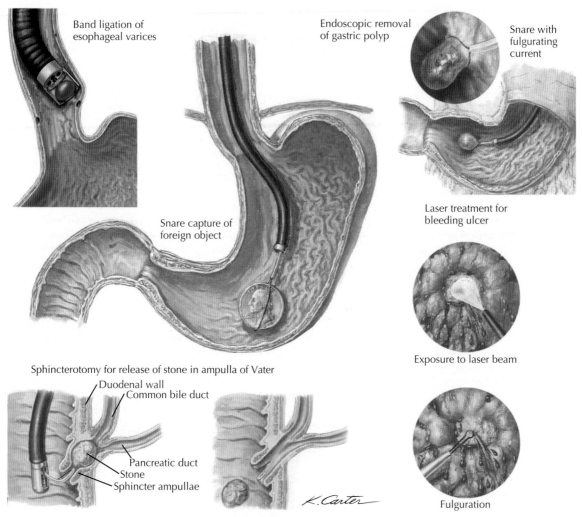

Band ligation of esophageal varices

Endoscopic removal of gastric polyp

Snare with fulgurating current

Snare capture of foreign object

Laser treatment for bleeding ulcer

Exposure to laser beam

Sphincterotomy for release of stone in ampulla of Vater

Duodenal wall
Common bile duct
Pancreatic duct
Stone
Sphincter ampullae

Fulguration

FIG. 45.1 **Potential Interventions in Therapeutic Endoscopy.**

Colonoscopy also may be indicated to evaluate an abnormality demonstrated radiologically (e.g., filling defect or stricture on barium enema or CT scan), unexplained iron-deficiency anemia, or to evaluate for anastomotic leak or patency in patients who have had operative interventions.

Screening and surveillance for colon cancer is a primary indication for colonoscopy (see Chapter 160 for further details). Current guidelines recommend screening colonoscopy in all adults over 50 years of age (if at average risk and asymptomatic) or earlier if there is a strong family history of colon cancer, a familial genetic syndrome (e.g., familial adenomatous polyposis), or for patients with inflammatory bowel disease or certain liver diseases (e.g., primary sclerosing cholangitis) who are at higher risk for development of malignancy. Therapeutic interventions include removal of foreign bodies, treatment of acute bleeding of lower gastrointestinal source, dilation of anastomotic or physiologic strictures, polypectomy (Fig. 45.2), decompression of acute megacolon or sigmoid volvulus, and palliative treatment of stenosing or bleeding malignant lesions (e.g., stent placement, electrocoagulation, or injection therapy). Colonoscopy is contraindicated if there is suspected or confirmed perforation, fulminant colitis, or active acute diverticulitis with high risk of perforation, or if consent cannot be obtained from the patient or designated proxy.

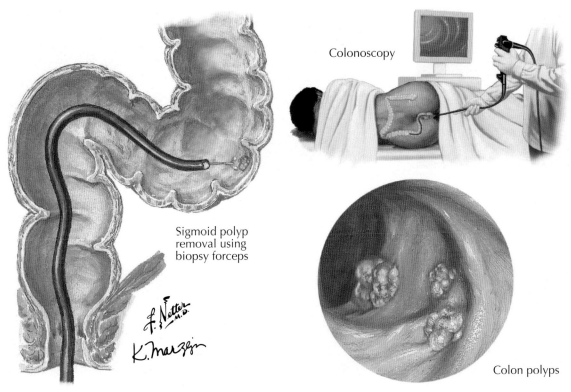

Colonoscopy

Sigmoid polyp
removal using
biopsy forceps

Colon polyps

FIG. 45.2 **Colonoscopy.**

COMPLICATIONS

Endoscopic procedures carry a small but significant risk of complications. The mortality rate is very low for both procedures (0.004% for upper endoscopy, 0.007% for colonoscopy). Complications of endoscopic procedures (EGD and colonoscopy) include cardiopulmonary complications of sedation, including hypoxemia, hypoventilation, hypotension, aspiration, and arrhythmias. These risks are higher with increased age and comorbidities. Bleeding and perforation are also possible and are more common when therapeutic interventions are performed. Infectious risk is low, although there have been reports of bacterial and viral pathogen transmission thought to be associated with improper equipment cleaning techniques.

Of note, colonoscopy also carries a risk of complications related to bowel preparation, including electrolyte disturbances, nausea, emesis, abdominal discomfort, and aspiration.

PREPARATION
Endoscopy

Patients should be made NPO (nil per os) at midnight prior to the day of planned endoscopy if the timing of the procedure is unknown. If timing is known, patients should take nothing by mouth for at least 8 hours prior to the planned procedure. Antibiotic prophylaxis is not indicated except for patients with cirrhosis and active variceal bleed (e.g., spontaneous bacterial peritonitis prophylaxis).

Preprocedure testing is not required for endoscopy in patients with low to average risk. If the patient has active bleeding or is on active anticoagulation, the gastroenterologist may request a recent hemoglobin/hematocrit and coagulation studies. Assessment should be done regarding the patient's risk for sedation and discussed with the anesthesiologist in advance if the patient is high risk (e.g., advanced heart failure or pulmonary disease, prior complications from sedation, prior difficult airway management)

Colonoscopy

Patients should consume a low-residue or clear liquid diet the day prior to colonoscopy. Patients should be made NPO at midnight or at least 8 hours prior to the planned procedure. To clean the colon for optimal visualization of potential lesions and interventions, patients must complete a bowel preparation in advance

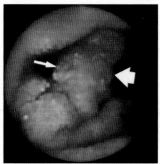

Capsule endoscopy demonstrating polypoid adenocarcinoma of the jejunum (*arrows*).

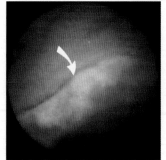

Capsule endoscopy demonstrating large jejunal ulcer (*arrow*).

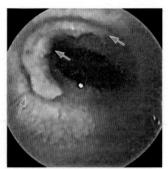

Large Crohn disease ulcer in ileum.

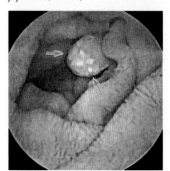

Duodenal polyp.

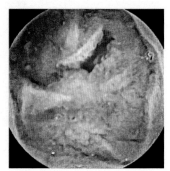

Small bleeding duodenal ulcer.

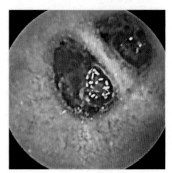

Opening to ileal diverticula.

FIG. 45.3 **Wireless Capsule Endoscopy.**

of their colonoscopy. Studies have shown that up to 25% of patients in the United States have inadequate or poor preparation prior to colonoscopy, which may lead to increased procedure time, complications, and higher risk of not identifying lesions. There are various preparations available with differences in volume, composition, and palatability. However, to optimize preparation quality, a split-dose regimen should be used with half of the prep beginning the night prior to the procedure and the remaining half taken within 5 hours of colonoscopy, to be completed at least 2 hours before the beginning of the procedure. Preprocedure testing and sedation assessment should be performed as indicated earlier.

RELATED PROCEDURES

- **Video capsule endoscopy:** A disposable capsule swallowed by the patient that transmits images to a data recorder. In particular, this is used to visualize the esophagus and small intestine (Fig. 45.3).
- **Enteroscopy:** A version of endoscopy that ventures deeper into the small bowel than an EGD. A variety of enteroscopes exist with different methods to achieve deeper intubation, each with the ability to perform diagnostic and therapeutic interventions.
- **Endoscopic ultrasound (EUS):** Use of endoscopy with an ultrasound transducer to better visualize structures adjacent to the gastrointestinal tract. Diagnostic and therapeutic interventions are possible, particularly biopsy of adjacent structures, including the pancreas.
- **Endoscopic retrograde cholangiopancreatography (ERCP):** Use of endoscopy to examine the biliary and pancreatic systems, often with injected contrast to directly visualize the ductal structures. Diagnostic and therapeutic interventions are possible through this method, including biopsy, cytology, stent placement, removal of choledocholithiasis, and sphincterotomy (see Chapter 130 for further information).
- **Flexible sigmoidoscopy:** A more flexible endoscopy that allows visualization of the rectum, sigmoid colon, and occasionally portions of the descending colon. Diagnostic and therapeutic interventions are possible through this method, including biopsy, hemostasis, and stent placement.

CHAPTER 46

Pulmonary Function Tests (PFTs)

CHRISTOPHER A. PUMILL • TALAL DAHHAN

INTRODUCTION

Pulmonary disease is one of the most burdensome illnesses in the United States, with asthma and chronic obstructive pulmonary disease (COPD) together taxing the US health care system nearly $40 billion per year. Approximately 17 million Americans are diagnosed with COPD, and it is the fourth most common cause of death in the United States. Additionally, asthma is one of the most common diseases from which children suffer and is a leading cause of school absences.

Pulmonary function tests (PFTs) provide an objective way of evaluating pulmonary function in an accurate, objective, and reproducible way. Testing aids in the screening, diagnosis, monitoring, and prognosis of a wide range of pulmonary diseases.

INDICATIONS

There are four main categories of indications for PFTs:

- Diagnosing disease: Physicians may perform PFTs in patients describing subjective pulmonary symptoms (e.g., cough, shortness of breath, dyspnea, wheezing), or those who have abnormal physical exam findings.
- Monitoring disease: PFTs are helpful in monitoring the progression of a disease, the assessment of prognosis, or to objectively measure the effect of a treatment. Of note, PFTs may be useful in patients with respiratory complaints apart from strict pulmonary disease, including cardiac, neuromuscular, or vascular diseases.
- Screening for disease: PFTs can help screen for pulmonary disease in high-risk individuals, such as smokers or patients with hazardous exposures.
- Perioperative assessment: PFTs are especially useful in surgeries requiring the removal of an entire lung or part of a lung, and other highly morbid abdominal or thoracic surgeries.

CONTRAINDICATIONS

Contraindications to PFTs include acute illnesses that may be aggravated by elevated intrathoracic pressure present during breath hold maneuvers. Examples include pneumothorax, recent myocardial infarction or unstable angina, recent thoracic/abdominal/ocular surgery, thoracic aortic aneurysm, and hemoptysis. PFTs performed during acute pulmonary illness, such as COPD exacerbation, are generally of no significant utility and are often postponed until a patient recovers. While not an absolute contraindication, practitioners should be cautious testing patients with neuromuscular disease, especially myasthenia gravis, as they are at high risk of respiratory failure after the vigorous breathing required when performing the test. β-Agonists should be used with caution in patients with a history of tachyarrhythmia or thyrotoxicosis.

PROCEDURE

The three main components of the PFT are **spirometry**, lung volumes, and diffusing capacity.

Spirometry

Spirometry is the first component performed, recording the total amount of air inhaled and exhaled and plotting this volume against time. Due to its ease of use, relative low cost, and utility in the diagnosis of obstructive disease, spirometry is often used in primary care offices. Spirometry allows the calculation of the **forced vital capacity (FVC), forced expiratory volume in 1 second (FEV$_1$),** and **maximum voluntary ventilation (MVV).**

FVC is obtained by measuring complete, forced exhalation from maximally inflated lungs. This measures the maximum ventilatory capacity of the lungs. FEV$_1$ is the amount of air exhaled during the first second of the FVC calculation (Fig. 46.1). These two values make up the **FEV$_1$/FVC ratio,** or the volume of air able to be forced out of the lungs in the first second as compared to the maximal possible exhalation volume. During spirometry, patients with an obstructive pattern (see "Interpretation" later) may undergo a bronchodilator challenge, usually with an inhaled β-agonist, to determine if some component of the obstruction is reversible.

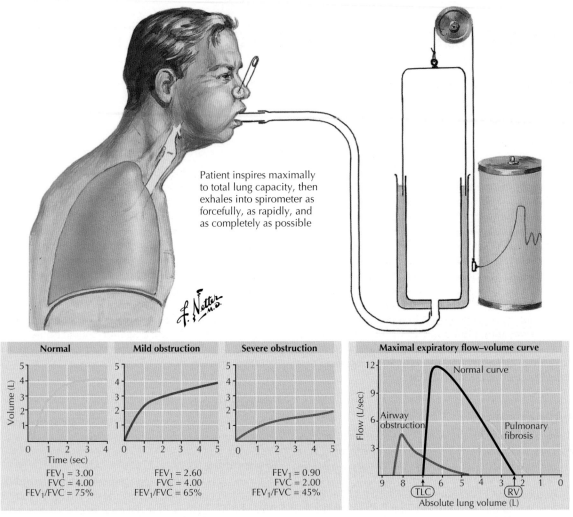

Patient inspires maximally to total lung capacity, then exhales into spirometer as forcefully, as rapidly, and as completely as possible

Normal	Mild obstruction	Severe obstruction
FEV$_1$ = 3.00	FEV$_1$ = 2.60	FEV$_1$ = 0.90
FVC = 4.00	FVC = 4.00	FVC = 2.00
FEV$_1$/FVC = 75%	FEV$_1$/FVC = 65%	FEV$_1$/FVC = 45%

Maximal expiratory flow–volume curve

Normal curve

Airway obstruction

Pulmonary fibrosis

FIG. 46.1 Forced Expiratory Volume Maneuver. *FEV$_1$*, Forced expiratory volume in 1 second; *FVC*, forced vital capacity; *RV*, residual volume; *TLC*, total lung capacity.

MVV measures the total ventilatory volume that a patient can produce in a set period of time, traditionally 1 minute. The patient is instructed to breathe as hard and as fast as possible for 10 to 15 seconds, and this volume of air is scaled to determine the MVV in 1 minute. The MVV can be used as an indicator of patient effort by comparing against reference standards. However, if the technician believes that the test is valid, a decreased MVV is a nonspecific marker of loss of respiratory muscle coordination, pathology in the chest wall muscula-ture, neurological/neuromuscular disease, or chronic deconditioning.

Flow-volume loops can be created by plotting the flow of air (in liters per second) on the y-axis, against the volume of air (in liters) on the x-axis. When graphed, the shape of the respiratory cycle is helpful in determining various pathologies (see Figs. 46.4 and 46.5 later). For example, in obstructive lung disease, there is difficulty with expiration, so there will be a scooped, prolonged expiratory phase. Flow-volume loops of restrictive lung disease appear similar to a normal loop with regard to flow (y-axis), but due to the restrictive nature of the disease they are shifted across the x-axis to represent decreased volume. While the information received from

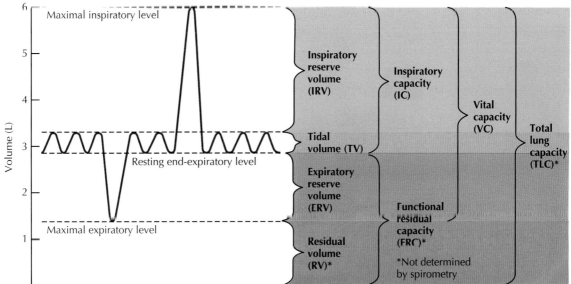

Inspiratory reserve volume (IRV): the additional volume that could be inhaled after a normal, quiet inspiration
Tidal volume (TV): the volume of air inhaled and exhaled during breathing. At rest, this is approximately 500 mL.
Expiratory reserve volume (ERV): the additional volume that could be exhaled after a normal, quiet expiration
Residual volume (RV): the volume remaining in the lung after maximal exhalation
Inspiratory capacity (IC): the maximum volume that can be inspired after expiration during normal, quiet breathing
Functional residual capacity (FRC): the volume remaining in the lung after expiration during normal quiet breathing
Vital capacity (VC): the maximum volume that can be exhaled after a maximal inspiration
Total lung capacity (TLC): the volume of air in the lung after maximal inspiration

FIG. 46.2 **Lung Volumes.**

both spirometry and flow-volume loops for restrictive and obstructive lung disease can be redundant, a flow-volume loop is most useful in determining various types of obstruction in the pulmonary system. Thus flow-volume loops are often used to differentiate between fixed, intrathoracic, and extrathoracic obstructions.

Lung Volumes

While spirometry is a relatively easy test that can be performed in the primary care setting, measuring lung volumes is significantly more complicated. These measurements are often obtained in dedicated laboratories with highly specialized equipment. Spirometry measures the inhaled and exhaled volumes in a patient and thus can only measure air that can be mobilized in the lungs. The lungs, however, must keep a **residual volume (RV)** of air to prevent total collapse of alveoli and distal airways. The RV and the FVC added together equal the **total lung capacity (TLC)** (Fig. 46.2).

There are three methods to calculate lung volumes:
• **Inert gas dilution** involves dissolving a small amount of inert gas, usually helium, into a patient's lungs.

After equilibration of the gas into the lungs, the total lung volume is calculated by using the original volume and concentration of the inert gas.
• **Nitrogen washout** technique. The TLC is calculated by measuring the concentration of expired nitrogen in the lungs both before and after inhaling pure (100%) oxygen. Knowing the concentration of nitrogen in room air allows the calculation of the TLC.
• **Body plethysmography** requires the use of a sealed chamber. The patient is then asked to inhale against a mouthpiece in a manner similar to panting. This changes the volume of the thoracic cavity, causing a corresponding change to the volume and pressure of the interchamber air. Using Boyle's law, $P_1V_1 = P_2V_2$, the clinician is able to calculate lung volumes from these interchamber air changes (Fig. 46.3).

As opposed to spirometry, which is most useful in diagnosing obstructive lung disease, the calculation of lung volumes is a valuable tool in the determination of restrictive lung disease. To be diagnosed with a restrictive lung disease, the TLC needs to be decreased. However, a decreased TLC is nonspecific to restrictive disease

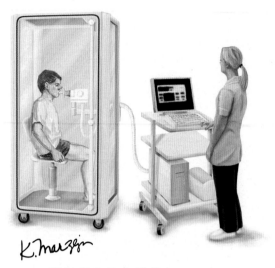

K. marzin

FIG. 46.3 **Body Plethysmography.**

and can be seen in other conditions, including chest wall pathology, pleural effusions, and neuromuscular disorders.

Diffusion Capacity

The final component of the PFT is the diffusion capacity, which is an objective measurement of how quickly a patient can absorb alveolar gases. It is often measured by using a small, safe amount of carbon monoxide (CO). CO is used, as it has one of the strongest affinities for hemoglobin. Reduction in the **diffusion capacity of the lung for carbon monoxide (D_LCO)** indicates dysfunction in the ability of a gas to properly pass from the alveoli spaces to pulmonary circulation.

INTERPRETATION

Spirometry

FEV_1 and FVC are perhaps the two most important clinical measurements in PFTs and the most reliable way to determine the difference between obstructive and restrictive pathology. While both the FEV_1 and FVC decline with age, the ratio should be preserved. In normal lungs, a majority of forcefully exhaled air should be exhaled within the first second—the particular normal is based on sex, age, weight, height, and ethnicity. Patients with a FEV_1/FVC ratio <70% show evidence of an **obstructive** process, as <70% of exhaled air is exhaled

in the first second. In COPD, the Global Initiative for Chronic Obstructive Lung Disease (GOLD) criteria uses the FEV_1 to grade the severity of obstruction (Fig. 46.4) (see Chapter 85 for further details).

Patients with decreased FEV_1 and FVC, but normal FEV_1/FVC ratio, may have a **restrictive** pulmonary process. This can be confirmed with lung volume testing (Fig. 46.5). Restrictive processes can be further delineated by D_LCO; intrapulmonary processes such as diffuse parenchymal lung diseases will have low D_LCO, but chest wall or neuromuscular disease will have normal D_LCO as a result of normal alveolar anatomy.

Testing for reversibility in obstructive lung disease allows the differentiation of asthma from other obstructive diseases such as COPD or bronchiectasis. If the FEV_1 increases by ≥12%, or if there is >200-mL increase in volume of the FEV_1 or FVC, it is a positive bronchodilator response, indicating reversible obstruction. If there is not a reversible component, then it is likely a fixed obstructive disease; examples include emphysema, chronic bronchitis, cystic fibrosis, bronchiectasis, bronchiolitis obliterans, and α1-antitrypsin deficiency.

Lung Volumes

A decreased TLC usually indicates a restrictive pulmonary process. In obstructive disorders, the TLC and RV are often increased, which indicates air trapping, a common phenomenon seen with disorders, including COPD and asthma.

Diffusion Capacity

A decreased D_LCO will be observed in disorders that result in destruction of pulmonary parenchyma (seen in pulmonary fibrosis), vascular abnormalities (pulmonary embolism, ventilation-perfusion [V/Q] mismatching, pulmonary hypertension), and reduction in the number of functional alveoli (lung resections, emphysema). Another common cause of decreased D_LCO is anemia, as a decreased quantity of circulating hemoglobin will also decrease the diffusion capacity. Thus it is always important to measure a patient's hemoglobin level when performing this test.

The measured D_LCO can be increased in certain cases. The most common causes of increased D_LCO include conditions with increased pulmonary circulation, such as left-to-right cardiac shunts, polycythemia, and asthma.

Lastly, the diffusion capacity also offers prognostic information for patients undergoing surgical resection of lung cancer. D_LCO calculated <40% of predicted is associated with decreased long-term survival.

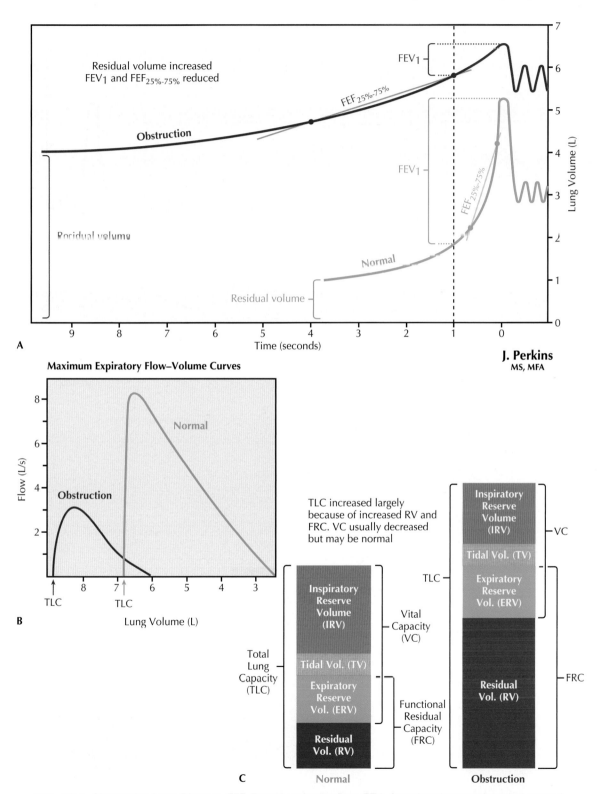

FIG. 46.4 **Obstructive Lung Disease.** *FEF,* Forced expiratory flow; *FEV₁,* forced expiratory volume in 1 second.

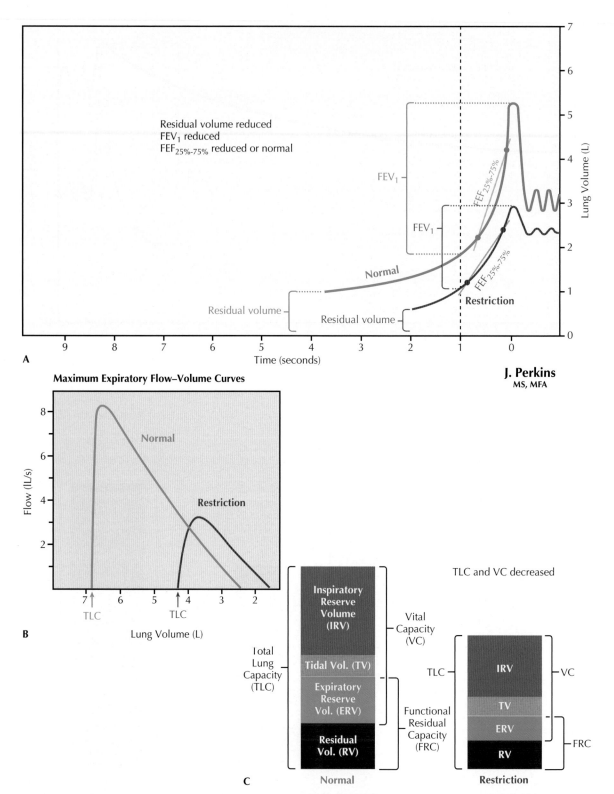

FIG. 46.5 **Restrictive Lung Disease.** *FEF,* Forced expiratory flow; *FEV₁,* forced expiratory volume in 1 second.

CHAPTER 47

Mechanical Ventilation

SARAH P. COHEN

INTRODUCTION

Mechanical ventilation is used to supplement and, at times, replace the functioning respiratory system. It is most commonly used in critically ill patients or for airway protection during a procedure. Less frequently, it is used long term for patients with chronic respiratory failure. Mechanical ventilation regulates both inspiration and expiration, most commonly through **endotracheal (ET) intubation.** Patients who are endotracheally intubated are presumed to be temporarily on ventilation; **tracheostomy** is required for long-term ventilation. For patients in whom ET intubation is not possible, **cricothyroidotomy** may be performed to allow mechanical ventilation.

Once mechanical ventilation has been initiated, oxygenation and ventilation can be managed by adjusting settings on the ventilator as described in the chapter.

INDICATIONS

Mechanical ventilation may be needed for one of three major reasons:

1. **Hypoxic respiratory failure.** This is typically due to pulmonary pathology such as pneumonia or acute respiratory distress syndrome (ARDS).
2. **Hypercarbic respiratory failure.** This could be from a primary pulmonary condition such as chronic obstructive pulmonary disease (COPD), respiratory muscle weakness as can be seen in muscular dystrophies or Guillain-Barré syndrome, or hypoventilation due to altered mental status.
3. Airway protection. This is used when a patient has a major central nervous system event (e.g., a brainstem stroke) or altered mental status that leads to loss of airway protective reflexes. This is also the indication for intubation during a procedure (e.g., in the operating room).

These are not mutually exclusive; many patients have combined hypoxic and hypercarbic respiratory failure or have respiratory failure and need airway protection.

INITIATION

ET intubation is needed to initiate mechanical ventilation. To proceed with that, **rapid sequence intubation (RSI)** procedure is usually followed. This process is composed of preoxygenation, deep sedation, and neuromuscular blockade (paralysis). Preoxygenation can be accomplished either passively with oxygen supplementation or via bag-valve-mask ventilation with 100% oxygen supplied. When the patient is adequately preoxygenated, deep sedation is then initiated, and paralysis is considered with a depolarizing (e.g., succinylcholine) or nondepolarizing (e.g., rocuronium, vecuronium) agent.

The laryngoscope blade is placed into the oropharyngeal cavity and manipulated such that the vocal cords are visible (the exact positioning depends on the type of laryngoscope), with careful attention paid to avoiding dental, maxillary, or mandibular trauma (Fig. 47.1). An ET tube is then passed through the vocal cords under direct visualization, the laryngoscope blade is removed from the oropharynx, and the balloon near the tip of the ET tube is inflated. Correct ET tube position is confirmed by auscultating bilateral lung sounds and ensuring absence of a gastric bubble sound on the upper stomach, as well as with color capnography, end tidal CO_2, and chest x-ray (though direct visualization of the tube passing through the cords is most important).

COMPLICATIONS

One of the most feared complications during ET intubation is unrecognized esophageal intubation, leading to gastric insufflation, which can cause aspiration of gastric contents in addition to absent pulmonary ventilation. Unrecognized esophageal intubation can be avoided using the confirmation methods described earlier. If the ET tube is cannulated too deep, it will preferentially go into the right mainstem bronchus, resulting in ventilation of only the right lung; this can be detected by auscultation or on chest x-ray and fixed by repositioning of the ET tube. Patients may aspirate, especially if the stomach was full due to recent PO intake or insufflation with air

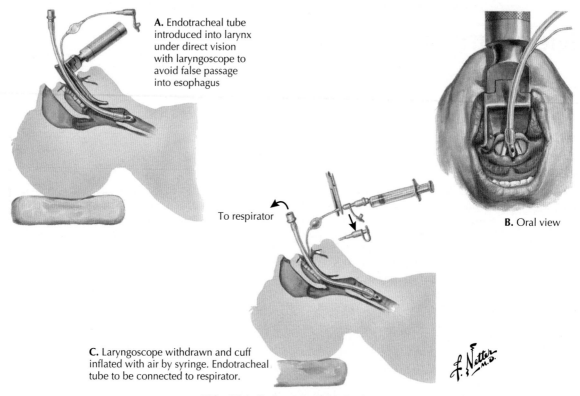

A. Endotracheal tube introduced into larynx under direct vision with laryngoscope to avoid false passage into esophagus

To respirator

B. Oral view

C. Laryngoscope withdrawn and cuff inflated with air by syringe. Endotracheal tube to be connected to respirator.

FIG. 47.1   **Endotracheal Intubation.**

during bag-mask ventilation prior to intubation. The act of ET intubation may lead to trauma to the oropharynx or vocal cords; severe trauma to the vocal cords during attempted intubation can lead to vocal cord edema resulting in inability to obtain an airway or ventilate, which can be fatal. Prolonged attempts at intubation without ventilation can also cause hypoxemia, which, if not recognized and managed emergently, can also be fatal (Fig. 47.2).

Mechanical ventilation with high pressures can lead to **barotrauma** of the lungs and may result in the development of a pneumothorax. Physicians must pay special attention to intrapulmonary pressures, including peak and plateau airway pressures, to prevent barotrauma and pulmonary damage. There is a higher incidence of pneumonia in patients being mechanically ventilated. Prolonged intubation can also cause damage to the vocal cords, and patients who require ventilation for more than 1 to 2 weeks typically undergo tracheostomy.

BASIC VENTILATOR MANAGEMENT

The first decision to make when initiating mechanical ventilation is the mode of ventilation. While pressure and volume are directly related, only one variable is directly controlled by the physician; these are **pressure control** and **volume control**, respectively. The provider then decides the frequency of breaths delivered per minute at a minimum; the patient may breathe faster than this preset rate. A common mode is assist control, in which the ventilator has a preset respiratory rate but will deliver a small amount of pressure support to overcome resistance from the ET tube should the patient trigger a breath on his or her own. Modes in which the patient triggers every breath are pure assist, or support, modes. The most common modes of mechanical ventilation are volume assist control, pressure assist control, and pressure support ventilation. Waveforms on the ventilator provide real-time information on the patient's respiratory status (Fig. 47.3).

Patients who are mechanically ventilated generally require sedation. The goals of sedation are to promote patient comfort and to avoid ventilator dyssynchrony, which occurs when a patient's own respiratory attempts are not coordinated well with the ventilator. When clinically appropriate, switching from an assist control mode of ventilation to a pressure support mode can improve patient–ventilator synchrony. Alternatively,

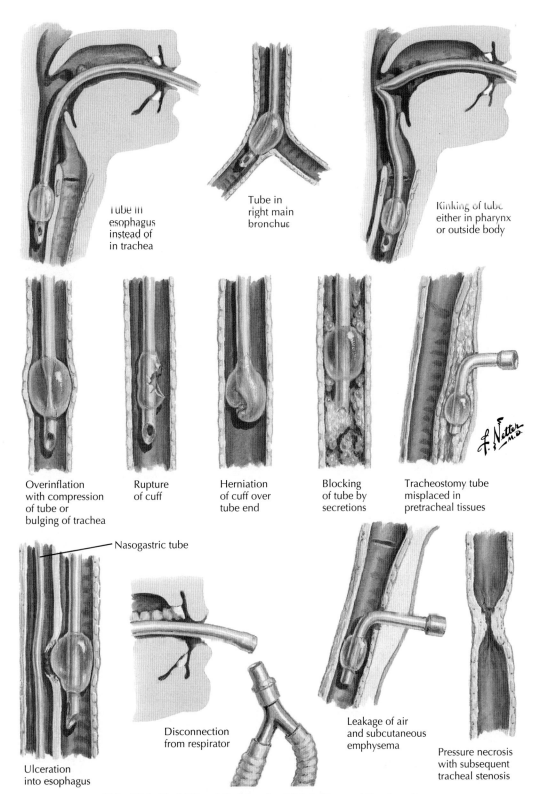

Tube in esophagus instead of in trachea

Tube in right main bronchus

Kinking of tube either in pharynx or outside body

Overinflation with compression of tube or bulging of trachea

Rupture of cuff

Herniation of cuff over tube end

Blocking of tube by secretions

Tracheostomy tube misplaced in pretracheal tissues

Nasogastric tube

Ulceration into esophagus

Disconnection from respirator

Leakage of air and subcutaneous emphysema

Pressure necrosis with subsequent tracheal stenosis

FIG. 47.2 **Morbidity of Endotracheal Intubation and Tracheostomy.**

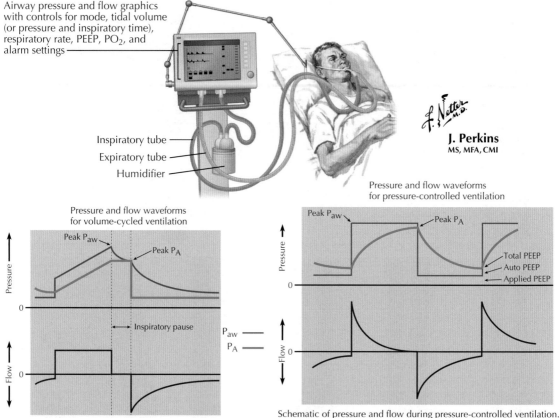

Airway pressure and flow graphics with controls for mode, tidal volume (or pressure and inspiratory time), respiratory rate, PEEP, PO₂, and alarm settings

J. Perkins
MS, MFA, CMI

Inspiratory tube
Expiratory tube
Humidifier

Pressure and flow waveforms for pressure-controlled ventilation

Pressure and flow waveforms for volume-cycled ventilation

Peak P_{aw}
Peak P_A
Inspiratory pause
P_{aw}
P_A

Peak P_{aw}
Peak P_A
Total PEEP
Auto PEEP
Applied PEEP

Schematic of pressure and flow during volume-cycled ventilation. The volume delivered is set by the operator; the resulting pressure is the dependent variable. The blue line shows ramped airway pressure (P_{aw}) applied during inspiration in response to a square-wave flow pattern shown in purple. The green line shows the change in alveolar pressure (P_A) with increasing lung volume. Application of a brief pause in flow at the end of inspiration allows demonstration of the plateau in P_{aw} and P_A.

Schematic of pressure and flow during pressure-controlled ventilation. The inflation pressure is set by the operator, the resulting volume delivered is the dependent variable. The blue line shows the square wave of airway pressure (P_{aw}) applied during inspiration, generated by the decelerating flow pattern shown in purple. The green line shows the change in alveolar pressure (P_A). At the end of the expiratory phase, the total positive end-expiratory pressure (PEEP) remaining in the alveoli is equal to the applied PEEP plus any residual pressure (auto PEEP) that results from incomplete emptying of the lung.

FIG. 47.3 Mechanical Ventilation.

the patient's sedation may be increased to improve synchrony with the ventilator. Though many patients require relatively deep sedation to tolerate mechanical ventilation via an ET tube, some patients can tolerate mechanical ventilation and achieve adequate synchrony with the ventilator while receiving minimal sedation. Patients who are being ventilated via a tracheostomy tube typically require less sedation than endotracheally intubated patients, and patients who are chronically mechanically ventilated via a tracheostomy generally do not require sedation when using their baseline ventilator settings.

Regardless of the mode of ventilation, the positive end-expiratory pressure (PEEP) and the fraction of oxygen

(FiO_2) must be set. Increasing PEEP and increasing FiO_2 are the primary ways to improve oxygenation in a mechanically ventilated patient.

PEEP is the amount of pressure still present in the lungs at the end of a breath. This end-expiratory pressure keeps alveoli open, preventing the development of atelectasis. The PEEP is usually set to no less than 5 cm H_2O; larger patients may require a higher PEEP to overcome the weight of their chest wall. The **FiO_2** is the fraction of oxygen present in inspired gas, typically varying from 21% (room air) to 100% oxygen. Efforts are made to keep the FiO_2 as low as possible while still maintaining aerobic respiration, as high levels of oxygen can lead to oxidative damage to lung tissues.

The primary determinant of ventilation, or removing CO_2, is **minute ventilation,** which is equal to respiratory rate multiplied by tidal volume. In assist control modes, a minimum respiratory rate is set. Classically, in pressure support ventilation, no respiratory rate is set; as such, the rate is entirely dependent on patient effort. The desired tidal volume is set directly in volume assist control ventilation. In pressure assist control or pressure support ventilation, an inspiratory pressure is set, and the resultant tidal volume is based on the patient's respiratory compliance (patients with less compliance require a higher inspiratory pressure to attain the same tidal volume). Increasing tidal volume (or inspiratory pressure) and the respiratory rate (in patients on assist control modes of ventilation) are the primary ways to improve ventilation in a mechanically ventilated patient.

As patients clinically improve, their respiratory function may progress to being able to breathe without requiring mechanical ventilation, necessitating weaning from mechanical ventilation. Supportive parameters, including FiO_2 and PEEP, are decreased as allowed by clinical status, generally to a goal of FiO_2 30% to 40% and PEEP 5 mm Hg (varies depending on body habitus). Once on minimal support, a **spontaneous breathing trial** may be attempted, in which sedation is decreased or paused and the patient triggers breaths on his or her own. The patient is then monitored for up to a few hours, and if his or her vital signs are stable and the tidal volumes are acceptable, the patient can then be considered for extubation. Patients who are intubated only for airway protection during a procedure, however, can usually be extubated shortly after the procedure without true weaning or spontaneous breathing trials.

CHAPTER 48

Echocardiography

LEILA HAGHIGHAT

INTRODUCTION

The use of ultrasound as a noninvasive means of evaluating cardiac structure and function was a revolutionary advancement in the late 20th century, providing greater detail regarding cardiac structure and function than physical exam and the electrocardiogram (ECG) alone. With the development of Doppler ultrasound in the 1980s, echocardiography became an invaluable method for evaluating cardiac function and hemodynamics without the invasiveness of cardiac catheterization. This chapter will cover primarily **transthoracic echocardiography (TTE)**, as opposed to **transesophageal echocardiography (TEE)** (Fig. 48.1). Both utilize the same principles, and while TEE offers greater resolution of cardiac structures (advantageous in, for example, diagnosing endocarditis), TTE is much more frequently used and can be performed readily at the bedside.

BASIC PRINCIPLES

Echocardiography utilizes sound waves generated from piezoelectric crystals within a transducer to generate images of the heart. Applying voltage to these crystals causes them to vibrate and emit a sound wave in the range of 1 to 10 MHz. When the sound wave bounces back from the structure being analyzed, it returns to the transducer, where the mechanical energy is converted back to electric energy and displayed on a screen. The time it takes for the sound wave to return determines the brightness of the display.

TTE, and indeed ultrasound, resolution depends on the wavelength of sound being transmitted, which in turn depends on the frequency of the probe selected. This relationship is summarized in the equation $c = f \times \lambda$, where c is the speed of light, f is the frequency of the sound wave, and λ is its wavelength. A higher frequency transducer produces a smaller wavelength and better image resolution.

Modern TTE uses a combination of various modalities, including the two-dimensional (2D) mode, M mode, and Doppler modalities. 2D imaging is the classic modality

of ultrasonography, while M (motion) mode pulses an ultrasound beam rapidly in a single plane through the heart. It results in a high-resolution plot of depth on the vertical axis against time on the horizontal axis. **Doppler** ultrasound uses the eponymous principle to calculate the velocity of blood moving through the heart based on the difference between the frequency of an emitted and reflected sound wave. The pressure gradient across a valve can then be calculated using the simplified Bernoulli equation $(P_1 - P_2) = 4V^2$, where P is pressure and V is velocity. When color mapping is applied to the Doppler modality, blood flow toward the transducer conventionally appears red, blood flow away from the transducer appears blue, and turbulent blood flow appears yellow or green (Fig. 48.2).

INDICATIONS

TTE is utilized to diagnose and monitor a diverse array of cardiac pathologies, including acute coronary syndrome, valvular disease, congestive heart failure, and pericardial effusion. Given the lack of radiation, TTE can be repeated as often as needed, allowing for long-term monitoring and comparison, as in patients receiving cardiotoxic chemotherapy. Because TTE is rapid and portable, it has a role in emergency situations for diagnosing life-threatening conditions such as cardiac tamponade, aortic dissection, myocardial infarction, and shock. Limitations to TTE are similar to those for ultrasound, in which dense structures preclude visualization of other deeper structures. These include acoustic shadowing from prosthetic valves, ventricular assist devices, large body habitus, calcification, and bones.

COMMON CARDIAC WINDOWS

Parasternal Long (Fig. 48.3)

The transducer is placed along the left sternal border at the level of the third to fourth intercostal space, pointing toward the patient's right shoulder. This view allows for assessment of left ventricular (LV) size and function;

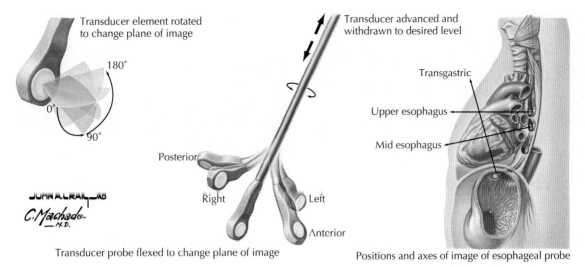

Transducer element rotated to change plane of image

180°

0°

90°

Posterior

Right

Left

Anterior

Transducer advanced and withdrawn to desired level

Transgastric

Upper esophagus

Mid esophagus

JOHN A.CRAIG—AD

C.Machado
M.D.

Transducer probe flexed to change plane of image

Positions and axes of image of esophageal probe

FIG. 48.1 **Transesophageal Echocardiography.**

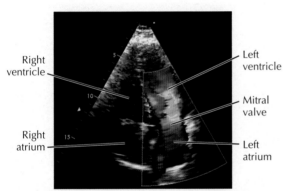

Right ventricle

Left ventricle

Mitral valve

Right atrium

Left atrium

Color enhancement in a four-chamber view.
Shows blood flow from left atrium to left ventricle through the open mitral valve. Blue is flow away from the transducer on the patient's skin, and red is toward the transducer. There is some turbulent/bidirectional flow in the left ventricle as evidenced by both the red and blue colors being present.

FIG. 48.2 **Doppler Color Mapping in Four-Chamber View.**

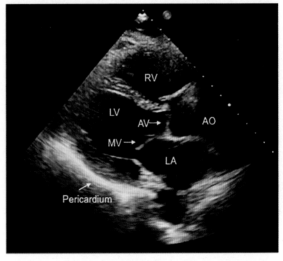

FIG. 48.3 **Parasternal Long View.** *AO,* Aortic outlet; *AV,* aortic valve; *LA,* left atrium; *LV,* left ventricle; *MV,* mitral valve; *RV,* right ventricle.

aortic and mitral valve opening, motion, and calcification; and pericardial fluid. Subtly tilting the transducer inferiorly provides views of the right heart, including the tricuspid valve.

Parasternal Short (Fig. 48.4)

From the parasternal long view, the transducer is rotated 90 degrees toward the patient's left shoulder and pointed downward toward the patient's left flank. This view shows

LV size and function, including an assessment of regional LV wall motion, and pericardial fluid.

Apical Four Chamber (Fig. 48.5)

The transducer is laid over the site of apical impulse with a tilt upward to cut through the long axis of the heart. Both atrial and ventricular sizes can be assessed, in addition to mitral and tricuspid valve motion and function.

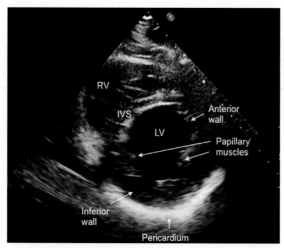

FIG. 48.4 **Parasternal Short View.** *IVS,* Interventricular septum; *LV,* left ventricle; *RV,* right ventricle.

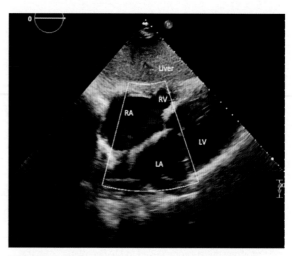

FIG. 48.6 **Subcostal View.** *LA,* Left atrium; *LV,* left ventricle; *RA,* right atrium; *RV,* right ventricle.

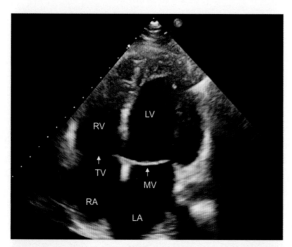

FIG. 48.5 **Apical Four-Chamber View.** *LA,* Left atrium; *LV,* left ventricle, *MV,* mitral valve; *RA,* right atrium; *RV,* right ventricle; *TV,* tricuspid valve.

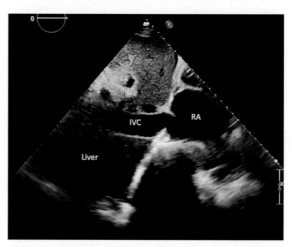

FIG. 48.7 **Subcostal Inferior Vena Cava** *(IVC)* **View.** *RA,* Right atrium.

Subcostal (Fig. 48.6)

The transducer is placed 2 to 3 cm below the xiphoid process, pointing toward the patient's left shoulder. Holding the transducer palm down facilitates cephalad angulation of the ultrasound beam. This view is similar to that of the apical four-chamber window but provides a better view of pericardial fluid.

Subcostal Inferior Vena Cava (IVC) (Fig. 48.7)

From the subcostal view, turning the transducer 90 degrees counterclockwise allows for visualization of the

inferior vena cava, which can be seen merging with the right atrium.

FINDINGS

Cardiac Function

The most popular method for assessing global function of the LV is based on a multisegment model put forth by the American Society of Echocardiography. The LV is divided into 17 segments, and each is given a score between 1 and 4, with a higher number signifying greater dyskinesia. Summing each segment and dividing by the number of segments yields the wall motion score

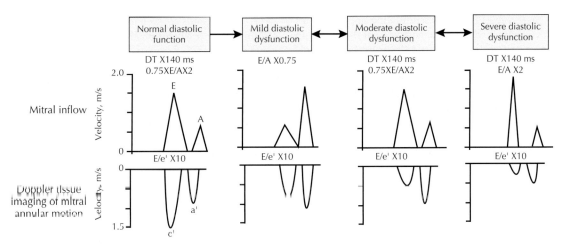

FIG. 48.8 **Doppler Criteria for Assessment of Diastolic Dysfunction.**

index (WMSI). A WMSI of 1 is considered normal, and a WMSI >1.7 is associated with physical exam findings of heart failure.

LV systolic function can be determined in multiple ways. On general inspection, good function is indicated by inward motion and thickening of the myocardium, downward motion of the mitral annulus, and uniform contractility of all wall segments. Calculating **LV ejection fraction (LVEF)** involves use of the Simpson biplane method. Manual tracing of the LV endocardial border in both two-chamber and four-chamber views generates volumes that are plugged into the equation $LVEF = (LVED_{vol} - LVES_{vol}) / LVED_{vol} \times 100$, where LVEF is ejection fraction, $LVED_{vol}$ is end diastolic volume, and $LVES_{vol}$ is end systolic volume. Generally, LVEF <55% is considered compromised. Additional quantifiers of LV function include stroke volume, cardiac index, contractility, and the Tei index, which evaluates for the combination of LV systolic and diastolic dysfunction.

Diastolic function can be assessed by calculating the E/A ratio, where E is the velocity of blood flow through the mitral valve during early diastole, and A is the velocity during late diastole and atrial contraction. Typically, the E/A ratio is between 1.2 and 1.5. However, as ventricular compliance worsens, the E wave decreases and the A wave increases with compensation from the atrium. This leads to a reversal of the normal E/A ratio and is classified as stage 1 diastolic dysfunction, or impaired LV relaxation. Over time, the atrium can no longer contract as effectively as before, decreasing the A velocity and returning the ratio close to normal—this is classified as stage 2 diastolic dysfunction. Progression of diastolic dysfunction leads to a restrictive pattern, classified as

stage 3 diastolic dysfunction, with an increased E/A ratio and steep descending slope of the E wave as it appears on Doppler ultrasound (Fig. 48.8).

Myocardial Infarction

Myocardial infarction (MI) may be first detected on TTE by the development and visualization of focal hypokinesis that occurs within seconds of infarction, even before chest pain and ECG changes. Additional evidence of MI includes thinning, paradoxical outward bulging, and increased echogenicity of the myocardial wall. The LVEF is the single greatest prognosticator of morbidity and mortality in acute MI. Secondary mechanical complications of MI that may be detected on TTE include acute mitral regurgitation with flailing of the mitral leaflet into the left atrium during systole because of acute papillary muscle dysfunction, ventricular septal defect formation, pseudoaneurysm with ventricular free wall perforation contained locally by adjacent pericardium, tamponade, and right ventricular infarction. Later complications of MI seen on TTE are LV remodeling, LV aneurysm with outpouching of all three cardiac layers, and LV thrombus that typically is adjacent to the endocardial border of a dyskinetic wall segment.

Cardiomyopathy

Each cardiomyopathy has characteristic findings on TTE. Dilated cardiomyopathy is identified based on an enlarged ventricular cavity with normal or thin walls plus systolic dysfunction, while restrictive and hypertrophic cardiomyopathies have normal to increased LV wall thickness plus impaired diastolic filling. **Amyloidosis,** a particular cause of restrictive cardiomyopathy, is associated with preserved LVEF and a scintillating appearance of the myocardium with biatrial enlargement that yields an owl-eyes pattern (see Chapter 147 for further details).

In **hypertrophic cardiomyopathy,** the LV cavity is often small and banana shaped, and LV systolic function is hyperdynamic. There can be asymmetric septal hypertrophy or diffuse concentric hypertrophy, systolic anterior motion of the mitral valve with a posteriorly directed jet of mitral regurgitation, and a resting LV outflow tract gradient >30 mm Hg. LV wall thickness can be markedly increased with LV wall thickness reaching 30 mm (normal up to 10 mm). Additional types of cardiomyopathy detectable on TTE include LV noncompaction and arrhythmogenic RV dysplasia.

Heart Failure

In the emergency room, TTE is useful to assess the dyspneic patient for possible exacerbation of heart failure (HF). Vertical hyperechogenic lines emanating from the pleura down to the end of the ultrasound screen are termed B lines. The presence of these lines has been shown to be more sensitive in detecting pulmonary edema than chest x-ray and correlate with levels of natriuretic peptides. In HF, TTE is also useful as an adjunct to ECG for assessing ventricular synchrony—asynchronous ventricles with QRS >130 milliseconds are seen in patients who could benefit from cardiac resynchronization therapy.

Pericardial Disease

Pericardial effusions appear as hypoechoic spaces between the visceral and parietal pericardium that persists throughout both diastole and systole. The appearance of such a small space only during systole may be a normal finding. Displacement of the aorta from the heart distinguishes pericardial from pleural effusion on TTE. The movement of both visceral and parietal pericardium in tandem, rather than a stationary parietal layer, differentiates pericardial effusion from constrictive pericarditis. A pericardial hematoma has a distinct echotexture, appearing more reticulated and echodense than an effusion. In cardiac tamponade, the right atrium inverts in late ventricular diastole when pressure in the chamber is the lowest, and pulsus paradoxus can be noted by a >10% decrease of the mitral E wave during inspiration.

Additional disease processes that may be identified using TTE include valvular heart disease, aortic disease (see Section 5), endocarditis (see Chapter 116 for further information), cardiac masses, and congenital heart disease.

CHAPTER 49

Arterial Blood Gas

STEFFNE KUNNIRICKAL

INTRODUCTION

Arterial blood gas (ABG) sampling is used to rapidly assess a patient's acid-base status, partial pressure of oxygen and carbon dioxide, and oxygen saturation. These parameters are particularly beneficial in the critical care settings in patients with a variety of respiratory and critical illnesses.

INDICATIONS

The indications for ABG sampling are very broad; if a patient is suspected of having significant derangements in oxygen and carbon dioxide gas exchange or **acid-base** balance, an ABG is generally recommended. Common indications for an ABG include:

- Identify and monitor respiratory, metabolic, or mixed acid-base disturbances
- Measure the partial pressure of oxygen and carbon dioxide
- Assess response to interventions, such as supplemental oxygen or **mechanical ventilation** in patients with respiratory failure, and diagnostic evaluations, such as exercise desaturation
- Monitor the severity and progression of previously diagnosed chronic diseases, such as chronic obstructive pulmonary disease (COPD)
- Determine the oxygen carrying capacity
- Quantify levels of carboxyhemoglobin and methemoglobin
- Obtain blood samples in an emergent setting when venous sampling is not possible

ABG sampling should be avoided in the following circumstances:

- Poor distal circulation: If there is poor distal perfusion or poor collateral circulation, sampling should be avoided in that particular limb to avoid the risk of ischemic injury.
- Local infection: If the selected puncture site appears infected, avoid that area and select an alternate site to prevent introduction of organisms into the bloodstream.

- Distorted anatomy: If the patient had previous surgical interventions, arteriovenous fistula, vascular grafts, stents, aneurysms, or malformations at the selected site, avoid puncture at that site.
- Severe peripheral vascular disease in the selected artery
- Active Raynaud syndrome

Supratherapeutic coagulopathy and infusion of thrombolytic agents are relative contraindications for arterial puncture. Therapeutic anticoagulation is not a contraindication for arterial puncture. In addition, arterial puncture should be avoided (if possible) in patients with platelets $<30 \times 10^3/\mu L$.

COMPLICATIONS

Life-threatening complications associated with ABG sampling are very rare. More common complications associated with ABG sampling include:

- Pain at the puncture site
- Bleeding or laceration at the puncture site, which can result in local hematoma and occlusion
- Arteriospasm
- Infection at the puncture site
- Air embolism or arterial thrombosis
- Damage to adjacent structures, such as nerves

PROCEDURE

Before the procedure, explain the indication and the risks and benefit of ABG sampling to the patient. This may not always be feasible, especially in critical care settings and during cardiopulmonary resuscitation. The procedure can be technically challenging in patients who are uncooperative, obese, or edematous, or in patients with severe contractures or poor pulses. An ultrasound-guided technique may be used in these instances (if necessary) to locate the artery and minimize complications.

Site Selection

Note that an ABG sample can be obtained from an indwelling arterial catheter if the patient has one. An

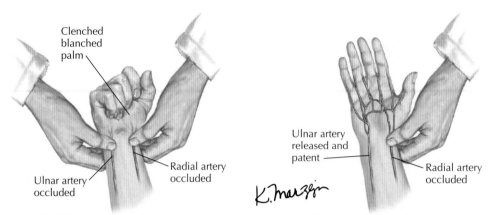

Clenched
blanched
palm

Ulnar artery
occluded

Radial artery
occluded

Ulnar artery
released and
patent

Radial artery
occluded

To perform a modified Allen test, position the hand above the heart and make a fist. Occlude the radial and ulnar artery at the same time, allowing for blood to drain out of the hand and leading to skin pallor. Then lower the hand, open the fist, and release the ulnar artery while maintaining occlusion at the radial artery. Blood flow should return to the palm within 6 seconds; if it takes longer, the Allen test is considered abnormal and the particular limb should be avoided for an arterial puncture.

FIG. 49.1 **Allen Test.**

arterial blood sample can be obtained from many sites, including the radial, femoral, brachial, dorsalis pedis, and axillary arteries. The **radial artery** is the most commonly used site, due to its easy accessibility and comfort of the patient. The radial artery can be palpated 2 to 3 cm proximal to the wrist crease, between the distal radius and the flexor carpi radialis tendon, with the wrist extended at 20 to 30 degrees. The needle can be inserted at a 45-degree angle to the skin.

The second most commonly used site is the brachial artery, which can be palpated between the medial epicondyle of the humerus and the biceps tendon in the antecubital fossa, with the arm extended, shoulder abducted, elbow extended, and forearm supinated. The needle should be inserted a few centimeters above the elbow crease at a 30-degree angle. The axillary artery is palpated in the axilla with the arm hyperabducted and externally rotated. The dorsalis pedis artery can be found lateral to the tendon of extensor hallucis longus. The needle should be inserted at a 30-degree angle at the midfoot. In patients with poor distal perfusion, large arteries, such as the femoral artery, are preferred because of relatively low risk of a hematoma or laceration compromising distal flow. The femoral artery is palpated between the pubis symphysis and the anterior superior iliac crest, 2 to 4 cm below the inguinal ligament. The needle should be inserted at an angle of 60 to 90 degrees.

Once a site has been selected, it is important to assess collateral circulation, as one of the complications of an arterial puncture is ischemia distal to the puncture site. If the radial artery is selected, a modified **Allen test** can be performed to assess collateral circulation via ulnar artery (Fig. 49.1). While the reliability of the Allen test is variable across multiple studies, it remains an important, easy-to-perform maneuver to assess collateral circulation, particularly in high-risk patients. With the larger vessels, such as the brachial and femoral arteries, assess the radial and pedal pulses, respectively, prior to puncture to ensure good circulation. If the dorsalis pedis artery is selected, occlude the artery and the nailbed of the great toe, then release the nailbed and assess the rapidity of return of blood flow.

Equipment

Many hospitals may have ABG sampling kits with all the necessary materials. If not, gather the following materials by the patient's bedside prior to the procedure: gloves, antiseptic solution, sterile gauze and bandage, bag with ice, and an ABG syringe. The ABG syringe is a preheparinized syringe and cap that may come with a protective needle and needle sleeve. Ensure that the heparin is completely flushed out or it may alter the pH of the sample. Leave the plunger depressed to allow blood to fill up during the procedure. A 22-gauge to 25-gauge needle may be used if none is provided in the kit.

Technique (Fig. 49.2)

- Gently palpate the pulse proximal to the selected puncture site using two fingers of the nondominant hand.
- Clean the selected puncture site with antiseptic skin solution (e.g., chlorhexidine or povidone-iodine solution). If needed, 1% to 2% lidocaine with epinephrine may be administered subcutaneously for anesthesia.

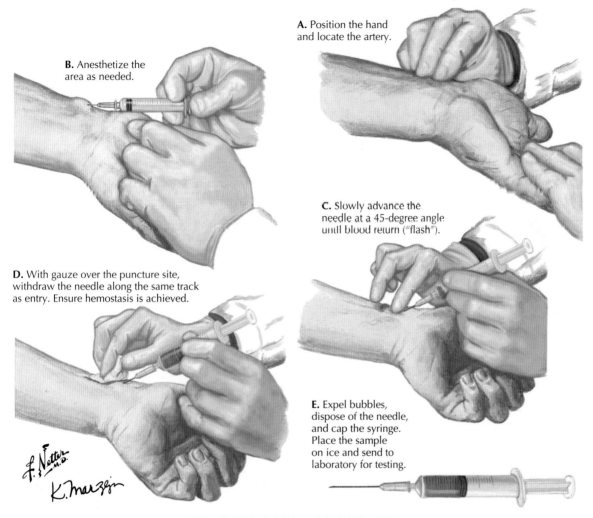

B. Anesthetize the area as needed.

A. Position the hand and locate the artery.

C. Slowly advance the needle at a 45-degree angle until blood return ("flash").

D. With gauze over the puncture site, withdraw the needle along the same track as entry. Ensure hemostasis is achieved.

E. Expel bubbles, dispose of the needle, and cap the syringe. Place the sample on ice and send to laboratory for testing.

FIG. 49.2 **Radial Artery Arterial Blood Gas.**

- Place the syringe in the dominant hand and, with the bevel facing up, insert the needle slowly at an angle appropriate for the selected artery. When the artery is punctured, a flash of pulsatile blood will be seen. The blood should fill into the syringe on its own, but in hypotensive patients or those with weak pulses, it may be necessary to pull back on the plunger to allow blood flow into the syringe. However, this may result in moving the needle tip, potentially preventing further sampling and injuring the artery and surrounding structures.
- If the blood flow stops at any point, the needle may have moved. Slowly withdraw the needle, as it may have gone "through-and-through" the arterial walls.

If there is still no blood return, withdraw the needle until the tip remains just underneath the skin before repositioning it for another attempt. If repeatedly unsuccessful, consider attempting the procedure at an alternate site, as even slight irritation can cause arterial spasm and prevent sampling.

- Once an adequate amount of blood has been withdrawn, remove the needle while simultaneously holding pressure at the puncture site with gauze. Hold pressure for 2 to 3 minutes or until the bleeding stops. It may be necessary to hold pressure for a longer time in patients with coagulopathy or on anticoagulation. Once hemostasis is ensured, apply a bandage over the puncture site.

- Cap and safely dispose of the needle.
- Hold the syringe upright, tap on it gently to allow air bubbles to move to the top from where it can be expelled. The presence of air bubbles can alter the results of the blood gas. Place the syringe cap on and roll the syringe between the hands to allow mixing. Place the sample in a bag of ice and send it to the laboratory for analysis.

After the procedure, monitor the patient for any signs of bleeding, hematoma, persistent pain, paresthesia, or limb ischemia.

ADDITIONAL TESTS

Since an ABG provides information regarding the physiologic state of a patient at the time of sampling, it is important to note the date, time, patient's body temperature, position, activity level, respiratory rate, sample site, supplemental oxygen flow, and mode of ventilation. The results should always be correlated with the clinical scenario (see Chapters 23 and 31).

CHAPTER 50

Central Venous Catheterization

SHARON ZHUO

OVERVIEW AND INDICATIONS

Central venous catheterization (CVC) is a commonly performed procedure in hospitalized patients, particularly for those patients in the intensive care unit. Common indications for CVC include delivery of caustic medications (most commonly vasopressors), monitoring of central venous pressure, and volume resuscitation. Specialized types of catheters can be used for hemodialysis and hemodynamic monitoring.

The choice of catheter is dependent on the specific patient need. Different catheters vary by length, gauge, and number of lumens. **Poiseuille's law** governs the flow rate *(Q)* through a catheter:

$$Q = \frac{\pi P r^4}{8 \eta l} \qquad \text{EQ. 50.1}$$

As the viscosity (η) of the infused fluid cannot change, the flow rate is directly proportional to the radius of the catheter *(r)* to the fourth power and inversely proportional to the length *(l)*. Therefore, for patients requiring rapid infusion of crystalloid or blood products, an introducer catheter (i.e., Cordis) should be considered due to its large gauge and short length, thus maximizing flow rate. A triple-lumen catheter, on the other hand, has a relatively smaller diameter with three distinct lumens within the catheter, which impedes the flow rate. It is, however, an ideal choice for patients who need multiple simultaneous infusions. Table 50.1 lists common types of catheters and their indications.

Other notable CVCs include **peripherally inserted central catheters (PICCs)**, which are longer central lines inserted through a peripheral vein on the arm and which course toward the cavoatrial junction. PICC lines are commonly used for long-term intravenous (IV) antibiotics, chemotherapy, or total parenteral nutrition. A **tunneled dialysis catheter (TDC)** (also called permacath) is a long-term indwelling catheter used for hemodialysis. As a tunneled catheter, the TDC traverses a subcutaneous tunnel before entering the vein. Their insertion is more technically involved but leads to lower rates of infection. A **port** is a subcutaneously implanted CVC used for the administration of chemotherapy. These catheters typically remain indwelling for an extended time and are inserted by specialists. This chapter focuses on temporary CVCs listed in Table 50.1, usually inserted at bedside.

CONTRAINDICATIONS

Most contraindications to CVC insertion are relative and depend on the urgency of the procedure. One common contraindication is thrombocytopenia or coagulopathy. If severe, periprocedural platelet or fresh frozen plasma transfusions can be considered. A different site for CVC placement should be chosen if there is venous thrombosis, stenosis, or altered anatomy such as traumatic injury. Overlying skin infection also should prompt alternate site selection.

SITES OF INSERTION

The three commonly used sites of insertion are the internal jugular, subclavian, and femoral veins (Fig. 50.1). Internal jugular vein access is often preferred due to compressibility and lower incidence of mechanical complications; subclavian insertion may be associated with lower rates of infection but has higher rates of **pneumothorax** and is relatively difficult to compress should bleeding occur. The femoral vein access is used as a last resort due to historically higher rates of infectious complications. The following section discusses the internal jugular approach, which is most commonly used.

PROCEDURE (INTERNAL JUGULAR VEIN APPROACH)

- After obtaining informed consent, place the patient in the supine, **Trendelenburg** position.
- Rotate the patient's head to face away from the site of catheter insertion. Use the ultrasound to locate the internal jugular vein, which lies in the triangle formed between the two heads of the sternocleidomastoid muscle and clavicle.

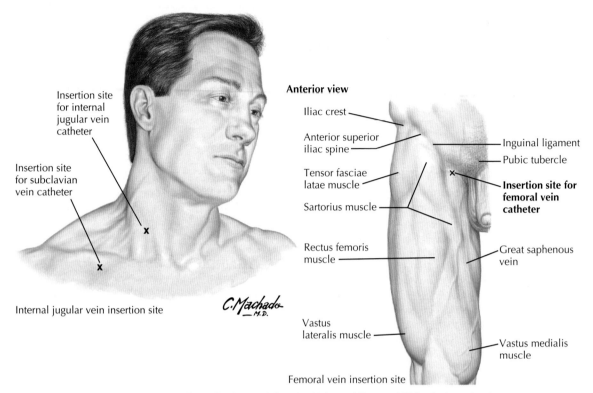

Insertion site for internal jugular vein catheter

Insertion site for subclavian vein catheter

Internal jugular vein insertion site

C. Machado M.D.

Anterior view

Iliac crest

Anterior superior iliac spine

Tensor fasciae latae muscle

Sartorius muscle

Rectus femoris muscle

Inguinal ligament

Pubic tubercle

Insertion site for femoral vein catheter

Great saphenous vein

Vastus lateralis muscle

Vastus medialis muscle

Femoral vein insertion site

FIG. 50.1 **Insertion Sites for Internal Jugular Vein and Femoral Vein Catheterization.**

TABLE 50.1
Common Types of Catheters and Their Indications

Catheter Type	Properties	Common Indications
Multilumen catheter (most commonly triple lumen)	Multiple lumens for simultaneous delivery of medications/fluids	Delivery of vasopressors or other medications, monitoring of central venous pressure
Dialysis catheter (Vascath, Trialysis)	Vascath: two lumens, used for temporary hemodialysis Trialysis: two lumens for hemodialysis with auxiliary lumen for infusion of medications/fluids	Hemodialysis
Sheath/introducer catheter (Cordis)	Short length, single large lumen	Rapid infusions (e.g., massive transfusion protocol), conduit for insertion of Swan-Ganz catheter, transvenous pacemakers, and inferior vena cava filters

- Using the ultrasound probe, scan along the length of the internal jugular vein for a location where it is farthest away from the carotid artery to avoid inadvertent arterial puncture. Typically, the artery runs medial and deep to the internal jugular vein. The artery will be pulsatile with thicker walls and will be difficult to compress. Indeed, compressibility is the most accurate sonographic determinant of vein versus artery, as pulsatility may radiate from artery to adjacent vein. Partially compressible veins may indicate presence of a thrombus. Make note of the ideal location of catheterization.
- Sterilize the area with chlorhexidine and drape the entire patient with a sterile drape.
- Infiltrate the skin and subcutaneous tissue with lidocaine.
- Using the nondominant hand, use the ultrasound to again visualize the vessel of interest. Using the dominant hand, advance the **introducer needle** at a 45-degree angle while drawing back on the syringe until blood return is visualized. Once blood returns, drop the ultrasound probe and steady the needle position. Drop the angle of the needle until almost parallel to the vessel while continuing to draw back on the syringe, ensuring continuous blood flow.
- Disconnect the syringe from the needle, making sure to hold the needle steady so as not to exit the vein. Thread the **guidewire** through the needle, aiming toward the ipsilateral nipple. Of note, it is of critical importance to hold the guidewire with one hand at all times to prevent dislodgement of the entire wire into the vein. Arrhythmias on the cardiac monitor indicate that the guidewire has been advanced too far with its tip in the right atrium or ventricle, and usually resolves when the wire is withdrawn slightly.
- Once the wire is inserted, remove the introducer needle. Use the ultrasound to confirm placement of the guidewire in the vein. If a blood gas machine is readily available, the oxygen saturation of the blood in the syringe can also be used to confirm that the blood is venous. Clinical judgment should always be used in interpretation of blood gases, as severe heart failure or sepsis can confound the results.
- After confirming wire position, use a scalpel to make a small incision in the skin along the path of the vein. This incision, or nick, facilitates insertion of the dilator. Insert the **dilator** over the wire and dilate 1 to 2 cm in depth. The dilator spreads subcutaneous tissue to allow for easier passage of the CVC, so it is not necessary to fully insert (hub) the dilator.
- Once the subcutaneous tissue is dilated, retract the dilator over the wire and introduce the central venous catheter over the wire to the desired depth (typically around 15 cm, depending on the patient's body habitus and specific insertion site/laterality). Remove the guidewire and, using a sterile flush, ensure that all lumens of the catheter draw back and flush smoothly. It is beneficial to flush each lumen before insertion over the guidewire to minimize chance of **air embolism.** Suture or staple the catheter in place to prevent dislodgement. Dress the insertion site with a chlorhexidine-impregnated dressing.
- Obtain a chest x-ray to confirm the correct position of the catheter and to rule out pneumothorax.

COMPLICATIONS

The rate of mechanical complications has decreased in recent years with the use of ultrasound guidance. Nevertheless, some common mechanical complications include bleeding, pneumothorax, inadvertent arterial puncture, catheter malposition, arrhythmias, and air embolism. Longer term complications include **central line–associated bloodstream infection (CLABSI)** and venous thrombosis.

Pneumothorax should be considered in the event of hypoxia or hypotension after CVC placement. If the patient is hemodynamically stable, obtain a chest radiograph or CT (see Chapter 39 for further details). If the pneumothorax is small, supportive management may be sufficient, while pigtail catheters or chest tubes may be required for larger pneumothoraces. Immediate needle decompression may be necessary in the event of hemodynamic collapse, particularly in ventilated patients more prone to developing tension pneumothorax. An air embolism may also present as hypoxia and hypotension; if suspected, place the patient in the left lateral decubitus and Trendelenburg position to prevent dislodgement of the air embolus from the right heart into the pulmonary arteries.

If arterial puncture occurs, immediately withdraw the introducer needle and apply direct pressure at the site of puncture to avoid a serious complication. Unrecognized dilatation and catheterization of the artery, however, can cause life-threatening bleeding and may require surgical intervention. This complication is rare and can be avoided by visualizing venous placement of the guidewire with ultrasound prior to dilatation/cannulation and measuring the oxygen saturation in the blood that is withdrawn.

As mentioned, later complications of CVC include CLABSI and venous thrombosis. The most common mechanism for CLABSI development is colonization of the catheter by skin flora, usually from the patient's skin, and occasionally from the hands of health care workers (Fig. 50.2). The CVC also serves as a nidus for infection

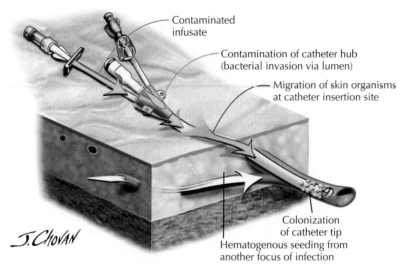

Contaminated infusate

Contamination of catheter hub (bacterial invasion via lumen)

Migration of skin organisms at catheter insertion site

Colonization of catheter tip
Hematogenous seeding from another focus of infection

J. CHOVAN

FIG. 50.2 **Development of a Central Line–Associated Bloodstream Infection.**

for bacteremia originating from other sites. CLABSI can be minimized by utilizing full barrier protection during CVC insertion, performing appropriate hand hygiene each time the catheter is accessed, and removing the catheter as soon as it is no longer clinically indicated.

Venous thrombosis can occur as a result of endothelial trauma caused by the CVC. Symptoms can range from mild localized edema to pulmonary embolus. Treatment includes removal of the catheter and possible anticoagulation if symptomatic.

CHAPTER 51

Lumbar Puncture

CHRISTOPHER BENTLEY TRANER

INTRODUCTION

Lumbar puncture (LP) has been a standard of medical practice since its introduction in 1894 by Heinrich Quincke. The typical LP involves obtaining a small sample of **cerebrospinal fluid (CSF)** from a patient for analysis. Done safely with knowledge of the anatomy, complications, procedural tasks, and postprocedure laboratory analysis involved, LP is an essential skill and tool for all trainees.

INDICATIONS

CSF provides a lens for clinicians to see into the physiology of the brain and central nervous system (CNS). The solute-poor, always-sterile fluid provides a cushion around the structures of the CNS. In the presence of a pathological condition, however, CSF can change drastically in ways that allow the clinician to discern the underlying pathology. Therefore the primary indication for LP is to evaluate the current makeup of CSF for the purpose of diagnosis and treatment. The practical indications for diagnostic LP fall into six broad categories: concern for infection, neuroinflammation, neoplasm, neurodegenerative disorders, hydrocephalus, and hemorrhagic stroke.

Meningoencephalitis should be suspected in patients who present with an array of symptoms, including high fever, altered mental status, nuchal rigidity, and severe headache. Regardless of whether infectious (including bacterial, viral, fungal, parasitic) or noninfectious (including hemorrhagic stroke, inflammatory conditions, and carcinomatous meningitis), early LP will shorten time to diagnosis and provide valuable information to rule in or rule out other diagnoses on a differential (see Chapter 113 for further details).

Inflammatory and autoimmune conditions feature neurological manifestations that prompt performing an LP, to narrow the diagnosis and rule out infectious causes. Some common clinical conditions that fall into this category include multiple sclerosis and related inflammatory disorders (such as **acute disseminated encephalomyelitis**

[ADEM] and **neuromyelitis optica [NMO]**), sarcoidosis, vasculitides (either as manifestations of a primary CNS angiitis or CNS manifestations of a systemic vasculitis), and medication-induced conditions. In these scenarios, the LP usually provides ancillary evidence when the clinical condition is already highly suspected.

Malignancy can have profound and devastating effects on the CNS. In patients in whom cancer is suspected, LP can elucidate neurological involvement. CSF cytology can be particularly helpful when **CNS lymphoma** or metastatic **leptomeningeal disease** is suspected. Rarely, CSF monoclonal gammopathy can be identified in patients with multiple myeloma. Patients presenting with an ever-increasing array of paraneoplastic and nonparaneoplastic autoantibody disorders may demonstrate CSF autoantibodies when not identified in serum.

LP may be useful in several other conditions not associated with acute or chronic cerebral infection or inflammation. Neurodegenerative disorders are increasingly recognized as having a host of CSF biomarker abnormalities. Evidence of Alzheimer disease and **Creutzfeldt-Jakob disease** can be identified using special biomarker assays for related protein abnormalities. Assessment may require special processing and should be done under the guidance of a neurologist. Patients highly suspected of having acute **subarachnoid hemorrhage (SAH)**, but without CT evidence to support the diagnosis, should undergo LP to exclude the small proportion with CT-negative SAH.

LPs can be diagnostic and therapeutic in several disorders. Many nervous system pathologies are marked by increased CSF production or decreased clearance and cause symptoms due to the high intracranial pressure (ICP) **(idiopathic intracranial hypertension [IIH])** or abnormal ventricular compliance **(normal pressure hydrocephalus [NPH])**. Patients with these disorders are treated with LP to mitigate symptoms. Serial LP can also serve as a treatment in other disorders associated with elevated CSF, including cryptococcal meningitis or (less commonly) neurosarcoidosis.

COMPLICATIONS

Performed by a skilled and knowledgeable clinician, the risks of performing LP are small. The most feared complication is brain herniation, which must be avoided by assessing the patient for signs of increased ICP, including **papilledema,** severe headache, depressed level of consciousness, and vomiting. Should LP be performed on a patient with an intracranial process that would alter fluid and anatomical dynamics with removal of fluid from the lumbar region, severe neurological morbidity and even mortality may follow. Nonetheless, LP may be used in some patients with these findings, but only under the guidance of a neurologist.

LP should never be performed in patients suspected of having elevated ICP, new seizures, or new focal neurological deficits, without first obtaining a CT of the head. Caution must be exercised in patients with thrombocytopenia or coagulopathy, including those on therapeutic anticoagulation, as they have higher risk of epidural or subdural spinal hematoma. Otherwise, bleeding risk is small and can be minimized by avoiding performing the procedure in patients with the issues mentioned; consult institutional guidelines for specific practices and cutoffs.

The most common complication of LP is postprocedural headache that typically is bilateral, begins after the LP, and, although is usually self-limited, may last several days afterward. It is thought that this complication is due to continued CSF leakage postprocedure secondary to dural puncture. The headache often is positional in nature and can be treated with rest, hydration, and pain medications with spontaneous resolution usually within a few days. Rarely a **blood patch** may need to be performed, typically under the guidance of an anesthesiologist.

It is not uncommon for patients to report some degree of transient (seconds-long) tingling during the procedure, likely as nerve roots are touched or are moved during needle insertion. Damage to a nerve root by needle puncture is possible, manifesting clinically as leg weakness or pain. In these cases, the needle should be immediately withdrawn and repositioned to avoid long-term neurological injury.

Other LP complications include soreness at the site of puncture once the effects of local anesthetics resolve. Infections at the site of puncture and postprocedure iatrogenic infections (e.g., meningitis) can occur but are quite rare presuming sterile technique is observed. An LP should never be attempted in patients with a skin infection overlying the procedure site or in patients in which epidural or spinal abscess is suspected.

PROCEDURE

The typical LP requires strict sterile technique and the use of basic equipment, including LP needle with stylet, collection tubes, sterile drapes and gloves, chlorhexidine or iodine for skin preparation, lidocaine, and anesthesia needle (Fig. 51.1).

Any patient undergoing LP should be properly positioned in either the lateral decubitus position (preferred, especially if intending to measure opening pressure) or sitting up at the edge of the procedure table. In either position, the patient should be encouraged to assume the fetal position, bringing the knees as close to the chest as possible to open the interspinous areas. A seated patient may hold on to a partner or lean over a table.

The spinal cord ends in most patients at the level of the L1/L2 vertebrae, and therefore L3/L4 and L4/L5 interspinous areas are usually safely targeted for LP without risk of spinal cord puncture. The clinician can palpate for the iliac crests bilaterally to typically identify the level of the L3/L4 spinous process interspace at midline. The clinician can either target this or a level below vertebra for proper introduction of the needle. In obese patients, palpation may be technically difficult, and either CT or ultrasound image guidance may prove useful to identify anatomic landmarks.

Once the desired site is marked and sterilely prepped, the following steps are taken:

- Inject lidocaine subcutaneously initially, followed by injection into deep tissue along the intended spinal needle tract. It is unlikely that the provided anesthetizing needle in most kits will reach into the spinal cord, but prior to each injection an attempt at aspiration should occur to additionally ensure that lidocaine is not introduced intravenously.
- When possible, an atraumatic needle (Sprotte) of 22 gauge or smaller should be used. If not available, a cutting tip (Quincke) needle with stylet in place should be inserted with the bevel orthogonal to the longitudinally oriented bands of the ligamentum flavum; that is, the bevel should be pointed superiorly with the patient in the lateral decubitus position or laterally with the patient in the seated position. The needle tip should be pointed toward the umbilicus, roughly at a 15-degree angle. The needle is advanced through the skin, subcutaneous tissue, interspinous ligament, ligamentum flavum, and finally the dura mater. Typically the clinician may feel a pop when passing through either the ligamentum flavum or the dura mater.
- As the needle is advanced, remove the stylet to check for CSF return. If no CSF is seen, patient and

1. Place patient in lateral recumbent position with thighs and neck flexed.

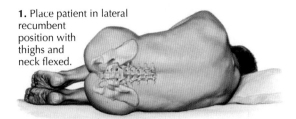

2. Palpate space between L3 and L4 and mark on patient.

Iliac crest

L4   L3

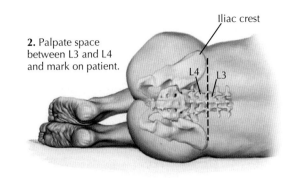

3–6. Use sterile gloves for remainder of procedure. Prepare puncture site with antiseptic solution. Clean skin in a circular fashion, starting centrally. Drape patient to create sterile work field. Anesthetize the area.

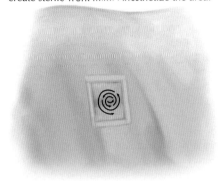

7. Stabilize the spinal needle on the index finger parallel to the bed.

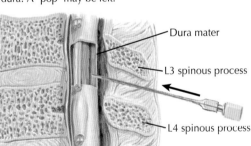

C. Machado
—M.D.

K. Marzejon

8. Slowly penetrate the subcutaneous tissue with the needle and then angle up slightly towards umbilicus.

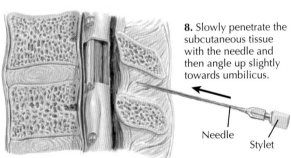

Needle

Stylet

9. Continue advancing needle until it pierces the dura. A "pop" may be felt.

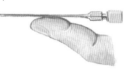

Dura mater

L3 spinous process

L4 spinous process

10–11. Once fluid is observed, the stylet may be withdrawn from the needle to allow for collection. The stylet may be removed incrementally to check for fluid return. If there is no fluid, replace stylet, move needle and recheck for fluid return. Repeat until fluid return occurs.

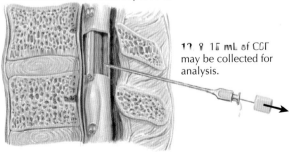

12. 8–15 mL of CSF may be collected for analysis.

13–14. Once samples are collected, replace stylet and remove needle. Apply sterile dressing.

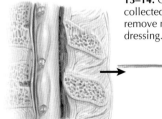

FIG. 51.1 **Performing a Lumbar Puncture.** *CSF,* Cerebrospinal fluid.

needle position and alignment should be reassessed, then advanced or withdrawn with a new trajectory attempted until the subarachnoid space is entered.

- Once CSF is seen, measure the opening pressure using a manometer (decubitus position only). It is not recommended that a seated patient be repositioned to a decubitus position once the needle is in the subarachnoid space, and vice versa, out of risk of injury with movement of the needle in the canal, as well as disruption of a sterile field.
- After pressure measurement is obtained, collect CSF for analysis. Typically, four small tubes of approximately 2 to 3 mL of fluid are collected. Although a number of studies may be intended, at least some of the CSF from tubes 1 and 4 (drawn in sequence) should have cell count performed, to distinguish a traumatic LP versus hemorrhagic CSF.
- Once collection is complete, replace the stylet into the needle and withdraw the entire apparatus. Once completely withdrawn, apply pressure to the site and cover with a bandage. Although patients have historically been asked to remain lying down for a minimum of 1 hour, it may be limiting strenuous activity; Valsalva may be more important to help prevent the risk of postprocedural headache.

POSTPROCEDURE ANALYSIS

As most LP procedures are done for diagnostic reasons, performing the correct tests on the CSF is crucially important. Every CSF analysis should include orders for measuring glucose and protein levels, as well as a cell count (cytology) and bacterial culture with Gram stain. Of note, as CSF glucose varies with serum glucose, clinicians should obtain a fingerstick blood glucose to properly interpret CSF glucose. Appropriate cultures can be ordered for suspected infections, including fungal and acid-fast bacilli cultures; other detection methods include viral polymerase chain reaction (PCR) detection, viral antibody screens, or pathogen antigen tests. Inflammatory condition tests may include not only cell counts but also electrophoresis of immunoglobulins, flow cytometry to analyze the inflammatory cells, or antibody detections specific for the condition of concern (e.g., c-ANCA, or PR3-ANCA, for granulomatosis with polyangiitis). If neoplasm or paraneoplastic etiologies are of concern, antibodies specific for the paraneoplastic syndrome can be detected, and cytology can be sent to the pathology lab to analyze for possible malignant cellular characteristics. A growing number of CSF biomarkers for degenerative disorders can help inform the diagnosis of a patient with cognitive impairment. Aside from laboratory tools, the patient's clinical picture should be reassessed serially after LP, particularly if done for the purposes of treatment and diagnostic workup. The astute clinician should always be sure to know which tests to order prior to performing the procedure.

CHAPTER 52

Thoracentesis

NEELIMA NAVULURI • TALAL DAHHAN

OVERVIEW

A thoracentesis is the withdrawal of pleural fluid through a needle or catheter to diagnose and treat **pleural effusions**. It allows for measurement of the cellular, chemical, and microbiological characteristics of the fluid, enabling categorization of pleural fluid as transudative or exudative. A diagnostic thoracentesis is indicated for patients with a pleural effusion of unknown etiology. A therapeutic thoracentesis is indicated in patients with respiratory symptoms from pleural effusion.

CONTRAINDICATIONS

Relative contraindications include patients on anticoagulation or those with coagulopathy or thrombocytopenia. Individualized decisions should be made regarding periprocedural platelets, fresh-frozen plasma, or reversal agents in patients with these conditions before proceeding to procedure. It is preferable to have platelet count >50,000/mL and international normalized ratio (INR) <1.5 and/or partial thromboplastin time (PTT) <30 seconds. Mechanical ventilation may increase the risk of tension pneumothorax and may be a relative contraindication depending on the clinical scenario. A thoracentesis needle should not pass through a site of cutaneous infection, such as cellulitis or herpes zoster, and should not be performed if a safe entry site cannot be identified.

PROCEDURE

Prior to starting the thoracentesis, the procedure should be explained to the patient, and informed consent should be obtained. A time-out should be taken prior to initiating the procedure to ensure the correct patient, procedure, and site. Thoracentesis is a sterile procedure requiring personal protective equipment, including sterile gloves, gown, and face shield. Prepackaged thoracentesis kits are available and often contain most of the materials required for the procedure. At minimum, an antiseptic solution, sterile gauze, drape, gloves, syringes, needles (22–25 gauge), and local anesthetic such as 1% to 2%

lidocaine are required to prep the area. A diagnostic thoracentesis requires an 18-gauge needle with over-the-needle catheter and large syringe, as well as sterile occlusive dressing and specimen tubes. Therapeutic thoracentesis also requires an over-the-needle catheter, three-way stopcock, high-pressure drainage tubing, and evacuated containers or sterile fluid collection bag; the latter is preferred to avoid rapid removal of fluid and monitor for complications.

Patients should be placed in a sitting position on the edge of the bed and have a bedside table in front of them, which they can lean forward over. If a patient is unable to sit up, then the procedure can be done in the recumbent or supine position, though this is technically more difficult.

The needle insertion site should be determined ideally by ultrasound guidance. On ultrasound, the skin and subcutaneous tissues are visualized as multiple layers of soft tissue echogenicity, and the pleura are represented by hyperechoic lines. A pleural effusion will manifest as an echo-free space (i.e., an area of black without stippling that lies between the chest wall, diaphragm, and lung surface) (Fig. 52.1). During respiration, there should be visualization of movement of the fluid or changes in the shape of effusion. Septations and debris may also be seen. If ultrasound is not available, the site can be determined based on diminished or absent breath sounds, dullness to percussion, or decreased or absent fremitus.

After choosing and marking a needle insertion site, the following steps are undertaken (Fig. 52.2):
- The intercostal site should be marked with marker or pressure imprint. Anesthetize the epidermis overlying the superior edge of the rib inferior to the intercostal space by injecting lidocaine at a shallow angle to the skin, creating a wheal. A neurovascular bundle runs along the inferior surface of each rib, so care should be taken to avoid this area. After creating the wheal, adjust the needle to be perpendicular to the skin and advance through the wheal into the dermis. Insert the needle along the projected track with alternating infusion of anesthetic and advancing the needle

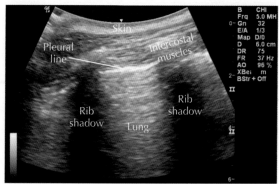

Left lower lung with ribs. Rib shadows form due to echo-dense ribs blocking ultrasound waves.

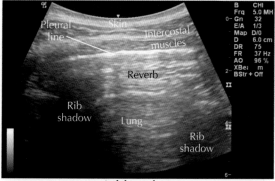

Left lower lung

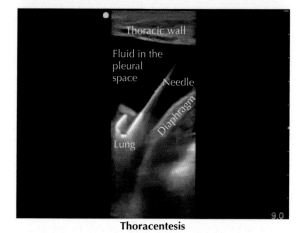

Thoracentesis

FIG. 52.1 **Ultrasound for Thoracentesis.**

under negative pressure to check for underlying vasculature.

- Once pleural fluid is aspirated, do not advance the needle further. Additional lidocaine should be injected into the area around the highly innervated parietal pleura to minimize discomfort. The depth of penetration should be noted on the needle to help guide the remainder of the procedure.
- Once the tract is anesthetized, use a scalpel or large-bore needle to make a small puncture ("nick") on the skin. This allows for easier entry of the thoracentesis catheter.
- Attach the large-bore needle with overlying catheter to a syringe and advance under negative pressure along the recently anesthetized track. Once pleural fluid is obtained, isolate the needle position and slide the catheter over the needle. Once the catheter is in place, remove the needle. The catheter hub should be covered with a gloved finger to prevent air entry, and a syringe, with or without stopcock, is attached to the catheter. Aspirate approximately 50 mL of fluid for diagnostic thoracentesis.
- If performing a therapeutic thoracentesis, a stopcock should be used. Once the syringe has been filled with 50 mL of fluid, close the stopcock to the patient. Connect the third stopcock port to the drainage tubing leading to either evacuated bottles or a drainage bag with a push/pull syringe and one-way valve. When ready to aspirate more fluid, open the stopcock to the patient and drainage system. It is recommended that no more than 1500 mL of fluid should be removed at one time. Coughing is a common symptom as lung reexpands and is to be expected. Indications to stop withdrawing fluid are coughing that does not resolve or significant chest pain.
- Once fluid has been obtained, instruct the patient to hold his or her breath at end expiration while the catheter is removed. If done with mechanical ventilation, remove the catheter during the expiratory phase. Cover the procedure site with an occlusive dressing. A postprocedure chest x-ray is often ordered to assess for complications.

COMPLICATIONS

Common complications include pain at the procedure site, cough, and localized infection. **Pneumothorax** is rare but does occur, and a postprocedure x-ray should be ordered if air was aspirated at any point during the procedure, multiple needle passes were needed, or the patient is critically ill or on mechanical ventilation. It also should be ordered if the patient has any chest pain, dyspnea, or hypoxemia (see Chapter 39 for details). Reexpansion pulmonary edema is another rare complication that may occur in the first 24 hours postprocedure; treatment is largely supportive. Rare complications include hemothorax, intraabdominal organ injury, and air embolism.

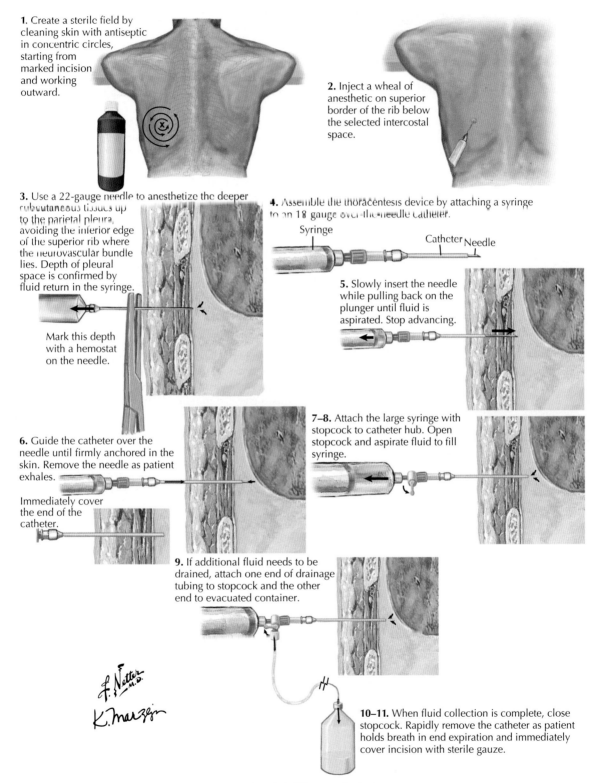

1. Create a sterile field by cleaning skin with antiseptic in concentric circles, starting from marked incision and working outward.

2. Inject a wheal of anesthetic on superior border of the rib below the selected intercostal space.

3. Use a 22-gauge needle to anesthetize the deeper subcutaneous tissues up to the parietal pleura, avoiding the inferior edge of the superior rib where the neurovascular bundle lies. Depth of pleural space is confirmed by fluid return in the syringe.

Mark this depth with a hemostat on the needle.

4. Assemble the thoracentesis device by attaching a syringe to an 18 gauge over-the-needle catheter.

Syringe

Catheter Needle

5. Slowly insert the needle while pulling back on the plunger until fluid is aspirated. Stop advancing.

6. Guide the catheter over the needle until firmly anchored in the skin. Remove the needle as patient exhales.

Immediately cover the end of the catheter.

7–8. Attach the large syringe with stopcock to catheter hub. Open stopcock and aspirate fluid to fill syringe.

9. If additional fluid needs to be drained, attach one end of drainage tubing to stopcock and the other end to evacuated container.

10–11. When fluid collection is complete, close stopcock. Rapidly remove the catheter as patient holds breath in end expiration and immediately cover incision with sterile gauze.

FIG. 52.2 **Thoracentesis.**

TABLE 52.1
Characteristics of Exudative Effusions on Pleural Fluid Analysis

Cause of Exudative Effusion	Pleural Fluid Analysis
Empyema	Positive pleural fluid culture, purulent fluid
Malignancy	Positive cytology; pleural fluid may be bloody
Tuberculosis (TB)	Adenosine deaminase >70; <40 excludes TB Yield of acid-fast bacilli on smear: 0%–10% Yield of acid-fast bacilli on culture: 11%–50% Yield of acid-fast bacilli on pleural biopsy: ~70%
Pancreatitis	Elevated pleural fluid amylase
Chylothorax	Triglycerides >110 mg/dL
Urinothorax	Pleural fluid/serum creatinine >1.0
Mesothelioma	Fibulin-3: Elevated in serum and/or pleural fluid Osteopontin: Can be elevated in serum
Hemothorax	Pleural fluid/serum hematocrit >0.5

DIAGNOSTIC TESTING

Pleural fluid should be sent, at a minimum, for protein and lactate dehydrogenase (LDH) levels. Serum protein and LDH levels should be obtained at around the same time to allow full evaluation by **Light criteria.** Patients with one or more of the following have an exudative effusion:

- Pleural fluid/serum protein ratio >0.5
- Pleural fluid/serum LDH ratio >0.6
- Pleural fluid LDH more than two-thirds the upper limit of normal serum LDH (the most valuable criterion of the three)

Light criteria carry a 98% sensitivity and 83% specificity, but notably may misidentify 25% of transudates as exudates.

Exudative effusions suggest the pleura is affected and is often from malignancy, infection (including bacterial pneumonia, tuberculosis [TB], and fungal infection), trauma, pancreatitis, pulmonary embolism, uremia, or connective tissue/autoimmune disease (systemic lupus erythematosus [SLE], rheumatoid arthritis).

Additional tests that should be sent, especially when an exudative effusion is suspected, include the following: glucose, pH, cell count, Gram stain, bacterial and fungal cultures, acid-fast bacilli stain, amylase (effusion due to pancreatic etiology), adenosine deaminase (ADA; this is elevated in tuberculous effusions), and cytology (Table 52.1).

Transudative effusions result from increased hydrostatic pressure or decreased oncotic pressure and do not involve pathology on the pleural surface. Common etiologies of transudative effusions include heart failure, cirrhosis, severe hypothyroidism, and nephrotic syndrome.

CHAPTER 53

Paracentesis

MONIKA LASZKOWSKA

INTRODUCTION

A paracentesis is a procedure in which a needle is inserted into the peritoneal cavity for diagnostic or therapeutic sampling of ascites. A diagnostic paracentesis is one in which a small amount of fluid is removed for diagnostic tests to assess the etiology of the ascites and to identify potentially life-threatening complications, such as **spontaneous bacterial peritonitis (SBP)**. This procedure should be performed in all patients presenting with new ascites, recurrent ascites, infectious symptoms such as fever or abdominal pain, or signs of decompensated liver disease (including encephalopathy, hyperbilirubinemia, or renal failure), which may be triggered by intraperitoneal infection. A therapeutic paracentesis is used to remove a larger volume of ascites for symptomatic improvement in patients who have significant abdominal swelling that causes pain/discomfort or negatively impacts respiratory status or ambulation.

COMPLICATIONS

Bleeding and infectious risks should be minimized if sterile technique is followed. Complications may arise due to fluid shifting from the intravascular to extravascular space and reaccumulating in the peritoneal space following removal of a large volume of ascites. The most dangerous of these is **hepatorenal syndrome (HRS)**. Given the high mortality rates associated with this complication, it is often recommended to administer **albumin** in patients with more than 5 L of ascites removed at one time (6–8 g albumin per liter of ascites fluid removed).

Other complications are rare and are usually associated with mechanical difficulties of the procedure, including persistent leakage of ascites fluid, formation of a hematoma or hemorrhage (e.g., due to injury to the **inferior epigastric artery**), as well as injury to intraabdominal organs.

While many patients with ascites have an elevated international normalized ratio (INR) and thrombocytopenia, these are not strict contraindications to performing a paracentesis. Often, the benefits of proceeding with a paracentesis outweigh risks. If there is a high level of concern, platelets and/or fresh frozen plasma can be transfused at the time of the procedure, though given that <1% of patients develop complications requiring transfusion postprocedurally, this is typically avoided if possible. The procedure should not be done in patients with disseminated intravascular coagulation or primary fibrinolysis.

When choosing an entry site, the skin should be inspected for blood vessels, abdominal-wall hematomas, and sites with cutaneous infection or surgical scars, as these should be avoided. Caution should also be used in patients with high risk for intraprocedural organ injury, such as those with hepatosplenomegaly, bowel obstruction, intraabdominal adhesions, or bladder distention. Ultrasound guidance should be used to identify these structures and adjust the procedure site to avoid such potential complications.

PROCEDURE

As with any procedure, informed consent should be obtained from the patient or appropriate health care proxy. All relevant risks should be discussed, including bleeding, infection, and possibility of injury to intraabdominal organs. All necessary materials should be gathered at the bedside. Many institutions have paracentesis kits with specialized devices, such as a retractable needle and blunt catheter, to reduce the risk of organ injury. If such a kit is not available, individual items should be collected and made easily accessible.

Once all materials have been gathered, position the patient supine in the bed. There are three possible sites for needle insertion during the procedure: in the midline below the umbilicus or in the right or left lower quadrant. In the midline approach, the ideal site is 2 cm below the umbilicus, as the linea alba has no major blood vessels, minimizing risk of bleeding complications. Alternatively, the needle can be inserted in the right or left lower quadrant, where the abdominal wall is thinner and the ascitic fluid pockets are deeper. To attempt this approach, one should palpate the anterior superior iliac spine and then palpate 2 to 4 cm medial and 2 to 4 cm cephalad to this site. Ensure the chosen site is lateral to the rectus sheath to avoid injury to the inferior epigastric artery. To make the rectus sheath easier to identify, ask the patient to tighten his or her abdominal muscles or cough. Once the patient is positioned, bedside ultrasonography should be used to confirm the presence of a safe ascites pocket that does not contain loops of bowel or adhesions that would put the patient at risk of viscous perforation (Fig. 53.1). Mark the appropriate site once identified.

After positioning the patient, sterile personal protective equipment, including sterile gown, gloves, and a facemask with a shield, should be worn. The skin at the marked site should be thoroughly cleaned with an antiseptic agent, such as chlorhexidine or an iodine-based solution, and then covered with a sterile drape. Once the patient and operator are fully draped and prepped, the following steps are taken (Fig. 53.2):

- Anesthetize the cutaneous tissue at the needle entry site using 5 to 10 mL of 1% or 2% lidocaine. With a small needle, inject a small amount of lidocaine just under the skin to form a wheal. After a few seconds, reposition the needle perpendicular to the skin and advance the needle through the anticipated needle track.
- As the needle is slowly advanced, gently pull back on the syringe plunger to ensure the needle is not in a blood vessel. If no blood returns, inject a small amount of lidocaine and then further advance the needle under negative pressure. This process should be repeated until ascites fluid flows back to the syringe while under negative pressure. Once the peritoneal cavity is reached, inject an additional ~3 mL lidocaine to anesthetize the peritoneal space and withdraw the needle.
- Once the tract is anesthetized, use a scalpel or large-bore needle to make a small puncture on the skin. This allows for easier entry of the paracentesis catheter.
- Gently advance the paracentesis needle with overlying catheter through the puncture site along the tract, applying negative pressure on the plunger of the attached syringe. The approach should follow either the angular technique (in which the needle is advanced at a 45-degree angle to the cutaneous tissues) or Z-tract technique (where the cutaneous tissue is pulled down prior to needle insertion). Both methods attempt to minimize leakage of ascites following the procedure.

Loops of bowel   Ascites fluid

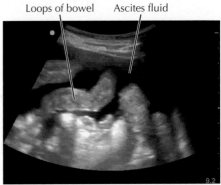

Abdominal ascites—no needle

Needle tip

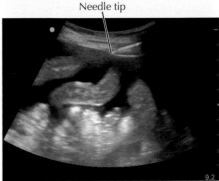

Visualization of advancing needle

Needle tip

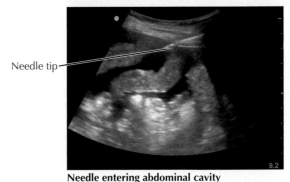

Needle entering abdominal cavity

FIG. 53.1 **Ultrasound in Abdominal Paracentesis.**

- There will be a loss of resistance once the needle enters the peritoneal space and ascites fluid fills the syringe. Stabilize the catheter in position and carefully withdraw the needle. A large syringe can be used to collect a diagnostic sample of the fluid. If a

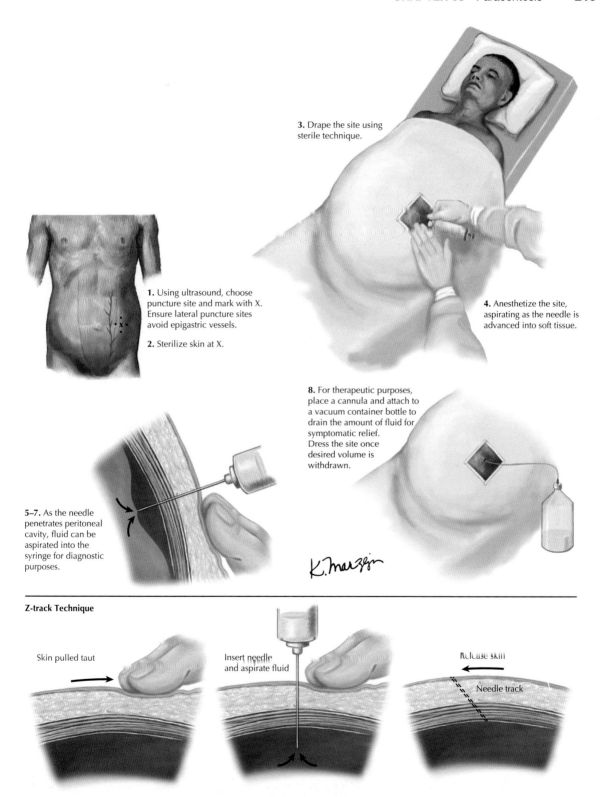

3. Drape the site using sterile technique.

1. Using ultrasound, choose puncture site and mark with X. Ensure lateral puncture sites avoid epigastric vessels.

2. Sterilize skin at X.

4. Anesthetize the site, aspirating as the needle is advanced into soft tissue.

8. For therapeutic purposes, place a cannula and attach to a vacuum container bottle to drain the amount of fluid for symptomatic relief. Dress the site once desired volume is withdrawn.

5–7. As the needle penetrates peritoneal cavity, fluid can be aspirated into the syringe for diagnostic purposes.

K. Marzejon

Z-track Technique

Skin pulled taut

Insert needle and aspirate fluid

Release skin

Needle track

FIG. 53.2 **Abdominal Paracentesis.**

large-volume paracentesis is required, tubing may be attached to the catheter, leading to a suction system such as an evacuated container or wall-suction device.
- Closely monitor the amount of fluid removed, and once the targeted volume has been reached, remove the catheter and apply a sterile occlusive dressing.

DIAGNOSTIC TESTING

Ascites fluid should be sent for analysis as soon as possible. Common tests to perform include cell count, Gram stain and culture, cytology, and protein and glucose levels. Further information on interpreting ascites test results may be found in Chapter 25.

CHAPTER 54

Renal Replacement Therapy

ANTHONY VALERI

INTRODUCTION

Renal replacement therapy (RRT) is used in the treatment of severe acute kidney injury (AKI) or end-stage renal disease (ESRD). It has several indications, typified by the mnemonic A-E-I-O-U:

- A: Correct *acid*-base abnormalities due to accumulating organic acids from protein metabolism.
- E: Correct *electrolyte* abnormalities, particularly hyperkalemia.
- I: Remove certain *intoxicants* or ingested substances that may be harmful to the body.
- O: Control salt and water balance by ultrafiltration of the plasma in volume *overload*. **Ultrafiltration** is the filtering of cell-free fluid from the blood to the dialysate compartment.
- U: Control and remove accumulating nitrogenous waste products generated from intermediary protein metabolism, which cause the symptoms of *uremia.*

In the case of ESRD, RRT typically becomes necessary when the glomerular filtration rate (GFR) is <10 to 15 mL/min/1.73 m² body surface area (BSA). Discussions for initiating dialysis should begin prior to the development of ESRD, typically when GFR is 20 to 30 mL/min, though those with more rapid functional decline may require earlier conversations.

Dialysis in any form achieves these objectives by **diffusive clearance,** choice of **dialysate,** and **convective clearance.** Diffusive clearance is the passive process whereby molecules diffuse along a concentration gradient across a semipermeable membrane between two fluid compartments—blood on one side of the membrane and a near physiological dialysate solution on the other. The two fluids pass through a cartridge, which contains the membrane typically arranged in long capillary tubes. Blood and dialysate flow in opposite directions, mimicking the concurrent exchange of the nephron to enhance diffusion. The dialysate solution is near, but not quite physiological, in some elements (e.g., potassium, bicarbonate, calcium, magnesium, phosphate); specific concentrations are chosen to create a more favorable concentration gradient across the membrane to correct deranged plasma concentrations (Fig. 54.1).

Convective clearance is the removal of molecules contained in the plasma across a semipermeable membrane as a result of ultrafiltration of the plasma. A hydrostatic pressure gradient across the pores of the membrane drives ultrafiltration and brings solutes along with water, termed **solvent drag.**

Clearance by diffusion or convection is roughly equivalent in terms of the clearance of small molecules (typically, those <500 g/mole), while convective clearance is better able to clear larger molecules. Alternatively, a longer duration of contact time between blood and the dialysis solution (e.g., nocturnal hemodialysis or short daily hemodialysis, described later) can provide better clearance for larger molecular weight nitrogenous waste products.

FORMS OF DIALYSIS

Two routes of dialysis encompass clinical practice: **peritoneal dialysis** and **hemodialysis.** In the setting of ESRD, adequacy of treatment is determined by the clearance of urea, which acts as a marker for small solute nitrogenous waste products.

In peritoneal dialysis, the dialysate solution is instilled via a catheter implanted subcutaneously through the abdominal wall into the peritoneal cavity. Blood flow through the mesenteric capillaries can exchange electrolytes and solutes across the peritoneal capillaries/connective tissue/peritoneal membrane with the dialysate solution by diffusion and convection. In place of a hydrostatic pressure gradient, a hypertonic glucose or poorly absorbed large carbohydrate polymer-containing dialysate creates an osmotic pressure gradient to drive convection of plasma water and, by solvent drag, electrolytes into the dialysate solution (Fig. 54.2).

Patients on peritoneal dialysis can undergo different modes of peritoneal dialysis. In continuous ambulatory peritoneal dialysis (CAPD), patients exchange their dialysate four times daily, leaving it to dwell in the peritoneum

Indications

- Metabolic acidosis that is refractory to medical treatment
- Electrolyte abnormalities, such as hyperkalemia, that are refractory to medical treatment
- Intoxication with dialysable drugs (e.g., salicylates, lithium)
- Volume overload that is refractory to diuretics
- Uremia and its complications (encephalopathy, pericarditis, bleeding)

In patients with chronic kidney disease:
- Glomerular filtration rate <10–15 mL/min/1.73 m^2
- Weight loss, anorexia, loss of appetite
- Any of the sequelae of impaired renal function listed above

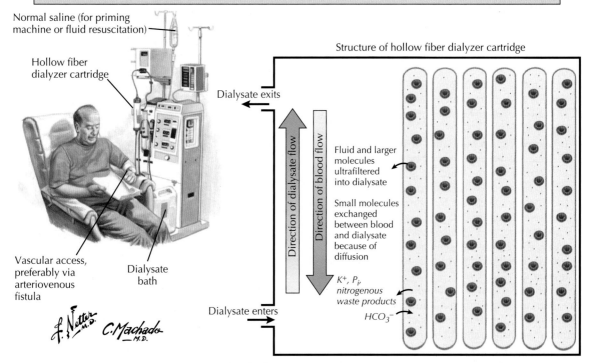

FIG. 54.1 **Overview of Hemodialysis.**

for 6 hours each dialysate, leading to near continuous dialysis. Automated peritoneal dialysis (APD) utilizes a cycler machine, which pumps the dialysis solution into the peritoneal cavity, allowing it to dwell for around 2 hours and then drain out before being replaced. APD typically occurs while the patient is sleeping. Finally, continuous cyclic peritoneal dialysis (CCPD) is essentially a combination of CAPD and APD, utilizing the cycler machine at night with one to two dialysate exchanges during the day to achieve additional clearance and sodium/water removal.

Hemodialysis is the most common route of dialysis, in which blood passes through a cartridge composed of

long capillary tubes made of a semipermeable membrane while a dialysate solution passes in a countercurrent direction on the other side. Hemodialysis typically utilizes a dialysis cartridge with about 1.5 to 2.2 m^2 effective surface area of contact between blood and the dialysate solution to maximize clearance.

Traditional, intermittent hemodialysis treatments are typically 3 to 4 hours per session, three times per week, to achieve adequate clearance of small molecular weight nitrogenous waste products. These sessions have higher flow rates, allowing for more effective clearance and greater fluid removal to facilitate longer breaks between sessions, but they require adequate blood pressure so

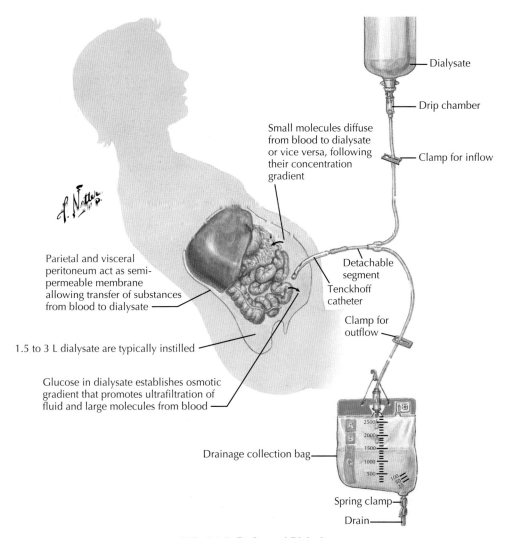

Dialysate

Drip chamber

Small molecules diffuse
from blood to dialysate
or vice versa, following
their concentration
gradient

Clamp for inflow

Parietal and visceral
peritoneum act as semi-
permeable membrane
allowing transfer of substances
from blood to dialysate

Detachable
segment

Tenckhoff
catheter

Clamp for
outflow

1.5 to 3 L dialysate are typically instilled

Glucose in dialysate establishes osmotic
gradient that promotes ultrafiltration of
fluid and large molecules from blood

Drainage collection bag

2500
2000
1500
1000
500
100
50
25

Spring clamp

Drain

FIG. 54.2 **Peritoneal Dialysis.**

the patient does not become hypotensive during treatment. Other forms of intermittent hemodialysis include nocturnal hemodialysis (8–10 hours per session, three to six times weekly at night with reduced blood and dialysate flows) and short daily hemodialysis (2–3 hours per session, five to six times weekly during daytime with reduced blood and dialysate flows).

For patients who are hemodynamically unstable, such as those requiring vasopressors or who require large amounts of fluid removal that may not be tolerated in normal sessions of 3 to 4 hours, **continuous renal replacement therapy (CRRT)** can provide slow, continuous treatment that allows for a slower rate of hourly fluid removal done over 24 hours. Although

CRRT allows for hour-by-hour control of fluid removal, it requires a dialysis catheter and can only be performed in hospitals.

The three forms of CRRT are:
1. **Continuous venovenous hemofiltration (CVVH):** Blood passes through a dialysis cartridge, and water in plasma is ultrafiltered across the semipermeable membrane. CVVH uses a high filtration rate to achieve convective clearance of sodium, water, and nitrogenous waste products. A physiological replacement solution is given to replace most of the sodium and fluid lost to limit the net rate of fluid removal; this replacement is titrated so as to remove a desired amount per hour.

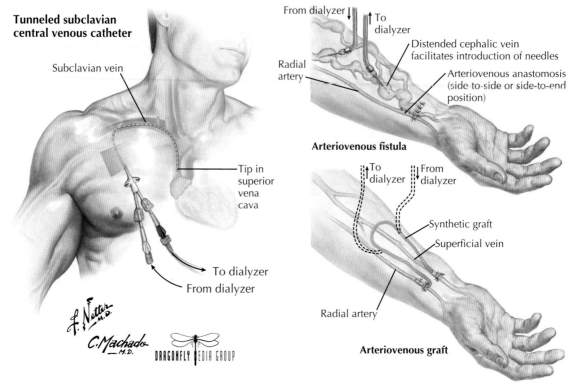

FIG. 54.3 **Vascular Access for Hemodialysis.**

2. **Continuous venovenous hemodialysis (CVVHD):** Similar to hemodialysis, blood passes through a dialysis cartridge in a countercurrent fashion with a physiological dialysate solution on the other side. This achieves diffusive clearance with a slower rate of ultrafiltration of plasma water across the membrane to achieve the desired rate of sodium and fluid removal.

3. **Continuous venovenous hemodiafiltration (CVVHDF):** Essentially a combination of CVVH using a high rate of plasma water ultrafiltration for convective clearance, and CVVHD using a physiologic dialysis solution, adding diffusive clearance.

DIALYSIS ACCESS

Patients undergoing peritoneal dialysis require a subcutaneously implanted catheter. As peritoneal dialysis often occurs at home and requires manipulation of medical technology outside of a health care setting, candidates for peritoneal dialysis are often highly motivated and able to understand and follow through on a set of instructions.

They should also have sufficient strength and dexterity, as errors manipulating the peritoneal catheter can lead to infection or dislodgement.

Patients undergoing hemodialysis typically have the surgical creation of an **arteriovenous fistula (AVF)** in one of two places: side-by-side anastomosis of the radial artery to the brachiocephalic vein at the wrist, or the brachial artery to the brachiocephalic or basilic vein at the elbow. After anastomosis, the vein enlarges and develops into a high-flow vessel lying just below the skin that is adequate for cannulation. Alternatively, an **arteriovenous graft (AVG)** is the surgical interposition of an artificial blood vessel (e.g., expanded polytetrafluoroethylene [ePTFE] graft) between the same artery and vein to create a high-flow blood vessel just below the skin for cannulation. Both AVF and AVG require time to mature (i.e., heal and adapt for dialysis) before use—typically 2 to 3 months for AVF and 2 to 3 weeks for AVG. On physical exam, AVF and AVG manifest as enlarged, tortuous vessels with a palpable thrill and auscultatable bruit; absence of these findings may indicate dysfunction or thrombosis of the fistula/graft (Fig. 54.3).

In CRRT, or in patients who have an acute need for hemodialysis, a large, dual-lumen central venous catheter is placed in the internal jugular, subclavian, or femoral vein to provide access to circulation with blood flow necessary for dialysis. Patients with need for dialysis but hope for renal recovery can receive a tunneled dialysis catheter. The tunneled catheter requires a more intensive procedure for placement but has fewer infectious/bleeding complications than a temporary central venous catheter, and patients can be discharged from the hospital with a tunneled catheter. No catheter-based access requires maturation before use.

CHAPTER 55

Cardiovascular System Anatomy Review

ARMAND GOTTLIEB

HISTOLOGY OF THE HEART

The heart sits inside the **pericardium,** which shields the heart from the rest of the mediastinum. The pericardium is composed of a thick, outer fibrous capsule fused to an inner, serous layer. The serous pericardium is divided into the outer, parietal pericardium and the visceral pericardium, which overlies the epicardium. Between these layers is the pericardial space, filled with a thin layer of serous fluid that lubricates sliding between the heart and the pericardium with each contraction (Fig. 55.1).

The heart itself is composed of three layers: **epicardium, myocardium,** and **endocardium.** The epicardium is a thin layer of mesothelial cells covering the heart; it contains the nerves and coronary arteries serving the heart itself. The thickest layer is the myocardium, which is the muscular layer of the heart. This layer is composed of cardiomyocytes, which are rich in glycogen and mitochondria to fuel the heart's heavy workload. As in skeletal muscle cells, muscle contraction is accomplished through the interaction of contractile proteins arranged into repeating units known as sarcomeres. Cardiomyocytes are also connected via intercalated discs that allow for ions to travel between cells and coordinate contraction. Indeed, these intercalated discs allow for electrical signals to propagate through muscular cardiac tissue, albeit at a slower rate than specialized conduction fibers described later. The myocardium is much thicker in the **ventricles** than the **atria,** as much greater pressures must be generated in the ventricles to move blood out to the body.

The endocardium covers the inner surfaces of the heart chambers and all four valves. The innermost layer is composed of a thin layer of squamous endothelial cells. Just below this layer lies the subendocardium, a layer of mixed connective tissues containing the cardiac conduction system.

CARDIAC CONDUCTION

All myocytes of the heart have an inherent rate of depolarization and will repeatedly contract and relax on their own. Specialized pacemaker cells and conduction fibers serve to set the rate and ensure synchronous contraction throughout the heart.

The **sinoatrial (SA) node** is a group of pacemaker cells in the right atrium that has the highest inherent depolarization rate in the heart; it is therefore able to determine the rate for the rest of the cardiomyocytes. From the SA node, an electrical impulse travels both cell to cell throughout the atria and through internodal pathways to reach the **atrioventricular (AV) node.** The atria are electrically isolated from the ventricles, and depolarization can only spread to the ventricles via the AV node.

The AV node causes a brief delay in electrical conduction, which allows for the ventricles to fill with blood. After this delay, depolarization travels from the AV node down the bundle of His to reach and depolarize the ventricles. These specialized conduction fibers make up the **His-Purkinje system,** allowing for rapid transmission of the electrical signal across the ventricles so that the myocytes contract within a very short time frame. The bundle of His branches into right and left bundles that serve the respective ventricles. The left bundle branch splits into anterior and posterior fascicles to ensure simultaneous contraction of myocytes within the large left ventricle (Fig. 55.2).

CARDIAC CHAMBERS

The heart is composed of four chambers: The left and right atria are the upper chambers, and the left and right ventricles are the lower chambers. The atria are relatively thin-walled structures that collect blood and

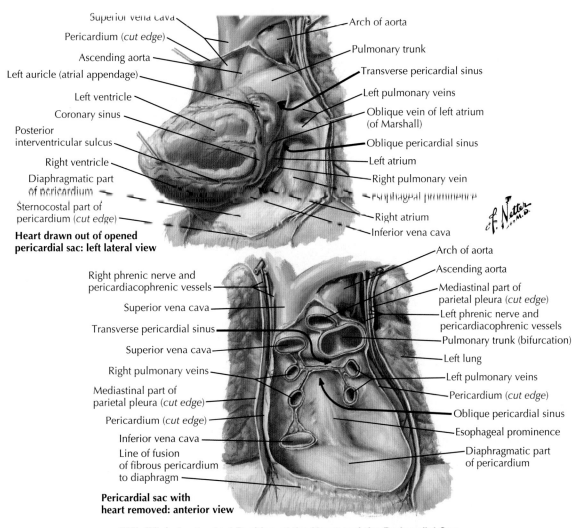

Heart drawn out of opened
pericardial sac: left lateral view

Superior vena cava
Pericardium (*cut edge*)
Ascending aorta
Left auricle (atrial appendage)
Left ventricle
Coronary sinus
Posterior interventricular sulcus
Right ventricle
Diaphragmatic part of pericardium
Sternocostal part of pericardium (*cut edge*)

Arch of aorta
Pulmonary trunk
Transverse pericardial sinus
Left pulmonary veins
Oblique vein of left atrium (of Marshall)
Oblique pericardial sinus
Left atrium
Right pulmonary vein
Esophageal prominence
Right atrium
Inferior vena cava

Pericardial sac with
heart removed: anterior view

Right phrenic nerve and pericardiacophrenic vessels
Superior vena cava
Transverse pericardial sinus
Superior vena cava
Right pulmonary veins
Mediastinal part of parietal pleura (*cut edge*)
Pericardium (*cut edge*)
Inferior vena cava
Line of fusion of fibrous pericardium to diaphragm

Arch of aorta
Ascending aorta
Mediastinal part of parietal pleura (*cut edge*)
Left phrenic nerve and pericardiacophrenic vessels
Pulmonary trunk (bifurcation)
Left lung
Left pulmonary veins
Pericardium (*cut edge*)
Oblique pericardial sinus
Esophageal prominence
Diaphragmatic part of pericardium

FIG. 55.1 **Anatomical Position of the Heart and the Pericardial Sac.**

then contract to fill their respective ventricles, which are thicker and more muscular. The right side of the heart collects deoxygenated blood returning from the body and, via the right ventricle, pumps the blood to the lungs for carbon dioxide removal and oxygenation. Oxygen-rich blood is then returned to the left side of the heart, where it can be ejected forcefully into the systemic circulation by the left ventricle for delivery to the body's tissues. Both the atria and the ventricles are separated by interatrial and interventricular septa, respectively, preventing the mixing of deoxygenated and oxygenated blood (Fig. 55.3).

Right Atrium and Ventricle

The superior and inferior venae cavae carry deoxygenated blood from the body and drain into the right atrium. Blood then passes through the **tricuspid valve** into the right ventricle. The inside of the right ventricle is covered with thick muscular ridges called trabeculae carnae. As the walls are relatively thin compared to the left ventricle, a band of tissue called the moderator band reinforces the right ventricle. Blood is then pumped across the **pulmonary valve** into the pulmonary arteries and the lungs.

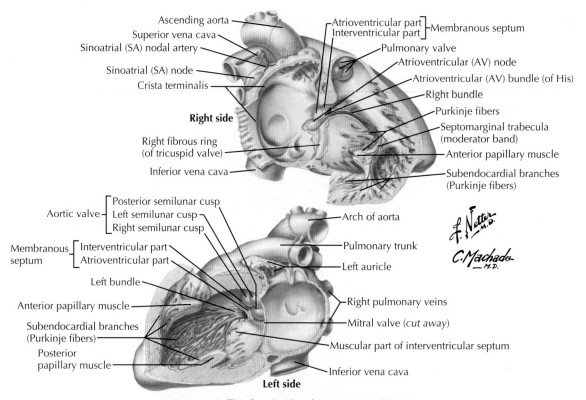

FIG. 55.2 The Conduction System of the Heart.

Left Atrium and Ventricle

Paired pulmonary veins from each lung combine and empty blood into the left atrium. Oxygenated blood passes across the **mitral valve** into the trabeculated left ventricle. The left ventricle is significantly thicker and more muscular than the right ventricle, as it must generate high pressures to move blood through the entire systemic circulation. With ventricular contraction, blood moves across the **aortic valve** and into the **aorta** for distribution to the body.

VALVES

To facilitate proper chamber filling and unidirectional blood flow, four cardiac valves exist. The atria are separated from the ventricles by AV valves: the tricuspid on the right and the mitral on the left. The aorta and pulmonary artery are separated from the ventricles by semilunar valves, so-called because of the half-moon shape of their cusps: the pulmonary valve on the right and the aortic valve on the left.

The tricuspid valve has three leaflets: anterior, posterior, and septal. The leaflets are connected by tough, fibrous chordae tendineae to three strong papillary muscles (also anterior, posterior, and septal) that contract to prevent backflow while blood is pumped forward out of the right ventricle. On the left side, the mitral valve has two leaflets (anterior and posterior), which are connected via chordae tendineae to papillary muscles, which contract to prevent backflow of blood from the left ventricle. The semilunar valves are not attached to muscular structures like the AV valves but instead are reinforced by folds of connective tissue.

CORONARY ARTERIES

The coronary arteries deliver blood to the cardiac tissue. The right and left coronary arteries have their openings in the most proximal root of the aorta, and blood is pumped into the coronary arteries immediately on contraction of the left ventricle. The **right coronary artery** supplies blood to the right side of the heart and inferior cardiac wall (named as such because of the heart's anatomical position within the chest). The right coronary artery often supplies the posterior descending artery, which brings blood to the posterior wall of the heart. The posterior

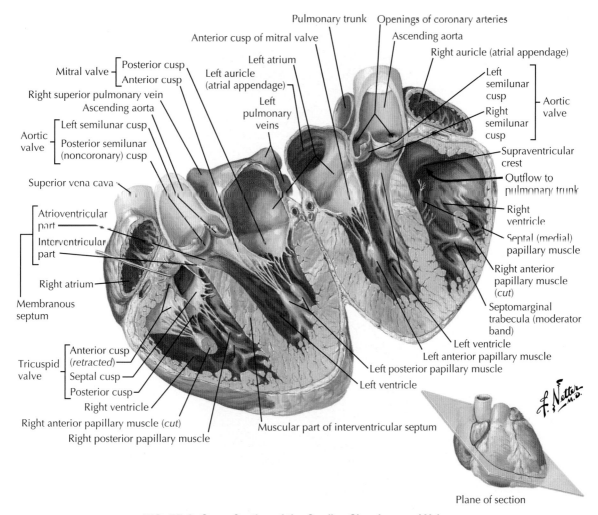

FIG. 55.3 Cross Section of the Cardiac Chambers and Valves.

descending artery arises from the right coronary artery in 70% of patients (termed right dominant); in 10%, it arises from the **left circumflex artery** (left dominant); in the remaining 20%, it is codominant, formed by anastomosis of the right coronary and left circumflex.

The left coronary artery supplies blood to the left side of the heart and the interventricular septum. The initial portion of the left coronary artery is the **left main coronary artery.** The left main coronary artery separates into two large branches, the **left anterior descending artery,** which supplies blood to the anterior and septal walls, and the left circumflex artery, which supplies blood to the lateral wall of the heart. The left circumflex further wraps around to the posterior of the heart where it anastomoses with branches from the right coronary

artery. Branches of the left anterior descending artery are termed diagonals and septals, and branches of the left circumflex are termed obtuse marginals. Deoxygenated blood from the myocardium enters the coronary veins, then the coronary sinus, which drains blood into the right atrium (Fig. 55.4).

VASCULAR ANATOMY

Arteries carry blood away from the heart to distant organs and tissues. Blood leaving the left ventricle enters the aorta, the largest artery in the body. The aorta initially travels superiorly (ascending aorta), then arches and descends (descending aorta) through the chest and into the abdomen. Three large vessels branch off the aortic

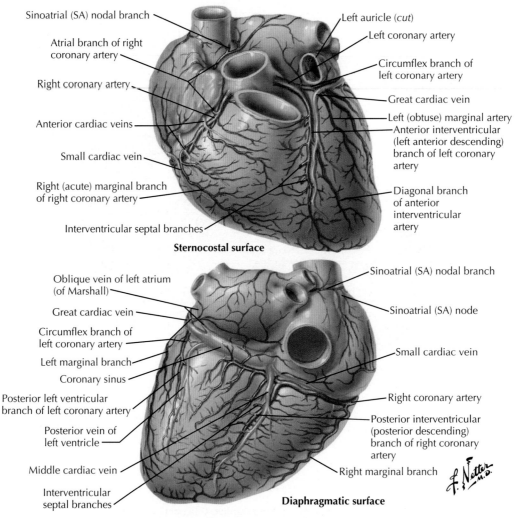

Sinoatrial (SA) nodal branch

Atrial branch of right coronary artery

Right coronary artery

Anterior cardiac veins

Small cardiac vein

Right (acute) marginal branch of right coronary artery

Interventricular septal branches

Left auricle (*cut*)

Left coronary artery

Circumflex branch of left coronary artery

Great cardiac vein

Left (obtuse) marginal artery

Anterior interventricular (left anterior descending) branch of left coronary artery

Diagonal branch of anterior interventricular artery

Sternocostal surface

Oblique vein of left atrium (of Marshall)

Great cardiac vein

Circumflex branch of left coronary artery

Left marginal branch

Coronary sinus

Posterior left ventricular branch of left coronary artery

Posterior vein of left ventricle

Middle cardiac vein

Interventricular septal branches

Sinoatrial (SA) nodal branch

Sinoatrial (SA) node

Small cardiac vein

Right coronary artery

Posterior interventricular (posterior descending) branch of right coronary artery

Right marginal branch

Diaphragmatic surface

FIG. 55.4 **Cardiac Vasculature.**

arch, supplying blood to the head and upper body—first the brachiocephalic trunk, then the left carotid artery, and finally the left subclavian artery. The brachiocephalic trunk, also known as the innominate artery, quickly splits to form the right subclavian and right carotid arteries.

Arterial walls are made up of three layers: an inner tunica intima, the middle tunica media, and an outer tunica adventitia. The aorta and other large arteries are called elastic arteries due to the thick elastic membranes that make up their tunica media. This helps maintain blood pressure between heart beats.

Most of the named arteries of the body are midsize muscular arteries. In both elastic and muscular arteries, the adventitia contains nerves and small blood vessels to feed the cells of the vessel walls. The media layer of muscular arteries is thick with smooth muscle, allowing for constriction when needed. The smallest arteries are called arterioles, which are significantly smaller and have only a thin layer of muscle in the media. However, due to the large total number of arterioles throughout the body, these vessels play a key role in regulating blood pressure by relaxing or constricting.

CHAPTER 56

Cardiovascular System Physiology Review

ARMAND GOTTLIEB

INTRODUCTION

The cardiovascular system is responsible for delivering blood to all tissues of the body. The heart serves as the pump, providing force to move blood throughout the body, while the arteries transport the blood to, and veins from, distant tissues. Through careful timing and regulation of pressures, this system constantly delivers oxygenated blood to the entire body to meet its metabolic demands.

THE CARDIAC CYCLE

The heart pumps blood through a series of electrical and mechanical events called the **cardiac cycle** (Fig. 56.1). The two primary divisions of the cardiac cycle are **diastole** and **systole.** Diastole refers to ventricular relaxation and filling with blood from the atria. Systole refers to ventricular contraction and forceful expulsion of blood from the heart.

Diastole begins with all the cardiac valves closed, as the ventricles relax after ejecting blood into the aorta and pulmonary vasculature. Ventricular pressures rapidly fall below atrial pressures, allowing the mitral and tricuspid valves to open and permitting the flow of blood from the atria to the ventricles. Ventricular volume and pressure gradually rise, and toward the end of ventricular diastole, the right and left atria contract (atrial systole), emptying blood into their respective ventricles.

Shortly after atrial systole, the ventricles themselves contract. The ventricular pressure quickly exceeds that in the atria, closing the tricuspid and mitral valves. This closure can be auscultated as the first heart sound, or **S1,** which marks the beginning of ventricular systole. The ventricles enter isovolumic contraction, in which cardiac valves remain closed but ventricular volume does not significantly change, leading instead to rapid escalation of ventricular pressure. Once ventricular pressure exceeds the pressure in the aorta and pulmonary arteries, the aortic and pulmonic valves open, and blood is ejected into the circulation.

The percentage of blood ejected from the left ventricle into the aorta with each ventricular systolic contraction, as compared to the total volume of blood in the left ventricle prior to systole (known as the left ventricular end-diastolic volume), is the **left ventricular ejection fraction (LVEF).** A normal LVEF is roughly 55% to 65%. After the ventricles have fully contracted and blood has been ejected into the pulmonary and systemic vasculatures, ventricular pressures fall in isovolumic relaxation, and once ventricular pressure falls below aortic and pulmonary arterial pressures, the semilunar (aortic and pulmonic) valves close. This closure can be auscultated as the second heart sound, or **S2.** Inspiration causes a decrease in intrathoracic pressure and therefore increased venous return to the right-sided chambers. This extra blood flow slightly delays closure of the pulmonic valve, producing what is called physiologic splitting of the second heart sound, or A2/P2. The heart is now in diastole, and the cardiac cycle repeats.

In various pathological states, including valvular or structural defects, abnormal blood flow can create additional sounds that may be auscultated. Depending on their quality and timing, these may be described as murmurs or gallops (see Chapter 22 for further details).

ELECTROPHYSIOLOGY

The coordinated contraction of cardiac tissue depends on the rapid transmission of electrical signals throughout the heart, and these electrical signals guide the action of the heart muscle cells during the cardiac cycle (Fig. 56.2).

Depolarization begins in the pacemaker cells of the **sinoatrial (SA) node,** and then travels cell to cell throughout the atria, causing atrial systole. When the signal reaches the **atrioventricular (AV) node,** it is delayed for completion of atrial systole and ventricular filling. The ventricles are electrically isolated from the atria, and depolarization can only spread to the ventricles through special conducting fibers emanating from the AV node. After this brief delay, the signal travels down

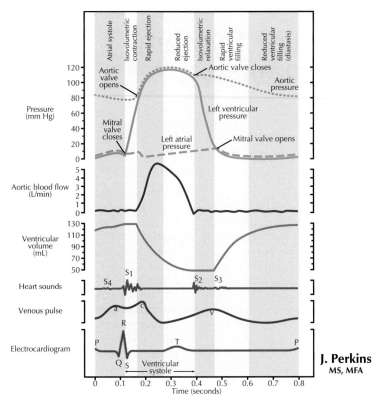

FIG. 56.1 **The Cardiac Cycle.**

J. Perkins
MS, MFA

the **bundle of His** and the **Purkinje fibers** to reach ventricular myocytes. By moving through these specialized rapid conducting fibers, depolarization reaches all ventricular myocytes within a short window of time, allowing for coordinated contraction and efficient expulsion of blood.

These electrical signals are relayed through what are known as **action potentials.** Cardiac muscle tissue is comprised of many bundles of contractile proteins called **sarcomeres** that produce coordinated muscle contraction in the presence of calcium. The action potential represents a series of movements of ions across the cardiac cell membrane, leading to the release of calcium from the sarcoplasmic reticulum and thus muscle cell contraction.

The action potential begins with the cell at rest. For cardiac muscle cells, this means the interior of the cell is negatively charged, or polarized, to −85 mV relative to the interstitial milieu. Positively charged ions leaving the cell polarize it to a negative voltage, while positively charged ions entering the cell depolarize it back toward neutrality. The five phases of an action potential are as follows:

- Phase 0: Sodium channels open and the cell is rapidly depolarized as positively charged sodium ions enter.
- Phase 1: Sodium channels close, and potassium channels begin to open. Positively charged potassium ions leave the cell, beginning the process of repolarization.
- Phase 2: Calcium channels open, and calcium influx electrically balances potassium efflux creating the so-called plateau phase. Increased intracellular calcium concentration triggers the release of calcium from the sarcoplasmic reticulum and leads to myocyte contraction. This process is called excitation-contraction coupling, as the electrical excitation of the heart causes mechanical contraction.
- Phase 3: More potassium channels open, and the efflux of potassium repolarizes the cell to baseline.
- Phase 4: The resting phase of the cell is at −85 mV. Sodium ions are pumped out of the cell, and potassium ions are brought in to maintain the cell's electrochemical gradients.

Electrocardiography is a commonly used tool to assess cardiac function. Whereas the action potential is a model of the electrical activity of a single cell, the electrocardiogram (ECG) measures the sum of all

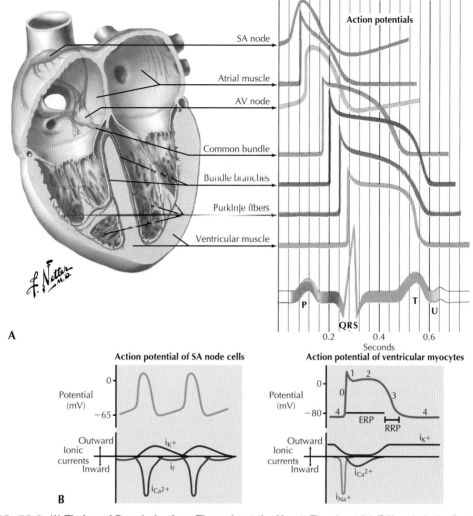

FIG. 56.2 (A) **Timing of Depolarizations Throughout the Heart.** The sinoatrial *(SA)* node is the first to depolarize, and this electrical current propagates throughout the conduction system. *AV,* Atrioventricular. (B) **Phases of the Action Potential.** The left graph depicts the unique action potential of the SA node. The "funny current" *(i_f)* is a mixed sodium-potassium current that slowly depolarizes SA node cells to ensure regular depolarizations, leading to a regular cardiac rhythm. The right graph depicts the timing of sodium, calcium, and potassium currents relative to voltage changes throughout a typical action potential. The cell is unable to depolarize to a new stimulus during the effective refractory period *(ERP),* but a large enough stimulus during the relative refractory period *(RRP)* can trigger depolarization.

electrical activity of the heart (see Chapter 38 for further details).

HEMODYNAMICS

Cardiac output (CO) and **mean arterial pressure (MAP)** are crucial parameters that describe tissue perfusion and the performance of the cardiovascular system.

Cardiac Output

CO measures the total volume of blood moving through the heart per unit time. It can be calculated by multiplying the stroke volume (SV) and the heart rate (HR).

$$CO = SV \times HR \qquad \text{EQ. 56.1}$$

The HR is determined by input from the autonomic nervous system. Increased sympathetic tone increases

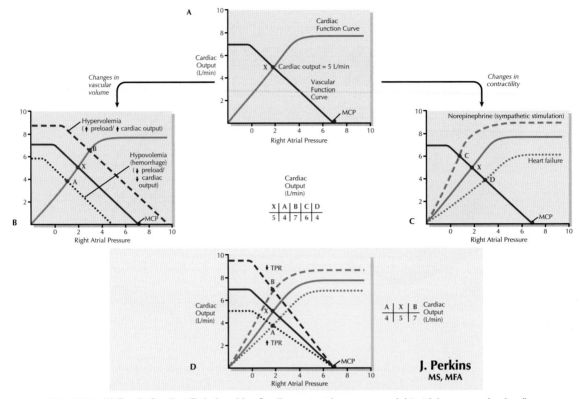

FIG. 56.3 (A) **Frank-Starling Relationship.** Cardiac output increases as right atrial pressure (preload) increases. Conversely, the vascular function curve demonstrates that, as right atrial pressure increases, cardiac output decreases as it becomes increasingly difficult for blood to return to the heart. The intersection of these curves determines the cardiac output for a given set of parameters. *MCP,* Mean circulatory pressure. (B) **Effect of Volume Status on Cardiac Output.** Changes in volume status (hypervolemia vs. hypovolemia) shift the intersection of the vascular function curve on the cardiac function curve. (C) **Effect of Contractility on Cardiac Output.** Changes in contractility (increased in sympathethic stimulation vs. decreased in heart failure) shift the intersection of the cardiac function curve on the vascular function curve. (D) **Combined Changes to the Cardiac and Vascular Function Curves.** *TPR,* Total peripheral resistance.

HR, while parasympathetic tone decreases HR. The SV can be calculated as the left ventricular end-diastolic volume minus the left ventricular end-systolic volume. SV therefore is the amount of blood ejected from the heart with each cycle and is a function of **contractility, preload,** and **afterload.**

Contractility is a measure of the forcefulness with which the myocardial fibers shorten and is mediated by catecholamines and sympathetic tone. SV rises with increases in contractility.

Preload and afterload refer to the pressures exerted on the ventricles before and after systole. Preload is the force of the blood filling the ventricle before systole (similar to end-diastolic pressure), stretching cardiac myocytes prior to contraction. According to the Frank-Starling relationship (Fig. 56.3), the greater the preload, the greater the SV.

Afterload is the force against which the ventricle must contract to move blood forward; this is aortic pressure for the left ventricle and pulmonary arterial pressure for the right ventricle. When the aortic pressure is high, the ventricle ejects relatively less blood into the systemic circulation, thus decreasing SV. Conversely, a relatively low aortic pressure provides less resistance to ventricular systole and blood flow out of the ventricle, increasing SV.

Mean Arterial Pressure

The cardiovascular system must maintain a MAP within a certain range to successfully perfuse the tissues of the body (Fig. 56.4). Analogous to Ohm's law that voltage = flow × resistance (V = I × R), MAP can be calculated as:

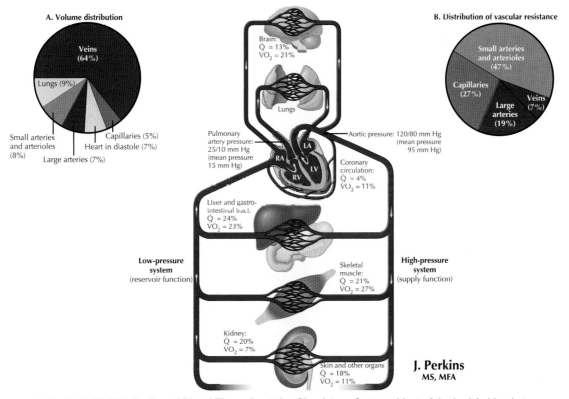

A. Volume distribution

Veins (64%)

Lungs (9%)

Small arteries and arterioles (8%)

Capillaries (5%)

Heart in diastole (7%)

Large arteries (7%)

B. Distribution of vascular resistance

Small arteries and arterioles (47%)

Capillaries (27%)

Large arteries (19%)

Veins (7%)

Brain:
$\dot{Q}$ = 13%
$\dot{V}O_2$ = 21%

Lungs

Pulmonary artery pressure: 25/10 mm Hg (mean pressure 15 mm Hg)

Aortic pressure: 120/80 mm Hg (mean pressure 95 mm Hg)

Coronary circulation:
$\dot{Q}$ = 4%
$\dot{V}O_2$ = 11%

Liver and gastrointestinal tract.
$\dot{Q}$ = 24%
$\dot{V}O_2$ = 23%

Low-pressure system (reservoir function)

High-pressure system (supply function)

Skeletal muscle:
$\dot{Q}$ = 21%
$\dot{V}O_2$ = 27%

Kidney:
$\dot{Q}$ = 20%
$\dot{V}O_2$ = 7%

Skin and other organs
$\dot{Q}$ = 18%
$\dot{V}O_2$ = 11%

J. Perkins
MS, MFA

FIG. 56.4 (A) **Distribution of Blood Throughout the Circulatory System.** Most of the body's blood at any given time lies in the veins, with smaller portions in arteries, capillaries, the heart, and lungs. (B) **Distribution of Vascular Resistance Throughout the Circulatory System.** Roughly half of the total vascular resistance comes from small arteries and arterioles. *LA,* Left atrium; *LV,* left ventricle; *Q,* percent of circulatory flow through each organ; *RA,* right atrium; *RV,* right ventricle; *VO₂,* percent of total body oxygen consumption by each organ.

$$MAP = Cardiac\ output\ (flow) \times Total\ peripheral\ resistance$$
EQ. 56.2

Total peripheral resistance (TPR) represents the resistance of the entire vasculature. The majority of vascular resistance comes from muscular arteries—specifically, the midsize arterioles—as opposed to thin-walled veins.

At a normal resting HR, about one third of the cardiac cycle is spent in systole and two-thirds is spent in diastole. MAP therefore can be estimated as:

$$MAP = 2/3\ Diastolic\ blood\ pressure + 1/3\ Systolic\ blood\ pressure$$
EQ. 56.3

MAP can be increased by either increasing CO or raising TPR through peripheral vasoconstriction. However, this relationship is complex, as changes in TPR may alter preload and afterload.

TPR is regulated primarily via short-acting baroreceptor reflexes and long-acting neurohormonal activation.

Baroreceptors are specialized, pressure-sensing cells located in the carotid sinus and aortic arch, which sense variations in the arterial pressure, relaying this information to the brainstem. From there, sympathetic and parasympathetic fibers convey adjustments in the HR, contractility, and vascular tone to help maintain a relatively constant MAP. A drop in arterial pressure sensed by the carotid sinus baroreceptors, for example, may result in compensatory increase in HR and myocardial contractility (leading to increased CO) and increased vascular tone.

Neurohormonal activation systems play a key role in maintaining blood pressure over the long term. These systems include the renin-angiotensin-aldosterone system and the secretion of antidiuretic hormone. These systems influence the amount of fluid retained by the kidney that influences circulating blood volume and pressure, and they have some important direct effects on peripheral vascular tone (see Chapter 93 for further details).

CHAPTER 57

Coronary Artery Disease and Stable Angina

JOSHUA LAMPERT

INTRODUCTION

The coronary arteries are epicardial blood vessels that deliver oxygenated blood to the myocardium. Over 15.5 million Americans have **coronary artery disease (CAD),** defined as the presence of atherosclerotic plaques in one or more coronary arteries. When CAD is severe enough to cause myocardial ischemia, patients may experience **angina pectoris,** often described as pain, tightness, fullness, or a squeezing sensation in the chest. Some patients, especially women, may experience atypical symptoms, such as epigastric pain or nausea.

Most coronary plaques are not flow limiting and do not cause angina. If a plaque becomes very large, however, it may interfere with myocardial perfusion during periods of high metabolic demand, such as aerobic exercise, and cause transient angina. Such angina is considered **stable,** in that it is associated with a predictable amount of exertion and reliably resolves with rest or nitroglycerin. Meanwhile, if a plaque of any size loses its structural integrity and exposes circulating blood to its contents, an overlying thrombus may form that abruptly reduces downstream perfusion, causing angina at rest or with minimal exertion. Such angina is considered **unstable** and is associated with acute myocardial infarction (MI).

This chapter will focus on the pathogenesis of CAD and the management of stable angina. For more details on unstable angina and MI, see Chapter 58.

PATHOPHYSIOLOGY

CAD was previously considered a simple disease of cholesterol deposition; however, more recent data indicate a major role for inflammation in its onset and progression. The initial event is likely the migration of low-density lipoprotein (LDL) cholesterol particles into the intima (Fig. 57.1). LDL binds to proteoglycans, coalesces into aggregates, and then undergoes oxidation. This oxidative stress, likely coupled with other factors (such as turbulent flow), prompts the overlying endothelial

cells to release cytokines, which attract monocytes that adhere to endothelial cells and then migrate toward the intima. The monocytes differentiate into macrophages and ingest oxidized LDL particles to become **foam cells.** As foam cells proliferate, a fatty streak becomes grossly apparent.

The foam cells further recruit macrophages and lymphocytes, and they also promote the migration of smooth muscle cells (SMCs) from the media to the intima (Fig. 57.2). SMCs produce extracellular matrix components such as collagen, forming a fibrous cap that separates the expanding plaque from the endothelium. SMCs can also become foam cells. Smoldering inflammation causes regional necrosis and apoptosis of foam cells, releasing lipids that coalesce to form a lipid core. As the plaque expands, it develops its own microcirculation that facilitates the ongoing influx of inflammatory cells, but which may also rupture and cause focal hemorrhages. Calcification may also occur.

The plaques that cause stable angina generally have thick fibrous caps. In contrast, those that cause unstable angina typically have thin caps, which can rupture in response to hemodynamic and inflammatory stress and expose the underlying lipid core to circulating blood.

RISK FACTORS

Almost all patients with CAD have at least one identified risk factor. The major modifiable risk factors are hypertension, hypercholesterolemia, diabetes, obesity, and smoking. The major nonmodifiable risk factors include male sex, age (≥45 for males, ≥55 for females), and a family history of premature CAD (i.e., MI or sudden death). CAD is considered premature when it occurs in men <55 years old or in women <65 years old. Additional risk factors include metabolic syndrome, chronic kidney disease, chronic inflammatory states (such as rheumatoid arthritis), mediastinal radiation, HIV infection, and psychological stress. Regular, moderate-intensity exercise

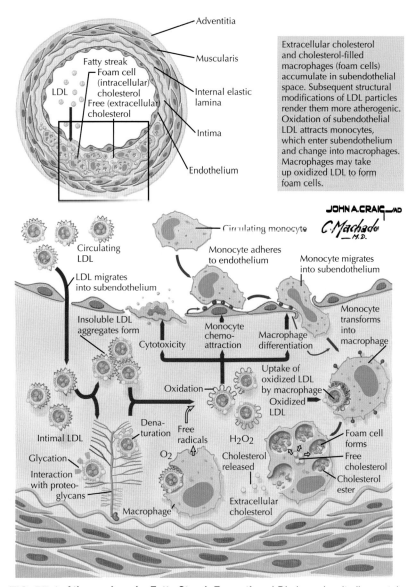

FIG. 57.1 **Atherosclerosis: Fatty Streak Formation.** *LDL,* Low-density lipoprotein.

and elevated serum high-density lipoprotein (HDL) concentrations (>60 mg/dL) both reduce the risk of CAD.

PRESENTATION AND EVALUATION

Angina is graded using the Canadian Cardiovascular Society system (Table 57.1). A classic history of angina in the presence of at least one risk factor is sufficient to

clinically diagnose CAD; however, further testing should be pursued to confirm the diagnosis, evaluate the disease burden, and determine overall risk.

The diagnostic test of choice is treadmill **exercise stress testing** (using the Bruce protocol) with electrocardiographic monitoring. The patient's exercise capacity, anginal symptoms, and ST segment response can be used to calculate a Duke treadmill score, which classifies

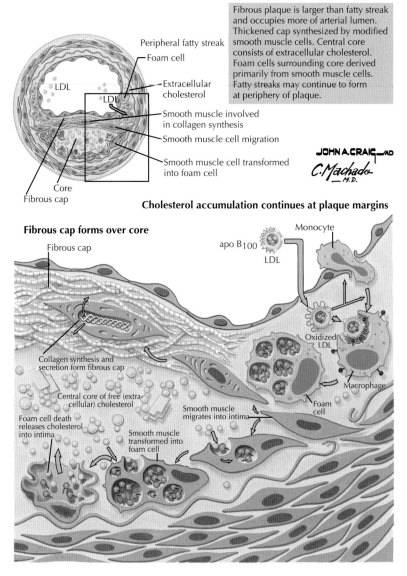

Peripheral fatty streak

Foam cell

Extracellular cholesterol

Smooth muscle involved in collagen synthesis

Smooth muscle cell migration

Smooth muscle cell transformed into foam cell

LDL

LDL

Core

Fibrous cap

Fibrous plaque is larger than fatty streak and occupies more of arterial lumen. Thickened cap synthesized by modified smooth muscle cells. Central core consists of extracellular cholesterol. Foam cells surrounding core derived primarily from smooth muscle cells. Fatty streaks may continue to form at periphery of plaque.

Cholesterol accumulation continues at plaque margins

Fibrous cap forms over core

Fibrous cap

Monocyte

apo B$_{100}$

LDL

Oxidized LDL

Macrophage

Collagen synthesis and secretion form fibrous cap

Central core of free (extra-cellular) cholesterol

Foam cell death releases cholesterol into intima

Smooth muscle transformed into foam cell

Smooth muscle migrates into intima

Foam cell

FIG. 57.2 Atherosclerosis: Fibrous Plaque Formation. *LDL*, Low-density lipoprotein.

patients into risk groups (low, moderate, and high). Patients with abnormal findings should undergo resting echocardiography to assess ventricular function.

If a patient has a high pretest probability of CAD, baseline electrocardiogram (ECG) abnormalities that preclude ST segment interpretation during stress, or an inability to exercise, an imaging-based stress test is more appropriate. Echocardiography can reveal stress-induced regional wall motion abnormalities, while nuclear imaging (single-photon emission computer tomography [SPECT] or positron emission tomography [PET]) can reveal stress-induced changes in perfusion and radiotracer distribution.

If the patient cannot exercise, pharmacological agents (such as regadenoson, adenosine, or dobutamine) are used to induce global coronary hyperemia and thereby identify territories with impaired perfusion. Because exercise capacity has prognostic significance, however,

TABLE 57.1
Canadian Cardiovascular Society Grading of Angina Pectoris

Grade	Description
Grade I	Ordinary physical activity, such as walking and climbing stairs, does not cause angina. Angina with strenuous or rapid or prolonged exertion at work or recreation.
Grade II	Slight limitation of ordinary activity. Walking or climbing stairs rapidly, walking uphill, walking or stair climbing after meals, or in cold, or in wind, or under emotional stress, or only during the few hours after awakening. Walking more than two blocks on the level and climbing more than one flight of ordinary stairs at a normal pace and in normal conditions.
Grade III	Marked limitation of ordinary physical activity. Walking one or two blocks on the level and climbing one flight of stairs in normal conditions and at normal pace.
Grade IV	Inability to carry on any physical activity without discomfort; anginal syndrome may be present at rest.

Reused with permission from Campeau L: Grading of angina pectoris, *Circulation* 54:522–523, 1976.

treadmill-based testing is preferred over pharmacological testing when possible.

TREATMENT

To reduce the risk of future cardiovascular events, all patients should be counseled regarding modifiable risk factors and prescribed low-dose aspirin (81 mg) and a high-dose statin (e.g., atorvastatin 40–80 mg or rosuvastatin 20–40 mg).

Patients with high-risk stress tests (e.g., high Duke treadmill score, large territories of ischemia, left ventricular dysfunction) should undergo invasive coronary angiography to further define the extent of CAD and determine the need for revascularization. In contrast, patients with intermediate or low-risk stress tests can generally defer angiography pending the response to antianginal medications.

High-risk angiographic findings include left main coronary disease, three-vessel disease, and two-vessel disease with a high-grade, proximal lesion of the left anterior descending (LAD) artery. Patients with such lesions should undergo revascularization, which offers a survival benefit over medical therapy. In contrast, patients without high-risk lesions should undergo revascularization only if their angina is refractory to medications, since there is less evidence of a survival benefit. **Coronary artery bypass grafting (CABG)** is preferred over **percutaneous coronary intervention (PCI)** in patients with complex or extensive disease (as determined using the SYNTAX score), especially in the presence of left ventricular dysfunction and/or diabetes mellitus.

The three main medication classes used to treat angina are β-blockers, nitrates, and calcium channel blockers. β-blockers are the most potent antianginal agents and have both negative inotropic and negative chronotropic effects that decrease myocardial oxygen demand in response to stress. Nitrates are available in short-acting forms (i.e., nitroglycerin), which are first-line therapy for acute anginal symptoms, and longer-acting forms, which are generally used as second-line agents. Ranolazine, a sodium channel antagonist, is a newer antianginal agent that is also effective as a second-line agent.

CHAPTER 58

Acute Coronary Syndromes

CHRISTOPHER R. KELLY

INTRODUCTION

An **acute coronary syndrome** (ACS) occurs when a sudden obstruction to coronary blood flow results in myocardial ischemia and, in many cases, infarction. The inciting event is usually the destabilization of an atherosclerotic plaque, which leads to the formation of an overlying thrombus.

The obstruction may be in a large coronary vessel or a small branch, may be complete or partial, and may be continuous or intermittent. These factors, in turn, give rise to a wide spectrum of possible clinical presentations, ranging from chest pain to complete hemodynamic collapse. As a result, the term "acute coronary syndrome" actually encompasses three different diagnoses on a spectrum of decreasing severity: ST-segment elevation myocardial infarction **(STEMI)**, non–ST-segment elevation myocardial infarction **(NSTEMI)**, and unstable angina **(UA)**.

STEMI is diagnosed when the presenting electrocardiogram (ECG) contains ST-segment elevations, generally indicating complete obstruction of a large vessel. NSTEMI is diagnosed when elevated serum biomarkers, such as **troponin**, indicate myocardial infarction (MI) but the ECG does not have ST-segment elevations, usually indicating partial, distal, or intermittent obstruction. Finally, UA is diagnosed when the overall clinical picture is consistent with acute myocardial ischemia but serum biomarkers do not indicate actual infarction.

Of note, UA and NSTEMI may also occur in the absence of an acute coronary event, a phenomenon known as type II MI or demand ischemia. An example is a patient with extremely high myocardial oxygen demand due to sepsis or a tachyarrhythmia who develops transient myocardial ischemia, usually on the background of stable coronary artery disease (CAD) (see Chapter 36 for details).

ACS is common and exacts a considerable toll on the US population. Each year, nearly 1 million Americans experience a new or recurrent MI. Approximately 15% do not survive. As a result, it is essential that all health care providers be familiar with the symptoms of ACS and capable of evaluating a suspected case.

PATHOPHYSIOLOGY

Coronary plaques are common and usually do not cause symptoms. Over time some plaques become large enough to limit myocardial perfusion during periods of high demand, causing chest pain with exertion that is relieved with rest (chronic stable angina) (see Chapter 57 for more details).

The plaques that cause ACS, however, are usually not large enough to cause exertion-related symptoms. Their distinguishing feature is a thin, unstable collagen cap that has been chronically weakened by macrophages and T cells in the lipid core.

In ACS, the collagen cap ruptures and exposes the underlying material to circulating blood. Circulating platelets bind to von Willebrand factor and collagen, prompting the release of signaling molecules that promote platelet activation (e.g., adenosine diphosphate [ADP]). Activated platelets assume a flattened shape, release thromboxanes that promote vasoconstriction and further platelet aggregation, become cross-linked by fibrinogen, and promote coagulation.

The final result is a platelet-rich clot that overlies the ruptured plaque and obstructs coronary flow, causing downstream myocardial ischemia (Fig. 58.1). Prolonged myocardial ischemia leads to infarction and may be associated with complications such as ventricular arrhythmia, papillary muscle rupture (resulting in acute mitral regurgitation), formation of a ventricular septal defect, and free wall rupture (Fig. 58.2).

Although most ACS events reflect destabilization of a plaque, other less common causes include coronary spasm (e.g., Prinzmetal angina, cocaine use), coronary embolism (e.g., infective endocarditis, prosthetic valve thrombosis, cardiac myxoma), coronary arteritis (e.g., Kawasaki syndrome), congenital coronary abnormalities, and generalized hypercoagulable state.

RISK FACTORS

ACS is more common with increasing age and rare before the fifth decade of life. Classical risk factors include

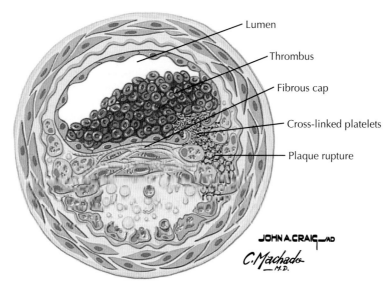

FIG. 58.1 **Cross Section of Coronary Artery With Ruptured Plaque.**

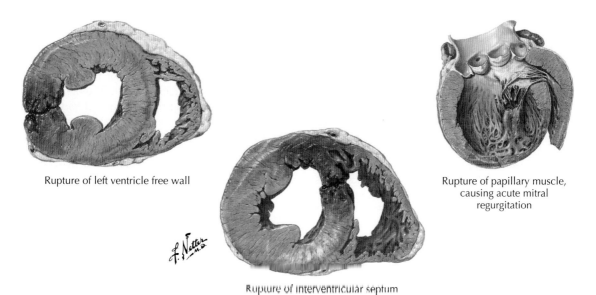

Rupture of left ventricle free wall

Rupture of papillary muscle, causing acute mitral regurgitation

Rupture of interventricular septum

FIG. 58.2 **Mechanical Complications of Myocardial Infarction.**

hypertension, hypercholesterolemia, diabetes, obesity, cigarette smoking, male gender, and a family history of CAD. The precise mechanisms linking these factors to the development of unstable atherosclerotic plaques are unclear; however, inflammation and dyslipidemia appear to have central roles. Given their shared risk factors and pathophysiology, cerebrovascular and peripheral arterial disease are strongly associated with CAD.

PRESENTATION, EVALUATION, AND DIAGNOSIS

A patient with possible ACS should undergo rapid evaluation that includes a focused history, physical exam, and 12-lead ECG (see Chapter 38 for more details).

A majority of patients with ACS present with chest pain (see Chapter 6 for differential diagnosis). Classically the pain is acute onset; compressive, viselike, or crushing; retrosternal with radiation to the neck, jaw, and arm on either or both sides; worse with exertion; and associated with diaphoresis and dyspnea. Some patients may report no prior chest pain, while others may report exertional pain that has become worse or more frequent. It is possible for symptoms to fluctuate as the underlying obstruction evolves and ischemia is either worsened or relieved (e.g., the thrombus expands or spontaneously breaks apart, or the affected vessel contracts or relaxes).

The clinical presentation of ACS, however, is famously protean. Some describe chest pain that is burning or knifelike and that originates from the epigastrium or right side. Others have no chest pain at all, instead experiencing dyspnea, nausea, or even belching as the dominant symptom. ACS should always be considered when patients with multiple risk factors report such symptoms.

The physical exam is generally nonspecific. Patients with large infarctions may have signs of heart failure (e.g., hypotension, hypoxemia, pulmonary rales). If the chest pain is positional or reproducible with palpation, ACS is less likely (but is not ruled out, especially if the patient has multiple risk factors).

The ECG should be compared with a prior baseline when possible. If the ECG meets criteria for abnormal ST-segment elevation (see Chapter 38 for more details) without an obvious alternate explanation, the presumptive diagnosis is STEMI, and immediate treatment is required.

If the ECG does not demonstrate ST-segment elevation, NSTEMI and UA remain possible. The ECG may have other evidence of ischemia (e.g., new ST-segment depressions or T-wave abnormalities) but may also be normal. In either case, a serum troponin concentration should be measured. If the troponin is elevated and another cause is not readily apparent (e.g., myocarditis, cardiac contusion), the presumptive diagnosis is NSTEMI. If the troponin is not elevated on serial measurements, but the overall presentation is consistent with acute myocardial ischemia, the diagnosis is UA. Of note, patients with infiltrative cardiomyopathies or end-stage renal disease may have chronic, mild elevations in serum troponin concentration. A rise and fall pattern in the troponin is more consistent with myocardial ischemia.

TREATMENT

If ACS is suspected, high-dose, crushed aspirin should be administered as soon as possible to inhibit thromboxane production and platelet aggregation. Nitroglycerin may be used to treat chest pain unless the patient is hypotensive, has recently used a phosphodiesterase inhibitor (e.g., sildenafil), or has evidence of inferior wall infarction (since the right ventricle may be involved, and a decrease in preload may cause hypotension). β-Blockers may be administered to reduce myocardial demand and suppress arrhythmias unless the patient is hypotensive, has bradycardia or heart block, or has evidence of acute heart failure.

Once ACS becomes the likely diagnosis, $P2Y_{12}$ inhibitors and anticoagulants may be given to further limit thrombus expansion. Inhibitors of the platelet $P2Y_{12}$ ADP receptor, which contributes to platelet activation, include both oral (ticagrelor, prasugrel, clopidogrel) and intravenous (cangrelor) agents. The anticoagulants used for ACS include unfractionated heparin, low molecular weight heparin, and bivalirudin. Of note, these agents are all contraindicated in patients with active bleeding. The exact timing and choice of agent is usually specified in local institutional protocols.

Patients with STEMI should undergo emergent cardiac catheterization to define and treat the coronary obstruction. If the hospital cannot perform percutaneous coronary intervention (PCI) (Fig. 58.3), the patient should be emergently transferred to a PCI-capable center. If transfer is not possible or a significant delay is anticipated, a fibrinolytic agent (e.g., tenecteplase, alteplase, streptokinase) may be administered instead. National guidelines recommend that the time from first medical contact (FMC) to coronary intervention be <90 minutes (or, if transfer to a PCI-capable facility was required, <120 minutes).

Patients with NSTEMI or UA should undergo immediate cardiac catheterization if they have refractory chest pain, hemodynamic instability, or recurrent ventricular

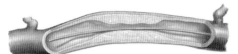

A guidewire is advanced through and beyond the obstruction.

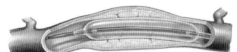

A balloon is advanced over the guidewire and inflated at the site of the obstruction, to facilitate stent insertion.

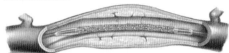

The initial balloon is removed, and a balloon-expandable stent is advanced to the site of the obstruction.

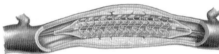

The balloon is inflated, and the stent expands.

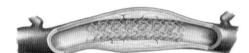

The stent provides a scaffold to maintain patency of the airway.

C. Machado
—M.D.

JOHN A. CRAIG—MD

D. Mascaro

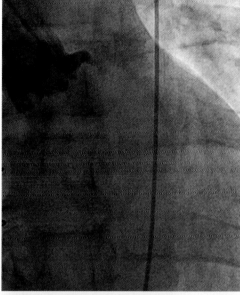

A complete obstruction of the left main coronary artery results in an abrupt termination of contrast opacification.

After the lesion is ballooned and dilated, contrast enters and opacifies the left anterior descending and left circumflex coronary arteries.

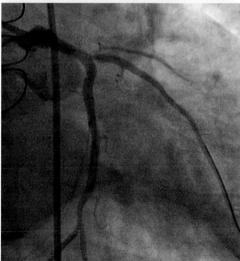

FIG. 58.3 **Percutaneous Coronary Intervention.**

arrhythmia, they should undergo urgent (within 24–48 hours) catheterization if they have high-risk features (i.e., ST-segment depression, elevated serum troponin, high TIMI or GRACE scores). Patients not meeting these criteria can be managed medically.

All patients with ACS should subsequently take aspirin for life and a P2Y$_{12}$ inhibitor for at least 1 year. Patients with recurrent ischemic events and a low risk for bleeding may benefit from more prolonged therapy with a P2Y$_{12}$ inhibitor. A high-intensity statin should be initiated as soon as feasible and continued indefinitely. β-Blockers and ACE inhibitors should be initiated for all patients without contraindications and are most beneficial among those with reduced left ventricular ejection fraction. Eplerenone is also beneficial for patients with reduced ejection fraction. Finally, all eligible patients should be referred for cardiovascular rehabilitation and receive annual influenza vaccination.

CHAPTER 59

Heart Failure

LAUREN K. TRUBY

INTRODUCTION

Heart failure (HF) is a clinical syndrome characterized by structural or functional impairment in the heart's ability to fill with, or eject, blood due to abnormalities of the pericardium, myocardium, cardiac valves, or great vessels. With more than 650,000 cases diagnosed annually, the risk of developing HF is 20% for a given adult over age 40 years in the United States. Over 5 million people in the United States currently are living with HF, which often manifests with symptoms of dyspnea, fatigue, limited exercise tolerance, and fluid retention, ultimately leading to the congestive signs of lower extremity and pulmonary edema. Despite significant advances in medical and surgical therapies for HF, the mortality remains at approximately 31% at 3 years.

While the majority of the following text pertains to **HF with reduced ejection fraction (HFrEF)**, special mention should be made of **HF with preserved ejection fraction (HFpEF)**. HFpEF is a clinical entity where patients have signs and symptoms of HF but have a normal or near normal ejection fraction. Most goal-directed medical therapy with proven benefits in HFrEF has not seen similar benefits in HFpEF, likely due to the heterogeneous nature of the condition, though trials are ongoing.

PATHOPHYSIOLOGY

HF can be conceptualized as a progressive disorder that follows an inciting event, one that impedes the heart's ability to generate force to contract normally. Regardless of the time course of the index event (abrupt or gradual), patients often remain asymptomatic for months to years while compensatory mechanisms sustain left ventricular (LV) function. These hormonally mediated compensatory mechanisms include activation of the renin-angiotensin-aldosterone system (RAAS) and increased production of endogenous vasodilators, such as **atrial natriuretic peptide (ANP)** and **brain natriuretic peptide (BNP)**. These mechanisms work to maintain cardiac output by increasing salt and water retention and counteracting peripheral vasoconstriction, respectively. This allows for relative preservation of LV function and maintenance of the asymptomatic or minimally symptomatic period described earlier. The transition from asymptomatic to symptomatic HF heralds the onset of LV remodeling, as these compensatory mechanisms eventually become increasingly maladaptive.

In general, the decreased force generated by the LV results in offloading of pressure in the carotid sinus, aortic arch, and LV. Decreased pressure in these areas results in loss of inhibitory parasympathetic stimuli and ultimately precipitates release of antidiuretic hormone, leading to increased free water reabsorption. Decreased pressure also increases efferent sympathetic activation, stimulating the heart, kidneys, and peripheral vasculature. Within the kidneys, activation of the RAAS pathway results in renin release and increased circulating levels of angiotensin II and aldosterone, increasing peripheral vascular resistance and free water retention. The RAAS hormones have direct and detrimental effects to the myocardium, over time causing cardiac myocyte hypertrophy, fibrosis, and (later) cell death (Fig. 59.1). Simultaneously, inflammatory markers, reactive oxygen species, and other maladaptive growth factors are stimulated; it is their overexpression, in combination with RAAS activation, that contributes to the progression of symptomatic HF.

CLINICAL PRESENTATION

Classically, HF symptoms are separated into left-sided and right-sided symptoms, depending on the affected ventricle. Symptoms also depend on the severity of HF and whether or not HF affects primarily systolic or diastolic ventricular function. Left-sided symptoms include fatigue, reduced exercise tolerance, and dyspnea; right-sided symptoms include lower extremity edema and abdominal discomfort/nausea. It must be noted, however, that the most common cause of right-sided (right ventricular [RV]) failure is LV failure, so patients with LV failure often develop right-sided symptoms, as well.

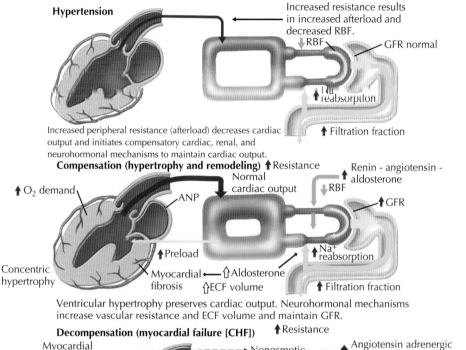

Hypertension

Increased resistance results in increased afterload and decreased RBF.

↓RBF

GFR normal

↑Na reabsorption

↑Filtration fraction

Increased peripheral resistance (afterload) decreases cardiac output and initiates compensatory cardiac, renal, and neurohormonal mechanisms to maintain cardiac output.

Compensation (hypertrophy and remodeling) ↑Resistance

↑O₂ demand

ANP

Normal cardiac output

Renin - angiotensin - aldosterone

↓RBF

↑GFR

↑Preload

Concentric hypertrophy

Myocardial fibrosis

⇑Aldosterone

⇑ECF volume

↑Na⁺ reabsorption

↑Filtration fraction

Ventricular hypertrophy preserves cardiac output. Neurohormonal mechanisms increase vascular resistance and ECF volume and maintain GFR.

Decompensation (myocardial failure [CHF]) ↑Resistance

Myocardial ischemia

Decreased output

Nonosmotic ↑AVP

Angiotensin adrenergic activity

↓RBF

GFR

↑Na⁺ reabsorption

↑Preload

Edema

Eccentric hypertrophy

Myocardial failure

↑ECF volume hyponatremia

↓Filtration fraction

C.Machado —M.D.

JOHN A. CRAIG—MD

Decreased output causes increased resistance and volume. This results in marked decrease in cardiac output, renal perfusion, and GFR.

FIG 59.1 **Hypertension and Heart Failure.** *ANP,* Atrial natriuretic peptide; *AVP,* arginine vasopressin; *CHF,* congestive heart failure; *ECF,* extracellular fluid; *GFR,* glomerular filtration rate; *RBF,* renal blood flow.

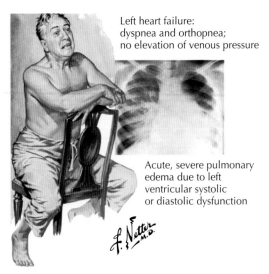

Left heart failure: dyspnea and orthopnea; no elevation of venous pressure

Acute, severe pulmonary edema due to left ventricular systolic or diastolic dysfunction

FIG. 59.2 **Pulmonary Edema in Heart Failure.**

Other symptoms may include orthopnea, paroxysmal nocturnal dyspnea, and chest pain/pressure (Fig. 59.2). Because of the abnormal remodeling of the myocardium, patients with HF are more susceptible to conduction disease; thus new-onset arrhythmias (atrial or ventricular) and associated symptoms may be their initial presenting complaint.

DIAGNOSIS AND EVALUATION

Despite impressive advances in noninvasive and invasive diagnostic testing, the cornerstone of diagnosis in HF remains the history and physical examination. A thorough history can provide clues to possible etiologies of HF, as well as an assessment of severity and duration. Interview questions should include inquiries regarding potential etiologies, including coronary artery disease (ischemic), family history, and alcohol use, as well as risk factors for HF such as uncontrolled hypertension or diabetes mellitus. Duration of illness should be elucidated, along with severity of symptoms. A thorough current (and in some cases, past) medication history should be obtained, as this could suggest a cause for the HF (e.g., chemotherapy-induced cardiomyopathy) or reason for decompensation (e.g., recent discontinuation of diuretic therapy). Adherence to the prescribed medical regimen and diet, particularly low salt, is equally important in discovering the underlying cause of changed clinical status.

Physical exam should include a full assessment of volume status, including measurement of jugular venous pressure, presence of hepatojugular reflex, and presence/extent of lower extremity edema. As can be expected, the cardiac and pulmonary exam are critical; the cardiac exam might reveal a diffuse and laterally displaced point of maximal impulse (PMI), suggesting cardiomegaly, with an S3 gallop signifying rapid ventricular filling. Pulmonary auscultation might reveal rales or wheezing suggestive of pulmonary edema. Examination of the peripheral pulses can provide clues as to the heart's ability to perfuse the body, as cool extremities may signify a state of poor forward flow leading to inadequate perfusion.

Initial laboratory evaluation should include a complete blood count, basic metabolic panel (including renal function), liver function tests, and screening for disorders of lipid metabolism and diabetes. A baseline electrocardiogram (ECG) should be performed. Although the usefulness in preventing readmission or predicting mortality has not been established, measurement of BNP or N-terminal pro-BNP should be performed both in the acute setting to inform therapeutic decision making and in the ambulatory setting to help confirm euvolemia. Caution, however, must be exercised in interpreting the results, as the history and physical exam remain the primary drivers of diagnosing HF. In the acute setting, markers of myocardial damage/injury (e.g., troponin) should also be measured. Patients with hypotension or signs of poor peripheral perfusion should have a lactate level checked.

All patients with new-onset HF or those presenting with suspected decompensated chronic HF should undergo noninvasive imaging with chest radiography and two-dimensional echocardiogram. Chest radiograph is useful in assessing possible alterative diagnoses, which could contribute to typical HF symptoms (e.g., pneumonia). It can also reveal cardiomegaly, chamber enlargement, or changes suggestive of pulmonary edema. Echocardiography is a cornerstone imaging modality for HF, as it can provide information on both systolic (especially ejection fraction) and diastolic function, as well as valvular competence and structural changes within the myocardium (see Chapter 48 for further details).

The role of invasive hemodynamic monitoring varies among centers, though it is utilized primarily at large academic medical centers that offer advanced and mechanical therapies for HF. In this setting, the use of pulmonary artery catheters has been associated with reduced mortality, particularly in patients with cardiogenic shock. Invasive monitoring can otherwise benefit those patients in whom volume status is difficult

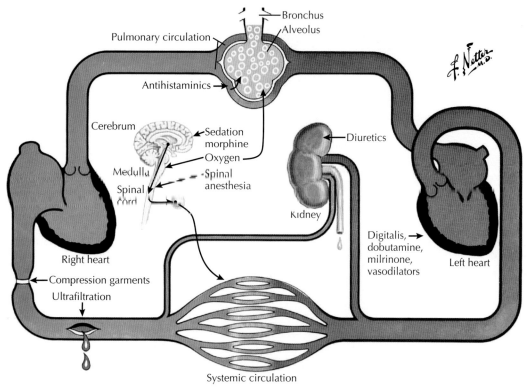

FIG. 59.3 **Treatment of Volume Overload in Heart Failure.**

to assess, in those who have worsening renal function or hypotension with ongoing diuresis despite persistent volume overload, or in those undergoing evaluation for advanced therapies, including mechanical circulatory support and transplant.

TREATMENT

American Heart Association/American College of Cardiology (AHA/ACC) guidelines for the treatment of HF are based on classification by symptom burden.

For those with AHA stage A HF (those at risk but without structural disease or symptoms of HF), comorbid conditions, including hypertension and hyperlipidemia, should be controlled. Once structural heart disease is present (stage B), pharmacological therapy targeted at preventing adverse remodeling and lowering mortality is initiated. For patients with HF with reduced ejection fraction, or those with recent myocardial infarction, medications with mortality benefit include:

- ACE inhibitors, such as enalapril or lisinopril
- Angiotensin II receptor blockers (ARBs), such as valsartan or candesartan
- β-blockers, such as carvedilol or metoprolol succinate
- Combination angiotensin receptor/neprilysin inhibitor, such as valsartan/sacubitril

Lipid-lowering therapy with statins should be utilized for primary or secondary prevention of coronary artery disease and ischemic cardiovascular events. Those patients with structural heart disease in combination with past or present symptoms of HF (stage C) should, in addition to the aforementioned measures, receive specific counseling on low-salt diet and be started on a loop diuretic if congestive symptoms are present (Fig. 59.3). In those patients with a significantly reduced ejection fraction (<35%), addition of an aldosterone antagonist (e.g., spironolactone, eplerenone) can further reduce morbidity and mortality.

For patients with a reduced ejection fraction (≤30%) despite optimal medical management for at least 6

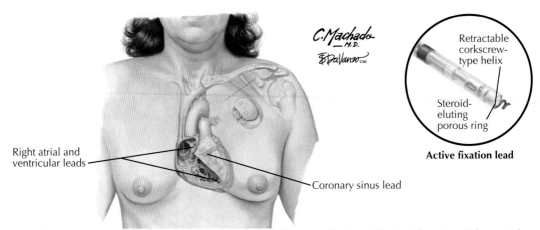

Cardiac resynchronization therapy involves placing three leads in the heart: one lead each in the right atrium, right ventricle, and coronary sinus, which acts on the left ventricle. The right atrial lead tracks atrial contraction to synchronize ventricular contraction via the other two leads.

FIG. 59.4 **Cardiac Resynchronization Therapy.**

months, placement of an **automated implantable cardiac defibrillator (AICD)** is recommended to reduce the risk of sudden cardiac death secondary to a malignant ventricular arrhythmia. If a patient has an ejection fraction ≤35% and a widened QRS >130 msec on ECG, he or she may also benefit from **cardiac resynchronization therapy** to improve ventricular synchrony and (subsequently) cardiac output (Fig. 59.4).

For those with refractory symptoms, advanced therapies such as inotropes, mechanical circulatory support with a ventricular assist device, or heart transplantation should be considered.

CHAPTER 60

Atrial Fibrillation

VEDRAN ORUC

INTRODUCTION

Atrial fibrillation (AF) is the most common arrhythmia in adults and is characterized by an irregularly irregular pulse arising from disorganized atrial electrical activity (Fig. 60.1). The loss of atrial contractility results in stasis of blood, which predisposes to thrombus formation and may result in thromboembolic complications such as stroke (Fig. 60.2). Meanwhile, constant stimulation of the atrioventricular (AV) node can cause difficult-to-control tachycardia. The prevalence of AF is estimated to be 3% among all adults older than 20 years, increasing to 12% among those aged 75 to 85 years.

AF is categorized as **paroxysmal** or **persistent** depending on whether it occurs continuously for >7 days. AF tends to progress from paroxysmal to persistent secondary to adverse cardiac remodeling. AF is categorized as permanent if no further attempts are planned to restore and maintain normal sinus rhythm.

AF is additionally categorized as **valvular** or **nonvalvular.** AF is valvular when associated with rheumatic mitral stenosis or mechanical heart valve replacement. Patients with valvular AF have a substantially greater risk of thrombus formation and embolism, along with more limited options for anticoagulation.

PATHOPHYSIOLOGY

AF is thought to occur when atrial ectopic focal discharges occur in conjunction with structural cardiac abnormalities that maintain the arrhythmia. The inciting ectopic foci are most commonly located in the left atrial myocardial sleeves, which extend into the pulmonary veins. The ectopic foci trigger a cascade of disorganized atrial depolarizations. In a structurally abnormal myocardium (i.e., with fibrotic changes from aging, inflammation, and environmental factors), electrical dissociation between muscle bundles creates areas of reentrant loops and rapid-firing foci, perpetuating and maintaining the disorganized electrical activation.

These electrical wave fronts interfere with the normal pacemaker activity of the sinoatrial (SA) node and chronically overstimulate the AV node. Although the refractory period of the AV node places an upper limit on the frequency of transmission to the ventricles, rapid conduction and tachycardia often occur.

The loss of organized atrial contraction and rapid depolarization of the ventricles interferes with diastolic filling. The effect on cardiac output is greatest in hypertrophic hearts dependent on diastolic filling to ensure adequate preload, such as those remodeled from chronic hypertension, hypertrophic cardiomyopathy, or restrictive cardiomyopathy.

Over time, AF causes pathological atrial remodeling, making restoration of sinus rhythm increasingly difficult. Even restoration of sinus rhythm may not result in recovery of normal atrial mechanical function. In addition, atrial myocardial damage leads to increased expression of prothrombotic factors. As a result, patients with AF have an increased long-term stroke risk even after restoration of normal sinus rhythm.

RISK FACTORS

The numerous risk factors for AF include increasing age, male gender, white race, hypertension, valvular heart disease, hyperthyroidism, diabetes mellitus, cardiac ischemia, heart failure, pulmonary embolus, infection, obesity, obstructive sleep apnea, surgery (both cardiac and noncardiac), electrolyte disturbances, family history, left ventricular hypertrophy, left atrial enlargement, and multiple environmental risk factors (including smoking, exercise, alcohol use, and illicit drug use).

PRESENTATION, EVALUATION, AND DIAGNOSIS

The most common presenting symptom is fatigue, though patients may experience palpitations, hypotension, syncope, stroke, chest pain, or heart failure. Physical examination reveals an irregular pulse with no repeating pattern (irregularly irregular), often with variability of the amplitude of the first heart sound owing to beat-to-beat

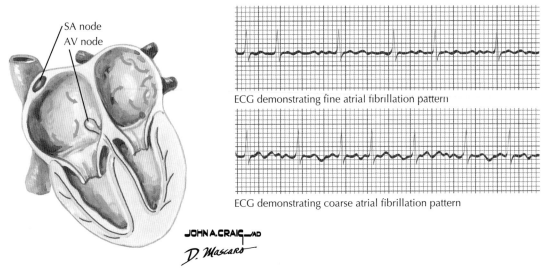

ECG demonstrating fine atrial fibrillation pattern

ECG demonstrating coarse atrial fibrillation pattern

JOHN A. CRAIG—AD

D. Mascaro

FIG. 60.1 **Atrial Fibrillation.** *AV,* Atrioventricular; *ECG,* electrocardiogram; *SA,* sinoatrial.

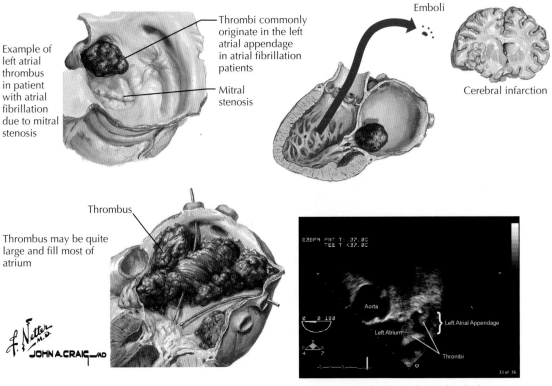

Example of left atrial thrombus in patient with atrial fibrillation due to mitral stenosis

Thrombi commonly originate in the left atrial appendage in atrial fibrillation patients

Mitral stenosis

Emboli

Cerebral infarction

Thrombus

Thrombus may be quite large and fill most of atrium

Transesophageal echocardiographic findings in a patient with atrial fibrillation, showing thrombi in the left atrial appendage and main left atrium

FIG. 60.2 **Thromboembolic Complications.**

variations in stroke volume. The diagnosis can be confirmed with an electrocardiogram (ECG).

When paroxysmal AF is suspected (i.e., a patient reports intermittent palpitations or has an unexplained thromboembolic stroke, but office-based ECGs are normal), ambulatory monitoring should be performed using Holter monitoring or implantable loop monitors. If AF is thought to be precipitated by exercise, stress testing can be informative.

Patients with a new diagnosis of AF require a complete history and physical to assess for comorbid cardiovascular conditions and determine thrombotic risk. An echocardiogram should be performed to evaluate ventricular function, determine atrial size, and assess for valvular pathology. Lab testing should include assessment of renal function to help guide anticoagulant choice, and of electrolytes and thyroid function to check for possible precipitants.

TREATMENT
General Guidelines

The treatment of AF is focused on reduction of risk factors for stroke and cardiovascular disease, anticoagulation to lower the risk of thromboembolic events, **rate control** as needed, and **rhythm control** for those who experience bothersome symptoms when in AF, are unable to tolerate rate control, or have an inadequate response to rate control.

Anticoagulation

Antithrombotic therapy is recommended for all patients with a significant stroke risk, regardless of the duration or persistence of AF, or of the decision to pursue a rate or rhythm control strategy. The decision to initiate anticoagulation, however, requires a discussion of the risks of both stroke and bleeding complications.

The stroke risk can be established using the CHA$_2$DS$_2$-VASc score (Table 60.1). Patients with a score of zero do not require oral anticoagulants unless there is a separate indication. Patients with a score ≥2 should receive anticoagulation unless the bleeding risk is high.

Patients with a score of 1 historically had an indeterminate risk/benefit, and were told to either take aspirin or anticoagulation. More recent data, however, and the development of **novel oral anticoagulants** (NOACs), which have a lower bleeding risk, have shifted the treatment toward anticoagulation, unless the score is due only to female gender.

Options for oral anticoagulation include **vitamin K antagonists** (warfarin) with a goal international normalized ratio (INR) of 2 to 3, direct thrombin inhibitors

TABLE 60.1
2009 Birmingham Schema Expressed as a Point-Based Scoring System, With the Acronym CHA$_2$DS$_2$-VASc

CHA$_2$DS$_2$-VASc Score	Points
Congestive heart failure (left ventricular ejection fraction ≤40%)	+1
Hypertension	+1
Age 65–74 years	+1
Age >75 years	+2
Diabetes mellitus	+1
Stroke/transient ischemia attack	+2
Vascular disease (coronary, peripheral)	+1
Sex (female)	+1

Modified from Lip GYH, Nieuwlatt R, Pisters R, et al: Refining clinical risk stratification for predicting stroke and thromboembolism in atrial fibrillation using a novel risk factor-based approach: the Euro Heart Survey on atrial fibrillation, *Chest* 137(2):263–272, 2010.

(dabigatran), and factor Xa inhibitors (apixaban, edoxaban, and rivaroxaban). For nonvalvular AF, the use of NOACs is preferred over warfarin due to ease of administration and equal to improved stroke prevention and bleeding rates. For valvular AF, warfarin remains the only effective oral agent. The efficacy of aspirin alone has been studied with mixed results, with only a single large study showing a stroke risk reduction with 325 mg daily. Likewise, the efficacy of aspirin and clopidogrel (dual antiplatelet therapy [DAPT]) was inferior to that of warfarin but with a similar bleeding risk.

Patients who have an indication for anticoagulation but high bleeding risk may be candidates for a left atrial appendage occlusion device to reduce the risk of stroke. A percutaneous **left atrial appendage occlusion device,** known as the Watchman device, has been approved for use in the United States, and some data indicate that it is noninferior to warfarin for long-term stroke reduction risk.

Rate Control

Multiple studies have compared rate and rhythm control strategies for AF and found equivalent outcomes for the general population. The rate control target for most patients is a resting heart rate <110 beats per minute (bpm), though a lower target may be reasonable in patients with symptoms at higher rates. In the absence of ventricular preexcitation, decompensated heart failure, or hypotension, β-blockers and calcium channel blockers

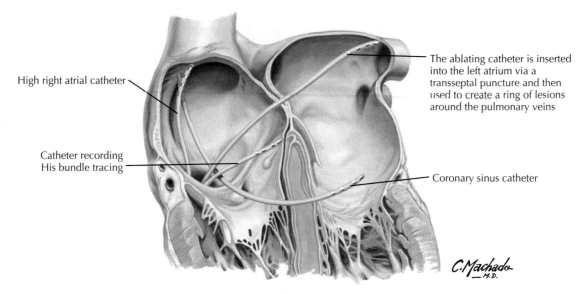

High right atrial catheter

The ablating catheter is inserted into the left atrium via a transseptal puncture and then used to create a ring of lesions around the pulmonary veins

Catheter recording
His bundle tracing

Coronary sinus catheter

FIG. 60.3 **Ablation of Atrial Fibrillation: Pulmonary Vein Isolation.**

are the first-line agents for rate control. For patients with decompensated heart failure or hypotension, digoxin or amiodarone may be preferred. For patients with preexcitation, AV nodal blocking medications are contraindicated, since they can cause unopposed conduction of atrial activity through the accessory tracts, which lack a refractory period.

Rhythm Control

Direct current cardioversion (DCCV) is indicated in all patients with hypotension, worsening heart failure, or myocardial ischemia who do not respond to, or are unable to tolerate, rate control medications.

Pharmacological rhythm control with class IC or III antiarrhythmics is indicated for patients who have bothersome symptoms from AF or who are unable to tolerate or achieve adequate rate control. Common contraindications to these medications include coronary artery disease, significant left ventricular hypertrophy (defined as left ventricular wall thickness ≥1.4 cm), and reduced left ventricular ejection fraction.

Patients with an elevated stroke risk, as described earlier, should receive indefinite anticoagulation regardless of whether a rate or rhythm control strategy is used. Furthermore, all patients should generally receive anticoagulation before and after elective cardioversion, whether pharmacological or electrical, because of an increased short-term risk of stroke secondary to short-term electromechanical dissociation in the atria postconversion. Prior to elective cardioversion, all patients should receive 3 weeks of effective anticoagulation or undergo a transesophageal echocardiogram to exclude thrombus in the left atrium. After cardioversion, all patients should receive at least 4 weeks of anticoagulation

Patients who are unable to tolerate pharmacological therapy or have inadequate control with at least one antiarrhythmic agent may be candidates for **catheter ablation** of AF through either **pulmonary vein isolation** (Fig. 60.3) or **AV nodal ablation** and insertion of a permanent pacemaker. These procedures do not, however, eliminate the need for anticoagulation. Additionally, recent randomized study has shown that catheter ablation may be beneficial compared to medical therapy in patients who have a reduced EF (<35%), though additional data is needed to better determine which subgroup of this population benefits most. Likewise, patients who are undergoing cardiac surgery for another indication may undergo a surgical ablation (e.g., Maze procedure) to improve rhythm control or surgical removal of the left atrial appendage to reduce thromboembolic risk.

CHAPTER 61

Pericarditis and Pericardial Effusions

WAQAS A. MALICK

INTRODUCTION

Diseases of the pericardium encompass a wide spectrum ranging from benign, self-limited pericarditis to life-threatening, acute cardiac tamponade. The etiologies of pericarditis are broad, and addressing the underlying cause remains an essential principle of management. Pericarditis and the associated symptoms can be managed with various antiinflammatory agents, but sequelae of pericarditis, most importantly pericardial effusion, may require more urgent or emergent management.

PATHOPHYSIOLOGY

Pericarditis is due to inflammation of the pericardium and results from a variety of causes. The most common etiology is idiopathic pericarditis, in which no clear causative factor is identified. The majority of these cases are thought to be due to viral illness or an autoimmune condition. Viruses that are associated with pericarditis include coxsackievirus, echovirus, adenovirus, human immunodeficiency virus (HIV), Epstein-Barr virus (EBV), cytomegalovirus (CMV), and varicella, among others. Other infectious causes include bacterial (tuberculosis being the most common cause in areas with high rates of *Mycobacterium* infection), fungal, or parasitic. Noninfectious causes are numerous and include:

- Autoimmune or rheumatological diseases, including systemic lupus erythematosus, rheumatoid arthritis, vasculitides, and systemic sclerosis
- Malignancy, often associated with pericardial effusions
- Uremia
- Hypothyroidism
- Postmyocardial infarction
- Radiation therapy
- Medication induced, including hydralazine, procainamide, isoniazid, and phenytoin

Under normal physiological conditions, the pericardial space contains about 30 to 50 mL of fluid. However, a larger volume of fluid may accumulate within this space, due to any of the aforementioned etiologies, and lead to the development of a **pericardial effusion.** Whether a pericardial effusion will have hemodynamically significant effects on a patient clinically depends on three factors: (1) the volume of fluid, (2) the rate at which the fluid accumulates, and (3) the stiffness (compliance) of the pericardium. For example, a sudden increase in the amount of fluid in the pericardial space, such as after trauma, can quickly lead to increased pressure in the pericardial space and hemodynamically significant cardiac tamponade. Alternatively, a slow accumulation of pericardial fluid over a prolonged period of time may not create significant hemodynamic effects, as the pericardium has time to stretch and accommodate the increase in volume (Fig. 61.1).

Hemodynamics play a vital role in the consequences of pericardial effusions. An increase in the volume of pericardial fluid leads to increased intrapericardial pressure; the more rapidly the volume accumulates, the more rapidly the pressure in the pericardial space increases. While the pericardium has some degree of compliance, eventually it will not be able to accommodate a growing pericardial effusion, which begins to impinge on the cardiac tissue itself. This impingement leads to external compression of the myocardium, impairing the heart's ability to relax during diastole and elevating the diastolic pressure. The diastolic pressure becomes equal to the intrapericardial pressure (known as equalization of pressures) and results in impaired diastolic filling; this, in turn, leads to an increase in venous pressures and decreased preload, which causes impaired contractility via the Frank-Starling curve. Increased venous pressures are transmitted to the systemic and pulmonary venous systems, and the decreased stroke volume will lead to activation of compensatory sympathetic responses to augment cardiac output. It is important to note that these effects rarely occur with a slow and gradual accumulation of pericardial fluid over a prolonged period of time (Fig. 61.2).

The pericardium itself can lose elasticity following episodes of pericarditis, and repeated episodes make this loss of compliance more likely. The loss of elasticity and resultant decreased compliance can lead to **constrictive**

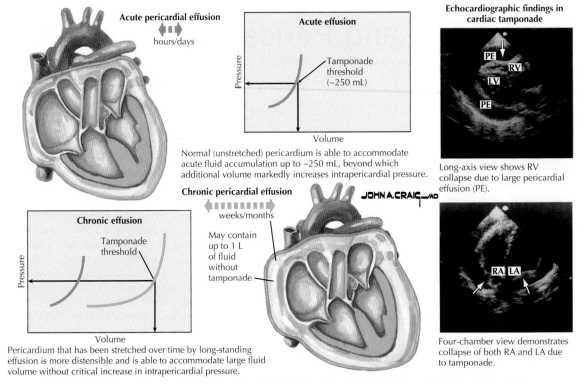

Acute pericardial effusion

hours/days

Acute effusion

Pressure

Tamponade threshold (~250 mL)

Volume

Normal (unstretched) pericardium is able to accommodate acute fluid accumulation up to ~250 mL, beyond which additional volume markedly increases intrapericardial pressure.

Chronic pericardial effusion

weeks/months

May contain up to 1 L of fluid without tamponade

Chronic effusion

Pressure

Tamponade threshold

Volume

Pericardium that has been stretched over time by long-standing effusion is more distensible and is able to accommodate large fluid volume without critical increase in intrapericardial pressure.

JOHN A.CRAIG—AD

Echocardiographic findings in cardiac tamponade

PE
RV
LV
PE

Long-axis view shows RV collapse due to large pericardial effusion (PE).

RA LA

Four-chamber view demonstrates collapse of both RA and LA due to tamponade.

FIG. 61.1 **Volume-Pressure Relationship of the Pericardium.** *LA,* Left artery; *LV,* left ventricle; *PE,* pericardial effusion; *RA,* right artery; *RV,* right ventricle.

pericarditis, in which a stiff pericardium impairs diastole by being unable to accommodate ventricular relaxation and filling. This results in greater interventricular dependence, altering cardiac hemodynamics and leading to hypotension, shortness of breath, and decreased exercise tolerance.

PRESENTATION, EVALUATION, AND DIAGNOSIS

The common presenting symptom for acute pericarditis is retrosternal chest pain. The pain is typically characterized as sharp and worse with inspiration, but improves with leaning forward. One may occasionally hear a friction rub in a patient with pericarditis, which is a low-pitched, grating sound present in both systole and diastole. A pericardial effusion, however, can muffle a friction rub, along with other normal heart sounds. **Cardiac tamponade** is the most feared complication of pericarditis with associated pericardial effusion. Cardiac tamponade is classically diagnosed with the triad of hypotension from

obstructive shock, muffled heart sounds, and elevated jugular venous pressure. Other concerning signs include tachycardia and pulmonary edema.

One important physical exam finding that should be regularly checked in patients with pericardial effusions is **pulsus paradoxus.** Humans experience physiologic variations in systolic blood pressure (SBP) with respiration, normally <10 mm Hg in SBP. Inspiration decreases intrathoracic pressure and leads to increased right ventricular filling, causing the interventricular septum to bow into the left ventricle and transiently decreasing cardiac output. In a patient with a pericardial effusion, this interventricular septal bowing is exaggerated by the inability of the right ventricle to expand into the pericardial space. This exaggerated interventricular bowing causes a greater decrease in SBP during inspiration; a pulsus paradoxus is defined by a fall in SBP >10 mm Hg during inspiration. While the presence of pulsus paradoxus is not entirely specific for the presence of cardiac tamponade, it does suggest that tamponade physiology is present. Furthermore, the absence of pulsus

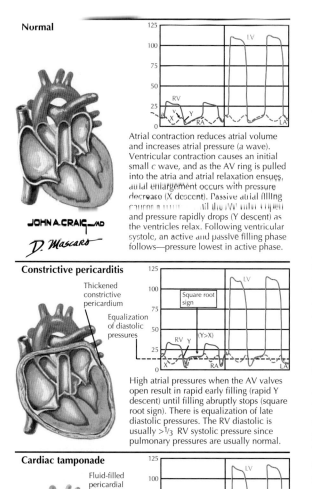

Normal

Atrial contraction reduces atrial volume and increases atrial pressure (a wave). Ventricular contraction causes an initial small c wave, and as the AV ring is pulled into the atria and atrial relaxation ensues, atrial enlargement occurs with pressure decrease (X descent). Passive atrial filling causes a rise until the AV valves open and pressure rapidly drops (Y descent) as the ventricles relax. Following ventricular systole, an active and passive filling phase follows—pressure lowest in active phase.

JOHN A. CRAIG—MD

D. Mascaro

Constrictive pericarditis

Thickened constrictive pericardium

Equalization of diastolic pressures

Square root sign

(Y>X)

High atrial pressures when the AV valves open result in rapid early filling (rapid Y descent) until filling abruptly stops (square root sign). There is equalization of late diastolic pressures. The RV diastolic is usually >1/3 RV systolic pressure since pulmonary pressures are usually normal.

Cardiac tamponade

Fluid-filled pericardial sac

Equalization of diastolic pressures

(X>Y)

High atrial pressure when the AV valves open in tamponade are met by the high pressures exerted on the ventricles by the pericardial fluid. Early filling is therefore blunted and the Y descent is less than the X descent. There is equalization of late diastolic pressures, and the pulmonary pressure is normal.

FIG. 61.2 Normal and Pathological Intracardiac Pressures. *AV*, Atrioventricular; *LA*, left artery; *LV*, left ventricle; *RA*, right artery; *RV*, right ventricle.

paradoxus does not always rule out tamponade, especially in patients with preexisting cardiac conditions, including aortic stenosis, pulmonary hypertension, or intracardiac shunting. The measurement can be trended over time in patients with pericardial effusions.

Diagnostic workup for pericarditis begins with an electrocardiogram (ECG), chest x-ray, and echocardiogram. For acute pericarditis, expected findings on ECG include diffuse ST elevations and PR depressions (Fig. 61.3). If acute pericarditis progresses to pericardial effusion or cardiac tamponade, the ECG findings change to show diffusely decreased QRS voltage or potential electrical alternans, in which the axis of the QRS complex varies from beat to beat, owing to the heart swinging back and forth within the effusion. A chest x-ray may show enlarged cardiac silhouette, and in tamponade, increased pulmonary vascular congestion. Echocardiograms are highly sensitive for pericardial effusions and can show evidence of hemodynamic compromise, including echocardiographic signs of pulsus paradoxus, increased ventricular interdependence, and chamber compression.

Pericardiocentesis is a critical tool in the diagnosis and management of pericardial effusions. Not every pericardial effusion requires drainage, and treatment can be directed at the underlying cause of the effusion should an etiology be readily identifiable. Echocardiography can visualize the most direct route of access to the effusion and confirm location for needle placement; following needle placement, a pigtail catheter can be left in place to ensure adequate drainage of the fluid. Pericardial fluid should be sent for Gram stain and culture (bacterial, fungal), acid-fast bacilli (AFB) stain and culture for tuberculous pericarditis, adenosine deaminase (also for tuberculous pericarditis), and cytology. Polymerase chain reaction (PCR) for concerning viruses may be useful (Fig. 61.4).

TREATMENT

Acute pericarditis without a significant effusion can be managed medically. The treatment of acute pericarditis is geared toward reducing inflammation of the pericardium and pain control. NSAIDs are used often as first-line agents, with ibuprofen, aspirin, and indomethacin all common choices. Patients with contraindications to NSAIDs may be treated with glucocorticoids, although the use of glucocorticoids is correlated with an increased risk of recurrence of pericarditis.

Colchicine may be used in combination with NSAIDs or as the primary agent for acute pericarditis, especially for cases of idiopathic or viral pericarditis.

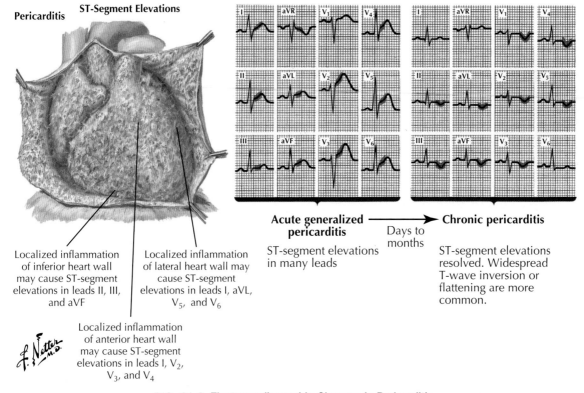

Pericarditis

ST-Segment Elevations

Acute generalized ——————→ **Chronic pericarditis**
pericarditis
Days to
months

Localized inflammation
of inferior heart wall
may cause ST-segment
elevations in leads II, III,
and aVF

Localized inflammation
of lateral heart wall may
cause ST-segment
elevations in leads I, aVL,
V_5, and V_6

Localized inflammation
of anterior heart wall
may cause ST-segment
elevations in leads I, V_2,
V_3, and V_4

ST-segment elevations
in many leads

ST-segment elevations
resolved. Widespread
T-wave inversion or
flattening are more
common.

FIG. 61.3 Electrocardiographic Changes in Pericarditis.

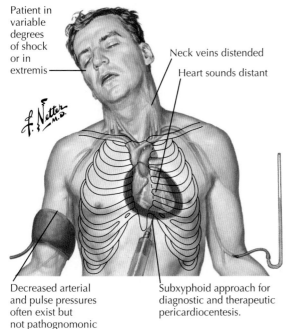

Patient in
variable
degrees
of shock
or in
extremis

Neck veins distended

Heart sounds distant

Decreased arterial
and pulse pressures
often exist but
not pathognomonic

Subxyphoid approach for
diagnostic and therapeutic
pericardiocentesis.

**FIG. 61.4 Cardiac Tamponade and
Pericardiocentesis.**

Notably, studies have shown that colchicine can not only reduce symptoms but also decrease the rate of recurrent pericarditis. While generally well tolerated, physicians must remain vigilant for bone marrow suppression that can result from overdose.

Patients with cardiac tamponade should undergo emergent pericardiocentesis to relieve obstructive shock; interim intravenous fluids can increase intraventricular pressure, allowing the ventricular wall to expand out against the intrapericardial pressure, thus improving preload and stroke volume. As noted, pericardiocentesis can also reveal the underlying etiology for the pericardial disease. For patients with symptomatic recurrent pericardial effusions, a pericardial window or pericardiotomy may be warranted.

For constrictive pericarditis, early disease may be treated with the antiinflammatories outlined earlier in an effort to decrease inflammation and preserve pericardial elasticity. Chronic constrictive pericarditis is ultimately best treated with surgical pericardiectomy.

CHAPTER 62

Aortic Stenosis

MOHSIN CHOWDHURY

INTRODUCTION

Aortic stenosis (AS) is the most common valvular heart disorder in developed countries. AS primarily affects older adults, with the prevalence rising from 0.2% in the sixth decade of life to 9.8% in the ninth decade. About one-quarter of the population older than 65 years has at least some aortic valve thickening and calcification.

AS is generally asymptomatic until it gradually becomes severe, at which point patients may experience angina, dyspnea, and syncope and are at increased risk of sudden death. No medical therapy has been shown to prevent or slow the progression of AS. Thus it is essential to identify those at risk, closely monitor disease severity and progression, and ensure timely valve replacement once indicated.

PATHOPHYSIOLOGY

The three primary causes of AS are calcific disease of a trileaflet valve, a congenitally abnormal valve (bicuspid or unicuspid) with superimposed calcification, and rheumatic heart disease (Fig. 62.1). Although rheumatic heart disease is rare in the developed world, it remains one of the most common causes of AS worldwide. Other rare causes include radiation exposure and metabolic diseases (e.g., Fabry disease).

The development of AS in a normal trileaflet valve can be divided into two stages. The early initiation phase is characterized by lipid accumulation and inflammation, as occurs with atherosclerosis. The later propagation phase consists primarily of calcification, which causes progressive stiffness and narrowing of the valve. The disease typically progresses over 10 to 15 years, presenting clinically between the ages of 60 and 80 years. The risk factors that can accelerate this process include male gender, older age, renal failure, hypercholesterolemia, diabetes mellitus, disorders of calcium metabolism, and smoking. Patients with unicuspid or bicuspid valves, meanwhile, usually experience an accelerated version of this process and present with symptoms between the ages of 40 and 60 years.

The left ventricular outflow tract (LVOT) obstruction caused by AS leads to an increase in left ventricular (LV) systolic pressure and a systolic pressure gradient between the LV and aorta. The LV develops concentric hypertrophy (i.e., the LV wall thickness increases) as a compensatory response, but eventually this becomes maladaptive, causing elevated LV end diastolic pressure, diastolic dysfunction, and heart failure. In the later stages of disease, myocardial contractility may also decrease, leading to systolic dysfunction and further worsening of heart failure.

The progressive mismatch between the high myocardial oxygen demand (due to the increase in LV mass, increase in LV systolic pressure, and prolongation of the systolic ejection phase) and reduced myocardial oxygen delivery (due to diminished coronary flow reserve and decreased diastolic perfusion pressure) may lead to myocardial ischemia and angina. Finally, if the AS is severe enough, the inability to increase cardiac output in response to physiological demand may result in exertional hypotension and syncope.

PRESENTATION, EVALUATION, AND DIAGNOSIS

The most common symptoms of AS are exertional dyspnea and lightheadedness. Oftentimes patients may not appreciate the severity of these symptoms due to the gradually progressive nature of the condition, instead attributing them to aging or unconsciously reducing their activity level to minimize their occurrence. As the disease progresses, patients may develop angina, syncope, and signs of more severe heart failure, such as paroxysmal nocturnal dyspnea and orthopnea.

On physical examination, patients with AS often have a number of characteristic findings:
- **Murmur:** The murmur of AS is characteristically described as a harsh, crescendo-decrescendo murmur best heard at the right second intercostal space with radiation to the carotid arteries. The peak onset of the murmur correlates with disease severity, with

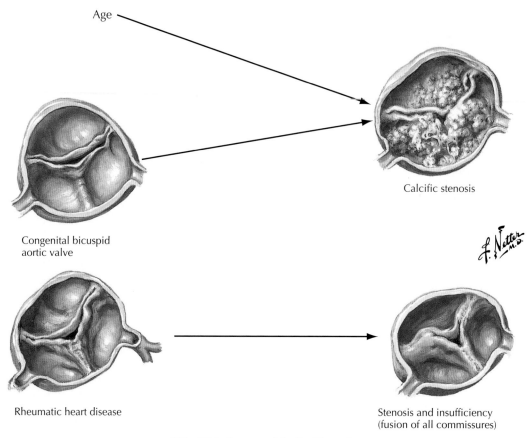

Age

Calcific stenosis

Congenital bicuspid
aortic valve

Rheumatic heart disease

Stenosis and insufficiency
(fusion of all commissures)

FIG. 62.1 **Causes of Aortic Stenosis.**

later-peaking murmurs reflecting more severe disease. An ejection click may be heard in patients with bicuspid aortic valve.

- **Pulsus parvus et tardus:** LVOT obstruction results in weak (parvus) and delayed (tardus) carotid pulsations. The amount of delay can be ascertained from simultaneous palpation of the carotid pulsations and the apical impulse.
- **Diminished or absent A2:** With severe disease, the S2 may be soft or absent, suggesting that the aortic valve is barely opening and closing.
- **Paradoxically split S2:** The splitting results from late closure of the aortic valve, reflecting prolongation of LV systole to generate adequate pressure.
- **Fourth heart sound (S4):** S4 is a low-frequency gallop sound that results from the vibration of the stiffened ventricular wall during atrial contraction.

Transthoracic echocardiography (TTE) is the primary diagnostic test for the diagnosis and evaluation of AS.

As summarized in Table 62.1, AS is staged according to symptoms, valve anatomy, valve hemodynamics, and LV characteristics (i.e., hypertrophy, dysfunction, wall thickness). Exercise testing is recommended in selected patients with asymptomatic severe AS (stage C) to confirm that they are truly asymptomatic. Exercise testing should not be performed in symptomatic patients.

On TTE the hemodynamic significance of AS is best characterized by the transaortic maximum velocity of blood flow and the transaortic mean pressure gradient; however, a subset of patients with AS have a low transaortic flow rate due to either LV systolic dysfunction, leading to low LV ejection fraction (LVEF), or significant LV hypertrophy, leading to a small cavity size and low stroke volume. These special subgroups of patients with low-flow/low-gradient AS are designated as stage D2 (if LVEF is reduced) or D3 (if LVEF is preserved) and pose additional diagnostic and management challenges.

TABLE 62.1
Stages of Aortic Stenosis

Stage	Description	Definition	Management
A	At risk (asymptomatic)	Bicuspid AV or aortic valve sclerosis V_{max} <2 m/s	Clinical monitoring
B	Progressive (asymptomatic)	Mild-to-moderate calcification or rheumatic changes with commissural fusion V_{max} 2.0–3.9 m/s or mean ΔP <40 mm Hg	Clinical monitoring and periodic echocardiographic monitoring every 3–5 years if V_{max} 2.0–2.9 m/s or mean ΔP <20 mm Hg (mild AS), or every 1–2 years if V_{max} 3.0–3.9 or mean ΔP 20–39 mm Hg (moderate AS) AVR if patient has moderate AS and is undergoing other cardiac surgery
C1	Asymptomatic severe AS with normal LVEF	Severe calcification or severely reduced leaflet opening LVEF ≥50% V_{max} ≥4 m/s or mean ΔP ≥40 mm Hg AVA typically is ≤1.0 cm²	Clinical monitoring and periodic echocardiographic monitoring every 6–12 months Exercise testing to confirm asymptomatic status AVR if V_{max} ≥5 m/s or ΔP ≥60 mm (low surgical risk patients), exercise testing positive, or undergoing other cardiac surgery (regardless of surgical risk)
C2	Asymptomatic severe AS with low LVEF	Severe calcification or severely reduced leaflet opening LVEF <50% V_{max} ≥4 m/s or mean ΔP ≥40 mm Hg AVA typically is ≤1.0 cm²	AVR
D1	Symptomatic severe high-gradient AS	Severe calcification or severely reduced leaflet opening LVEF ≥50% V_{max} ≥4 m/s or mean ΔP ≥40 mm Hg AVA typically is ≤1.0 cm²	AVR
D2	Symptomatic severe low-gradient/ low-flow AS, with reduced LVEF	Severe calcification or severely reduced leaflet opening LVEF <50% AVA ≤1.0 cm² with V_{max} <4 m/s or mean ΔP <40 mm Hg, or AVA ≤1.0 cm² and V_{max} ≥4 m/s or mean ΔP ≥40 mm Hg on dobutamine stress echocardiography (any dose)	AVR
D3	Symptomatic severe low-gradient/ low-flow AS with normal LVEF	Severe calcification or severely reduced leaflet opening LVEF ≥50% AVA ≤1.0 cm² with V_{max} <4 m/s or mean ΔP <40 mm Hg, but with an indexed AVA ≤0.6 cm²/m² with stroke volume index of <35 mL/m² when patient is normotensive	AVR if AS is most likely cause of symptoms

AS, Aortic stenosis; *AV,* aortic valve; *AVA,* aortic valve area; *AVR,* aortic valve replacement; *ΔP,* transaortic pressure gradient; *LVEF,* left ventricular ejection fraction, *V_{max},* maximum aortic velocity.
Reused with permission from Kanwar A, Thaden JJ, Nkomo VT: Management of patients with aortic valve stenosis, *Mayo Clin Proc* 93(4):488–508, 2018.

Balloon-Expandable Valve

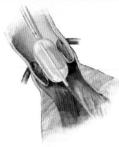

A. Initial aortic balloon valvuloplasty

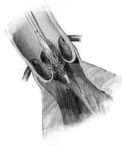

B. Positioning of stented valve

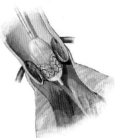

C. Inflation of balloon with stented valve

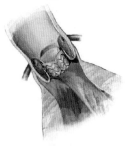

D. Final position of stented valve

Self-Expanding Valve

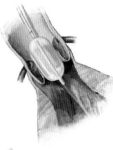

A. Initial aortic balloon valvuloplasty

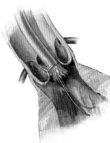

B. Positioning of stented valve still in sheath

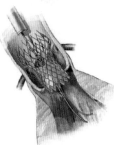

C. Withdrawal of sheath. Self-expanding prosthesis

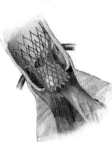

D. Final position of stented valve

FIG. 62.2 **Transcatheter Aortic Valve Replacement.**

TREATMENT

The only definitive therapy for AS is aortic valve replacement (AVR). Table 62.1 summarizes the indications for AVR. The specific method of AVR (i.e., surgical or transcatheter) depends on the patient's overall surgical risk, as assessed using the Society of Thoracic Surgeons Predicted Risk of 30-Day Mortality (STS-PROM) score, patient preference, and heart team (cardiac surgeon, interventional cardiologist, imaging cardiologist, cardiac anesthesiologist, geriatrician) assessment. Although transcatheter aortic valve replacement (TAVR) (Fig. 62.2) with either a balloon-expandable or self-expanding valve is approved in patients with low surgical risk (i.e., STS-PROM <4%), younger age patients with low surgical risk typically undergo surgical valve replacement as long-term durability of transcatheter valve is still unknown. Patients with intermediate to high surgical risk (i.e., STS-PROM ≥4%) typically undergo TAVR if there is reasonable expectation of survival of >12 months.

Patients who do not require intervention should undergo regular monitoring to reassess stenosis severity (see Table 62.1). Medications have not been shown to prolong life in patients with AS and have limited utility in treating symptoms. Diuretics, ACE inhibitors, β-blockers, and vasodilators should be carefully used to treat symptoms of heart failure, and aggressive diuresis and preload reduction should be avoided since patients with AS are preload dependent.

CHAPTER 63

Mitral Regurgitation

NIDHI TRIPATHI

INTRODUCTION

A normally functioning mitral valve allows for unidirectional blood flow from the left atrium into the left ventricle. More than a mild amount of retrograde flow is considered pathological, and although moderate mitral regurgitation can be tolerated indefinitely, severe mitral regurgitation may lead to left ventricular remodeling, reduced cardiac output, neurohumoral activation, left ventricular damage, heart failure, and death.

Mitral regurgitation occurs either due to primary disruption of the mitral valve apparatus or as a secondary consequence of a cardiomyopathy. The mitral valve apparatus consists of the mitral valve annulus, the anterior and posterior leaflets, the chordae tendineae, and the papillary muscles. The most common etiology for primary mitral regurgitation in the developed world is degenerative mitral valve disease, including mitral valve prolapse. **Mitral valve prolapse** is a form of myxomatous valve degeneration, in which the valve leaflets become enlarged and the chordae tendineae elongated, leading to prolapse of the leaflets into the left atrium during ventricular systole. While generally benign, progressive degeneration can lead to mitral regurgitation (Fig. 63.1). Additional etiologies include rheumatic heart disease, infective endocarditis, trauma, acute myocardial ischemia, and mitral annular calcification.

Secondary mitral regurgitation is a consequence of remodeling of the left ventricle due to coronary artery disease, nonischemic dilated cardiomyopathies, hypertrophic cardiomyopathy, or long-term right ventricular pacing. The left ventricle supports the mitral valve apparatus via the papillary muscle and chordae tendineae, so that any remodeling of the left ventricle may also affect the ability of the mitral valve leaflets to coapt, or close.

Mitral valve regurgitation can present as acute, chronically compensated, or chronically decompensated, and the evaluation and treatment must be tailored to the phase of the disease.

PATHOPHYSIOLOGY

Acute, chronically compensated, or chronically decompensated mitral regurgitation share the common feature of left ventricular volume overload. During diastole, the left ventricle is filled both with the normal pulmonary venous return from the left atrium and the volume of regurgitated blood from the prior beat.

Acute primary mitral regurgitation is caused by abrupt compromise of the mitral valve apparatus. In this situation, the left ventricle is suddenly overwhelmed with extra volume, resulting in sarcomeric stretch, increased end diastolic volume, and sympathetic activation. Although the ejection fraction is generally preserved, or even elevated because of increased contractility and the decreased resistance of the left atrium, the forward cardiac output remains low, as more than 50% of the blood volume in the left ventricle is ejected retrograde. In acute mitral regurgitation, the left atrial compliance is usually normal, resulting in elevated filling pressures from the extra regurgitant volume. These elevated pressures, in turn, cause pulmonary venous congestion, pulmonary edema, and acute hypoxemia. Severe, acute primary mitral insufficiency may result in shock.

Chronic primary mitral regurgitation occurs when regurgitation worsens gradually over time. In this situation, the left heart undergoes gradual remodeling in response to volume overload, including eccentric hypertrophy of the left ventricle and dilation of the left atrium. As the left ventricular end diastolic volume increases, left ventricular contractility is initially preserved, and systemic cardiac output is maintained despite a large regurgitant volume. Because the left atrium is dilated, filling pressures remain normal, and pulmonary edema is avoided. Therefore, even with exercise, patients in a chronic compensated state may remain asymptomatic. However, prolonged volume overload eventually leads to contractile dysfunction and pulmonary congestion, and patients present with heart failure symptoms such

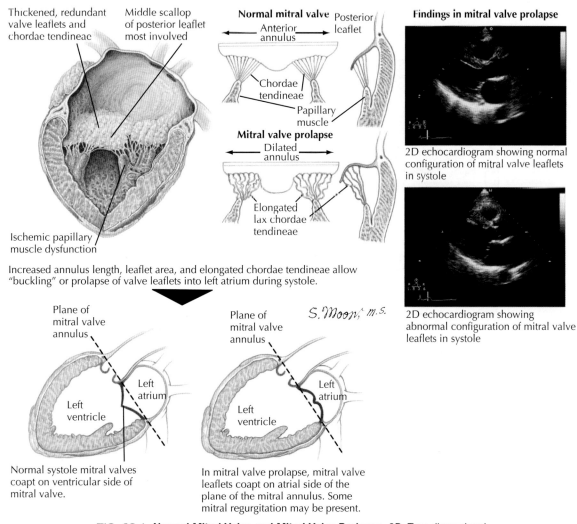

Thickened, redundant valve leaflets and chordae tendineae

Middle scallop of posterior leaflet most involved

Ischemic papillary muscle dysfunction

Normal mitral valve
Anterior annulus
Posterior leaflet
Chordae tendineae
Papillary muscle

Mitral valve prolapse
Dilated annulus
Elongated lax chordae tendineae

Findings in mitral valve prolapse

2D echocardiogram showing normal configuration of mitral valve leaflets in systole

2D echocardiogram showing abnormal configuration of mitral valve leaflets in systole

Increased annulus length, leaflet area, and elongated chordae tendineae allow "buckling" or prolapse of valve leaflets into left atrium during systole.

S. Moon, M.S.

Plane of mitral valve annulus
Left ventricle
Left atrium

Plane of mitral valve annulus
Left ventricle
Left atrium

Normal systole mitral valves coapt on ventricular side of mitral valve.

In mitral valve prolapse, mitral valve leaflets coapt on atrial side of the plane of the mitral annulus. Some mitral regurgitation may be present.

FIG. 63.1 **Normal Mitral Valve and Mitral Valve Prolapse.** *2D,* Two-dimensional.

as shortness of breath, orthopnea, and lower extremity edema.

Secondary mitral regurgitation is caused by compromise of the papillary muscles or chordae tendineae due to a primary left ventricular pathology. Ventricular dilation or segmental wall motion abnormalities change the geometry of both the left ventricle and the papillary muscles that are attached to the left ventricular walls, and this change in geometry prevents adequate coaptation of the mitral leaflets. With time, this leads to worsening left ventricular dilation and worsening mitral regurgitation—in effect, mitral regurgitation begets mitral regurgitation.

RISK FACTORS

Acute mitral regurgitation may be a result of dysfunction or rupture of the papillary muscles due to acute myocardial ischemia, or acute rupture of a chordae due to endocarditis, acute on chronic degenerative disease, or blunt chest wall trauma. With ischemia, the posteromedial papillary muscle is involved more frequently than the anterolateral papillary muscle because it is only supplied by the right coronary artery, whereas the anterolateral papillary muscle has a dual blood supply. Chronic compensated mitral regurgitation may be due to primary valvular pathology, most commonly mitral

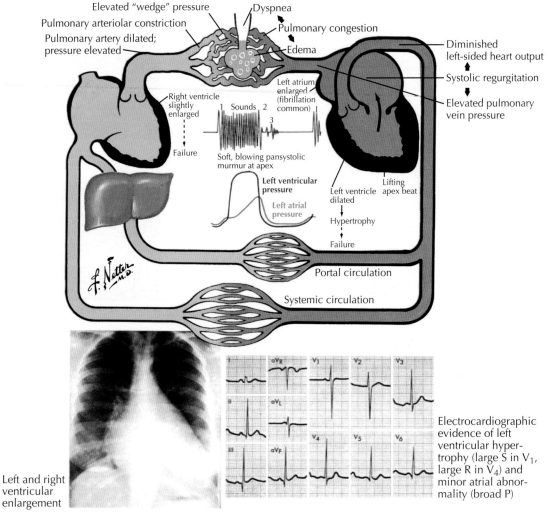

FIG. 63.2 **Pathophysiology and Symptoms of Mitral Regurgitation.**

valve prolapse, or secondary regurgitation due to a cardiomyopathy as described previously.

PRESENTATION, EVALUATION, AND DIAGNOSIS

Mild to moderate mitral regurgitation is generally asymptomatic, but severe mitral regurgitation can lead to symptoms typically associated with left ventricular dysfunction such as dyspnea on exertion, orthopnea, and paroxysmal nocturnal dyspnea. If chronic and severe, pulmonary hypertension and right heart failure may develop, resulting in ascites and edema. While patients with chronic decompensated mitral regurgitation

may have an insidious onset of the abovementioned symptoms, patients suffering from acute severe mitral regurgitation often may present with acute respiratory distress and shock (Fig. 63.2).

On physical exam, the reduced anterograde stroke volume tends to reduce blood pressure and pulse pressure, but this is not a consistent finding as some patients are hypertensive upon presentation. A holosystolic, blowing murmur may be appreciated at the cardiac apex with radiation to the axilla. However, the murmur may be subtle or absent in acute severe mitral regurgitation, as the pressure gradient between the ventricle and atrium dissipates early in systole with a normally compliant left atrium. Severe mitral regurgitation may be accompanied by an S3 gallop as the large volume of the left atrium empties into the ventricle and a split S2 due to early closure of the aortic valve as less blood moves through the valve and instead contributes to the large regurgitant fraction.

Electrocardiogram (ECG) findings are nonspecific but may include left atrial enlargement and left ventricular hypertrophy in chronic mitral regurgitation. Atrial fibrillation may be a consequence of left atrial enlargement from chronic mitral regurgitation. ECGs should be carefully evaluated for ischemic changes, especially when acute severe mitral regurgitation is suspected.

The diagnosis of mitral regurgitation is made with echocardiography, which both quantifies the degree of mitral regurgitation and identifies the mechanism of regurgitation (primary vs. secondary). Transthoracic echocardiography is performed first, but if the mitral valve is inadequately visualized or the mechanism is unclear, transesophageal echocardiography can provide greater clarity.

TREATMENT
Acute Mitral Regurgitation

Severe acute mitral regurgitation due to abrupt disruption of the mitral valve apparatus is a surgical emergency. Medical therapy and circulatory support devices (intraaortic balloon pump) can be used as temporary measures until a definitive surgical intervention can be performed. Vasodilators such as nitroprusside or nicardipine decrease aortic pressure and thereby preferentially direct blood flow anterograde, as opposed to retrograde into the left atrium, but their use may be limited by systemic hypotension.

Intraaortic balloon pumps (IABPs) are mechanical counterpulsation devices placed in the descending aorta that are frequently used with acute mitral regurgitation. The balloon inflates during diastole, augmenting diastolic pressure and thus coronary perfusion, and deflates during systole, thereby reducing afterload and promoting forward flow (Fig. 63.3). Again, placement of an IABP is only a temporary measure until a patient can undergo surgical repair or replacement of the mitral valve. In both acute and chronic primary mitral regurgitation, the preferred surgical treatment is **mitral valve repair**, but mitral valve replacement may be required if repair is not feasible.

Chronic Primary Mitral Regurgitation

The primary treatment for chronic primary mitral regurgitation is mitral valve repair when there is evidence of systolic dysfunction (ejection fraction <60%), severe ventricular dilation, or clinical decompensation.

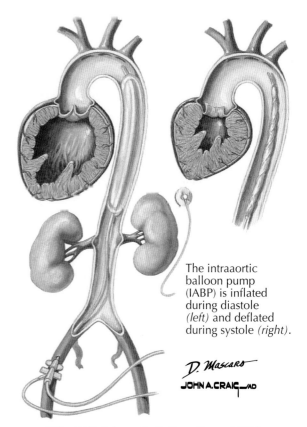

The intraaortic balloon pump (IABP) is inflated during diastole *(left)* and deflated during systole *(right)*.

D. Mascaro

JOHN A.CRAIG—AD

FIG. 63.3 **Intraaortic Balloon Pump (IABP).**

Blood pressure control is recommended in hypertensive patients, but there is a limited role for vasodilator therapy in normotensive and asymptomatic patients, as this has not been shown to slow the progression of disease. In those patients with severe ventricular dysfunction who are unable to undergo surgery, initiation of heart failure therapy, including β-blockers, ACE inhibitors or angiotensin receptor blockers (ARBs), and aldosterone antagonists, is reasonable.

Chronic Secondary Mitral Regurgitation

The treatment of chronic secondary mitral regurgitation is directed at treatment of the underlying disease and left ventricular dysfunction (β-blockers, ACE inhibitors/ARBs, spironolactone, diuretics). The benefit of mitral valve repair or replacement is less clear with secondary mitral regurgitation, as the primary pathology does not lie with the valve itself. It can be considered in severely symptomatic patients with chronic severe mitral regurgitation despite optimal heart failure therapy or in those who are undergoing cardiac surgery for other indications.

A less-invasive mechanical mitral valve repair option, originally developed to treat severe primary mitral regurgitation in patients at prohibitive surgical risk, is now available for patients with chronic and severe secondary mitral regurgitation under select circumstances. Recent evidence suggests that carefully selected patients with severe secondary mitral regurgitation who undergo percutaneous mitral valve repair with a device called a **MitraClip** experience decreased mortality, decreased rates of hospitalization, and improvement in functional capacity. The MitraClip is a device that is inserted via a catheter through the femoral vein, across the intraatrial septum, and into the left atrium to the position of the mitral valve. The malcoapting mitral valve segments are clipped together creating a double orifice mitral valve and to close the regurgitant orifice, thus reducing the degree of mitral regurgitation. This approximates the surgical Alfieri stitch. The patients enrolled in the early trials with the MitraClip were on maximally tolerated medical therapy for heart failure with reduced ejection fraction, as well as cardiac resynchronization therapy if clinically indicated. They were evaluated by a multidisciplinary team of advanced heart failure cardiologists, interventional cardiologists, and cardiothoracic surgeons to ensure maximal medical therapy, as well as technical feasibility of percutaneous mitral valve repair prior to intervention. The number needed to treat to prevent one death at 24 months was six, and the MitraClip device has now been approved for use in patients with severe secondary mitral regurgitation.

CHAPTER 64

Aortic Dissection

CHRISTOPHER R. KELLY • WILL HINDLE-KATEL

INTRODUCTION

Aortic dissection is a condition in which blood passes through a tear in the intimal layer of the aortic wall, entering the medial space and establishing a **false lumen** (Fig. 64.1). Because progressive expansion of the false lumen can compromise flow through the true lumen, end-organ ischemia and life-threatening complications may occur.

Aortic dissections are categorized based on their anatomical location using the **DeBakey** or **Stanford** system (Fig. 64.2). The DeBakey system classifies dissections as follows:

- **Type I:** Dissection originates in the ascending aorta (proximal to the brachiocephalic artery) and propagates to the aortic arch and descending aorta.
- **Type II:** Dissection originates in the ascending aorta, without further propagation.
- **Type III:** Dissection originates in the descending aorta (distal to the left subclavian artery) and propagates distally. Type IIIa dissections are confined to the thoracic aorta, while type IIIb dissections extend below the diaphragm.

Meanwhile, the Stanford system classifies type A dissections as those that involve the ascending aorta and type B dissections as those that do not.

Related conditions include aortic **intramural hematoma,** in which blood collects within the aortic wall but no intimal tear is apparent, and penetrating atherosclerotic ulcer, in which a lesion extends through the intimal layer. Together with aortic dissection, these conditions constitute the acute aortic syndromes.

Aortic dissection is a relatively uncommon event, and its exact incidence is unknown because many patients may suffer fatal complications prior to medical evaluation. Nonetheless it has been estimated to affect 100,000 people per year, at a median age of 63 years.

PATHOPHYSIOLOGY

The aortic wall contains three main layers: the **intima,** which consists of endothelial cells and a basement membrane; the **media,** which contains concentrically arranged elastic fibers and smooth muscle cells bounded by internal and external laminae; and the **adventitia,** which contains the vasa vasorum and consists mostly of collagenous fibers.

An aortic dissection begins with a tear in the intima that allows blood to flow into the medial layer and establish a false lumen. Such tears occur because of degradation or dysfunction of connective tissue in the aortic wall and/or increased aortic wall stress.

Aortic wall abnormalities may result from genetic conditions or acquired risk factors. The predisposing genetic conditions include Marfan syndrome (fibrillin deficiency), Ehlers-Danlos syndrome (collagen mutation), Loeys-Dietz syndrome (transforming growth factor-β [TGF-β] mutation/overactivation), Turner syndrome, bicuspid aortic valve disease, and familial thoracic aortic aneurysm disease. Acquired risk factors include inflammatory aortitis (e.g., Takayasu arteritis), tobacco use, and pregnancy. Many of these conditions are also associated with aortic aneurysm (see Chapter 65), which significantly increases the risk of dissection. Less often, patients may have a recent history of invasive aortic manipulation (e.g., cardiac catheterization) with undetected aortic wall injury.

Meanwhile, increased aortic wall stress generally reflects chronic uncontrolled hypertension, which is present in three-quarters of patients with aortic dissection; however, it can also result from conditions such as cocaine/methamphetamine use, weightlifting, pheochromocytoma, acute deceleration injury (e.g., motor vehicle accident), and aortic coarctation.

Once initiated, the dissection can propagate anterograde or retrograde and can involve branch vessels. As the false lumen expands, flow through the true lumen becomes compromised, and end-organ injury can occur. Dissection of the aortic root, for example, can lead to occlusion of a coronary artery (usually the right coronary artery) and myocardial infarction. Dissection into one or both carotid arteries can cause acute ischemic stroke.

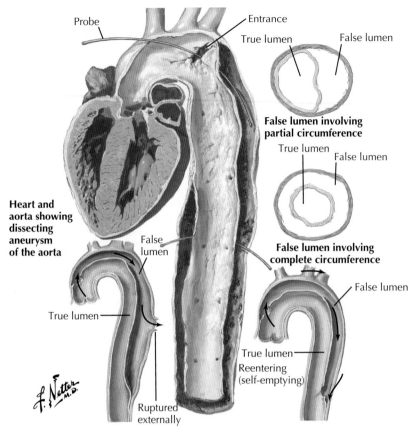

FIG. 64.1 **Aortic Dissection.**

The false lumen can dissect back into the true lumen at one or more locations, or it can extend through the adventitial layer and cause overt aortic rupture. The false lumen can also thrombose and stabilize.

PRESENTATION, EVALUATION, AND DIAGNOSIS

Almost all patients with acute aortic dissection present with severe, sudden-onset pain described as tearing, ripping, stabbing, or sharp. Pain can occur throughout the length of the aorta and often localizes to the site of dissection. Patients with type A dissections, for example, generally present with anterior chest pain, while patients with type B dissections may present with chest, back, or abdominal pain. Some patients may experience migratory pain as the dissection propagates, or they may experience temporary relief of pain if the pressure in the false lumen falls (e.g., from dissection back into the true lumen).

Although pain is nearly universal, the severity and associated features are variable, and so a high degree of clinical suspicion is required for those with risk factors for dissection, given the potentially catastrophic complications.

Additional symptoms generally reflect end-organ ischemia. Neurological symptoms can include stroke, syncope, spinal cord ischemia, and peripheral neuropathy. Cardiovascular complications can include aortic valve insufficiency (from distortion of the aortic root), pericardial effusion and tamponade (from transudation of fluid through the thin wall of the false lumen, or from overt false lumen rupture, into the pericardial space), and myocardial infarction (generally from dissection of the right coronary artery). Mesenteric, renal, and limb ischemia may also occur. Hypotension at presentation is a grave prognostic sign and typically reflects cardiac tamponade (the most common cause of death), severe aortic insufficiency, or aortic rupture.

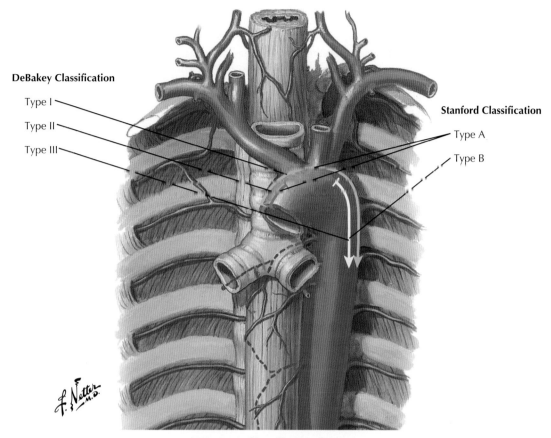

DeBakey Classification

Type I

Type II

Type III

Stanford Classification

Type A

Type B

FIG. 64.2 **Classification Systems.**

Given these symptoms, all patients with risk factors for aortic dissection and a characteristic pain syndrome should be evaluated for pulse deficits/blood pressure differential (with a difference of ≥20 mm Hg between arms considered significant), neurological deficits, and potential cardiac complications (i.e., auscultation for aortic insufficiency).

The laboratory evaluation of aortic dissection is typically nonspecific. The serum D-dimer concentration is almost always elevated, but official guidelines do not recommend testing as part of the diagnostic algorithm since there are no validated clinical criteria to determine when a negative test can safely rule out disease.

All patients suspected of having dissection should have an electrocardiogram to assess for myocardial ischemia. Given the infrequency of dissection-related coronary events, however, the finding of ST-segment elevations should prompt urgent treatment for an acute coronary syndrome rather than aortic imaging, unless the patient has risk factors for dissection or other suggestive symptoms (e.g., new focal neurological deficit).

Patients with low or intermediate probability of aortic dissection should undergo chest x-ray. An abnormal aortic contour or mediastinal widening is present in ~80% of cases, but these findings have low specificity. Patients at high risk for dissection, or with abnormal findings and/or ongoing concern, should undergo prompt CT angiography, which offers sensitivity and specificity rates of >95%. Transesophageal echocardiogram is preferred in unstable patients and can accurately diagnose dissections of the ascending aorta and arch, though it is less sensitive for more distal lesions.

TREATMENT

To reduce shear stress and limit further propagation of the dissection, patients should receive intravenous β-blockers with the goals of lowering the heart rate to

<70 beats per minute (bpm) and the systolic blood pressure to 100 to 120 mm Hg. If β-blockers achieve the goal heart rate but not blood pressure, additional short-acting antihypertensive agents may be administered.

All patients with acute dissection should be emergently evaluated by a multidisciplinary team to determine the need for intervention and to establish a treatment plan. Typically, patients with type A dissection require emergency surgical repair, while patients with type B dissections receive medical management in the absence of complications, such as critical ischemia, refractory symptoms, extension of dissection, and inability to control blood pressure.

Surgical repair typically involves excision of the entire affected portion of the aorta and reimplantation of the major vessels into a graft. If the root is involved, it may be necessary to resuspend or replace the aortic valve. Endovascular graft stenting, with exclusion of the affected portion of the aorta, may be an option for type B dissections.

Patients who survive aortic dissections require regular monitoring and lifelong β-blockade therapy to control blood pressure and reduce aortic shear stress. Over the long term, the 10-year survival following acute dissection is 30% to 60%, with most mortality occurring in the first 30 days.

CHAPTER 85

Aortic Aneurysm

JONAH RUBIN

INTRODUCTION

An aortic aneurysm (AA) is an abnormal widening of the aorta over 50% of the expected diameter at a given location, which weakens the vessel wall and predisposes it to rupture (Fig. 65.1). A true aneurysm involves all three layers of the blood vessel (the intima, media, and adventitia).

An AA is classified as either **thoracic (TAA)** or **abdominal (AAA),** and can be further described as fusiform (dilation of the entire circumference) or saccular (asymmetric outpouching). An **ascending TAA** is located between the aortic root and the innominate artery, while a **descending TAA** is located between the left subclavian artery and diaphragm; both may also extend into the aortic arch and involve the brachiocephalic vessels. An AAA is located below the diaphragm. An aneurysm that involves both the thoracic and abdominal aorta is classified as thoracoabdominal.

AAs are typically asymptomatic until they rupture, with devastating results. It is therefore imperative to identify, monitor, and treat aneurysms before complications occur.

PATHOPHYSIOLOGY

The degradation or abnormal production of elastin, collagen, and smooth muscle cells predisposes to aneurysm formation. Such disturbances arise primarily in association with traditional risk factors for atherosclerosis, including age (>50–60 years), cigarette smoking, hypertension, and hyperlipidemia. Surprisingly, there is a negative association between diabetes and AA. The reason for this is under investigation, but possibilities include increased cross-linking of collagen in the aortic wall induced by advanced glycation, which confers protection from degradation. Plasmin, an inducer of matrix metalloproteases that degrade collagen, is also suppressed in diabetes.

TAAs may also result from infection, genetic disorders, vasculitis, and trauma. The most common pathogens associated with infective, or mycotic, TAAs are *Streptococcus* and *Salmonella,* although other bacteria and even fungi may also be responsible. In the past, syphilis *(Treponema pallidum)* accounted for a large number of mycotic aneurysms, usually of the ascending aorta. Genetic disorders associated with AA (usually ascending) include Marfan syndrome, Ehlers-Danlos syndrome (type IV), Loeys-Dietz syndrome, bicuspid aortic valve, Turner syndrome, and familial TAA. Several different vasculitides can cause TAA; the most common are Takayasu and giant cell arteritis. Finally, traumatic chest injury may lead to a true full-thickness aneurysm in rare cases, usually in the descending aorta.

PRESENTATION, EVALUATION, AND DIAGNOSIS

Most AAs are asymptomatic and are discovered either during screening or incidentally when an echocardiogram, CT of the chest, or MRI of the chest is performed for another indication (Fig. 65.2). Screening for TAAs is typically limited to those with predisposing genetic disorders or a first-degree relative with TAA. Screening for AAAs using ultrasound is recommended in men aged 65 to 75 who have ever smoked (>100 cigarettes during their lifetime).

Large AAs occasionally do cause symptoms. TAAs can cause pain or symptoms of mass effect, including dysphagia (from esophageal compression), hoarseness (from compression of the recurrent laryngeal nerve), cough and shortness of breath (from compression of the tracheobronchial tree), and superior vena cava syndrome. Ascending TAAs can cause aortic regurgitation and heart failure. Large AAAs may cause noticeable abdominal pulsations or pain in the flank or lower back.

If TAA is identified, the patient should undergo echocardiography to assess for the presence of a bicuspid valve. Patients who present at a young age and/or have first-degree relatives with TAA should be referred for genetic screening.

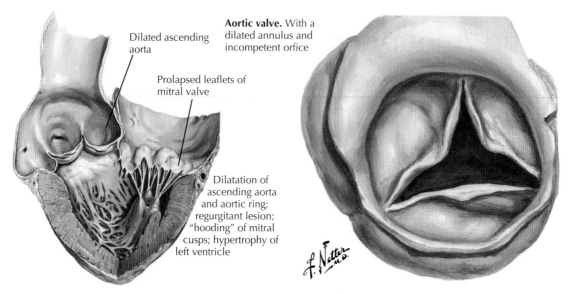

Dilated ascending aorta

Aortic valve. With a dilated annulus and incompetent orfice

Prolapsed leaflets of mitral valve

Dilatation of ascending aorta and aortic ring; regurgitant lesion; "hooding" of mitral cusps; hypertrophy of left ventricle

FIG. 65.1 **Ascending Aortic Aneurysm.**

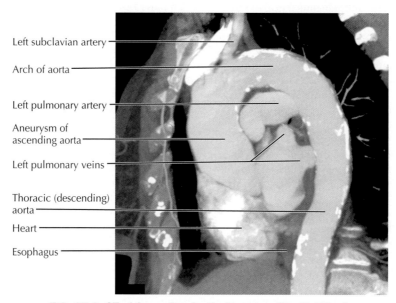

Left subclavian artery

Arch of aorta

Left pulmonary artery

Aneurysm of ascending aorta

Left pulmonary veins

Thoracic (descending) aorta

Heart

Esophagus

FIG. 65.2 **CT of Ascending Aortic Aneurysm (Sagittal View).**

MANAGEMENT
Medical
Patients with TAAs should receive β-blockers to control their blood pressure and slow aneurysm expansion, based primarily on studies showing benefit among patients with Marfan syndrome. Patients with AAAs should also have strict blood pressure control, although no specific agent has proven superior to others. The benefits of other agents, including antiplatelet agents, ACE inhibitors, angiotensin receptor blockers, statins, and doxycycline, are under active investigation but have thus far not been clearly established. Most patients, however, have atherosclerosis and therefore warrant treatment with aspirin and statins. Finally, all patients should receive smoking cessation counseling when appropriate.

- All symptomatic or ruptured aneurysms, provided there is a reasonable chance of recovery
- Ascending TAAs that are sporadic (not associated with a genetic syndrome) and are ≥5.5 cm or growing >5 mm per year
- Ascending TAAs that are associated with bicuspid aortic valve and are ≥4.5 cm, if surgical intervention is indicated for aortic valve disease, or ≥5 cm, if there is a family history of dissection
- Descending TAAs that are sporadic and are ≥5.5 cm (if endovascular repair is possible) or ≥6 cm (if open repair is necessary)
- TAAs that are genetically mediated (Marfan syndrome, Loeys-Dietz syndrome, etc.) and are ≥4–5 cm, depending on the specific condition
- AAAs that are ≥5.5 cm, or growing >5 mm per 6 months

AAA, Abdominal aortic aneurysm; *TAA*, thoracic aortic aneurysm.

Surgical

Surgical intervention is indicated when the risk of aneurysm rupture exceeds the risk associated with intervention. The risk of AAA rupture, for example, is <1% when the diameter is <4 cm but rises to >10% when the diameter exceeds 6 cm. Several factors are taken into consideration when determining the need for surgical intervention for an AA, including size, rate of growth, symptoms, etiology, and genetics (Box 65.1). The decision to intervene is made in collaboration with thoracic surgeons.

Patients with ascending TAAs require open surgery. If the root is involved but the aortic valve leaflets are in good condition, the aortic valve can be resuspended within a prosthetic graft (David procedure). If the valve also requires replacement, a composite graft-valve conduit can be used. If the aortic arch is involved, the brachiocephalic vessels must be reimplanted into a multibranched graft.

In contrast, patients with descending TAAs and AAAs generally undergo endovascular aneurysm repair (EVAR) when possible, in which a stent graft is implanted to exclude the aneurysmal segment from the circulation. Although EVAR is associated with shorter hospitalizations and less morbidity than open surgery, these benefits are partially offset by the greater need for frequent post-operative imaging surveillance studies and subsequent procedures to address complications such as endoleaks, which occur when the aneurysmal segment continues to receive perfusion (i.e., because of a leak at one end of the graft, from collateral perfusion through a branch vessel, or from leak through the graft) and therefore remains at risk of rupture.

Surveillance

Patients with AA who do not meet the criteria for surgical intervention should undergo regular surveillance. For TAAs, the preferred modalities are CT or MRI; however, echocardiography may be used to monitor ascending TAAs. Ideally, the same imaging modality should be used each time, and in the same center, so that images can be directly compared for changes. For AAAs, the preferred imaging modality is ultrasound. Annual imaging is generally adequate unless the AA is approaching the threshold for intervention, at which point a more appropriate interval is every 3 to 6 months.

CHAPTER 66

Hypertension

MERILYN S. VARGHESE

INTRODUCTION

Hypertension, commonly referred to as high blood pressure, is a condition in which the arterial pressures in the body are elevated. Hypertension is extremely common in the United States, affecting one in three adults, and the majority of adults with hypertension are unaware that they have this condition. Variation in blood pressure throughout the day is a normal phenomenon. Blood pressure can be temporarily increased in response to numerous factors, including stress, medications, sleeping patterns, or fluid/sodium intake in a patient without chronic hypertension. Persistent, uncontrolled elevation of blood pressure, however, can lead to dangerous complications.

Hypertension over time increases the risk of ischemic heart disease, stroke, and chronic kidney disease, and it is the major risk factor for intracranial hemorrhage. Normotensive men at 50 years of age live about 7 years longer than their hypertensive counterparts. Similar findings have also been observed in women. Thus timely diagnosis and treatment can potentially prevent these fatal complications.

PATHOPHYSIOLOGY

Primary (essential) hypertension refers to hypertension that cannot be attributed to another cause (Fig. 66.1). The underlying etiology for primary hypertension is multifactorial. Blood pressure is affected and regulated by a multitude of factors, including the sympathetic and parasympathetic nervous system, the renin-angiotensin-aldosterone system (RAAS), circulating cytokines, and glucocorticoids. The causes of the development of elevated blood pressures within the cardiovascular system are secondary to this complex interplay. Regardless, once the body's vasculature is subjected to sustained, higher pressures, the vessels themselves will remodel to accommodate the higher pressure, leading to deleterious effects on end organs such as the kidneys, brain, and retina. Similarly, owing to increased afterload, the left ventricle will remodel and hypertrophy.

Secondary hypertension refers to hypertension that is attributable to another cause. Known etiologies of secondary hypertension include:

- Renovascular hypertension, in which the renal arteries are narrowed, restricting blood flow to the kidneys. This restricted blood flow induces the RAAS to increase blood pressure in an effort to improve renal perfusion, thus leading to hypertension. In young females fibromuscular dysplasia, and in older adults atherosclerosis, can result in renal artery stenosis.
- Chronic kidney disease can lead to overactivation of certain hormonal systems, the RAAS in particular, contributing to elevated blood pressures.
- Pheochromocytoma, a tumor of the adrenal gland, produces supraphysiological levels of catecholamines (primarily epinephrine and norepinephrine). These elevated levels lead to episodes of dangerously elevated blood pressure.
- Medications, including steroids and oral contraceptives. Illicit drugs such as cocaine and amphetamines can also lead to hypertension.
- Cushing disease.
- Hyperthyroidism.
- Aortic coarctation, where narrowing of the proximal descending thoracic aorta may lead to elevated blood pressure in the upper extremities and lower blood pressure in the lower extremities.

RISK FACTORS

A combination of environmental and genetic factors is associated with the risk of developing hypertension. These risk factors include older age (especially in patients >65 years), being overweight or obese, family history of hypertension, African American race, diabetes, physical inactivity, and increased salt consumption.

PRESENTATION, EVALUATION, AND DIAGNOSIS

The majority of patients with hypertension are asymptomatic. In a minority of cases, a patient can present with life-threatening elevations in blood pressure—a condition termed **hypertensive emergency**. Current guidelines encourage blood pressure checks yearly in patients >18 years of age. History and physical exam

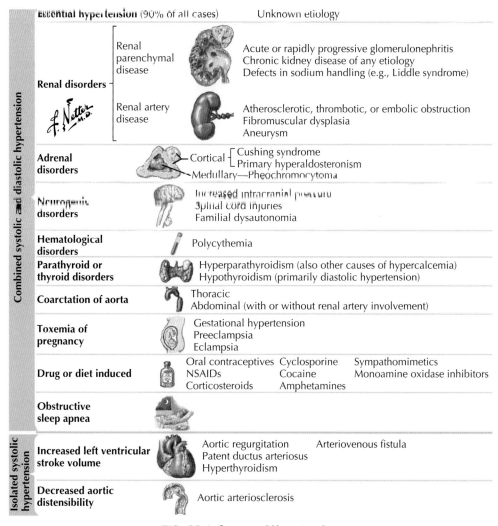

FIG. 66.1 Causes of Hypertension.

are important to help evaluate for secondary causes of hypertension.

To diagnose hypertension, patients do not necessarily need to have their blood pressures measured in an office setting. Ambulatory blood pressure monitoring allows for patients to have their blood pressure monitored at home, multiple times throughout the day, providing more data with which to make the diagnosis. In addition, ambulatory monitoring can be helpful for patients who are suspected of having so-called white coat hypertension, in which the stress of being in a clinical setting (i.e., seeing a clinician's white coat) leads to elevated blood pressure.

To diagnose hypertension in an office setting, a patient must have elevated blood pressure readings at two distinct office outpatient visits. Blood pressure should be measured with the patient seated and relaxed for at least 5 to 10 minutes prior to the measurement. Blood pressure should be taken in both arms to note any differences. In addition, care should be taken to ensure the right-size cuff is used for the patient; an overly large cuff can lead to a falsely lower blood pressure measurement, while an overly tight cuff can lead to a falsely higher blood pressure measurement.

The physical exam for systemic effects of hypertension (in the absence of emergency) is grossly nonspecific.

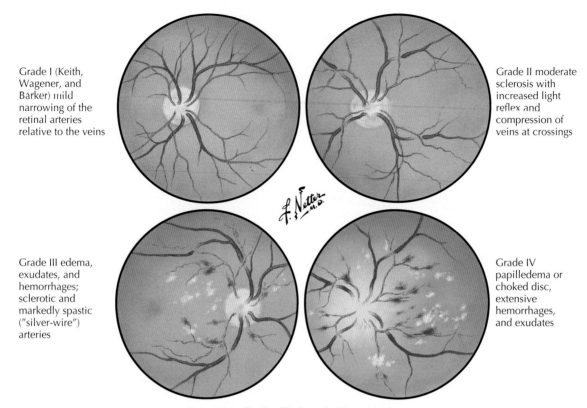

Grade I (Keith, Wagener, and Barker) mild narrowing of the retinal arteries relative to the veins

Grade II moderate sclerosis with increased light reflex and compression of veins at crossings

Grade III edema, exudates, and hemorrhages; sclerotic and markedly spastic ("silver-wire") arteries

Grade IV papilledema or choked disc, extensive hemorrhages, and exudates

FIG. 66.2 **Ocular Findings in Hypertension.**

Fundoscopic exam can reveal atrioventricular (AV) nicking, cotton-wool spots, or papilledema (Fig. 66.2). An S4 may be appreciated on cardiac auscultation. Abdominal exam should include auscultation for renal bruits, which would prompt evaluation for renovascular hypertension.

Guidelines regarding the definition and treatment of hypertension are regularly revised based on available data and expert opinion. Per the Eighth Joint National Committee (JNC8) guidelines, a systolic blood pressure ≥140 mm Hg, or a diastolic blood pressure ≥90 mm Hg, in adults <60 years of age is diagnostic of hypertension. In adults >60 years of age, a less stringent diagnostic criterion of ≥150 systolic or ≥90 diastolic has been recommended. However, the 2015 SPRINT trial showed that more stringent goals (<120/80 mm Hg) have mortality benefit in selected patients, and its applicability to the general population remains under evaluation. In 2017, the American College of Cardiology released its guidelines for the management of hypertension; these can be found in the online Further Readings.

When diagnosing hypertension, the vast majority of patients will have primary hypertension, so specific testing for secondary causes of hypertension is not routinely indicated. Workup at diagnosis can include basic metabolic panel (including electrolytes and creatinine), lipid profile, and a urinalysis to assess for proteinuria. An electrocardiogram (ECG) should also be obtained once the diagnosis is made to evaluate for any changes that would indicate cardiac disease, such as left ventricular hypertrophy (Fig. 66.3).

TREATMENT

Perhaps the most important initial intervention for hypertension is lifestyle change. Weight loss in obese and overweight individuals can be highly effective, as is a salt-restricted diet. Current recommendations suggest that individuals with hypertension should consume <1500 mg/day of sodium chloride. Smoking is another modifiable risk factor that, although it may not lower blood pressure directly, can decrease the risk of coronary artery disease.

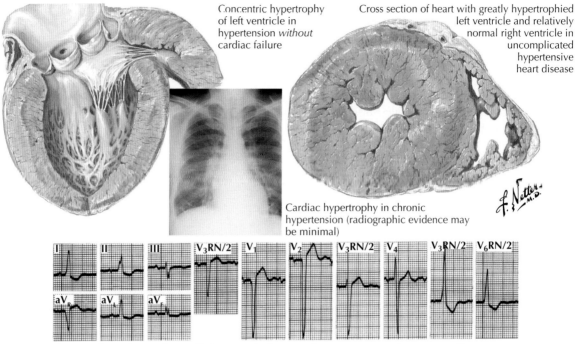

Concentric hypertrophy of left ventricle in hypertension *without* cardiac failure

Cross section of heart with greatly hypertrophied left ventricle and relatively normal right ventricle in uncomplicated hypertensive heart disease

Cardiac hypertrophy in chronic hypertension (radiographic evidence may be minimal)

Electrocardiographic evidence of left ventricular hypertrophy may or may not be present (tall R waves in V_4, V_5, and V_6; deep S waves in V_3R, V_1, V_2, III, and aV_R; depressed ST and inverted T in V_5, V_6, I, II, aV_L, and aV_F)

FIG. 66.3 **Heart Disease in Hypertension.**

Multiple classes of blood pressure medications are in use; the most commonly used medications include **calcium channel blockers (CCBs), ACE inhibitors, angiotensin receptor blockers (ARBs), thiazide diuretics,** and **β-adrenergic blockers.** Other secondary and less commonly used medications for management of hypertension include nitrates (e.g., isosorbide mononitrate), direct vasodilators (e.g., hydralazine), and α-adrenergic blockers (e.g., clonidine). The use of each class of medications should be based on individual patient characteristics and comorbidities. Upon initiating an antihypertensive, blood pressure should be reassessed within a month to assess response. If not at goal, an antihypertensive from a second, nonrelated class should be started, as this has been shown to be more effective than simply increasing the dose of a single medication.

CCBs block uptake of calcium in the muscular arterial wall, decreasing their contraction and resulting in vasodilation. CCBs have few restrictions based on comorbidities but can lead to peripheral edema. Peripherally acting (dihydropyridine) CCBs do not affect the heart directly and include amlodipine and nifedipine. Centrally acting (nondihydropyridine) CCBs can affect calcium mobilization in the cardiac tissue, decreasing inotropy and chronotropy; these include verapamil and diltiazem.

ACE inhibitors act on RAAS, preventing the conversion of angiotensin I to the potent vasoconstrictor angiotensin II. Side effects of ACE inhibitors include renal dysfunction and hyperkalemia (from decreased aldosterone). A moderate reduction in renal function of no greater than 30% increased creatinine is considered acceptable. Some patients will develop cough due to buildup of bradykinins from ACE inhibition, and they should be switched from an ACE inhibitor to an ARB. Another adverse reaction to ACE inhibitors related to increased kinin activity is angioedema, which should also prompt discontinuation of the drug. Examples of ACE inhibitors include lisinopril and enalapril.

ARBs also work on RAAS, inhibiting the angiotensin receptor. ARBs still can lead to renal dysfunction and hyperkalemia but, by not directly affecting ACE, do not have the same risk of angioedema or cough seen in

ACE inhibitors. For diabetic patients, ACE inhibitors and ARBs have a protective effect on development of renal dysfunction and are often the first prescribed. Examples of ARBs include losartan and valsartan.

Thiazide diuretics act on the nephron and inhibit Na^+Cl^- transporters in the distal convoluted tubule. Thiazides can cause hyponatremia, hyperuricemia, and hypercalcemia. Examples of thiazides include hydrochlorothiazide (HCTZ) and chlorthalidone. For African Americans, thiazides and CCBs are more effective than ACE inhibitors and ARBs.

β-adrenergic blockers act primarily on either $\beta1$-adrenergic or $\beta2$-adrenergic receptors. $\beta1$ receptors increase chronotropy (heart rate) and inotropy (contractility), so blocking these decreases cardiac output and thus arterial pressure. $\beta2$ receptors mediate smooth muscle relaxation, and while blocking them can produce a mild vasoconstrictive effect, this is overshadowed by effects on $\beta1$. Notably, some β-blockers, including labetalol and carvedilol, also act on $\alpha1$ receptors, which mediates vasoconstriction; blockade of these receptors leads to vasodilation.

CHAPTER 67

Hyperlipidemia

ANKEET S. BHATT

INTRODUCTION

Hyperlipidemia refers to elevated levels of lipids and cholesterol in the serum. Hyperlipidemia is a major risk factor for the development and progression of atherosclerosis and obstructive coronary artery disease. Lipids are formed from the combination of cholesteryl esters and triglycerides and are packaged into molecules called lipoproteins. Lipoproteins contain a lipid core surrounded by hydrophilic phospholipids and proteins referred to as **apolipoproteins.** Apolipoproteins are cell surface proteins that aid in targeting and uptake of lipids in several tissues.

Five major classes of lipoproteins exist and can be characterized in order of increasing density: **chylomicrons, very low-density lipoproteins (VLDLs), intermediate-density lipoproteins (IDLs), low-density lipoproteins (LDLs), and high-density lipoproteins (HDLs).** Lower density lipoproteins structurally have higher triglycerides-to-protein ratios than higher density lipoproteins.

The term hyperlipidemia usually corresponds to high levels of circulating total cholesterol and LDL in the serum. Hyperlipidemia is common, with data from the Centers for Disease Control and Prevention reporting that over 30% of the US population has elevated LDL levels, and less than one-third of patients have adequate control of their lipids through diet, exercise, or pharmacological treatment. As a result, an understanding of the mechanisms of hyperlipidemia, its clinical presentation, and available treatment options is essential for health care professionals.

PATHOPHYSIOLOGY

Lipid formation, circulation, breakdown, and regeneration require complex pathways that principally involve the gastrointestinal (GI) tract, the liver, and peripheral tissues (Fig. 67.1).

The exogenous pathway is the major pathway in which dietary fat intake is incorporated into lipids. Dietary fats are absorbed in the small intestine and packaged into triglyceride-rich chylomicrons, which enter the serum. Circulating chylomicrons are transported to muscle and adipose tissues, where the enzyme lipoprotein lipase (LPL) catalyzes the release of free fatty acids, which then enter body tissues. Chylomicron remnants return to the liver for further processing, where some are incorporated into bile acids and secreted into the duodenum, completing the exogenous pathway.

The endogenous pathway is the major mechanism by which the liver repackages and recycles lipid molecules. Chylomicron remnants are repackaged by the liver into VLDL, which is secreted by the liver into the bloodstream. As VLDL approaches target peripheral tissues, it delivers free fatty acids into these tissues, and thereby gradually increases in density and transforms sequentially into IDL, and later LDL. LDL is recycled by the liver though receptor-mediated endocytosis, repackaged with higher levels of triglycerides, and released into the serum as VLDL.

Reverse cholesterol transport refers to the net movement of cholesterol from peripheral tissues to the liver. The process lays the foundation for the beneficial effects of HDL; HDL accepts cholesterol from peripheral tissues and esterifies it. HDL then exchanges esterified cholesterol for triglycerides drawn from LDL and IDL. Cholesterol esters in LDL and IDL can then be taken up by the liver and excreted into the bile.

RISK FACTORS

Identifiable risk factors for the development of hyperlipidemia include both modifiable risk factors and predisposing conditions. Dietary intake of saturated fat can increase circulating levels of LDL. Obesity, large waist circumference (>40 inches in males and >35 inches in females), smoking, and high fasting blood sugars are also established risk factors. Regular, moderate-intensity aerobic exercise can increase HDL levels and facilitate removal of cholesterol from the circulation.

Familial hypercholesterolemia is an inherited syndrome comprising multiple genetic defects that affect cholesterol metabolism. Familial hypercholesterolemia

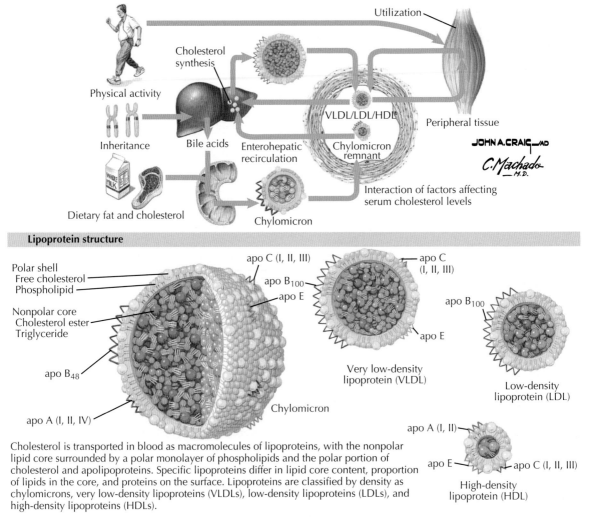

Cholesterol is transported in blood as macromolecules of lipoproteins, with the nonpolar lipid core surrounded by a polar monolayer of phospholipids and the polar portion of cholesterol and apolipoproteins. Specific lipoproteins differ in lipid core content, proportion of lipids in the core, and proteins on the surface. Lipoproteins are classified by density as chylomicrons, very low-density lipoproteins (VLDLs), low-density lipoproteins (LDLs), and high-density lipoproteins (HDLs).

FIG. 67.1 **Cholesterol Synthesis and Metabolism.**

has an overall prevalence of 1 in 250 to 500 people. Common and recognized genetic alterations involve the LDL receptor on hepatocytes. These genetic mutations alter the configuration of the LDL receptor on hepatocytes, impairing the liver's ability to remove circulating LDL. Patients with familial hypercholesterolemia often have extremely high LDL levels with associated accelerated atherosclerosis and higher rates of coronary artery disease, myocardial infarction, peripheral artery disease, and stroke.

PRESENTATION, EVALUATION, AND DIAGNOSIS

Evaluating and screening for hyperlipidemia in a patient should include a complete history and physical

examination, laboratory assessment, and as-needed imaging. In the majority of cases, hyperlipidemia, like hypertension, may be asymptomatic; therefore clinical suspicion and a careful history are needed to identify those at risk. Important historical points to elicit include dietary fat/sugar intake, frequency/duration of exercise, and social and family history. A family history of early coronary artery disease, peripheral artery disease, cerebrovascular disease, and myocardial infarction should raise clinical suspicion of potential familial hypercholesterolemia.

Physical exam findings may be present in a minority of patients with hyperlipidemia and include fatty skin deposits, called xanthomas, and ring formation in the cornea margin, called corneal arcus. In addition, history of angina or claudication, and/or bruits (carotid/

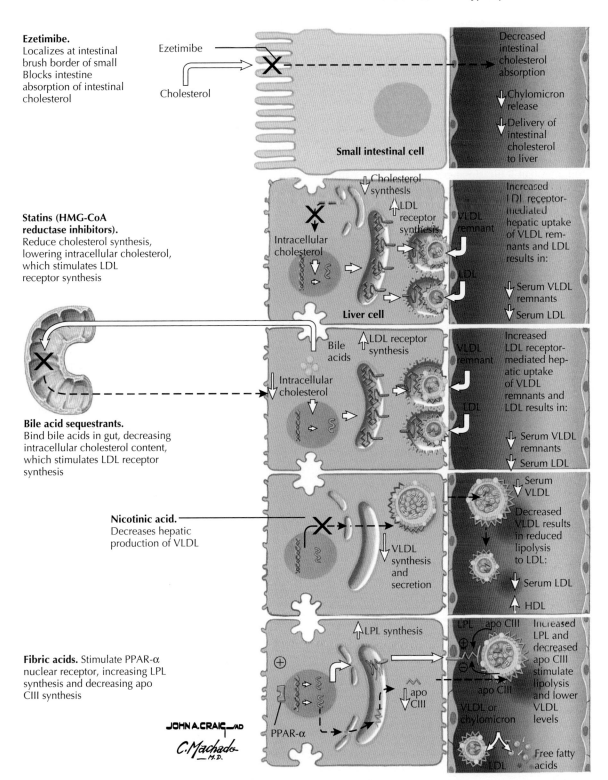

Ezetimibe.
Localizes at intestinal brush border of small intestine Blocks absorption of intestinal cholesterol

Ezetimibe

Cholesterol

Small intestinal cell

Decreased intestinal cholesterol absorption

↓ Chylomicron release

↓ Delivery of intestinal cholesterol to liver

Statins (HMG-CoA reductase inhibitors).
Reduce cholesterol synthesis, lowering intracellular cholesterol, which stimulates LDL receptor synthesis

↓ Cholesterol synthesis

↑ LDL receptor synthesis

Intracellular cholesterol

Liver cell

VLDL remnant

LDL

Increased LDL receptor-mediated hepatic uptake of VLDL remnants and LDL results in:

↓ Serum VLDL remnants

↓ Serum LDL

Bile acid sequestrants.
Bind bile acids in gut, decreasing intracellular cholesterol content, which stimulates LDL receptor synthesis

Bile acids

↑ LDL receptor synthesis

↓ Intracellular cholesterol

VLDL remnant

LDL

Increased LDL receptor-mediated hepatic uptake of VLDL remnants and LDL results in:

↓ Serum VLDL remnants

↓ Serum LDL

Nicotinic acid.
Decreases hepatic production of VLDL

↓ VLDL synthesis and secretion

↓ Serum VLDL

Decreased VLDL results in reduced lipolysis to LDL:

↓ Serum LDL

↑ HDL

Fibric acids. Stimulate PPAR-α nuclear receptor, increasing LPL synthesis and decreasing apo CIII synthesis

↑LPL synthesis

⊕

↓ apo CIII

PPAR-α

LPL   apo CIII
⊕
⊖
apo CIII

VLDL or chylomicron

LDL

Increased LPL and decreased apo CIII stimulate lipolysis and lower VLDL levels

Free fatty acids

JOHN A. CRAIG—MD

C. Machado —M.D.

FIG. 67.2 **Mechanisms of Lipid-Lowering Agents.** *HDL,* High-density lipoprotein; *LDL,* low-density lipoprotein; *LPL,* lipoprotein lipase; *PPARα,* peroxisome proliferator-activated receptor; *VLDL,* very low-density lipoprotein.

femoral) heard on exam, should prompt evaluation for hyperlipidemia.

Laboratory evaluation should include a complete lipid profile inclusive of total cholesterol, LDL, HDL, and triglycerides. A total cholesterol level ≥240 mg/dL is consistent with the diagnosis of hyperlipidemia. If possible, patients should obtain lab work after at least 12 hours of fasting, as triglyceride levels rise acutely after meals. LDL can be measured directly or calculated based on the specific assay used. Further testing, including apolipoprotein-B measurement and LDL peak particle diameter, may be useful in specialized circumstances.

Imaging studies frequently performed in the evaluation of hyperlipidemia involve imaging of arteries to detect the presence of atherosclerosis. This can be accomplished through a fundoscopic exam, ultrasound examination of the carotid arteries or abdominal aorta, or CT scanning of arteries in the chest and pelvis.

TREATMENT

Treatment for hyperlipidemia has traditionally focused on lowering the LDL (often LDL-C, or calculated LDL), as strong data exist that elevated LDL-C is associated with increased cardiovascular risk. Debate continues regarding the optimum goal and monitoring of hyperlipidemia, especially whether to treat based on specific LDL-C levels, certain cardiovascular risk factors, or a combination of both (Fig. 67.2).

The hallmark of treatment for hyperlipidemia are the statins. Statins inhibit HMG-CoA reductase, the rate-limiting enzyme in hepatic cholesterol synthesis. Statins are categorized by intensity, with high-intensity statins (atorvastatin 40–80 mg daily, rosuvastatin 20–40 mg daily) producing on average reductions of LDL ≥50%. The 2019 American College of Cardiology/American Heart Association (ACC/AHA) guidelines on management of blood cholesterol recommend moderate to high-intensity statin therapy in populations with the following: (1) known atherosclerotic cardiovascular disease (ASCVD),

(2) LDL ≥190 mg/dL, (3) diabetics age 40 to 75 years, and (4) estimated 10-year ASCVD risk of ≥7.5%. In patients age >75 years, clinical assessment and shared risk discussion should be made. These guidelines categorize primary prevention patients by risk level using the ASCVD risk calculator. Patients started on statin therapy should have liver function tests assessed periodically, as statins can lead to transaminitis in about 1% to 2% of patients. Myopathy and (in rare cases) myositis and rhabdomyolysis can occur with statin therapy, but the prevalence of severe myositis is low at <1%. The dose response and tolerance of statins should be assessed in about 4 to 12 weeks after therapy initiation or dose change.

Other infrequently used lipid-lowering agents include bile acid–binding agents (cholestyramine, colestipol, colesevelam), niacin, and fibrates. While these drugs may lower circulating lipid levels, they have not systematically been shown to improve clinical outcomes in terms of primary and secondary prevention of cardiovascular disease. They are also associated with significant GI side effects. Ezetimibe, a cholesterol absorption inhibitor, added to moderate-intensity statin in patients with previous myocardial infarction may improve cardiovascular outcomes compared to moderate-intensity statin alone, but these patients should preferentially be on high-intensity statin therapy if tolerated.

Newer therapeutic drugs available for the treatment of hyperlipidemia include proprotein convertase subtilisin/kexin type 9 (PCSK9) inhibitors. PCSK9 inhibitors accelerate the endocytosis of the LDL:LDL-receptor complex into the liver and allow for the rapid recycling of the LDL receptor to the surface of hepatocytes, where it can accept circulating lipids. These drugs allow for greater extraction of lipids from the circulation and can lead to reductions in LDL ≥40% above the reductions achieved by optimal statin therapy alone. These drugs were first validated in familial hyperlipidemia syndromes and are now approved as add-on therapy to statins in very high-risk patients who do not achieve adequate LDL reduction with statin and ezetimibe therapy alone.

CHAPTER 68

Pancreas Anatomy and Physiology Review

SARA J. CROMER

ANATOMY

The pancreas is a retroperitoneal organ that lies transversely within the posterior abdominal cavity, posterior to the stomach and transverse colon and anterior to the lumbar spine at L1–L2, and serves both **exocrine** and **endocrine** functions. It is anatomically divided into the pancreatic head, neck, body, and tail, which stretch from the curve of the duodenum at the head to the gastric pylorus at the neck, and to the splenic hilum and splenorenal ligament at the tail. The superior mesenteric artery and vein pass behind the neck of the pancreas, and the pancreatic head includes a posterior uncinate process that passes between the superior mesenteric vessels. The **main pancreatic duct (duct of Wirsung)** stretches the entire length of the pancreas and joins the common bile duct to terminate at the **ampulla of Vater.** Ductal secretions are regulated by the sphincter of Oddi at the major duodenal papilla in the second (descending) segment of the duodenum. Many people also have an accessory pancreatic duct (duct of Santorini), located dorsal to the main pancreatic duct within the pancreatic head, which usually drains through the minor papilla also into the second segment of the duodenum.

Blood supply to the pancreatic head includes the superior pancreaticoduodenal artery arising from the celiac trunk and the inferior pancreaticoduodenal artery arising from the superior mesenteric artery. Blood supply to the pancreatic body and tail is provided by pancreatic branches of the superior mesenteric and splenic arteries. Pancreatic innervation is provided by parasympathetic nerve fibers from the celiac branch of the posterior vagal trunk (Fig. 68.1).

EXOCRINE PANCREAS

The majority of pancreatic tissue is histologically divided into lobules of acinar cells serving an exocrine function, draining into ductules and eventually into the main and accessory pancreatic ducts. The exocrine pancreas plays a critical role in the postpyloric digestion of carbohydrates, proteins, and fats by secreting digestive enzymes as well as bicarbonate. Upon ingesting a meal, enteroendocrine cells in the duodenum and jejunum, termed **I cells,** release **cholecystokinin (CCK),** which activates adenylate cyclase within pancreatic acinar cells. Meanwhile, gastric emptying results in **secretin** release from duodenal **S cells,** mobilizing intracellular calcium through a Gq-G protein–coupled receptor (GPCR) pathway.

CCK and secretin work synergistically in acinar and centroacinar cells, respectively, resulting in the release of digestive enzymes, including α-amylase, trypsin, chymotrypsin, carboxypeptidase, and pancreatic lipase, as well as bicarbonate. This bicarbonate both neutralizes gastric acid and provides the optimum pH for digestive enzyme function.

ENDOCRINE PANCREAS

Although composing less than 5% of the pancreas by mass, the endocrine pancreas plays an indispensable role in the regulation of metabolism. The endocrine functions of the pancreas are localized to small clusters of cells known as pancreatic islets, or **islets of Langerhans.** The most prominent cells within these islets are β **cells,** which produce **insulin,** and α **cells,** which produce **glucagon.** However, recent research has also demonstrated the existence of less common δ **cells;** γ,

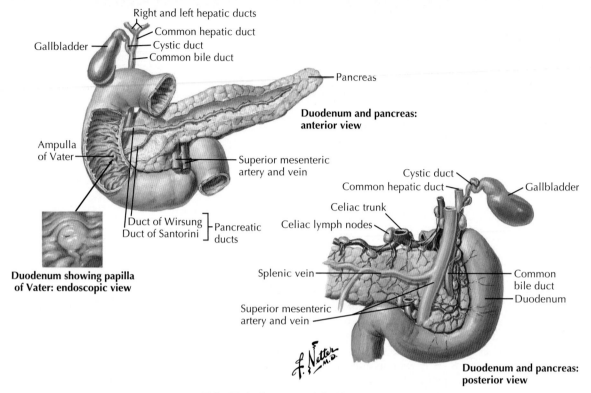

FIG. 68.1 **Anatomy of the Pancreas.**

or **PP (pancreatic polypeptide), cells;** and ε cells. All of these less common cell types secrete hormones that regulate digestion and energy homeostasis.

The β cell synthesizes and secretes insulin. Glucose in the blood moves freely into β cells by facilitated diffusion through bidirectional GLUT2 transporters. As intracellular glucose levels rise, glucokinase initiates glycolysis in a concentration-dependent manner and raises intracellular adenosine triphosphate (ATP). This ATP closes potassium ion channels, allowing potassium to build up within the cell. As the membrane potential rises, voltage-gated calcium channels open, leading to rapid influx of calcium and exocytosis of vesicles containing insulin, thus leading to insulin release within the blood. Of note, insulin release can be regulated by several other signaling pathways including acetylcholine activation of a Gq GPCR pathway; cholecystokinin, glucagon, or incretin activation of a Gs GPCR; and somatostatin activation of a Gi GPCR (Fig. 68.2).

Insulin, in turn, plays a number of critical roles within the body; its main actions, however, are to increase glucose uptake by tissues and thus lower blood glucose, halt catabolism, and promote anabolism. Insulin binding

to dimeric insulin receptors results in formation of a tyrosine kinase, which activates insulin receptor substrate 1 (IRS1). The insulin receptor–IRS1 complex is the active intracellular arm of insulin signaling.

Insulin upregulates the glucose transporter GLUT4 on the luminal surface of endothelial cells in adipose tissue and striated muscles, allowing for facilitated diffusion of glucose into these cells during periods of hyperglycemia. Insulin also activates lipoprotein lipase in adipocytes, which, combined with increased intracellular glucose, results in triglyceride synthesis and storage. In hepatocytes and myocytes, insulin activates glycogen synthase, resulting in storage of excess glucose as glycogen. Other effects of insulin, through numerous and diverse signaling mechanisms, result in cell proliferation and division, consistent with the overarching anabolic effects of the hormone (Fig. 68.3).

The pancreatic α cells synthesize and secrete glucagon. Regulation of glucagon secretion is not entirely understood; however, secretion is known to be stimulated by hypoglycemia and epinephrine. Inhibitory triggers include somatostatin, insulin, **glucagon-like peptide-1 (GLP1),** and increased serum levels of catabolic products

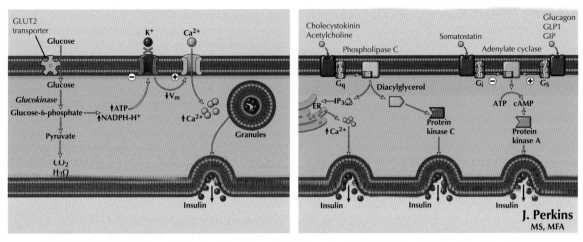

FIG. 68.2 **Mechanisms of Insulin Secretion.** *ATP*, Adenosine triphosphate; *cAMP*, cyclic adenosine monophosphate; *ER*, endoplasmic reticulum; *GLP1*, glucagon-like peptide-1; *IP₃*, inositol triphosphate; *NADPH*, nicotinamide adenine dinucleotide phosphate.

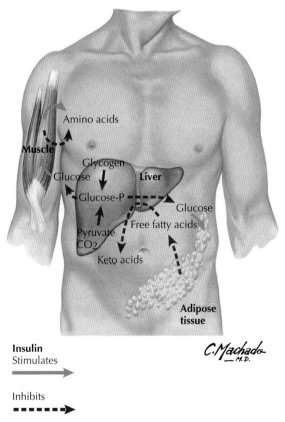

Insulin
Stimulates

Inhibits

FIG. 68.3 **Actions of Insulin.**

such as free fatty acids, ketoacids, and urea. Glucagon responds to periods of fasting by mobilizing stored energy sources. It activates glycogen phosphorylase, resulting in consumption of hepatic glycogen via glycogenolysis, and stimulates hepatic gluconeogenesis. Glucagon further stimulates proteolysis and lipolysis, releasing glycolytic intermediates that can enter the Krebs cycle for gluconeogenesis in the liver or participate in ketogenesis. This process provides nonglucose energy sources for most tissues while allowing tissues such as the brain and red blood cells, which preferentially use glucose over other fuel molecules, to continue glucose-dominant metabolism.

δ cells exist with low frequency in pancreatic islets but are also found in intestinal mucosa. δ cells secrete somatostatin, which plays a complex role in moderating metabolic responses. It decreases release of growth hormone, gastrin, and gastric acid, and decreases fasting insulin levels in the serum.

γ cells secrete PP, which autoregulates pancreatic exocrine and endocrine functions. Though its exact role in digestion remains unclear, PP is known to increase with fasting, hypoglycemia, and protein intake; it decreases with somatostatin or intravenous glucose administration. PP also stimulates gastric enzyme secretion, opposes the action of CCK, and may decrease appetite.

Finally, ε cells secrete **ghrelin.** Ghrelin is stimulated by fasting and plays a complex role in weight balance by altering the sensations of hunger and satiety, as well as the balance of fat and carbohydrate storage. Ghrelin and ghrelin analogues result in weight gain, disproportionately weighted toward adipose tissue.

REGULATION OF METABOLISM

The exocrine and endocrine functions of the pancreas intersect to optimize the body's response to energy intake, creating a number of feedback loops similar to those seen in other hormonal pathways of the body. When the stomach empties into the duodenum, CCK and secretin stimulate release of digestive enzymes and bicarbonate from the exocrine pancreas. Among these, α-amylase breaks down polysaccharides into a variety of monosaccharides, which trigger the release of incretins, hormones that augment insulin release. The most studied incretins, GLP1 from intestinal L cells and gastric inhibitory peptide (also known as glucose-dependent insulinotropic peptide [GIP]) from intestinal K cells, have become major drug targets in recent years, as has **dipeptidyl peptidase-4 (DPP4)**, which is the enzyme responsible for their inactivation.

While incretins augment insulin release in response to a meal, they also serve to slow gastric emptying and promote satiety, creating a negative feedback loop. Similarly, when β cells release insulin in response to rising serum glucose, they also release amylin, another hormone that slows gastric emptying, induces satiety, and suppresses appetite.

Taken in its entirety, the exocrine and endocrine pancreas work in conjunction to promote digestion and regulate metabolism, responding to fed and fasting states with complex hormonal pathways. These hormones create stable fuel sources by storing and mobilizing energy molecules as needed based on the environment.

CHAPTER 69

Diabetes Mellitus

BEVERLY G. TCHANG

INTRODUCTION

Diabetes mellitus is a chronic disease characterized by insulin insufficiency, insulin resistance, and its subsequent comorbidities. According to 2014 census data, it affected 29.1 million adult Americans, or 9.3% of the US population, from 2009 to 2012. More than 1.5 million new cases were diagnosed in 2012. Diabetes has been associated with multiple complications, including hypertension, cardiovascular disease, stroke, blindness, kidney disease, and amputations.

Diabetes has traditionally been classified into two types (type 1 and type 2), but the spectrum of disease has expanded to include prediabetes, gestational diabetes mellitus (GDM), and mature-onset diabetes of the young (MODY), among many other subtypes discovered in recent decades. This chapter aims to provide an introduction to the pathophysiology of diabetes that will serve as the foundation for understanding the clinical evaluation and management of diabetes types 1 and 2.

PATHOPHYSIOLOGY

The pathophysiology of diabetes varies with type. **Type 1 diabetes mellitus (T1DM)** is characterized by the autoimmune-mediated destruction of β-islet cells in the pancreas, usually leading to complete insulin deficiency. A number of autoantibodies have been implicated in this process, including anti-GAD65, antiislet cell, antizinc transporter, and antiinsulin. The etiology of this autoimmunity is still to be fully elucidated but is thought to be a combination of genetic predisposition and environmental factors.

In contrast to T1DM, **type 2 diabetes mellitus (T2DM)** is characterized by insulin resistance, reduced (but not absent) insulin secretion, and excessive hepatic glucose production. Multiple studies have suggested mechanisms involving proinflammatory cytokines, dysregulated adipose tissue, and downregulation of insulin receptor expression or intracellular signaling.

Whether it is absolute insulin deficiency (as in T1DM) or relative insulin insufficiency (as in T2DM), the body is unable to take up glucose from the bloodstream due to impaired glucose transporter proteins. Without glucose, the body perceives an overall state of fasting that stimulates hepatic glucose production (Fig. 69.1). The subsequent increase in serum glucose also increases serum osmolality, resulting in glucosuria and polyuria, which lead to overall body volume depletion that then stimulates thirst and polydipsia. If the body persists in this fasting state, it will enter into a state of starvation and initiate processes that provide an alternate source of energy, such as fatty acid oxidation, protein catabolism, and ketosis (see Chapter 70). Overall, without sufficient insulin to mediate peripheral tissue uptake of glucose, the body falls into an energy-deficient state, which manifests clinically as weight loss. The persistent elevation in serum glucose also causes inflammation to the endothelial lining of vessels, resulting in multiorgan damage on microvascular and macrovascular scales (Fig. 69.2).

RISK FACTORS

Risk factors for T1DM include being part of certain ethnic groups with a greater predisposition to T1DM through the inheritance of various immune system modulators, known as human leukocyte antigen (HLA) groups. HLA-DQ, HLA-DR, and HLA-DP are associated with T1DM and tend to cluster in those of European ancestry. As autoimmune diseases tend to occur together, having other autoimmune diseases such as hypothyroidism, systemic lupus erythematous, rheumatoid arthritis, celiac disease, vitiligo, and alopecia may predispose certain individuals to T1DM.

Risk factors for T2DM are far more heterogeneous and include the following:
- Overweight (body mass index [BMI] ≥25 kg/m^2) or obesity (BMI ≥30 kg/m^2)
- Physical inactivity
- First-degree relative with diabetes
- High-risk race/ethnicity (e.g., African American, Latino, Native American, Asian American, Pacific Islander)

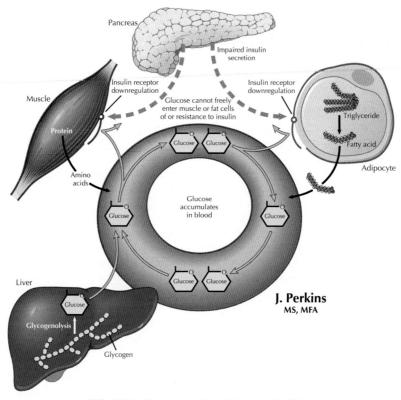

FIG. 69.1 **Pathogenesis in Diabetes Mellitus.**

- Women who delivered a baby weighing >9 lb or were diagnosed with GDM
- Women with polycystic ovary syndrome (PCOS)
- Hypertension
- High-density lipoprotein (HDL) cholesterol level ≤35 mg/dL or a triglyceride level ≥250 mg/dL
- Hemoglobin **A1c** (glycated hemoglobin, or A1c) ≥5.7%
- History of cardiovascular disease

PRESENTATION, EVALUATION, AND DIAGNOSIS

T1DM most commonly presents in childhood but can also present in late adulthood due to development of autoimmunity with age. T2DM can present at any time in life. While it used to be considered an adult-onset disease, rates of childhood T2DM have been increasing. Both T1DM and T2DM can present with similar symptoms: polyuria, polydipsia, nausea, anorexia, and weight loss. Both can also present asymptomatically with elevated blood glucose or A1c found during routine medical examination. Patients with long-standing, poorly controlled diabetes are more likely to present with complications such as diabetic neuropathy, nephropathy, retinopathy, or cardiovascular disease. Although classically associated with T1DM, diabetic ketoacidosis (DKA) can occur in either T1DM or T2DM. T2DM patients are more likely to present with the metabolic syndrome than T1DM patients.

The history of a patient with suspected diabetes should include questions regarding symptoms listed earlier, as well as elicitation of any complications of diabetes. Physical exam should evaluate for any signs of end-organ damage (i.e., blurry vision, digital numbness, foot ulcers) and signs of conditions associated with insulin resistance (i.e., hypertension, obesity, acanthosis nigricans). To establish the diagnosis of diabetes, a patient must fulfill one of the following criteria, as set forth by the American Diabetes Association (ADA):

- Fasting plasma glucose ≥126 mg/dL
- Two-hour plasma glucose after a 75-g oral glucose tolerance test ≥200 mg/dL
- A1c ≥6.5%
- Random plasma glucose ≥200 mg/dL with classic symptoms of hyperglycemia or hyperglycemic crisis

Diabetic retinopathy

Diabetic retinopathy can be easily detected during a dilated eye examination and is the leading cause of blindness among adults in the United States. Visual loss can be prevented with early recognition and treatment of retinopathy.

Nonproliferative retinopathy (early stage)

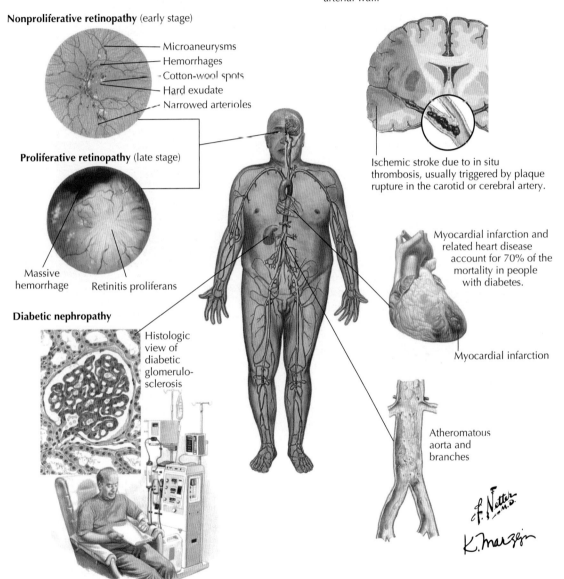

- Microaneurysms
- Hemorrhages
- Cotton-wool spots
- Hard exudate
- Narrowed arterioles

Proliferative retinopathy (late stage)

Massive hemorrhage   Retinitis proliferans

Diabetic nephropathy

Histologic view of diabetic glomerulosclerosis

Diabetes mellitus is the leading cause of end-stage renal disease in the Western world.

Cerebrovascular disease

The high incidence of vascular complications among patients with diabetes is related not only to blood glucose elevations, but also to the frequent association of dyslipidemia, hypertension, a procoagulant state, and the tendency to form unstable plaques in the arterial wall.

Ischemic stroke due to in situ thrombosis, usually triggered by plaque rupture in the carotid or cerebral artery.

Myocardial infarction and related heart disease account for 70% of the mortality in people with diabetes.

Myocardial infarction

Atheromatous aorta and branches

FIG. 69.2 Microvascular and Macrovascular Complications of Diabetes Mellitus.

A1c provides an estimate of the average glucose concentration over 3 months, slightly less than the average lifespan of a red blood cell. It is a less sensitive test for the diagnosis of diabetes as compared to the serum glucose criteria. In addition, A1c should be interpreted with caution in patients with hemoglobinopathies, anemias, or conditions associated with varied red blood cell turnover rate (i.e., recent blood transfusion, pregnancy, erythropoietin therapy, or hemolysis).

TREATMENT

Treatment for diabetes depends on the type of diabetes and the setting (inpatient vs. outpatient). In T1DM, the guiding principle is that these patients are entirely reliant on insulin. The standard of care is a basal-bolus regimen, in which a long-acting insulin is given to cover endogenous glucose production, while a short-acting insulin is given to cover any carbohydrate-rich food intake. Most patients are prescribed a long-acting insulin that is only administered once a day and a short-acting insulin that is taken three times a day with meals. Some patients utilize a continuous subcutaneous insulin infusion (CSII) pump to do both (Fig. 69.3).

The dose of insulin prescribed depends on a number of factors. The initial dose for long-acting insulin is usually weight based. Short-acting insulin is administered based on a patient's insulin sensitivity factor (ISF) and insulin-to-carb ratio (ICR). An ISF of 1:50 indicates that 1 unit of insulin will decrease the patient's blood glucose by 50 mg/dL. An ICR of 1:30 indicates that 1 unit of insulin will cover 30 g carbohydrates. T1DM patients are taught to use ISF to correct hyperglycemia and to use ICR with carbohydrate counting to cover each meal. Of note, while the ISF and ICR are concepts that can theoretically be applied to T2DM patients, such strict calculations are generally not required for their management. Regarding noninsulin agents, only pramlintide, a subcutaneously injected amylin analogue, is FDA-approved for use in T1DM. Other noninsulin agents are either still under investigation or not recommended.

In T2DM patients, diet and lifestyle modifications remain first-line treatment. ADA guidelines recommend reduction in carbohydrate intake, 150 minutes per week of physical activity, and at least 5% weight loss. After this, metformin as monotherapy is highly recommended given its known long-term safety profile and microvascular disease benefits, which has been demonstrated in seminal randomized controlled trials like the UKPDS-34. After metformin, second-line or combination therapies are largely driven by patient preference or comorbidities. When considering adding a second agent, it is important

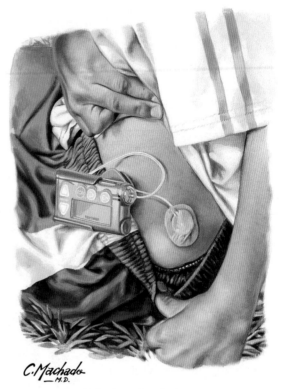

FIG. 69.3 **Insulin Pump.**

to take into account each agent's effect on weight, renal impairment, and hypoglycemia risk. Table 69.1 summarizes noninsulin treatments for T2DM. Bariatric surgery has also been shown to be an effective management option obtaining near to complete remission of diabetes. With both T1DM and T2DM, ADA guidelines state a goal A1c <7% based on landmark clinical trials such as ACCORD and ADVANCE to reduce risk of microvascular complications. Outpatient care for any diabetic patient should include regular A1c checks, microalbuminuria screening for nephropathy, ophthalmology evaluation for retinopathy, and foot exams or podiatry visits.

Inpatient care for the patient with diabetes is beyond the scope of this chapter, but the following are a few guiding principles:

- Current ADA guidelines recommend a goal random blood glucose of 140 to 180 mg/dL for general inpatient floors; this is largely supported by a meta-analysis of multiple trials, including the NICE-SUGAR trial, which suggested an association between increased mortality and tighter glycemic control.
- Metformin is commonly held upon admission given its reported history of association with lactic acidosis,

TABLE 69.1
Noninsulin Medications in Type 2 Diabetes Mellitus (T2DM)

Name	Route	Mechanism	Advantages	Disadvantages
Biguanides (metformin, metformin XR)	PO	• Inhibits gluconeogenesis • Increases insulin-mediated glucose utilization	• Low risk of hypoglycemia • Weight loss • Cheap	• Gastrointestinal side effects • Concern in renal impairment • Concern for lactic acidosis
Sulfonylureas (glyburide, glipizide, glimepiride)	PO	• Stimulates pancreatic insulin release	• Long-acting forms available • Cheap	• Weight gain • Risk of hypoglycemia • Concern in renal impairment and elderly (age >65)
GLP1 receptor agonists (semaglutide, liraglutide, dulaglutide, exenatide)	SQ PO	• Agonist for glucagon-like peptide-1, which stimulates pancreatic insulin release • Slows gastric emptying, inhibiting postmeal glucagon release and reducing food intake	• Weight loss • Improved CV outcomes in patients with CV disease • Low risk of hypoglycemia	• Gastrointestinal side effects
DPP4 inhibitors (sitagliptin, saxagliptin, linagliptin)	PO	• Inhibits dipeptidyl peptidase-4, which metabolizes GLP1	• Low risk of hypoglycemia • Weight neutral	• Possible increased risk of heart failure with saxagliptin (not necessarily class effect)
Thiazolidinedione (pioglitazone)	PO	• Increases insulin sensitivity to increase glucose utilization, decreases glucose production	• Improved lipid profile	• Increased risk of fluid retention, heart failure • Increased risk of fractures • Weight gain
SGLT2 inhibitors (empagliflozin, dapagliflozin, canagliflozin)	PO	• Inhibits sodium-glucose cotransporter-2 in kidneys, increasing renal excretion of glucose	• Weight loss • Improved CV outcomes in patients with CV disease	• Urinary tract infections • Vulvovaginal candidiasis • Risk of euglycemic DKA
Meglitinides (repaglinide, nateglinide)	PO	• Blocks ATP-dependent potassium channels in β cells, stimulating insulin release		• Weight gain • Dosing with every meal • Avoid in renal impairment
Pramlintide	SQ	• Synthetic analog of human amylin that slows gastric emptying, suppresses appetite, and inhibits postmeal glucagon release	• Weight loss	• Risk of hypoglycemia • Multiple injections per day
Acarbose	PO	• Blocks α-glucosidase, an intestinal enzyme that releases glucose from carbohydrates	• Weight neutral • Insulin sensitizer • Cheap • Can use with some degree of renal impairment	• Flatulence, diarrhea

ATP, Adenosine triphosphate; *CV,* cardiovascular; *DKA,* diabetic ketoacidosis; *PO,* per os (by mouth); *SQ,* subcutaneous.
Data from Nathan DM, Buse JB, Davidson MB, et al: Medical management of hyperglycemia in type 2 diabetes: a consensus algorithm for the initiation and adjustment of therapy: a consensus statement of the American Diabetes Association and the European Association for the Study of Diabetes, *Diabetes Care* 32(1):193–203, 2009.

especially in patients with preexisting renal disease, although this side effect of metformin is rarely seen.

- T1DM patients are a special population in that long-acting insulin must never be withheld. While this is not often a problem in the outpatient setting, providers can fall into pitfalls when a T1DM patient is admitted to the hospital and insulin is held in anticipation of NPO (nothing by mouth) status or a procedure. Even in these scenarios, basal insulin should be administered to cover endogenous glucose production and may be given at a reduced dose.
- Consider obtaining expert assistance for the patient on enteral/parenteral feedings or the patient with steroid-induced hyperglycemia.

CHAPTER 70

Diabetic Ketoacidosis and Hyperosmolar Hyperglycemic State

JOSHUA R. COOK

DIABETIC KETOACIDOSIS

Pathophysiology

Understanding the nexus between insulin deficiency, hyperglycemia, and fatty acid metabolism that produces **diabetic ketoacidosis (DKA)** requires two key insights. First, the relationship between insulin level and its effect on target tissues exists on a dose-response spectrum. Activating glucose uptake by skeletal muscle requires 10-fold greater insulin concentrations than those required to inhibit adipose tissue lipolysis to the same degree. Therefore, particularly in type 2 diabetes mellitus (T2DM), ambient levels of insulin generally suffice to prevent excessive fatty acid efflux from adipose tissue even as blood glucose levels rise. However, in cases of near total insulin deficiency, often in type 1 diabetes mellitus (T1DM), not enough insulin circulates to block lipolysis.

The second key insight is that DKA does not hinge solely on insulin deficiency. Rather, an imbalance between the activity of insulin and its counterregulatory hormones—in particular, glucagon—is essential to the development of DKA. DKA less commonly develops in cases of simultaneous insulin and glucagon depletion, such as following pancreatectomy; conditions in which levels of glucagon or other counterregulatory hormones are increased (e.g., infection or stress), or in which insulin levels are acutely decreased (e.g., poor adherence to diabetes therapy), set the stage for DKA.

Insulin and glucagon act in two main ways to regulate ketogenesis. First, in the total absence of insulin, glucagon may act unopposed to stimulate adipocyte lipolysis, shunting the resultant glycerol and fatty acids to the liver for conversion into acetyl-CoA. Second, insulin and glucagon coordinately regulate the fate of acetyl-CoA; insulin favors the complete oxidation of acetyl-CoA to form adenosine triphosphate (ATP) or the synthesis of new fatty acids, while glucagon stimulates the partial oxidation of acetyl-CoA to the ketone bodies, acetoacetic acid, and β-hydroxybutyric acid. Ketone bodies, intended as emergency fuel for neurons in starvation, are weak acids that titrate serum bicarbonate and result in considerable metabolic acidosis. Ketones also are osmotically active; in concert with concomitant hyperglycemia, they draw water out of cells and ultimately, through osmotic diuresis, out of the body, leading to profound volume depletion (Fig. 70.1).

Presentation, Evaluation, and Diagnosis

Symptoms of DKA typically present acutely over 1 to 2 days. In addition to signs of hyperglycemia, including blurred vision, polyuria/polydipsia, and polyphagia, DKA often is associated with significant abdominal pain, nausea, and vomiting, which can exacerbate volume depletion. Other associated symptoms include weakness, fatigue/malaise, or, in cases of significant hyperosmolality, altered mental status, though this is far more common in a **hyperosmolar hyperglycemic state (HHS)**. Physical examination may reveal fruity, acetone-like breath; rapid, deep breathing (termed **Kussmaul breathing**) to compensate for underlying metabolic acidosis; and signs of volume depletion.

In cases of suspected DKA, a fingerstick blood glucose (FSBG) should be checked, along with a urinalysis, to evaluate for glycosuria and ketonuria. Of note, although hyperglycemia is generally present, presenting blood glucose levels may range from only 250 to 400 mg/dL despite severe ketosis. Euglycemic DKA can occur in patients taking SGLT2 inhibitors. This stands in contrast to HHS, in which blood glucose levels tend to be much higher. Basic chemistries quantify the anion gap and degree of metabolic acidosis, and elevated levels of serum β-hydroxybutyric acid further support the diagnosis. Physicians should evaluate for any underlying physiologic stressor that may have triggered DKA.

Treatment

DKA is a medical emergency; as such, its treatment has become protocol driven to minimize time to resolution

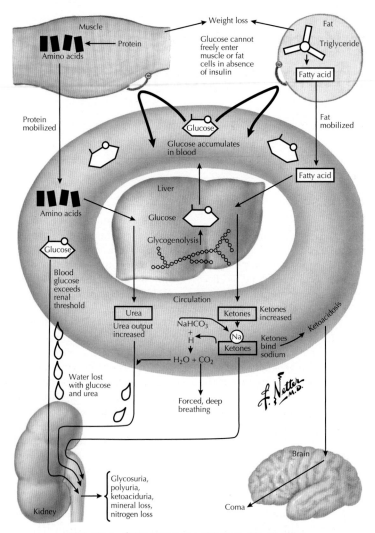

FIG. 70.1 **Consequences of Insulin Deprivation.**

and opportunities for error. Treatment is directed toward correcting ketosis and its associated anion gap, hyperglycemia, and volume depletion. The ultimate goal of DKA therapy is replacing deficient insulin, classically with a regular insulin drip at a rate substantially higher than that required for treatment of hyperglycemia alone, typically 0.1 U/kg/hr. Insulin replacement shuts off unchecked lipolysis both via direct effects on the adipocyte and by inhibition of pancreatic glucagon secretion. Insulin also stimulates glucose uptake by skeletal muscle and adipose tissue and decreases hepatic glucose production, thus improving hyperglycemia.

The regular insulin drip is maintained not until resolution of hyperglycemia, but until the cessation

of ketone production, as ketones and their associated acidosis pose the gravest threat to the patient. This cessation is quantified by a normalized, or closed, anion gap. Once the anion gap closes and the patient is able to eat, patients should receive a long-acting, basal insulin, such as insulin glargine or neutral protamine Hagedorn (NPH) insulin, to prevent the gap from reopening. The insulin drip is maintained for a 2-hour overlap period following the administration of long-acting insulin to allow the insulin to take effect. Any patient in whom DKA is diagnosed can be assumed to require long-term insulin therapy.

Volume depletion in DKA requires aggressive fluid resuscitation that should be initiated even before the

TABLE 70.1
Diagnostic Criteria for Hyperosmolar Hyperglycemic State (HHS)

Parameter	Value	Parameter	Value
Plasma glucose	≥600 mg/dL	Serum β-hydroxybutyrate	<3 mmol/L
Arterial pH	>7.30	Effective serum osmolality[a]	>320 mOsm/kg
Serum bicarbonate	>18 mEq/L	Anion gap	Variable
Urine or serum ketones	Negative or small	Mental status	Most with stupor, coma

[a]Per the American Diabetes Association definition, excludes the usual contribution of blood urea nitrogen to the calculation.
Data from American Diabetes Association: Hyperglycemic crises in diabetes, *Diabetes Care* 27:S94–S102, 2004. https://doi.org/10.2337/diacare.27.2007.394, Umpierrez GE: Hyperosmolar hyperglycemic state: a historic review of the clinical presentation, diagnosis, and treatment, *Diabetes Care* 37(11):3124–3131, 2014. https://doi.org/10.2337/dc14-0984.

insulin drip, typically via continuous infusion of normal saline or half-normal saline, although lactated Ringer may also be used in the setting of worsening hyperchloremia. Two potential dangers arise in the course of treating DKA, both of which can be avoided by customizing the resuscitation fluid. First, a constant infusion of insulin can lead to hypoglycemia, especially considering that the total dose of insulin required to close the anion gap may be greater than that needed to correct hyperglycemia alone. DKA treatment guidelines recommend adding 5% to 10% dextrose to the replacement fluid once the serum glucose reaches 250 mg/dL, with a goal blood glucose between 70 and 150 mg/dL. Treatment with an insulin drip also can result in hypokalemia, due to insulin stimulation of the plasma membrane Na^+-K^+ ATPase. Serum potassium should be monitored and supplemented with potassium chloride every 2 to 4 hours while the insulin drip is running. Of note, profound hypokalemia on presentation requires supplementation prior to starting the insulin drip, as lower levels are associated with cardiac arrhythmias.

Once these derangements are corrected, treatment can shift to initiating basal-bolus insulin therapy and patient education regarding strict adherence to their insulin regimen.

HYPEROSMOLAR HYPERGLYCEMIC STATE
Pathophysiology
Like DKA, the **hyperosmolar hyperglycemic state**—also referred to as HHS—confers significant morbidity. Unlike DKA, the pathophysiology of HHS arises purely from extreme hyperglycemia. HHS requires a considerable degree of insulin resistance and develops primarily in patients with T2DM who still have some minor endogenous insulin reserve, recalling the dose-response spectrum of insulin's downstream metabolic activities.

As in DKA, conditions in which levels of glucagon and counterregulatory hormones are increased predispose to the development of HHS. Medications that predispose to hyperglycemia, including glucocorticoids or thiazide diuretics, may also trigger decompensation to HHS.

In HHS, plasma glucose levels are generally higher than those in DKA, over 600 mg/dL by definition but sometimes over 1000 mg/dL. As glucose is osmotically active, this extreme hyperglycemia draws water out of the intracellular compartment and overwhelms the resorptive capacity of the proximal convoluted tubule, resulting in massive glycosuria and profound volume depletion. The underlying condition predisposing to HHS may impinge upon the patient's ability to access fluids, particularly in the elderly, worsening the downward spiral as the ensuing hypovolemia depresses renal function further and exacerbates hyperglycemia. Profound hypovolemia in combination with ongoing cellular fluid shifts impairs cerebral perfusion, resulting in progressive decline in mental status leading to obtundation and coma.

Presentation, Evaluation, and Diagnosis
Although coma is the most classic feature of HHS, less than one-third of patients are comatose on presentation. Nevertheless, serum osmolality >320 mOsm/kg—a defining criterion of HHS—is very commonly associated with some degree of mental status alteration, from mild inattentiveness to obtundation and coma. Focal neurological symptoms can also present in HHS, which may be due to wholesale central nervous system (CNS) fluid shifts or to specific cranial nerve palsies; seizures may also occur. The other major presenting feature of HHS is volume depletion due to polyuria with insufficient, albeit in many cases increased, fluid intake. Exam features range from dry mucous membranes and axillae to poor skin turgor or, in severe cases, hypovolemic shock. Although abdominal pain and nausea/vomiting

are common presenting symptoms in DKA, they are not classic manifestations of HHS. Finally, as there is no prominent acid-base disturbance in HHS, these patients will not exhibit Kussmaul breathing.

The American Diabetes Association has established a system of criteria for the diagnosis of HHS. Many of these criteria can distinguish HHS from DKA, although overlap syndromes may exist (Table 70.1).

Treatment

As in DKA, HHS treatment centers on correcting hyperglycemia and volume depletion, albeit without a need to improve a significant acid-base abnormality. Insulin and fluids are the mainstays of treatment, but there have been no prospective, randomized trials on particular insulin protocols. Many practitioners utilize a regular insulin-based regimen similar to that used for DKA, but the end goals are correction of altered mental status, hyperosmolality, and hyperglycemia, not closure of anion gap. Excessively rapid correction of hyperglycemia—and therefore hyperosmolarity—may precipitate cerebral edema, so expert opinion tends to favor initial correction of blood glucose to around 300 mg/dL. Once patients are able to eat and drink reliably, they can be converted to intermittent insulin dosing and their blood glucose further treated to euglycemia. Volume repletion remains an equally important facet of HHS treatment, with normal saline or lactated Ringer commonly utilized, and electrolyte abnormalities frequently monitored and corrected. Finally, patients with significant alteration in mental status may require intubation for airway protection.

CHAPTER 71

Thyroid and Parathyroid Glands Anatomy and Physiology Review

MICHELE YEUNG

THYROID GLAND

Anatomy and Histology

The thyroid gland is a butterfly-shaped organ located anterior to the trachea and inferior to the larynx. The thyroid consists of two lateral lobes that are connected by a narrow band of tissue called the isthmus. The lobes extend superiorly to the midthyroid cartilage and laterally to the common carotid arteries. The isthmus typically sits overlying the second and third tracheal rings. Normal anatomical variants of the thyroid gland do occur, including an absent isthmus or an extra lobe known as the **pyramidal lobe.** The pyramidal lobe is found in over 50% of the population, and when present, is located superior to the isthmus. It is a remnant of the thyroglossal duct, as the primitive thyroid gland descends from the base of the tongue to its final location in the neck during embryonic development (Fig. 71.1).

A fibrous capsule covers the thyroid gland. Several key structures are located nearby and thus important to consider in the setting of surgery on the thyroid gland, such as parathyroid glands (see "Parathyroid Glands" later) and the **recurrent laryngeal nerve.** The recurrent laryngeal nerve provides sensory and motor innervation to the larynx. Therefore surgical injury can lead to symptoms ranging from hoarse voice to stridor. The thyroid gland's blood supply comes primarily from the right and left superior and inferior thyroid arteries. The superior thyroid arteries originate from the external carotid arteries, and the inferior thyroid arteries originate from the thyrocervical trunk. The lymphatic drainage of the thyroid mainly involves the deep cervical lymph nodes in the central compartment.

Microscopically, the thyroid is composed of follicles. Each follicle is composed of a single layer of follicular cells surrounding a lumen filled with colloid, a proteinaceous store of the thyroid hormone precursor, **thyroglobulin.** In addition to thyroid follicular cells, the thyroid gland also contains parafollicular, or C, cells. **Parafollicular cells** make up only 2% to 4% of the

organ's cells. They are nestled in the connective tissue between thyroid follicles.

Thyroid Hormone Synthesis and Regulation

The main function of the thyroid gland is to produce adequate amounts of thyroid hormone. Thyroid hormone affects virtually every organ system in the body, including the heart, central nervous system, autonomic nervous system, bone, gastrointestinal tract, and overall metabolism.

The binding of **thyrotropin (thyroid-stimulating hormone [TSH])** to the thyrotropin receptor (TSHR) on the basolateral aspect of the thyroid follicular cells stimulates the uptake of iodide via the sodium/iodide (Na/I) transporter. This allows iodide to be actively transported across the cell membrane. Once inside, iodide rapidly diffuses to the apical surface of the cells, where it is transported by pendrin, a membrane iodide-chloride transporter into the colloid of the follicle. **Thyroid peroxidase (TPO)** rapidly oxidizes iodide and covalently binds it to the tyrosyl residues of thyroglobulin within the colloid. This forms the thyroid hormone precursor molecules, monoiodotyrosine (MIT) and diiodotyrosine (DIT). **Triiodothyronine (T_3)** is made by coupling one MIT and one DIT molecule, while **thyroxine (T_4)** is made by coupling two DIT molecules. These reactions are also catalyzed by the enzyme TPO. The newly formed hormones remain in the colloid center of the thyroid follicles until TSH binds to its receptor, triggering the endocytosis of iodinated thyroglobulin molecules back into the follicular cell. There, lysosomal enzymes break down the iodinated thyroglobulin molecule, releasing free T_3 and T_4 molecules to enter circulation (Fig. 71.2).

In the bloodstream, <1% of the circulating T_3 and T_4 remains unbound. Unbound, free T_3 and T_4 can freely cross the lipid layer of cell membranes. The remaining 99% of circulating T_3 and T_4 is bound to either specialized transport proteins called thyroxine-binding globulins (TBGs), albumin, or other plasma proteins.

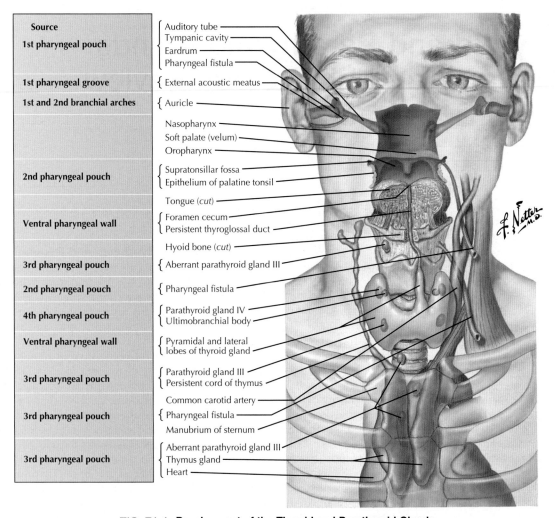

Source	
1st pharyngeal pouch	{ Auditory tube Tympanic cavity Eardrum Pharyngeal fistula
1st pharyngeal groove	{ External acoustic meatus
1st and 2nd branchial arches	{ Auricle
	Nasopharynx Soft palate (velum) Oropharynx
2nd pharyngeal pouch	{ Supratonsillar fossa Epithelium of palatine tonsil
	Tongue (cut)
Ventral pharyngeal wall	{ Foramen cecum Persistent thyroglossal duct
	Hyoid bone (cut)
3rd pharyngeal pouch	{ Aberrant parathyroid gland III
2nd pharyngeal pouch	{ Pharyngeal fistula
4th pharyngeal pouch	{ Parathyroid gland IV Ultimobranchial body
Ventral pharyngeal wall	{ Pyramidal and lateral lobes of thyroid gland
3rd pharyngeal pouch	{ Parathyroid gland III Persistent cord of thymus
	Common carotid artery
3rd pharyngeal pouch	{ Pharyngeal fistula
	Manubrium of sternum
3rd pharyngeal pouch	{ Aberrant parathyroid gland III Thymus gland Heart

FIG. 71.1 Development of the Thyroid and Parathyroid Glands.

This packaging prevents their free diffusion into body cells. When serum levels of T_3 and T_4 are low, bound T_3 and T_4 are released from these plasma proteins and readily cross the membrane of target cells. T_3 is more potent than T_4, and many cells convert T_4 to T_3 through the removal of an iodine atom.

The release of T_3 and T_4 from the thyroid gland is tightly regulated by TSH. Low blood levels of T_3 and T_4 stimulate the release of **thyrotropin-releasing hormone (TRH)** from the hypothalamus, which triggers secretion of TSH from the anterior pituitary. In turn, TSH stimulates the thyroid gland to secrete T_3 and T_4. The levels of TRH, TSH, T_3, and T_4 are regulated by a classic negative feedback system in which increasing levels of T_3 and T_4 decrease the production and secretion of TSH.

Thyroid parafollicular cells, together with the parathyroid glands, tightly regulate serum calcium homeostasis. They secrete the hormone **calcitonin** in response to elevations in blood calcium levels. Calcitonin decreases serum calcium by inhibiting the activity of osteoclasts and increasing calcium excretion in the urine.

PARATHYROID GLANDS
Anatomy and Histology

The parathyroid glands are small structures, about the size of a grain of rice, usually found embedded on the posterior surface of the thyroid gland. A thick, connective tissue capsule separates these glands from the thyroid tissue. Most patients have four parathyroid glands,

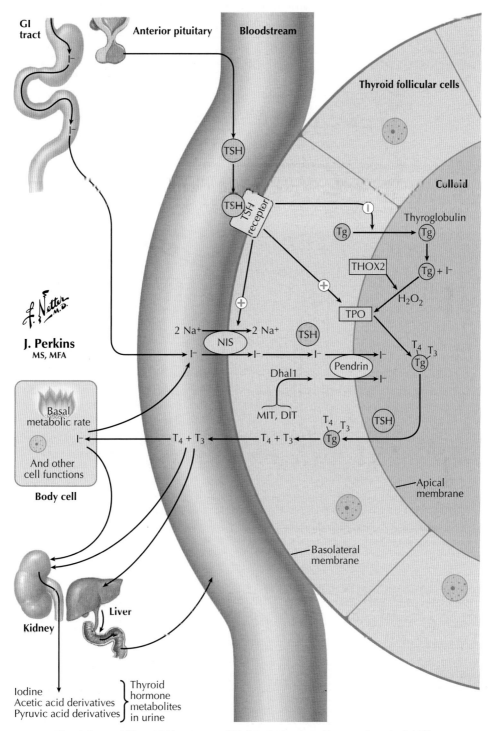

FIG. 71.2 Physiology of Thyroid Hormones. *DIT,* Diiodotyrosine; *GI,* gastrointestinal; *MIT,* monoiodotyrosine; *NIS,* sodium/iodide symporter; *THOX2,* thyroid oxidase 2; *TPO,* thyroid peroxidase; *TSH,* thyroid-stimulating hormone.

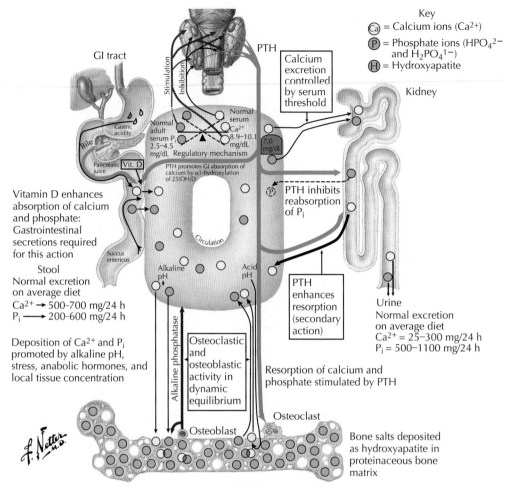

Key
Ⓒa = Calcium ions (Ca²⁺)
Ⓟ = Phosphate ions (HPO₄²⁻ and H₂PO₄¹⁻)
Ⓗ = Hydroxyapatite

PTH

Calcium excretion controlled by serum threshold

Kidney

GI tract

Stimulation Inhibition

Gastric acidity

Bile

Pancreatic juice Vit. D

Normal adult serum P 2.5–4.5 mg/dL

Normal serum Ca²⁺ 8.9–10.1 mg/dL

7.0 mg/dL

Regulatory mechanism

PTH promotes GI absorption of calcium by α1-hydroxylation of 25(OH)D

PTH inhibits reabsorption of Pᵢ

Ⓟ

Vitamin D enhances absorption of calcium and phosphate: Gastrointestinal secretions required for this action

Succus entericus

Circulation

Alkaline pH

Acid pH

PTH enhances resorption (secondary action)

Urine
Normal excretion on average diet
Ca²⁺ = 25–300 mg/24 h
Pᵢ = 500–1100 mg/24 h

Stool
Normal excretion on average diet
Ca²⁺ → 500–700 mg/24 h
Pᵢ → 200–600 mg/24 h

Deposition of Ca²⁺ and Pᵢ promoted by alkaline pH, stress, anabolic hormones, and local tissue concentration

Alkaline phosphatase

Osteoclastic and osteoblastic activity in dynamic equilibrium

Resorption of calcium and phosphate stimulated by PTH

Osteoclast

Osteoblast

Bone salts deposited as hydroxyapatite in proteinaceous bone matrix

Matrix growth requires protein, vitamin C, anabolic hormones (androgens, estrogen, IGF1) ≤ stress of mobility. Matrix resorption favored by catabolic hormones (11-oxysteroids [cortisol], thyroid), parathyroid hormone ≤ immobilization

FIG. 71.3 Physiology of Parathyroid Hormone. *GI*, Gastrointestinal; *IGF1*, insulin-like growth factor-1; *PTH*, parathyroid hormone.

divided into two pairs based on location, although variation in number is common. Usually, two superior parathyroid glands are located on the posterior-lateral surface of the middle to superior thyroid lobe, and two inferior parathyroid glands are found near the inferior poles of the thyroid gland. Migration patterns during embryogenesis can cause the parathyroid glands to exhibit a range of anatomical variations. This variation in individuals increases the risk of damaging or inadvertently removing the parathyroid glands during a thyroidectomy.

The superior parathyroid glands receive most of their blood supply from the inferior thyroid artery. For 15%

to 20% of patients, the superior parathyroid glands are also supplied by branches of the superior thyroid artery. The inferior parathyroid glands receive their blood supply from the inferior thyroid artery. Similar to the thyroid, the lymphatic vessels of the parathyroid glands drain into the deep cervical lymph nodes and paratracheal lymph nodes.

The parathyroid glands contain two main cell types: **chief cells** and oxyphil cells. The chief cells synthesize and secrete **parathyroid hormone (PTH),** the major hormone involved in the regulation of blood calcium levels. The oxyphil cells have no recognized endocrine function.

Maintaining calcium homeostasis

The parathyroid glands maintain calcium homeostasis through the production and secretion of PTH. PTH secretion is regulated by the change in extracellular calcium concentration, which is detected by the calcium-sensing receptor (CaSR) on the surface of parathyroid cells. To a smaller degree, PTH secretion is also regulated by extracellular phosphate, calcitriol, and fibroblast growth factor-23 (FGF23). PTH is essential for the maintenance of calcium homeostasis. A negative feedback loop regulates the levels of PTH, with rising blood calcium levels inhibiting further release of PTH from the parathyroid glands.

PTH acts directly on the bone and kidneys, and indirectly on the gastrointestinal tract. At the bone, PTH indirectly causes the release of calcium from the bones. Stimulation is indirect because only osteoblasts have PTH receptors. PTH binds to receptors on osteoblasts, which leads to an increase in expression of **receptor**

activator of nuclear factor κB ligand (RANKL). The binding of RANKL to its receptor on osteoclast precursors stimulates them to fuse and mature into osteoclasts, which ultimately enhances bone resorption.

PTH has two main roles in the kidney: increasing reabsorption of calcium and blocking phosphate reabsorption from the tubules. PTH also works at the proximal tubule to upregulate translation of α1-hydroxylase, the enzyme responsible for forming the biologically active form of vitamin D (1,25-dihydroxyvitamin D [calcitriol]). Calcitriol binds to receptors in the bone and participates with PTH to stimulate osteoclastic bone resorption (Fig. 71.3).

While PTH has no direct effects on the gastrointestinal tract, it does exhibit effects indirectly through the action of calcitriol. Calcitriol binds to receptors on the cells in the small intestine to increase calcium and phosphate absorption.

CHAPTER 72

Hypothyroidism

ABHINAV NAIR

INTRODUCTION

Hypothyroidism, characterized by a deficiency in thyroid hormone, is one of the most common endocrine disorders. It can result from a defect anywhere along the hypothalamic-pituitary-thyroid (HPT) axis; primary thyroid gland dysfunction is the most common cause, though infrequently the culprit is a central process. Diagnosis of clinical hypothyroidism requires identification of a constellation of symptoms compatible with the disease and initiation of hormone replacement therapy to mitigate symptoms.

Approximately 0.1% to 0.2% of the population is estimated to have overt hypothyroidism, although 4% to 10% may have subclinical disease. Women are over five times as likely to be hypothyroid, and the incidence increases significantly with age, although there is some controversy related to normal, age-related increases in thyroid-stimulating hormone (TSH), which may confound the picture.

PATHOPHYSIOLOGY

Measuring thyroid function takes into account both clinical symptoms and levels of thyroid-related hormones, primarily TSH. Although not required for a diagnosis of hypothyroidism, levels of the thyroid hormones triiodothyronine (T_3) and thyroxine (T_4) may influence treatment decisions, especially in cases with minor elevations of TSH or in the setting of critical illness. Free thyroxine (FT_4) is that component of thyroxine that is not protein bound and is biologically active, making it a meaningful measure of clinical thyroid status.

In **primary hypothyroidism,** decreased concentrations of T_3 and T_4 cause a compensatory increase in TSH; therefore overt hypothyroidism is diagnosed by elevated TSH (often >10 mU/L) and low FT_4. **Subclinical hypothyroidism** is diagnosed in patients with elevated TSH but normal FT_4 levels; these patients usually lack the classic signs and symptoms of hypothyroidism.

As iodine is critical for the production of thyroid hormone, iodine deficiency is the leading cause of hypothyroidism worldwide. In iodine-sufficient regions, such as the United States, or in countries that enrich their food with iodine, **chronic autoimmune thyroiditis (Hashimoto thyroiditis)** is the most commonly implicated etiology. Hashimoto thyroiditis can feature both cell-mediated and antibody-mediated destruction of thyroid tissue. Histology reveals lymphocytic infiltration, and the overwhelming majority of patients with overt hypothyroidism will have elevated autoantibodies, most commonly the thyroid peroxidase (TPO) antibody. Routine measurement of thyroid autoantibodies is not recommended for diagnosis and is used only in the context of subclinical disease or in the presence of goiter to predict disease progression.

Central hypothyroidism is characterized by abnormal hypothalamic-pituitary function, leading to inadequate stimulation of the thyroid gland. This defect can arise either from decreased thyroid-releasing hormone (TRH) at the level of the hypothalamus or decreased TSH secretion from the anterior pituitary. Patients with central hypothyroidism have signs and symptoms of hypothyroidism and typically present with low FT_4 levels, but TSH levels can be either low, normal (inappropriately), or slightly elevated (generally <10 mU/L). Patients with central hypothyroidism will often present with other endocrine abnormalities suggestive of central dysfunction, such as hypogonadism and hypocortisolism.

Euthyroid sick syndrome, or nonthyroidal illness syndrome, denotes changes in thyroid function tests during critical illness. Nearly three-quarters of hospitalized patients can develop abnormalities in the HPT axis, which resolve following resolution of the acute, nonthyroidal illness. T_3 levels decline first, followed by total T_4 and later TSH. Free T_4 tends to be preserved in the acute stages of nonthyroidal illness, and low free T_4 is an overall poor prognostic sign. Symptom history and physical exam are key for distinguishing abnormalities in thyroid function tests that result from euthyroid sick syndrome from abnormalities signifying true, overt hypothyroidism, but these entities are often hard to distinguish in hospitalized patients. It may be helpful to measure **reverse** T_3, which is elevated in cases of nonthyroidal illness while low in true hypothyroidism.

RISK FACTORS

Aside from iodine deficiency and chronic autoimmune thyroiditis, alternate etiologies of primary hypothyroidism include medications (e.g., lithium, amiodarone, immunomodulators), environmental toxins (e.g., polybrominated diphenyl ether [PBDE] flame retardants), infiltrative diseases (e.g., amyloidosis, hemochromatosis), or congenital abnormalities of the thyroid gland. Certain patients with hypothyroidism may have been previously hyperthyroid and underwent thyroidectomy or radioiodine ablation, resulting in hypothyroidism. External neck radiation is another well-known iatrogenic cause. Patients with a history of pituitary masses, infarction, surgery, or radiotherapy are at risk for developing central hypothyroidism.

The time course of progression in hypothyroidism is variable and often dependent on the underlying cause. While formal, randomized control studies are lacking, many believe in screening for hypothyroidism as a cost-effective prevention strategy in women >50 years of age. The American Thyroid Association and American Association of Clinical Endocrinologists recommend screening anyone at risk, including prior head/neck radiation, prior thyroid surgery, family history of thyroid disease, and personal history of autoimmune diseases (including type 1 diabetes).

PRESENTATION, EVALUATION, AND DIAGNOSIS

Hypothyroidism may present very heterogeneously, and as such there is a lack of specificity in its clinical manifestations. As every cell requires thyroid hormone to function, slowing of the body's metabolic processes contributes to the most common symptoms: fatigue, cold intolerance, weight gain, cognitive slowing, menstrual irregularities, dry skin, brittle nails, thinning hair, and constipation. Patients may have bradycardia, diastolic hypertension, slow movements, and delayed reflexes. Deposition of extracellular glycosaminoglycans (GAGs) in the interstitial spaces can cause dry skin, throat hoarseness, tongue enlargement, and nonpitting edema. Hematological changes include hypercoagulability (from acquired von Willebrand syndrome) and macrocytic anemia. Laboratory testing may also reveal hypercholesterolemia (low-density lipoprotein [LDL]), increased serum creatine kinase from muscle strain, and hyponatremia from decreased free water clearance (Fig. 72.1).

Ultimately, the clinical severity depends on the extent of hormone deficiency, the acuity of its decline, and its duration or chronicity. **Myxedema coma** is the most feared complication and often arises from severe long-standing disease exacerbated by an acute stressor, essentially a clinical diagnosis of decompensated, severe hypothyroidism. While the diagnosis reflects dysfunction in multiple organ symptoms, the hallmarks include altered mental status and hypothermia. It is a medical emergency with a high mortality rate and as such requires early recognition and aggressive therapy.

Overall, given the clinical variability of presentations, diagnosis of hypothyroidism depends primarily on laboratory testing. TSH is the preferred screening test; if >10 mU/L, the diagnosis of hypothyroidism is made. Patients with elevated TSH that is <10 mU/L should have their FT_4 level checked, and if central hypothyroidism is suspected, FT_4 is the screening test of choice as TSH can be variable.

TREATMENT

Unless an individual's overt, primary hypothyroidism is transient or reversible (e.g., medication induced), lifelong therapy is often indicated with thyroid hormone replacement. Daily oral synthetic T_4 supplementation with **levothyroxine** is the standard treatment of choice, as T_4 is converted to T_3 throughout the body in a regulated manner by various deiodinase enzymes. Initial dosing is weight based, (approximately 1.6 µg/kg) but an individual's requirements may vary widely. Patients with known coronary artery disease and tachyarrhythmias should start at lower doses (generally 25 µg/day) and then uptitrated to lessen the risk of cardiac ischemic events. To aid in absorption, tablets should not be taken in close proximity to meals, and especially not taken together with foods or medications that contain iron or calcium, as these greatly hamper levothyroxine absorption. It is best to take levothyroxine immediately after waking in the morning.

Patients should notice clinical improvements within the first few weeks of levothyroxine initiation, but steady state is not reached until 6 weeks. Dosing is titrated to achieve normal TSH levels, but dose adjustments and repeat TSH measurements generally should not be more frequent than every 4 to 6 weeks as it takes at least that long to reach steady state. Prescribers should always make dose adjustments with regard to clinical symptoms, making attempts to avoid overreplacement and subclinical hyperthyroidism, which may manifest with atrial fibrillation or accelerated bone loss in postmenopausal women, especially as TSH falls to the 0.1-mIU/L range.

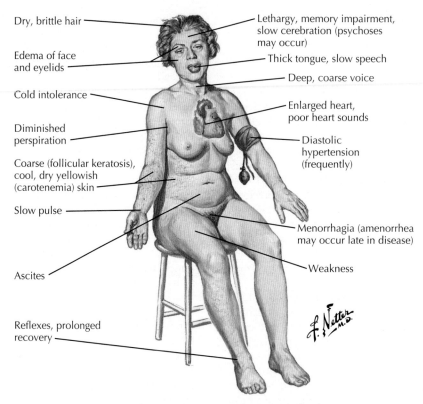

Dry, brittle hair

Edema of face and eyelids

Cold intolerance

Diminished perspiration

Coarse (follicular keratosis), cool, dry yellowish (carotenemia) skin

Slow pulse

Ascites

Reflexes, prolonged recovery

Lethargy, memory impairment, slow cerebration (psychoses may occur)

Thick tongue, slow speech

Deep, coarse voice

Enlarged heart, poor heart sounds

Diastolic hypertension (frequently)

Menorrhagia (amenorrhea may occur late in disease)

Weakness

FIG. 72.1 Clinical Manifestations of Hypothyroidism.

Patients with subclinical hypothyroidism should have repeat TSH and FT$_4$ levels drawn approximately 6 weeks following diagnosis, as some patients will have normalized lab values. Patients with central hypothyroidism should undergo laboratory investigation and, if appropriate, MRI imaging of the pituitary gland, as it is vital not to start levothyroxine on any patient with concomitant adrenal insufficiency prior to cortisol replacement. In central hypothyroidism, levothyroxine is titrated to target free T$_4$ levels at the upper half of the normal range. TSH is not useful to measure in these patients, owing to the central basis of hypothyroidism.

CHAPTER 73

Hyperthyroidism and Thyrotoxicosis

TARIQ CHUKIR

INTRODUCTION

Hyperthyroidism is a state of increased synthesis and secretion of thyroid hormones. **Thyrotoxicosis,** meanwhile, is a clinical state characterized by elevated thyroid hormones due to any cause. Thyroxine (T_4), the main circulating form of thyroid hormone, is a prohormone for triiodothyronine (T_3), the biologically active form of thyroid hormone. The estimated prevalence of thyrotoxicosis in the United States is 1.3%.

ETIOLOGIES AND PATHOPHYSIOLOGY

Thyrotoxicosis can be caused by several disorders. **Graves disease** is the most common cause of thyrotoxicosis, accounting for 50% to 80% of cases. Graves disease involves circulating immunoglobulin G (IgG) autoantibodies that bind and activate the thyrotropin receptor, resulting in follicular hypertrophy and hyperplasia with a subsequent increase in thyroid hormone production (T_4 and T_3), which can lead to hyperthyroidism. The female-to-male ratio of patients with Graves disease ranges from 5:1 to 10:1, with most cases diagnosed between ages 40 and 60 years (Fig. 73.1).

Solitary **toxic adenoma** and **toxic multinodular goiter (MNG)** are the second most common causes of thyrotoxicosis. Thyrotoxicosis is mediated through the autonomous overproduction of thyroid hormones, independent of the thyroid-stimulating hormone (TSH), by one or more nodules (Fig. 73.2).

Thyroiditis refers to a group of conditions in which the destruction of thyroid cells causes the release of preformed thyroid hormone into the circulating bloodstream. Notably, this is not synonymous with hyperthyroidism, due to oversecretion of thyroid hormone seen in cases of Graves disease and toxic adenoma(s), as the thyroid hormone was produced appropriately but was released inappropriately from damaged thyroid cells (Fig. 73.3). It accounts for 10% of thyrotoxicosis cases. The clinical course of thyroiditis is characterized by an initial thyrotoxic phase lasting 1 to 3 months, followed by a euthyroid phase. Although some patients experience a temporary or permanent hypothyroid state, return to a euthyroid phase within 12 to 18 months after the onset of symptoms does occur in most patients. Thyroiditis can be divided into two categories based on its presentation: painful thyroiditis and painless thyroiditis.

Painful thyroiditis includes subacute thyroiditis and suppurative thyroiditis. Subacute thyroiditis, also known as subacute granulomatous or de Quervain thyroiditis, is thought to be caused by a viral infection, such as from adenovirus, coxsackie virus, Epstein-Barr virus, influenza, or HIV. Suppurative thyroiditis normally is caused by bacterial pathogens; however, fungal, mycobacterial, and parasitic pathogens are also reported causes. In contrast to subacute thyroiditis, suppurative thyroiditis is rare, as the thyroid is resistant to bacterial infections due to its capsule, rich supply of blood, high iodine content, and extensive lymphatic drainage network.

Painless thyroiditis includes silent thyroiditis, **postpartum thyroiditis,** drug-induced thyroiditis, and **Riedel thyroiditis.** Silent thyroiditis, also known as **subacute lymphocytic thyroiditis,** is likely autoimmune in nature. Postpartum thyroiditis is the development of thyroid dysfunction within 12 months after pregnancy.

Several medications have been implicated in the development of thyroiditis, such as amiodarone, immunotherapy, lithium, and interferon-α. Immunotherapy-induced thyroiditis occurs in patients following their exposure to inhibitors of cytotoxic T-lymphocyte–associated antigen-4 (CTLA4) and programmed cell death-1 or its ligand (PD1/PD-L1), with reported incidence rates of 5% to 20%. Riedel thyroiditis is a rare condition characterized by progressive fibrosis of the thyroid gland; its pathophysiology is unclear, although it may involve IgG4 plasma cell accumulation.

A common cause of thyrotoxicosis is iatrogenic intake of thyroid hormone, which is characterized by low serum thyroglobulin levels. Rarely, thyrotoxicosis results from a TSH-producing pituitary adenoma, or the **struma ovarii** syndrome, in which an ovarian teratoma produces thyroid hormone.

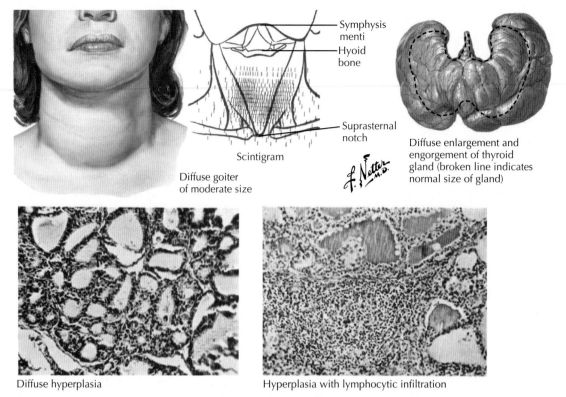

Symphysis menti

Hyoid bone

Suprasternal notch

Scintigram

Diffuse goiter of moderate size

Diffuse enlargement and engorgement of thyroid gland (broken line indicates normal size of gland)

Diffuse hyperplasia

Hyperplasia with lymphocytic infiltration

FIG. 73.1 **Graves Disease.**

RISK FACTORS

The prevalence of thyrotoxicosis increases with age and is more prevalent in women. The risk of Graves disease is increased in patients with a family history of the disease or a family history of other autoimmune conditions. Solitary toxic adenoma or toxic MNG is more prevalent in areas of low iodine intake. The risk factors for suppurative thyroiditis include preexisting thyroid disease, congenital anomalies, and immunosuppression. Women who have elevated antithyroid peroxidase (anti-TPO) antibodies, a personal history of type 1 diabetes mellitus or thyroid disease, or a family history of thyroid disease are at increased risk for the development of silent and/or postpartum thyroiditis.

PRESENTATION, EVALUATION, AND DIAGNOSIS

The clinical presentation of thyrotoxicosis is broad and ranges from patients having almost no symptoms to those with **thyroid storm,** the most severe and life-threatening presentation. Symptoms of thyrotoxicosis include anxiety,

tremor, palpitations, heat intolerance, weight loss, fever, difficulty sleeping, diarrhea, apathy, diaphoresis, and/or menstrual irregularities. Thyroid storm is a state of severe hyperthyroidism in which the body cannot compensate for hyperadrenergic symptoms, resulting in end-organ damage.

The findings seen in thyrotoxicosis on physical examination may be notable for goiter, tachycardia, hyperreflexia, lid retraction, and lid lag, all symptoms of sympathetic overactivation. In contrast to these clinical findings, pretibial myxedema and exophthalmos are specific clinical features of Graves disease because they are immune mediated (Fig. 73.4).

In the absence of pituitary disease, the optimal test for diagnosing thyrotoxicosis is the level of TSH, as a subnormal value is highly sensitive and specific. The total T_4 laboratory test measures the level of T_4 bound to thyroid-binding globulin (TBG) in addition to the level of free T_4. Many conditions alter the TBG levels (e.g., pregnancy raises it, while nephrotic syndrome lowers it); therefore testing both the levels of total T_4 and free T_4 is recommended. An isolated elevation in levels of

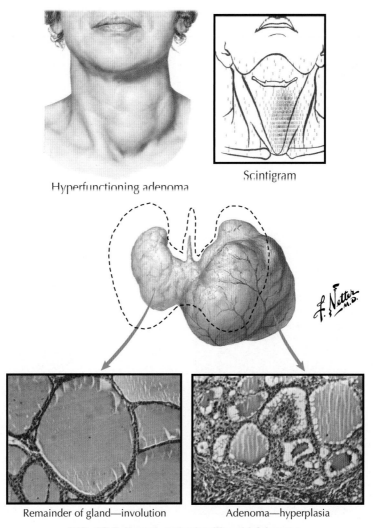

Hyperfunctioning adenoma

Scintigram

Remainder of gland—involution

Adenoma—hyperplasia

FIG. 73.2 **Hyperfunctioning Thyroid Adenoma.**

T_3 can be observed in patients with T_3 thyrotoxicosis, so measuring TSH with concurrent T_4, free T_4, and total T_3 is advised.

Further biochemical testing and imaging are needed to differentiate the cause of thyrotoxicosis. The gold standard test to distinguish causes of hyperthyroidism is the **radioactive iodine uptake (RAIU) scan,** which uses the ^{123}I isotope to measure areas of hyperactivity within the thyroid gland. The test will show elevated uptake in a homogenous pattern in Graves disease; patchy, focal uptake in toxic adenoma; and low uptake in thyroiditis. Medications with high concentrations of iodine (e.g., amiodarone) or the administration of iodinated contrast limit the use of RAIU scans. RAIU

scan is contraindicated in pregnancy. The diagnosis of Graves disease also can be confirmed by the detection of thyrotropin receptor antibodies (TRAbs) (e.g., thyroid-stimulating immunoglobulin [TSI] or thyrotropin-binding inhibitory immunoglobulin [TBII]). Increased vascularity on Doppler imaging is nonspecific but also suggests Graves disease.

TREATMENT

The therapeutic approach to managing thyrotoxicosis consists of symptom control and a definitive treatment regimen that targets the underlying etiology. β-blockers can be used on an as-needed basis to effectively improve

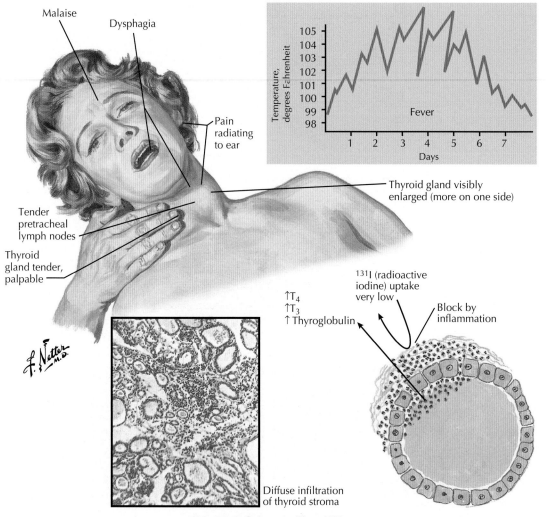

Malaise

Dysphagia

Pain radiating to ear

Temperature, degrees Fahrenheit

105
104
103
102
101
100
99
98

Fever

1   2   3   4   5   6   7

Days

Thyroid gland visibly enlarged (more on one side)

Tender pretracheal lymph nodes

Thyroid gland tender, palpable

↑T₄
↑T₃
↑ Thyroglobulin

¹³¹I (radioactive iodine) uptake very low

Block by inflammation

Diffuse infiltration of thyroid stroma

FIG. 73.3 **Subacute Thyroiditis.**

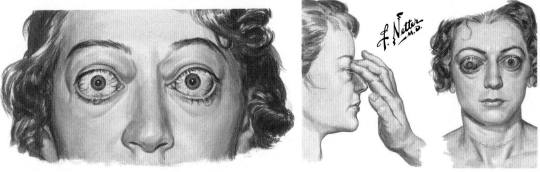

Moderately severe ophthalmopathy

Testing for resiliency

Severe progressive ophthalmopathy

FIG. 73.4 **Graves Ophthalmopathy.**

the symptoms of thyrotoxicosis by decreasing both the sympathetic stimulation and the conversion of T_4 to T_3.

Graves disease can be managed with medical therapy, **radioactive iodine ablation,** or surgery. **Thionamides,** such as methimazole and propylthiouracil (PTU), decrease the synthesis of thyroid hormones by inhibiting the organification of iodide and the coupling of iodothyronines. PTU also prevents the peripheral conversion of T_4 to T_3. Methimazole is generally preferred over PTU due to its rapid action, simple administration with one daily dose, and lower incidence of hepatotoxicity. PTU is preferred for women in their first trimester of pregnancy due to the risk of teratogenicity with methimazole. In addition to hepatotoxicity, agranulocytosis is a rare but severe adverse event of thionamides, with an estimated incidence rate of 0.1% to 0.3%. The relapse rate for patients treated with medical therapy is 30% to 60%.

Radioactive iodine ablation is a safe and effective intervention used to treat Graves disease. Permanent hypothyroidism should develop following radioactive iodine ablation, for which lifelong thyroid hormone supplementation is required. Radioactive iodine ablation therapy is contraindicated in patients who present with severe ophthalmopathy, and during pregnancy and lactation. The estimated relapse rate in patients treated with radioactive iodine ablation is 21%. Surgical intervention through total thyroidectomy is indicated for patients with obstructive goiter, severe ophthalmopathy, those planning pregnancy in the near future, and those who fail or have adverse reactions to thionamides. Total thyroidectomy results in permanent hypothyroidism, and these patients require lifelong thyroid hormone.

The therapeutic options for toxic adenoma or toxic MNG include temporary use of thionamides for symptom control followed by surgery to remove the thyroid lobe that contains the adenoma(s). Hemithyroidectomy will leave these patients with a 50% chance of being hypothyroid so they may or may not need thyroid hormone supplementation with levothyroxine postsurgically. If patients are elderly or cannot tolerate surgery, they can remain on thionamide therapy lifelong instead of undergoing surgery.

The treatment of patients with thyroiditis involves administering β-blockers and antiinflammatory agents on an as-needed basis to reduce thyrotoxic symptoms and pain. NSAIDs are considered first-line medications for thyroiditis-associated pain. Steroids are reserved for severe and/or NSAID-refractory cases.

CHAPTER 74

Hyperparathyroidism

ZOË LYSY

INTRODUCTION

Hyperparathyroidism can be characterized as primary, secondary, or tertiary, depending on its etiology. This chapter will mainly cover primary hyperparathyroidism (PHPT), which is a primary endocrine disorder. **Secondary hyperparathyroidism** occurs with a physiologically appropriate elevation in **parathyroid hormone (PTH)** to low calcitriol, low calcium (Ca), or elevated phosphorus levels. **Tertiary hyperparathyroidism** is the result of prolonged secondary hyperparathyroidism, usually in setting of chronic kidney disease (CKD), and can persist even post renal transplant when renal function has normalized.

PHPT is a condition characterized by dysregulation of the normal feedback mechanism between serum Ca and PTH. Normally, concentrations of PTH and Ca are inversely correlated, such that lowering of serum Ca is met with a rise in PTH (to reestablish normal Ca levels) and inversely, elevation in serum Ca leads to suppression of PTH (until normal Ca levels are reestablished). There is individual variability in responses of PTH to Ca partly determined by the **Ca sensing receptor (CaSR),** which is responsible for Ca detection by the parathyroid gland. PTH in turn acts on the gut, kidney, and activation of vitamin D to regulate serum calcium levels.

Primary hyperparathyroidism can occur in the setting of either normal or elevated PTH, depending on the respective Ca level. For example, an elevated PTH is considered abnormal in the setting of normal Ca, and a normal PTH is considered inappropriately normal when Ca is elevated. Like many endocrine conditions relying on feedback loops, the level of Ca must be considered when determining whether hyperparathyroidism is present. This is also an important distinction from secondary hyperparathyroidism, where the PTH elevation is physiologically appropriate as in the setting of hyperphosphatemia, low vitamin D, hypocalcemia, or CKD.

PATHOPHYSIOLOGY

It is important to make the pathophysiological distinction between primary, secondary, and tertiary hyperparathyroidism. Secondary hyperparathyroidism is characterized by an appropriate (physiological) elevation in PTH. This most commonly occurs in the setting of **25-hydroxyvitamin D (25[OH]D)** deficiency. Another common etiology is in CKD (estimated glomerular filtration rate [eGFR] <60) where an interplay of phosphate retention, decreased calcitriol production, hypocalcemia, and CaSR setpoint shift results in secondary hyperparathyroidism. Tertiary hyperparathyroidism occurs when secondary hyperparathyroidism is prolonged and results in autonomous, dysregulated PTH secretion, unresponsive to Ca levels. The main biochemical distinction between these two entities is the presence of elevated Ca in tertiary hyperparathyroidism, not explained by exogenous Ca supplementation, while hypocalcemia is often present in secondary hyperparathyroidism due to decreased gastrointestinal (GI) absorption from impaired calcitriol synthesis and impaired renal Ca absorption.

The main cause of primary hyperparathyroidism is autonomous secretion from one or more parathyroid glands. Excess PTH secretion occurs via one of three pathological conditions: parathyroid adenoma, hyperplasia, or carcinoma. The majority (80%–85%) of cases are single adenomas. Multiple adenomas range between 2% and 15% of cases, whereas hyperplasia accounts for 2% to 20% of cases, of which up to 26% have concurrent multiple endocrine neoplasia **(MEN1 or MEN2A syndrome).** Parathyroid carcinomas account for <1% of cases (Fig. 74.1).

One additional disease to note is **familial hypocalciuric hypercalcemia (FHH),** a rare form of familial, autosomal dominant hyperparathyroidism. FHH features inactivating mutations of the CaSR present on the parathyroid gland and renal tubules. In this condition, higher Ca levels are required to suppress PTH (resulting in rightward shift of Ca/PTH curve), and there is an increase in the tubular reabsorption of Ca (hypocalciuria). This presents with mild elevation in Ca and high PTH as a higher setpoint of Ca is required for PTH to be suppressed.

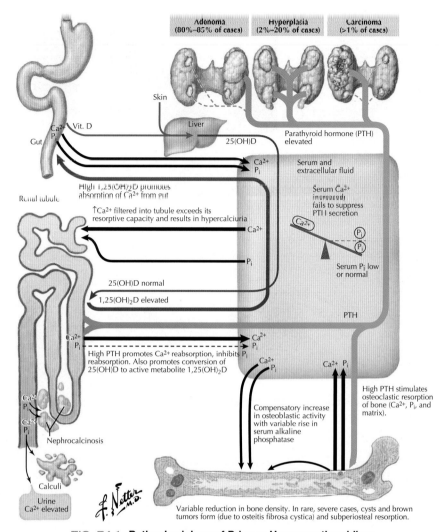

FIG. 74.1 **Pathophysiology of Primary Hyperparathyroidism.**

Other familial forms of primary hyperparathyroidism occur as part of MEN1 or MEN2A syndromes, where they occur as a clinical spectrum with other endocrine neoplasias. Other inherited conditions include familial isolated hyperparathyroidism (FIHP) and hyperparathyroidism jaw-tumor syndrome (HPT-JT). These conditions typically present with parathyroid hyperplasia.

PRESENTATION, EVALUATION, AND DIAGNOSIS

The most common presentation of primary hyperthyroidism is mild elevation of Ca on routine lab work; 85% of patients are asymptomatic. Other manifestations of hyperparathyroidism occur predominantly in the bones and the kidneys, organs on which PTH acts. Symptoms in hyperparathyroidism result primarily from hypercalcemia, classically described by the mnemonic "bones, stones, groans, and moans," reflecting both effects of elevated PTH and ensuing hypercalcemia:

- *Bone* pain in the setting of osteitis fibrosa cystica, in which increased osteoclastic activity leads to demineralization of bone and formation of cyst-like, brown tumors (fibrous tissue that are not true tumors)
- Kidney *stones* (nephrolithiasis from hypercalciuria)
- Abdominal *groans* (constipation, nausea from hypercalcemia)

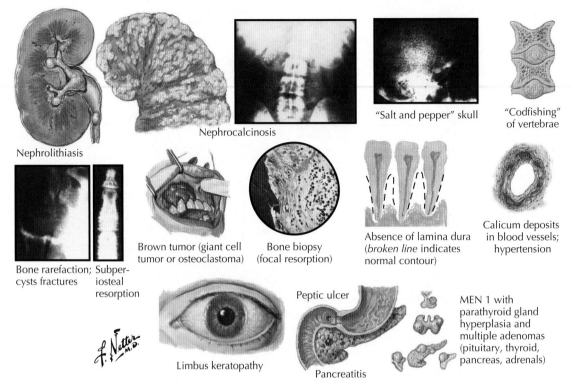

Nephrolithiasis

Nephrocalcinosis

"Salt and pepper" skull

"Codfishing" of vertebrae

Bone rarefaction; Subper-cysts fractures iosteal resorption

Brown tumor (giant cell tumor or osteoclastoma)

Bone biopsy (focal resorption)

Absence of lamina dura (*broken line* indicates normal contour)

Calicum deposits in blood vessels; hypertension

Limbus keratopathy

Peptic ulcer

Pancreatitis

MEN 1 with parathyroid gland hyperplasia and multiple adenomas (pituitary, thyroid, pancreas, adrenals)

FIG. 74.2 **Pathology and Clinical Manifestations of Primary Hyperparathyroidism.** *MEN1*, Multiple endocrine neoplasia-1.

- Psychiatric *moans* (lethargy, fatigue, depression, cognitive impairment)

Other manifestations of hyperparathyroidism include osteoporosis, disproportionately affecting cortical bone, proximal muscle weakness, and gradual deterioration in renal function. There is observational data regarding cardiac and vascular changes in this condition, as well as increase in fracture rates (typically vertebral, though distal forearm, hip, pelvic, and rib fractures have also been reported) (Fig. 74.2).

Special attention should be paid to obtaining a complete drug history, especially for use of lithium and thiazide diuretics. Lithium shifts the Ca/PTH curve rightward by decreasing sensitivity of PTH gland to negative feedback from Ca. Thiazide diuretics can unmask PHPT by reducing urine Ca excretion, thereby raising Ca.

PTH and Ca levels are essential for making the diagnosis of hyperparathyroidism. Laboratory findings in hyperparathyroidism include elevated PTH (in the setting of normal or elevated Ca) or normal PTH (in the setting of elevated Ca, in which PTH is inappropriately normal). Ca must be measured at the same time to ensure proper interpretation of PTH levels. As with normal evaluation of Ca, levels must be adjusted in the case of abnormal albumin levels; ionized Ca can be utilized as well.

Concomitant laboratory investigations are conducted to identify the pathophysiology of the hyperparathyroidism, which in turn will dictate management. 25(OH)-vitamin D is the most accurate measure of total body vitamin D stores, and levels must be obtained to ensure elevation in PTH is not secondary (when vitamin D levels are <50 mmol/L). Renal function and phosphate levels should be drawn to rule out secondary hyperparathyroidism (from CKD or hyperphosphatemia). Urinary Ca excretion is measured to distinguish primary hyperparathyroidism (in which Ca excretion in urine is elevated) from FHH, where the Ca-to-creatinine (Cr) ratio (Ca:Cr) is usually <0.01.

Further testing can examine the impact of hyperparathyroidism, which in turn will dictate management. A dual-energy x-ray absorptiometry (DEXA) scan is measured at baseline to determine extent of osteoporosis and bony disease. Renal imaging is performed in

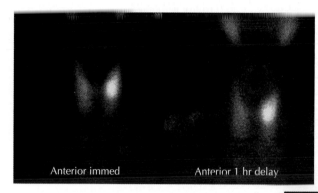

Technetium 99m sestamibi scan demonstrating an abnormal focus of radiotracer accumulation seen in the left side of the neck on immediate and 1 hour delayed images.

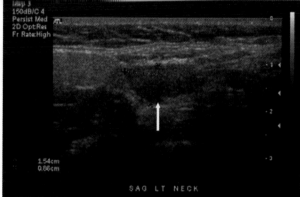

Static sonographic image in the sagittal plane demonstrating a homogeneous, hypoechoic mass inferior to the left lobe of the thyroid gland that corresponded to a left inferior parathyroid adenoma.

FIG. 74.3 **Preoperative Imaging of Neck: Sestamibi Scintigram and Sonogram.** (Reused with permission from Delaney C editor: *Netter's surgical anatomy and approaches*, Philadelphia, 2013, Elsevier.)

all patients, as nephrolithiasis can be asymptomatic, but if present, is a criterion for parathyroidectomy. Evaluation of renal function can demonstrate acute kidney injury from polyuria seen in hypercalcemia or obstructive nephrolithiasis, and the presence of known CKD in the setting of elevated PTH raises suspicion for secondary hyperparathyroidism. Tertiary hyperparathyroidism can present after persistent secondary hyperparathyroidism.

Once confirmation of PHPT has been made on investigations, the next step is localization of the pathology in the parathyroid gland by performing a nuclear uptake scan of the parathyroid, called a **sestamibi scan.** Sestamibi is a coordination complex of technetium-99m to six MIBI ligands and is taken up by parathyroid adenoma(s) or parathyroid hyperplasia responsible for most cases of PHPT. This should be undertaken when physicians suspect either PHPT or tertiary hyperparathyroidism (Fig. 74.3). Imaging is typically not undertaken for secondary hyperparathyroidism, where the goal is to reverse the underlying driver of the elevation in PTH (hyperphosphatemia, hypovitaminosis D, CKD).

TREATMENT

The definitive management of PHPT is parathyroidectomy. The surgical strategy and extent of parathyroidectomy depends on results of the sestamibi scan (single adenoma vs hyperplasia). Patients undergoing parathyroidectomy must be monitored for postprocedural hypocalcemia and voice changes that may result from injury to the recurrent laryngeal nerve. Management of secondary hyperparathyroidism is targeted at correcting the underlying driver of the hyperparathyroidism. Hence the distinction between the two is fundamental to guide treatment. Similarly, in drug-induced hyperparathyroidism, the causative agent is stopped (if possible); in FHH, typically management is conservative (observation).

Patients with symptomatic PHPT should undergo surgery. For patients with asymptomatic hyperparathyroidism, guidelines suggest parathyroidectomy if the following occur:
- Ca >1 mg/dL above upper limit of normal
- Decline in renal function (eGFR <60)
- On DEXA, bone mineral density (BMD) <-2.5 on T (or Z) score and/or prior atraumatic vertebral fracture

- Age <50
- 24-hour urine for Ca >400 mg/day or presence of nephrolithiasis/nephrocalcinosis on imaging

In asymptomatic patients who do not meet previous criteria for surgical consideration or who are poor surgical candidates, physicians must monitor Ca and renal function regularly, as well as BMD every 1 to 2 years to ensure they do not progress to indications for surgical intervention. Fortunately, many patients (as many of 30% of all PHPT patients) remain stable for decades without medical or surgical intervention. Nevertheless, physicians should encourage patients to receive adequate hydration, physical activity to prevent bone resorption, and adequate dietary Ca and vitamin D intake. Physicians should counsel avoidance of a high-Ca diet (>1000 mg/day) and drugs with hypercalcemia as a side effect.

In symptomatic patients who cannot undergo surgery, medical therapy includes bisphosphonates and calcimimetics such as cinacalcet, which mimic the action of Ca in tissues, essentially tricking the body into thinking adequate Ca is present and decreasing the stimulation for PTH secretion. Calcimimetics already are recommended for treatment of secondary hyperparathyroidism in patients with CKD; however, they are often difficult to tolerate at therapeutic doses due to nausea.

CHAPTER 75

Osteoporosis

KAHLI E. ZIETLOW

INTRODUCTION

Osteoporosis is characterized by decreased bone mass and disruption of bony microarchitecture, leading to fragility and predisposing to fracture. This occurs most commonly in postmenopausal women, when decreased levels of circulating estrogen result in higher rates of bone resorption. However, this disorder is also common in older men, particularly those with predisposing conditions or risk factors.

One in three postmenopausal women and one in five older men will experience an osteoporotic fracture, and this incidence is expected to climb as the population ages. The high disease prevalence leads to significant worldwide morbidity. Because this disorder is clinically silent until fractures occur, it is also widely underdiagnosed. However, osteoporosis is both treatable and, to some extent, preventable, highlighting the importance of appropriate screening, diagnosis, and management.

PATHOPHYSIOLOGY

Maintenance of bone mass is a dynamic, ongoing process. Remodeling occurs in response to the continuous microtrauma bones undergo with routine physical activity. Existing bone is resorbed by **osteoclasts,** and new bone is deposited by **osteoblasts.** As we age, this balance shifts such that bone resorption outpaces deposition. Bone mass peaks around age 30, and inadequate peak bone mass is a risk factor for later development of osteoporosis. Nutrition, physical activity, use of tobacco and alcohol, certain medications, and genetic factors all ultimately contribute to one's peak bone mass.

Bone remodeling is a complex process regulated by multiple exogenous and endogenous hormones. As part of this regulatory process, osteoblasts secrete receptor activator of nuclear factor-κB ligand (RANKL) and osteoprotegerin (OPG). RANKL binds to RANK on osteoclast cells, promoting osteoclast differentiation and thus bone resorption, while OPG binds and inactivates RANKL. After menopause, there is a dramatic increase in bone resorption, due to estrogen's regulatory effects on RANKL/OPG. This accounts for the high prevalence of osteoporosis in postmenopausal women, although younger women and men are also susceptible to osteoporosis, particularly if they have a low peak bone mass and/or exposure to risk factors.

RISK FACTORS

Age and menopause are the greatest risk factors for osteoporosis. Other risk factors include alcohol use, smoking, poor nutrition, physical inactivity, low body mass index (BMI), hypogonadism, and family history of osteoporosis and/or fragility fractures. Numerous medications can increase the risk of osteoporosis; in particular, glucocorticoids promote bone resorption and inhibit bone deposition through a variety of mechanisms, including inducement of osteoblastic apoptosis. Other medications that increase risk of osteoporosis include antiepileptics, thiazolidinediones, heparin, cyclosporine, tacrolimus, selective serotonin reuptake inhibitors, antimetabolite drugs such as methotrexate, aromatase inhibitors, gonadotropin-releasing hormone agonists, antiandrogens, and high-dose progesterone. There is increasing evidence that proton-pump inhibitors decrease absorption of calcium and may increase risk of osteoporosis (Fig. 75.1).

PRESENTATION, EVALUATION, AND DIAGNOSIS

Osteoporosis is asymptomatic unless patients experience a fracture. When fractures occur with minimal trauma, such as falling from standing height or even sneezing, these low-impact fractures are referred to as **fragility fractures,** a hallmark of osteoporosis. The most common sites of fracture are at the spine, hip, and distal radius (also known as a Colles fracture), although virtually any bone is susceptible (Fig. 75.2).

Presentation of vertebral fractures is highly variable and may present with acute, severe back pain, radiculopathy, or may be clinically silent. Sometimes, the only

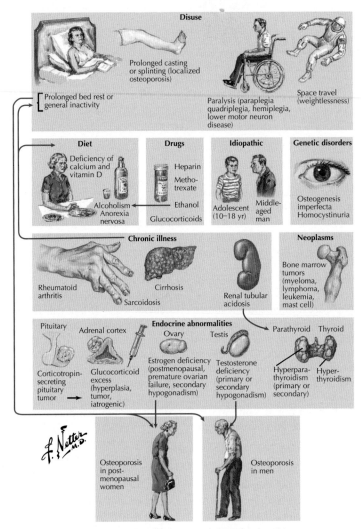

FIG. 75.1 **Risk Factors for Osteoporosis.**

manifestation of vertebral fracture(s) is loss of height or development of kyphosis (Fig. 75.3). Femoral head and distal radial fractures typically present with acute pain at the involved site. Hip fractures are associated with significant morbidity and loss of function; 1-year mortality following hip fracture is as high as 25%.

Osteoporosis is typically diagnosed via **dual energy x-ray absorptiometry (DEXA),** an imaging technique that allows for estimation of **bone mineral density (BMD).** BMD is measured in comparison to a reference population of young, healthy adults to create a T score. In men and postmenopausal women, a T score ≤2.5 standard deviations below the mean BMD of the reference population meets criteria for osteoporosis. A T score

between -1.0 and -2.5 meets criteria for **osteopenia,** an intermediate stage of low BMD. T scores should not be applied to premenopausal women, as the relationship between BMD and fracture risk in this population is less certain. As BMD by DEXA is not a perfect measure of bone quality, anyone who suffers a fragility fracture also meets criteria for osteoporosis.

As many as 40% of postmenopausal women meet criteria for osteoporosis. Because this disease is widely prevalent and treatable, the US Preventative Task Force (USPTF) recommends that all women ≥65 years of age, as well as younger women whose risk is equal to or greater than that of a 65-year-old Caucasian female, should undergo screening via DEXA scan. The USPTF

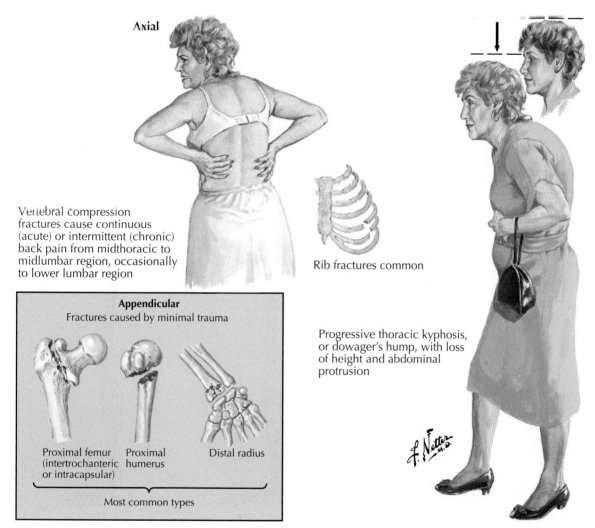

Axial

Vertebral compression fractures cause continuous (acute) or intermittent (chronic) back pain from midthoracic to midlumbar region, occasionally to lower lumbar region

Rib fractures common

Appendicular
Fractures caused by minimal trauma

Proximal femur (intertrochanteric or intracapsular)

Proximal humerus

Distal radius

Most common types

Progressive thoracic kyphosis, or dowager's hump, with loss of height and abdominal protrusion

FIG. 75.2 **Clinical Manifestations of Osteoporosis.**

does not make recommendations for screening men. However, current evidence supports screening men >70 years of age, and younger men with multiple risk factors for osteoporosis. Anyone who suffers a fragility fracture should undergo DEXA scan to evaluate their BMD, more to establish a baseline BMD prior to osteoporosis treatment than to make a diagnosis of osteoporosis, as the occurrence of a fragility fracture already meets the definition of osteoporosis.

Once low bone density or fragility fracture is diagnosed, physicians should evaluate for contributing factors: secondary causes of osteoporosis and alternate diagnoses. In addition to osteoporosis, the differential for apparent low-trauma fractures includes malignancy, osteomalacia, renal osteodystrophy, Paget disease, and

physical abuse. A careful history and physical exam, including an evaluation of the patient's nutritional status, physical activity level, and medication list, can help assess for etiologies of secondary osteoporosis. In addition, basic chemistries (including calcium and phosphorus), vitamin D, parathyroid hormone (PTH), complete blood count, liver function tests, and a thyroid-stimulating hormone should be checked. Elevated urine calcium can reveal evidence of hypercalciuria.

TREATMENT

All patients >50 years of age with a BMD T score ≤−2.5 meet criteria for osteoporosis and should be offered pharmacological treatment, as should anyone >50 years

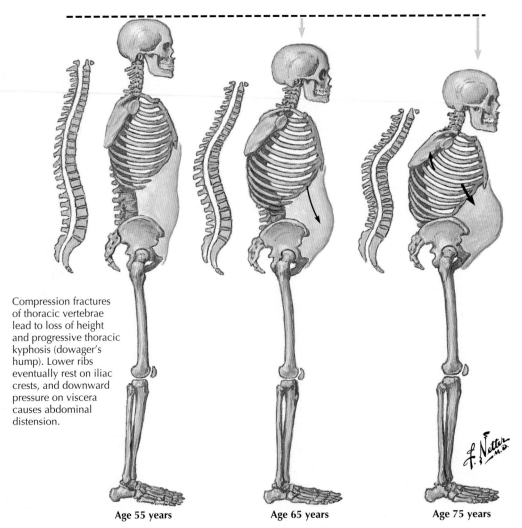

Compression fractures
of thoracic vertebrae
lead to loss of height
and progressive thoracic
kyphosis (dowager's
hump). Lower ribs
eventually rest on iliac
crests, and downward
pressure on viscera
causes abdominal
distension.

Age 55 years   Age 65 years   Age 75 years

FIG. 75.3 **Progressive Spinal Deformity in Osteoporosis.**

of age with a history of fragility fracture. Pharmacological therapy is also offered to those at high risk of clinically significant fracture. We can assess fracture risk via the **Fracture Risk Assessment Tool (FRAX)**. The FRAX is an assessment model available online that calculates the 10-year risk of hip fracture and combined risk of other osteoporotic fracture, based on BMD from the patient's DEXA scan and other readily available clinical data. Anyone with ≥3% risk of hip fracture and/or 20% risk of osteoporotic fracture may be offered pharmacological treatment, although pharmacotherapy for prevention of fractures is less effective in patients without a diagnosis of osteoporosis. Note that the FRAX tool is not validated in premenopausal women or men aged ≤40 years.

Lifestyle counseling should be offered to anyone with low BMD, including osteopenia. All patients should be counseled to ingest 1200 mg of elemental calcium daily; if unable to obtain this via their diet, they should also take calcium supplementation. Additionally, patients with low BMD should take 800 IU of vitamin D daily. Patients should engage in a combination of strength-training and weight-bearing exercises. Fall precautions, including physical therapy and balance training, are particularly important for elderly and frail patients with osteoporosis to prevent fractures. All patients should be counseled to limit alcohol intake and stop smoking, if applicable.

For patients who require pharmacological treatment, **bisphosphonates** are first-line agents. There are numerous bisphosphonates available on the market, both as oral and intravenous formulations with variable dosing schedules. These medications have a high affinity for the bone, where they are absorbed and prevent osteoclast-mediated bone resorption. As a class, the oral formulations of these medications may irritate the esophagus (gastroesophageal reflux disease [GERD], esophagitis) and are contraindicated in patients with esophageal disorders. Patients with GERD whose symptoms are controlled on medications can safely take bisphosphonates. Bisphosphonates are contraindicated in patients with estimated glomerular filtration rate (eGFR) <35 ml/min/1.73 m². Osteonecrosis of the jaw and atypical femoral fractures are well-known but extremely rare side effects of bisphosphonates. If possible, dentoalveolar surgery should be avoided while on these medications. Patients who take bisphosphates should be given a drug holiday after 5 years of therapy to mitigate risk of atypical femur fracture. Additionally, any patient on bisphosphonates who experiences new hip or groin pain should be evaluated for atypical femur fracture. Patients with preexisting hypocalcemia and/or vitamin D deficiency should have this corrected before starting bisphosphonate therapy, as bisphosphonates can contribute to hypocalcemia.

For patients in whom bisphosphonates are contraindicated, or for those who experience progressive decline in BMD despite treatment with bisphosphonates, alternate pharmacological agents are available based on comorbidities and patient preference. For those with esophageal side effects, bisphosphonates can be dosed intravenously on an annual basis. Teriparatide and abaloparatide are PTH analogues that stimulate bone formation and are taken as a daily injection. Denosumab is an anti-RANKL antibody, injected monthly. Selective estrogen receptor modulators (SERMs), such as raloxifene, can improve BMD, although only at the spine. Some side effects of SERMs include hot flashes and increased risk of thromboembolic events. Bisphosphonates, PTH analogues, and denosumab can also be used to treat osteoporosis in men. Additionally, testosterone replacement should be considered in men with hypogonadism. There are little data to guide treatment of premenopausal osteoporosis, but secondary causes such as nutritional deficiencies, hypoestrogenism, and hyperparathyroidism should be thoroughly ruled out in this patient population.

Adrenal Glands Anatomy and Physiology Review

SARA J. CROMER

INTRODUCTION

The adrenal glands are small, pyramidal-shaped endocrine glands, each weighing 4 to 5 g at adulthood and located just superior to the upper pole of the bilateral kidneys. A thin capsule overlies each adrenal gland. Due to distinct embryological origins, the gland itself can be divided into an outer cortex (from mesoderm origin) and an inner medulla (of neural crest origin) (Fig. 76.1).

The adrenal glands receive a rich blood supply derived from the superior, middle, and inferior adrenal (or suprarenal) arteries, which flow from the inferior phrenic artery, abdominal aorta, and renal artery, respectively. The right adrenal gland drains via the right adrenal vein directly into the inferior vena cava (IVC), whereas the left adrenal vein drains first into the left renal vein and then into the IVC.

The **adrenal cortex** is divided into three zones—the **zona glomerulosa, zona fasciculata,** and **zona reticularis**—which produce different hormones utilizing enzymes present in each zone (Fig. 76.2). It is important to note that all hormones synthesized in the adrenal cortex are **steroid hormones** derived from a cholesterol molecule. Because the adrenal cortex uses cholesterol as a substrate for hormone synthesis, cortical cells are lipid-rich on histology. Steroid hormones are lipophilic, so large proportions of these hormones are protein bound within the serum. As steroids, they take their effect within the nucleus of target cells, where they bind intracellular receptors, which act as hormone-dependent transcription factors, altering deoxyribonucleic acid (DNA) expression and taking action over hours to days.

MINERALOCORTICOIDS

The outermost zone of the adrenal cortex, the zona glomerulosa, produces hormones known as **mineralocorticoids.** These hormones, including **aldosterone,** the primary mineralocorticoid, increase the reabsorption of sodium and water in the kidneys, thereby increasing extracellular volume. Aldosterone secretion is regulated by the **renin-angiotensin-aldosterone system (RAAS).**

RAAS begins with increased production of renin, a hormone secreted by the juxtaglomerular apparatus of the kidney. Renin secretion can be stimulated by multiple physiologic changes: baroreceptors in the afferent arteriole sensing decreased renal perfusion pressure (secondary to true hypovolemia/hypotension or other causes of decreased renal blood flow such as renal artery stenosis); the macula densa sensing decreased sodium delivery to the distal nephron; or sympathetic neurons activating beta-1 receptors in the juxtaglomerular apparatus. Renin converts angiotensinogen to angiotensin I, which is then converted to angiotensin II by angiotensin converting enzyme (ACE) in the lungs. Angiotensin II causes vasoconstriction, increasing blood pressure in the setting of hypovolemia, and promotes secretion of aldosterone from the adrenal gland. Of note, aldosterone secretion is also stimulated, to a much lesser extent, by hyperkalemia, hyponatremia, and elevation in adrenocorticotropic hormone (ACTH) (Fig. 76.3).

Aldosterone acts on the nuclear mineralocorticoid receptor to upregulate epithelial sodium channels (ENaCs) and basolateral sodium-potassium pumps. These proteins increase reabsorption of sodium and water from renal tubular epithelial cells in the distal convoluted tubule and cortical collecting ducts, thereby increasing extracellular volume. This sodium reabsorption is paired to potassium and hydrogen ion secretion (to maintain charge balance) via Na-K pumps within principal cells and H+ ATPase action within intercalated cells, respectively. Lesser, although synergistic, effects of aldosterone include increased absorption of sodium and water in the colon and decreased secretion of sodium and water from salivary and sweat glands.

GLUCOCORTICOIDS

The middle zone of the adrenal cortex is the zona fasciculata, which produces **glucocorticoids,** most notably

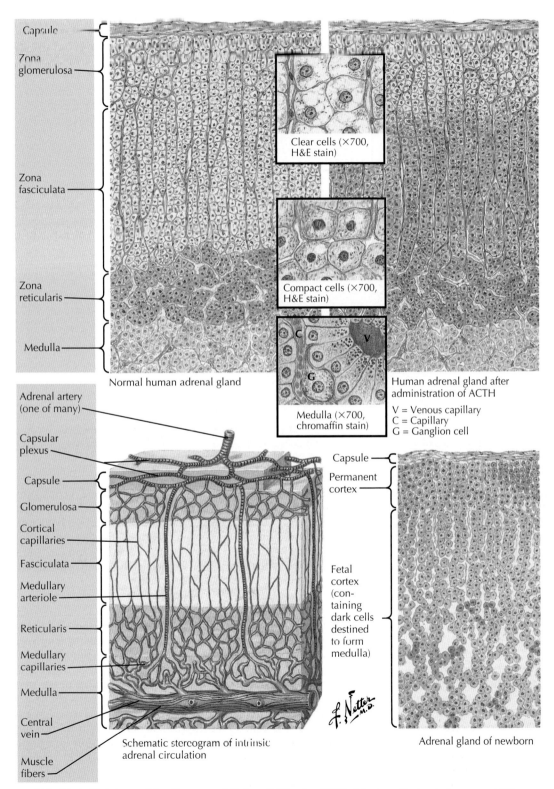

Capsule

Zona glomerulosa

Zona fasciculata

Zona reticularis

Medulla

Clear cells (×700, H&E stain)

Compact cells (×700, H&E stain)

C = Capillary

G = Ganglion cell

V = Venous capillary

Medulla (×700, chromaffin stain)

Normal human adrenal gland

Human adrenal gland after administration of ACTH

V = Venous capillary
C = Capillary
G = Ganglion cell

Adrenal artery (one of many)

Capsular plexus

Capsule

Glomerulosa

Cortical capillaries

Fasciculata

Medullary arteriole

Reticularis

Medullary capillaries

Medulla

Central vein

Muscle fibers

Schematic stereogram of intrinsic adrenal circulation

Capsule

Permanent cortex

Fetal cortex (containing dark cells destined to form medulla)

Adrenal gland of newborn

FIG. 76.1 **Histology of the Suprarenal (Adrenal) Glands.** *ACTH,* Adrenocorticotropic hormone; *H&E,* hematoxylin and eosin.

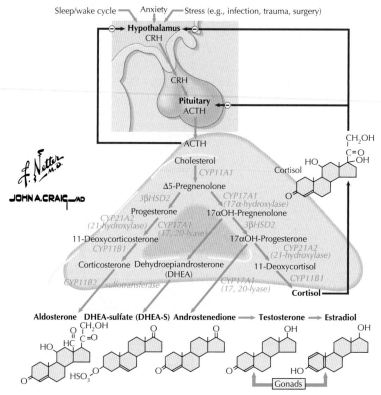

FIG. 76.2 Adrenal Cortical Hormones. *ACTH,* Adrenocorticotropic hormone; *CRH,* corticotropin-releasing hormone; *3βHSD2,* 3β-hydroxysteroid dehydrogenase; *CYP11B1,* steroid 11β-hydroxylase; *CYP11B2,* aldosterone synthase.

cortisol. Glucocorticoid synthesis and secretion are mediated primarily by ACTH produced in the anterior pituitary gland, which itself is regulated by secretion of corticotropin-releasing hormone (CRH) from the hypothalamus. CRH, ACTH, and cortisol are secreted in a circadian fashion with peak serum levels occurring in the early morning and trough levels occurring in the evening.

Glucocorticoids have a variety of functions within the body and are often secreted in response to a stressor. Acutely, glucocorticoids increase glycogenolysis in both liver and muscle tissue, but if fasting is prolonged, they can prepare the body for a starvation state by promoting hepatic gluconeogenesis, using amino acids from muscle breakdown and fatty acids from lipolysis as alternative energy sources. They also induce the upregulation of antiinflammatory molecules, which can impair an individual's immune response; specifically, glucocorticoids moderate the immune response by stabilizing lysosomal membranes, preventing release of proteolytic enzymes, and decreasing capillary permeability and leukocyte

chemotaxis. Chronic glucocorticoid excess can also lead to atrophy of lymphoid tissues, further impairing immune responses, as well as increased bone turnover and thinned skin/easy bruisability. Of note, cortisol also has mild mineralocorticoid activity and can contribute to the hypertension frequently seen in hypercortisolism.

ADRENAL ANDROGENS

The innermost zone of the cortex, the zona reticularis, produces male sex hormones, including dihydroepiandrosterone (DHEA), dihydroepiandrosterone-sulfate (DHEA-S), androstenedione, and 11-hydroxyandrostenedione, as well as small quantities of estrogen and progesterone. While these hormones all have weak effects and play a role in early sexual development and puberty in both sexes, they take their main effect through peripheral or extraadrenal conversion to testosterone in men and, via aromatase, estrogen in women. The zona reticularis is also stimulated, in part, by secretion of ACTH.

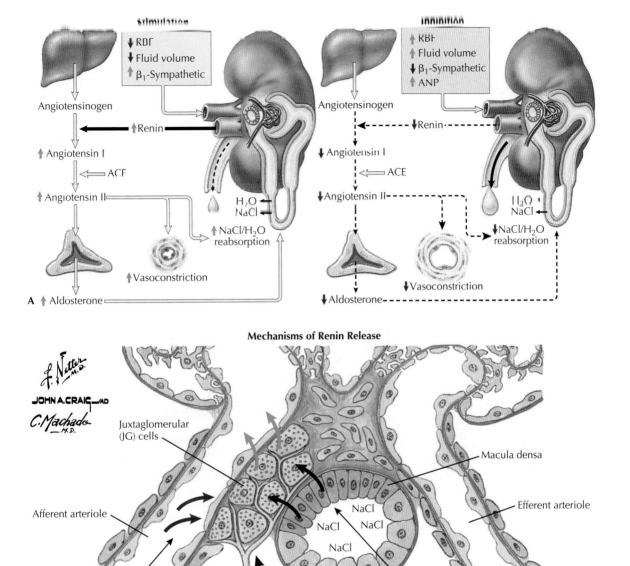

FIG. 76.3 Regulation of the Renin-Angiotensin-Aldosterone System. *ANP,* Atrial natriuretic peptide; *RBF,* renal blood flow.

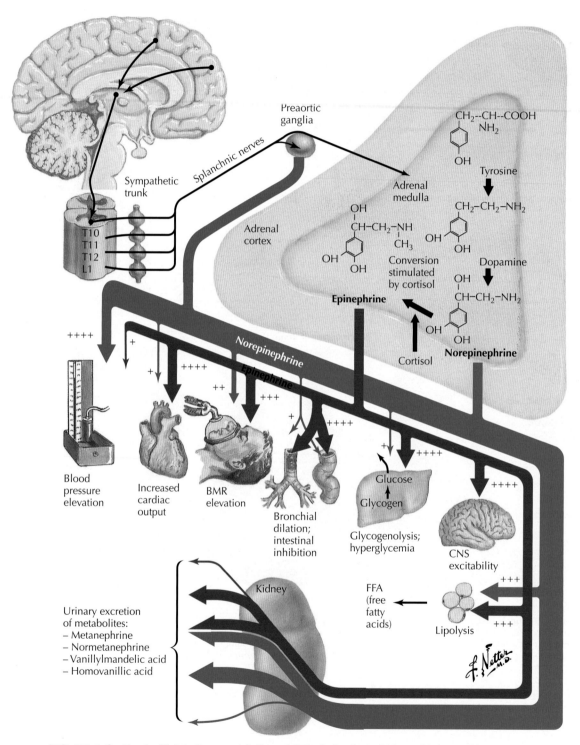

FIG. 76.4 Synthesis, Metabolism, and Action of Catecholamines. Refer to Chapter 18 for further information on catecholamine activity. *BMR,* Basal metabolic rate; *CNS,* central nervous system.

CATECHOLAMINES

The adrenal medulla differs from the adrenal cortex in that it secretes nonsteroidal catecholamine hormones, synthesized by chromaffin cells. The adrenal medulla is often considered to be an extension of the sympathetic nervous system, as it originates from embryonic neural crest cells and is regulated by acetylcholine release from preganglionic sympathetic nerves arising from the intermediolateral horn of the spinal cord. The medulla releases **catecholamines**, including ~80% **epinephrine**, also known as adrenaline, 20% **norepinephrine**, also known as noradrenaline, and trace amounts of dopamine, in the setting of a sympathetic nervous system activation from a stressor. These hormones bind to adrenergic and dopaminergic receptors throughout the body, regulating the fight-or-flight response by increasing heart rate, respiratory rate, and peripheral vascular resistance, among other effects (Fig. 76.4).

Of note, other sites of chromaffin cells exist throughout the body, mostly in midline complexes, including the paraaortic organ of Zuckerkandl. These cell clusters are believed to arise from neural crest cells that have failed to successfully migrate to the adrenal medulla.

CHAPTER 77

Cushing Syndrome

BENJAMIN D. GALLAGHER

INTRODUCTION

Cushing syndrome refers to a constellation of signs and symptoms attributable to glucocorticoid excess. Today the most common cause of **hypercortisolism** is iatrogenic, as corticosteroids are routinely prescribed for a variety of medical problems. This chapter discusses the endogenous causes of Cushing syndrome.

PATHOPHYSIOLOGY

Endogenous hypercortisolism is due either to excess adrenocorticotropic hormone (ACTH) production (80% of cases) or to autonomous production of cortisol by one or both adrenal glands (20%). ACTH-dependent causes include pituitary corticotroph adenomas (known as **Cushing disease,** 70% of all cases) and extrapituitary tumors (known as ectopic ACTH syndrome, 10%). Most cases of ectopic ACTH syndrome are caused by small cell lung cancer or carcinoid tumors. The most common cause of ACTH-independent Cushing syndrome is a benign adrenocortical adenoma. Less common are adrenocortical carcinoma (ACC) and bilateral adrenal hyperplasia.

Cushing syndrome is a rare condition, with an incidence of 0.2 to 0.5 per million person-years. There is an overall female-to-male predominance of 3 : 1, but this varies by etiology. While Cushing disease favors women over men by 5 : 1 and is usually diagnosed in the third or fourth decade of life, ectopic ACTH syndrome is most common in older men, mainly owing to the increased incidence of lung cancer in this group. The leading cause of death in Cushing syndrome is cardiovascular disease, with serious infections and venous thromboembolic events also contributing significantly to mortality.

PRESENTATION, EVALUATION, AND DIAGNOSIS

Because glucocorticoids act on every tissue in the body, the signs and symptoms of Cushing syndrome are myriad. Perhaps the most notable is weight gain around the abdomen (central obesity), with associated fat accumulation in the cheeks (moon facies) and dorsocervical fat pads (buffalo hump), as well as supraclavicular fullness. Thinning of the skin, easy bruisability, facial plethora, and thick, violaceous striae are common dermatological manifestations. The catabolic effects of excess cortisol cause proximal muscle weakness, and decreased bone formation and increased bone resorption result in early-onset osteoporosis and increased predisposition to fracture. Glucose intolerance and frank diabetes mellitus may occur and are attributable to increased gluconeogenesis and the insulin resistance that comes with obesity. Compared to the general population, patients with Cushing syndrome have a 10-fold higher risk of venous thromboembolic events due to increased synthesis of coagulation factors and impaired fibrinolysis (Fig. 77.1).

Although the mechanisms are poorly understood, Cushing syndrome is associated with neuropsychiatric disturbances, immunosuppression, and menstrual irregularities. When glucocorticoid levels exceed the capacity of 11β-hydroxysteroid dehydrogenase in the kidney to inactivate cortisol to cortisone, signs of mineralocorticoid excess (including hypertension, edema, hypokalemia, and metabolic alkalosis) develop.

Hyperpigmentation occurs only in ACTH-dependent Cushing syndrome, as ACTH is secreted as part of the precursor polypeptide pro-opiomelanocortin (POMC), which also includes the melanocyte-stimulating hormone (MSH). This is most often seen in the ectopic ACTH syndrome, where ACTH levels can be quite high. Since the adrenals are the major source of androgens in women but not men, women alone may experience symptoms of androgen excess, such as hirsutism and acne. This is especially pronounced in cases of ACC, where the tumor may produce adrenal androgens as well as cortisol.

Many of the features of Cushing syndrome are non-specific and common in the general population, making the diagnosis a challenging one. The rapid development of severe manifestations of multiple symptoms is most suggestive of true hypercortisolism. Easy bruising, facial plethora, proximal myopathy, striae, and unexplained

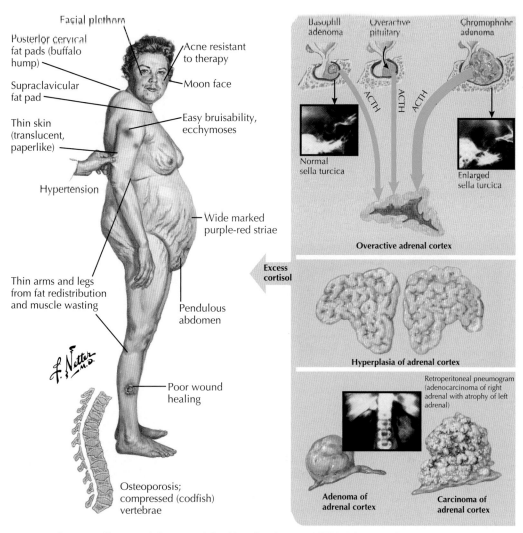

FIG. 77.1 Signs and Causes of Cushing Syndrome. *ACTH*, Adrenocorticotropic hormone.

osteoporosis are thought to have the best discriminatory value in making the diagnosis.

Patients suspected of having Cushing syndrome should undergo one of three available screening tests to confirm hypercortisolism: the 24-hour urine free cortisol test, the late-night salivary cortisol test, and the overnight 1-mg **dexamethasone suppression test.** The results of the urine test represent total cortisol excretion over a 24-hour period, whereas the saliva test is a measure of cortisol at its daily nadir (so that an elevated level signifies cortisol excess). If either of these cortisol based assays is chosen as the initial test, at least two samples should be obtained due to the variability of cortisol levels in Cushing syndrome. In the dexamethasone suppression

test, the patient takes 1 mg dexamethasone at bedtime, and the serum cortisol is measured the following day at 8:00 a.m. (when cortisol is at its daily peak). In normal subjects, dexamethasone suppresses the a.m. cortisol level, but patients with Cushing syndrome fail to suppress due to autonomous cortisol. The dexamethasone suppression test assumes the patient has a typical day/night, awake/asleep cycle and may need to be modified in those with irregular sleep patterns, such as nightshift workers.

Patients with one positive screening test should undergo one of the other tests for confirmation. If the initial screening test is negative but suspicion for Cushing syndrome is high, it is reasonable to perform a different

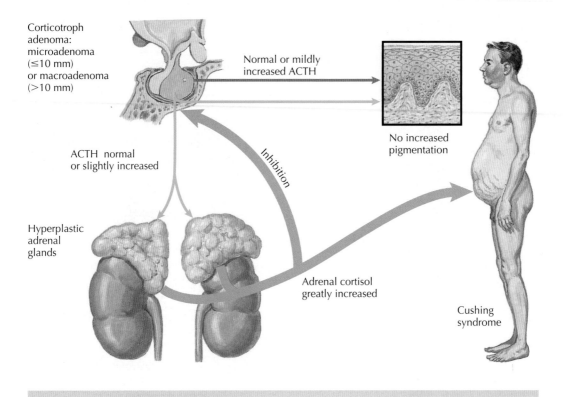

Corticotroph adenoma: microadenoma (≤10 mm) or macroadenoma (>10 mm)

Normal or mildly increased ACTH

No increased pigmentation

ACTH normal or slightly increased

Inhibition

Hyperplastic adrenal glands

Adrenal cortisol greatly increased

Cushing syndrome

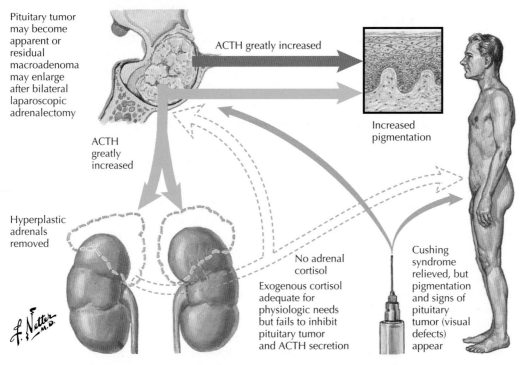

Pituitary tumor may become apparent or residual macroadenoma may enlarge after bilateral laparoscopic adrenalectomy

ACTH greatly increased

Increased pigmentation

ACTH greatly increased

Hyperplastic adrenals removed

No adrenal cortisol

Exogenous cortisol adequate for physiologic needs but fails to inhibit pituitary tumor and ACTH secretion

Cushing syndrome relieved, but pigmentation and signs of pituitary tumor (visual defects) appear

FIG. 77.2 **Nelson Syndrome.** *ACTH,* Adrenocorticotropic hormone.

test. Patients with discrepant results on two tests, or with two negative tests despite high clinical suspicion, should undergo further evaluation under the guidance of an endocrinologist.

Once the diagnosis of Cushing syndrome has been established, the next step is to determine its etiology by measuring the plasma ACTH level. Patients with suppressed ACTH have ACTH-independent Cushing syndrome and should undergo cross-sectional imaging of the adrenal glands. Patients with elevated ACTH levels in the setting of hypercortisolism have either Cushing disease or ectopic ACTH production. Differentiating between these two diagnoses can be challenging. While the vast majority will have Cushing disease, pituitary MRI is only 50% sensitive in detecting corticotroph adenomas, which can be quite small, and given the high prevalence of clinically insignificant microadenomas in the general population, an adenoma should not be deemed causative unless it measures >6 mm.

Three noninvasive biochemical tests are also available. In the modified low-dose dexamethasone suppression test, the patient takes 2 mg dexamethasone (divided dosing over 48 hours) and cortisol is measured in the morning, 6 hours after the last dose of dexamethasone. This test may have improved specificity to the traditional 1-mg dexamethasone suppression test. In the high-dose dexamethasone suppression test, the patient takes 8 mg dexamethasone at bedtime, then the serum cortisol is measured the following day at 8:00 a.m. Because patients with Cushing disease are only relatively resistant to negative feedback inhibition, their a.m. cortisol will be suppressed to at least 50% of the baseline morning cortisol value, whereas in patients with extrapituitary sources of ACTH, the a.m. cortisol will either fail to suppress or will suppress but by <50% of the baseline morning cortisol value. The high-dose dexamethasone suppression test, however, has fallen out of favor in recent years due to significant overlap in pituitary and ectopic tumor responses to high-dose dexamethasone.

The corticotropin-releasing hormone (CRH) stimulation test involves measuring the change in serum ACTH and cortisol following administration of CRH. Corticotroph adenomas remain sensitive to CRH, so ACTH and cortisol levels will increase in Cushing disease, but this is not seen in ectopic ACTH syndrome because the extrapituitary tumor is completely autonomous and thus unresponsive to CRH. The CRH stimulation test, however, is difficult to administer from a practical perspective due to lack of availability of CRH preparations.

The gold standard test for differentiating between pituitary and ectopic Cushing syndrome is **inferior petrossal sinus sampling (IPSS)**. During this procedure, catheters are introduced into the inferior petrossal sinuses bilaterally (where the pituitary gland drains) to measure the ACTH levels at baseline and in response to CRH stimulation. Because IPSS is invasive and available only at specialized centers, many clinicians pursue it only if biochemical tests suggest Cushing disease and pituitary MRI shows no adenoma or shows an adenoma that is <6 mm in size.

If the evaluation points to the ectopic ACTH syndrome, imaging should be pursued to search for an extrapituitary tumor; most often chest imaging has the highest yield in these cases.

TREATMENT

The first-line treatment for all types of Cushing syndrome is surgical. Patients with adrenocortical adenomas or ACC should undergo unilateral adrenalectomy, and those with bilateral adrenal hyperplasia necessitate bilateral adrenalectomy, provided cortisol production is elevated bilaterally, which can be assessed by adrenal vein sampling. In the ectopic ACTH syndrome, the culprit tumor should be resected.

The standard of care for Cushing disease is transsphenoidal surgery (TSS) (selective adenomectomy), which leads to remission in 80% of microadenomas but <50% of macroadenomas. The success of Cushing disease remission is also highly dependent on the skill and experience of the neurosurgeon; ideally, these patients will be directed to a center or surgeon with experience in Cushing disease surgeries.

If TSS is unsuccessful or relapse occurs, second-line options include repeat surgery, radiation, and medical therapy; medical therapy includes steroidogenesis inhibitors (ketoconazole, metyrapone, etomidate), adrenolytics (mitotane), antipituitary drugs (pasireotide, cabergoline), and glucocorticoid receptor antagonists (mifepristone). In refractory cases of Cushing disease, bilateral adrenalectomy may be pursued for refractory symptoms. The resulting loss of negative feedback from adrenal cortisol production may lead to corticotroph adenoma growth, extreme ACTH elevation, and marked hyperpigmentation, a condition known as Nelson syndrome (Fig. 77.2).

All patients who undergo surgery for Cushing syndrome require glucocorticoid replacement until the suppressed hypothalamic-pituitary adrenal (HPA) axis recovers (usually several months to 1 year), while those undergoing bilateral adrenalectomy require lifelong glucocorticoid and mineralocorticoid replacement.

CHAPTER 78

Adrenal Insufficiency

RICHARD K. KIM

INTRODUCTION

Adrenal insufficiency (AI) occurs when the adrenal glands are unable to produce adequate amounts of steroid hormones. There are three types of AI corresponding to the hypothalamic-pituitary-adrenal (HPA) axis: primary, secondary, and tertiary. Damage or suppression of the adrenal glands can be insidious or acute, creating presentations that are either diagnostically confusing or medically emergent. The diagnosis of AI is classically associated with weakness, anorexia, and orthostatic hypotension. Low random or morning cortisol may trigger further laboratory testing and imaging of the HPA axis to confirm the etiology.

Primary AI, or **Addison disease,** is rare in the United States, occurring in 1 in 25,000 people. The most common cause of primary AI worldwide is tuberculosis. Secondary AI is more common and often iatrogenic from exogenous steroid administration. Cardiac and infectious complications, as well as delay in diagnosis and treatment, can result in significant morbidity and death.

PATHOPHYSIOLOGY

Chronic, primary AI is most commonly due to autoimmune destruction of the adrenal gland **(autoimmune adrenalitis)** via autoantibodies to 21-hydroxylase and 17-hydroxylase, enzymes critical in the synthesis of steroid hormones. In tuberculosis and fungal disease, granulomatous inflammation directly destroys steroidogenic cells. While the adrenals have a rich blood supply, hemorrhage and ischemia can also cause primary AI. Growth of metastatic carcinoma, commonly from breast, lung, and renal cancers, can perturb glandular structure, causing endocrine dysfunction. Glucocorticoid, mineralocorticoid, and androgen insufficiency can all occur, but >90% of the glands must be involved for symptoms of chronic disease to manifest.

In secondary AI, the anterior pituitary fails to produce adrenocorticotropic hormone (ACTH). In tertiary AI, the hypothalamus does not make corticotropin-releasing hormone (CRH). Both cause atrophy of the zona fasciculata and low cortisol production. Unlike primary chronic AI, only glucocorticoid deficiency is present in secondary and tertiary AI. As mentioned earlier, the majority of cases are from the use of synthetic glucocorticoids, but pituitary disease, surgery, autoimmune destruction of corticotrophs, and/or irradiation can also cause ACTH/CRH insufficiency.

Acute AI is either insufficient or absent steroid production in response to stress. The body can adapt to chronic AI, but can succumb to acute AI if homeostasis is perturbed by any inflammatory stressor that mandates immediate increases in steroid output. Long-term corticosteroid administration causes suppression of the HPA axis and adrenal atrophy. Withdrawal of exogenous steroids or failure to increase doses during acute stress in a steroid-dependent patient can induce acute AI or **adrenal crisis.**

Any critical illness that causes significant hypotension and/or shock may cause adrenal hypoperfusion and infarction. In particular, **Waterhouse-Friderichsen syndrome** occurs when overwhelming bacterial sepsis, most commonly from *Neisseria meningitidis*, leads to septic shock and direct bacterial seeding of adrenal vessels. This, in turn, triggers disseminated intravascular coagulation, leading to massive adrenal hemorrhage and adrenocortical insufficiency (Fig. 78.1).

RISK FACTORS

Autoimmune adrenalitis is more common in females and children. In adults, it most commonly presents between ages 30 and 50. Personal or family history of autoimmune disease, including type 1 diabetes, Hashimoto thyroiditis, vitiligo, pernicious anemia, and antiphospholipid syndrome, is associated with earlier presentation of Addison disease. Other risk factors include exogenous steroid dependence, tuberculosis exposure, HIV/AIDS, and cancer. Deposition diseases, including hemochromatosis, amyloidosis, and sarcoidosis, are associated with primary chronic AI. Anticonvulsant

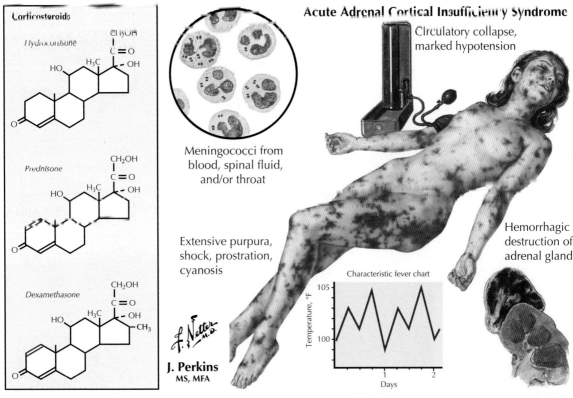

FIG. 78.1 Waterhouse-Friderichsen Syndrome.

medications and the anesthetic etomidate are especially associated with adrenal suppression. Secondary AI is becoming an increasingly known side effect of novel monoclonal antibody-based chemotherapeutic agents such as ipilimumab.

PRESENTATION, EVALUATION, AND DIAGNOSIS

In chronic primary and secondary AI, anorexia, fatigue, and orthostatic hypotension are common. Nausea and vomiting may be present, in addition to myalgias and arthralgias. Laboratory abnormalities include hyponatremia and hyperkalemia. Primary AI also presents with cutaneous and mucosal hyperpigmentation; ACTH and melanocyte-stimulating hormone (MSH) share the same precursor molecule, and upregulated ACTH production in response to adrenal insufficiency leads to concomitant increased MSH, in turn causing the abovementioned skin changes (Fig. 78.2). Physicians should look for signs and symptoms of other autoimmune disorders that

may be present, such as the autoimmune polyendocrine syndrome type 2, which is characterized by primary AI, primary hypothyroidism, and type 1 diabetes.

Patients in acute adrenal crisis may present with abdominal, flank, or back pain in the setting of fever, hypotension not responsive to intravenous (IV) fluids, and hypoglycemia. Altered mental status is common.

In the hospitalized patient, random serum cortisol can be obtained for initial evaluation. Any value >20 µg/dL may reflect intact adrenal function. Early a.m. serum cortisol is better and more sensitive because it should be elevated during the waking process. A value <5 µg/dL is strongly suggestive of AI; values <10 µg/dL are also suggestive but warrant a **cosyntropin stimulation test (CST)**. Of note, cortisol measurements may be inaccurate in patients with abnormalities in albumin or cortisol-binding globulin (CBG), including those with cirrhosis or nephrotic syndrome, or women taking oral contraceptives (which raise CBG levels). Free cortisol levels and measurement of CBG can be considered if available. If AI is high on the differential and immediate

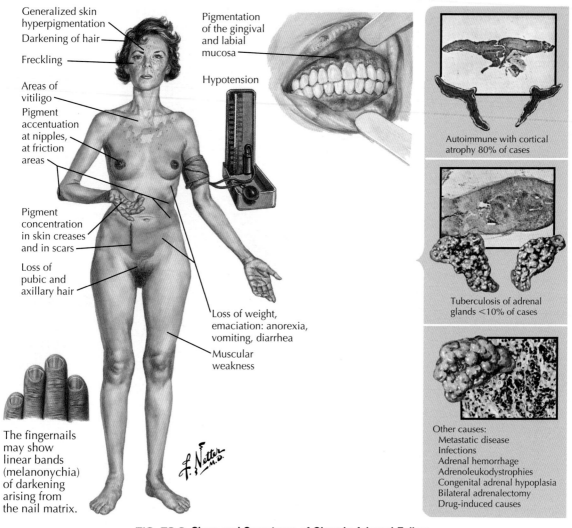

Generalized skin hyperpigmentation

Darkening of hair

Freckling

Areas of vitiligo

Pigment accentuation at nipples, at friction areas

Pigment concentration in skin creases and in scars

Loss of pubic and axillary hair

The fingernails may show linear bands (melanonychia) of darkening arising from the nail matrix.

Pigmentation of the gingival and labial mucosa

Hypotension

Loss of weight, emaciation: anorexia, vomiting, diarrhea

Muscular weakness

Autoimmune with cortical atrophy 80% of cases

Tuberculosis of adrenal glands <10% of cases

Other causes:
Metastatic disease
Infections
Adrenal hemorrhage
Adrenoleukodystrophies
Congenital adrenal hypoplasia
Bilateral adrenalectomy
Drug-induced causes

FIG. 78.2 **Signs and Symptoms of Chronic Adrenal Failure.**

steroids are planned, a concomitant serum ACTH level can be obtained; ACTH is elevated in primary AI and decreased in secondary/tertiary AI.

To perform a CST, the patient receives ACTH 250 μg, either intravenously or intramuscularly. Cortisol levels are measured at 30 and 60 minutes following ACTH administration. A poststimulation cortisol value >20 μg/dL confirms intact adrenal function. In early acute secondary or tertiary AI, this value may be falsely negative because the adrenal glands may still respond. For a hemodynamically unstable patient, dexamethasone should be used for steroid replacement because it interferes less with most cortisol assays and facilitates

CST if needed. However, any steroid administration for more than a few days or at higher than physiological replacement doses may interfere with testing results.

Septic patients may have reduced cortisol responses to the CST between 30 and 60 minutes, but such a diagnosis of "relative AI" remains controversial. While the CST helps to predict mortality from sepsis, it does not predict benefit from corticosteroid supplementation.

CT of the adrenal glands can be considered if primary AI is suspected, particularly in acute AI or in HIV/AIDS patients with higher risks of infection. Pituitary MRI may detect lesions if secondary AI, independent of exogenous steroids, is suspected. The adrenal glands may appear atrophic on imaging. In cases of prolonged secondary or tertiary AI due to lack of pulsatile stimulation by ACTH.

TREATMENT

In acute adrenal crisis, volume resuscitation with isotonic saline and IV hydrocortisone is needed. Dosing and frequency of hydrocortisone usually starts at 50 to 100 mg every 6 hours, tapered over 3 to 5 days. In an unstable patient with suspected AI, dexamethasone can be used instead so that subsequent diagnostic workup can avoid cortisol cross-reactivity.

There is a lack of consensus regarding hydrocortisone supplementation in septic shock. Although the Surviving Sepsis Campaign continues to recommend its use in refractory shock, the largest randomized controlled trials had divergent conclusions on exogenous steroidal effect on septic shock prevention, morbidity, and mortality. Use of hydrocortisone remains institution and patient specific.

Primary chronic AI merits replacement of both glucocorticoids and mineralocorticoids. Glucocorticoids include hydrocortisone, prednisone, and dexamethasone, while fludrocortisone supplements mineralocorticoid activity. The glucocorticoids prednisone and hydrocortisone have mineralocorticoid activity at higher than physiological replacement doses, whereas dexamethasone does not have mineralocorticoid activity at any dose. Consequently, patients with primary AI may be able to forego fludrocortisone doses in temporary situations, such as stress, when they are taking supraphysiological hydrocortisone or prednisone. Secondary chronic AI warrants only glucocorticoid replacement because mineralocorticoid function is under the regulation of the renin-angiotensin-aldosterone system (RAAS) in the zona glomerulosa. Physiological daily cortisol secretion is equivalent to 10 to 25 mg/day of hydrocortisone or 4 to 7 mg/day of prednisone. Because glucocorticoids are metabolized by the cytochrome P450 system, higher doses are needed for patients taking P450 inducers, such as rifampin and phenytoin. Lower doses are needed for those taking P450 inhibiting medications, such as protease inhibitors. Close monitoring by a primary care physician and an endocrinologist should focus on evidence of underreplacement (weakness, dizziness) or overreplacement (cushingoid features, osteoporosis).

Because of a dysfunctional HPA axis, patients under physiologic stress may require additional doses of steroids, termed stress dosing. Optimal stress dosing for chronic AI patients suffering from acute illness has not been established. One common practice involves doubling or tripling the maintenance doses of outpatient steroids with gradual tapering to baseline as the patient improves. As an example, maintenance doses are used during pregnancy, but stress doses are used during labor and delivery.

Surgery is an acute stressor meriting consideration for perioperative steroid supplementation in patients with chronic AI. There is a lack of consensus on how patients at risk for adrenal crisis should be identified, but any patient receiving the equivalent of greater than prednisone 5 mg/day for >3 weeks within the previous year is considered at risk. Superficial surgeries, such as dental procedures or biopsies, may not require supplementation. Optimal supplemental dosing of steroids is also debated. For now, minor procedures merit hydrocortisone 25 mg IV; moderate procedures merit hydrocortisone 50 to 75 mg IV tapered over 1 to 2 days. Major surgeries warrant hydrocortisone at 100 to 150 mg IV tapered over 1 to 2 days.

CHAPTER 79

Adrenal Masses

JUDITH KIM

INTRODUCTION

With the widespread use of cross-sectional imaging, including CT and MRI, physicians are increasingly encountering adrenal masses. Increased detection of these masses has led to the adoption of a new diagnosis, termed **incidentaloma,** for those incidentally found masses >1 cm in diameter. Adrenal masses are seen in about 1% to 9% of the population, based on findings of autopsy studies, with the prevalence increasing with age.

An adrenal mass can have a variety of clinical presentations and effects. A mass can be benign and further delineated as either nonfunctional or functional based on potential hormone secretion. Alternatively, a mass may be a malignant tumor, either a primary adrenal carcinoma (which may or may not secrete hormones) or metastasis from another primary malignancy. Given the importance for eventual treatment or surveillance, it is crucial to be able to identify any potential malignancy and/or hormone-producing mass.

EVALUATION, DIAGNOSIS, AND TREATMENT

Benign Masses

The majority of adrenal masses are benign. Most are nonfunctional, adrenocortical adenomas, but ~10% secrete excess hormones. All patients with an adrenal mass should undergo biochemical testing for aldosterone hypersecretion (the most common abnormality, also known as Conn syndrome), **Cushing syndrome,** and **pheochromocytoma.**

Up to 6.7% of adrenal incidentalomas produce cortisol, leading to subclinical or clinical Cushing syndrome. Patients typically lack overt Cushing syndrome features but are more likely to have hypertension, dyslipidemia, diabetes, and atherosclerosis. An overnight dexamethasone suppression test can confirm adrenocorticotropic hormone (ACTH)–independent cortisol production, and Cushing syndrome can be diagnosed with further testing. Patients with excess endogenous glucocorticoid production should be considered for unilateral adrenalectomy,

particularly in younger patients or those with disorders due to the excess cortisol (see Chapter 77 for further information). Note that these patients are often adrenally insufficient after unilateral adrenalectomy due to suppression of cortisol production by the uninvolved adrenal gland, which will eventually resume cortisol production, often several months after surgery.

Pheochromocytomas comprise about 3% of adrenal incidentalomas. Pheochromocytomas may have characteristic features on imaging, including size >3 cm, higher attenuation, increased vascularity, and slow washout of contrast. All adrenal incidentalomas should be assessed for catecholamine excess; however, when the pretest probability of a pheochromocytoma is high based on imaging, plasma fractionated metanephrines should be measured. Plasma metanephrines have a high sensitivity but lower specificity; for those with lower probability of a pheochromocytoma, a 24-hour collection of urinary fractionated metanephrines and catecholamines may be preferred. Pheochromocytomas should be resected promptly, as even clinically silent pheochromocytomas can lead to significant cardiovascular complications (Fig. 79.1).

Aldosteronomas comprise <1% of adrenal masses. Patients who have hypertension and an adrenal incidentaloma, or hypertension with hypokalemia, should be ruled out for an aldosteronoma. Initial evaluation begins with checking the plasma aldosterone concentration (PAC) and the plasma renin activity (PRA). A PAC-to-PRA ratio >20 is suggestive of primary aldosteronism but is not diagnostic unless the patient also presents with spontaneous hypokalemia, undetectable renin, and aldosterone concentration >20 ng/dL. If the patient does not fit these criteria, the next diagnostic step is to administer oral sodium chloride (NaCl) and measure urine aldosterone secretion. In primary aldosteronism, urine aldosterone would remain elevated despite oral sodium loading. Adrenal vein sampling can be performed to distinguish a unilateral aldosteronoma from bilateral hyperplasia if there is concern on imaging for bilateral adrenal abnormalities or if the patient is

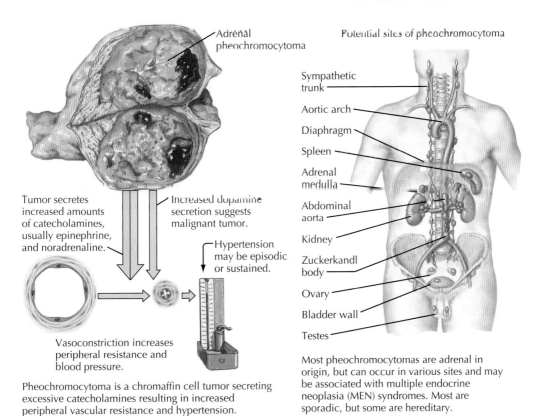

Adrenal pheochromocytoma

Potential sites of pheochromocytoma

Tumor secretes increased amounts of catecholamines, usually epinephrine, and noradrenaline.

Increased dopamine secretion suggests malignant tumor.

Hypertension may be episodic or sustained.

Vasoconstriction increases peripheral resistance and blood pressure.

Pheochromocytoma is a chromaffin cell tumor secreting excessive catecholamines resulting in increased peripheral vascular resistance and hypertension.

Sympathetic trunk

Aortic arch

Diaphragm

Spleen

Adrenal medulla

Abdominal aorta

Kidney

Zuckerkandl body

Ovary

Bladder wall

Testes

Most pheochromocytomas are adrenal in origin, but can occur in various sites and may be associated with multiple endocrine neoplasia (MEN) syndromes. Most are sporadic, but some are hereditary.

Clinical features of pheochromocytoma

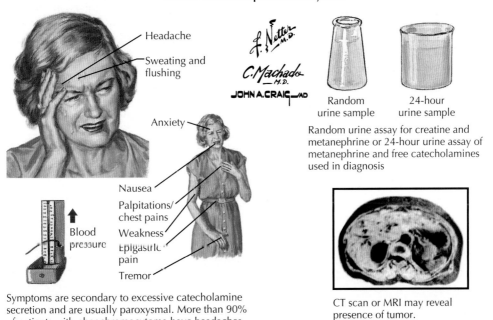

Headache

Sweating and flushing

Anxiety

Nausea

Palpitations/ chest pains

Weakness

Epigastric pain

Tremor

Blood pressure

Random urine sample

24-hour urine sample

Random urine assay for creatine and metanephrine or 24-hour urine assay of metanephrine and free catecholamines used in diagnosis

CT scan or MRI may reveal presence of tumor.

Symptoms are secondary to excessive catecholamine secretion and are usually paroxysmal. More than 90% of patients with pheochromocytoma have headaches, palpitations, and sweating alone or in combination.

FIG. 79.1 **Pheochromocytoma.**

older, which confers a higher chance of incidentalomas than aldosteronoma. Unilateral adrenalectomy is the preferred treatment for patients with an aldosteronoma, but medical management is preferred in those with bilateral adrenal cortical hyperplasia as the etiology of hyperaldosteronism.

If testing for hormonal excess is negative, then the adrenal mass is thought to be a benign, nonfunctional adrenal mass. In these cases, repeat imaging after 6 to 12 months should be performed to evaluate for possible development of malignancy, and repeat hormonal testing should be performed every 1 to 3 years. Physicians may repeat the dexamethasone suppression test yearly for 4 years if initial evaluation is negative, as abnormal adrenal function may not be present at baseline and could be detected on subsequent testing; the utility of such testing is unknown.

Malignant Masses

Malignancy comprises a minority of adrenal masses. About 2% to 5% are found to be primary adrenal cancer, and about ~0.7% to 2.5% are nonadrenal metastases to the gland.

Adrenocortical carcinoma (ACC) is a rare diagnosis with an incidence of one to two cases per million per year. It can develop at any age, though peaks before 5 years of age and in the fourth to fifth decade of life. It is more commonly seen in women than men. Patients can present with abdominal pain or flank pain due to mass effect, or with symptoms related to adrenal hypersecretion of cortisol, androgens, estrogens, or aldosterone. About 60% of ACC cases present clinically with hormonal excess, most commonly Cushing syndrome, though virilization, feminization, or hyperaldosteronism may be evident depending on the hormone secreted. Other tumors are nonfunctioning or have subclinical production of hormones that does not lead to overt symptoms.

ACC can typically be distinguished from a benign adenoma based on imaging phenotype. ACC is significantly associated with larger mass diameter, and 90% are >4 cm in diameter. Compared to an adenoma, an ACC typically appears irregular, vascular, and heterogeneous. On noncontrast enhanced CT, an ACC has higher attenuation (measured by >10 Hounsfield units). Furthermore, on delayed contrast-enhanced CT, a washout of >50% at 10 minutes after contrast administration is reported to be 100% sensitive and specific for adenoma rather than carcinomas, pheochromocytomas, and metastases. Patients who are diagnosed with ACC should undergo prompt surgical adrenalectomy, as the disease can progress rapidly, and medical oncological treatments are not sufficient to cure it.

More common than ACC, the other type of malignant adrenal mass is adrenal metastases. Usually, the primary cancer has already been diagnosed by the time an adrenal mass is found. Fine-needle aspiration biopsy of a nodule can be used to differentiate metastasis from a primary adrenal process, but this should only be done in conjunction with an endocrine surgeon and medical endocrinologist, as suspected ACCs are never to be biopsied due to risk of spreading ACC within the peritoneum. However, a biopsy is thought to not be necessary in patients with a primary cancer with known metastases.

Bilateral Adrenal Masses

Adrenal masses can occur bilaterally in up to 15% of patients with an adrenal incidentaloma. The most common diagnoses are metastatic disease, congenital adrenal hyperplasia, bilateral cortical adenomas, and infiltrative disease of the adrenal glands. Patients with bilateral masses may have adrenocortical hypofunction, and screening for hypofunction should be performed based on clinical judgment.

CHAPTER 80

Pituitary Gland Anatomy and Physiology Review

YING L. LIU

ANATOMY

The pituitary gland, known as the master regulatory gland, oversees the homeostatic regulation of several metabolic and reproductive processes. It is located at the base of the skull in the **sella turcica** and consists of two lobes: the larger anterior lobe (also known as the adenohypophysis) and the smaller posterior lobe (also known as the neurohypophysis). The anterior lobe originates from the oropharynx **(Rathke pouch)** and grows upward toward tissue of neural origin that forms the posterior lobe. The **pituitary stalk** connects the pituitary to the hypothalamus above it and contains axons and nerve terminals that originate in the hypothalamus and transmit signals to the posterior lobe. The pituitary stalk also contains the **hypophyseal portal system,** which transmits hormones synthesized in the hypothalamus to the anterior pituitary.

The sella turcica is covered by dura called the **diaphragma sella** and sits within the cavernous sinus, which also contains cranial nerves (CN) III, IV, and VI, as well as CN V1 and V2. In addition, the optic chiasm sits above the diaphragma sella. Given the location and surrounding nerves, growths (adenomas) or inflammation (hypophysitis) of the pituitary gland can cause nerve compression, resulting in extraocular muscle dysfunction (CN III, IV, or VI), ipsilateral facial pain (CN V1 and V2), or bitemporal hemianopsia (optic chiasm compression) (Fig. 80.1).

PHYSIOLOGY

The secretion of pituitary hormones is tightly controlled by regulatory signals originating in the hypothalamus along with negative feedback signals from downstream-affected glands, such as the thyroid or adrenals. This intricate regulatory system is termed the **hypothalamic-pituitary axis,** and any perturbations to this tightly regulated axis can lead to disease states.

Posterior Pituitary (Fig. 80.2)
Oxytocin

Oxytocin is a nine–amino acid peptide synthesized in the hypothalamic neurons and transported via pituitary stalk axons to the posterior pituitary, where it is released in the blood. Oxytocin stimulates milk secretion from the mammary ducts and stimulates uterine smooth muscle contractions during childbirth. Oxytocin also plays a role in maternal behavior and infant bonding. The release of oxytocin occurs by stimulation of the nipples, and oxytocin release is inhibited by several factors, including other sex hormones and stress. Pitocin, a synthetic form of oxytocin, can be used to induce uterine contractions.

Antidiuretic hormone

Antidiuretic hormone (ADH), or **vasopressin,** is a nine–amino acid peptide synthesized in the hypothalamus, packaged via neuronal axons to the posterior pituitary and secreted to the bloodstream. ADH regulates water content in the body by binding to receptors on the cells of the collecting duct of the kidney and facilitating water reabsorption through aquaporins, which are membrane channels in the kidney tubules. Secretion of ADH is tightly regulated by plasma osmolarity, which is sensed by osmoreceptors in the hypothalamus, which stimulate secretion of ADH when plasma osmolality rises above a certain setpoint and suppress secretion when it falls below a setpoint. Although plasma osmolality is the most sensitive regulator of ADH, large decreases in blood pressure/plasma volume can stimulate stretch receptors in the heart/large arteries and result in ADH secretion.

Two diseases related to disordered ADH secretion are **syndrome of inappropriate ADH secretion (SIADH)** and **diabetes insipidus (DI).** SIADH, characterized by excess ADH secretion, results from myriad etiologies, including surgery, central nervous system (CNS) disturbances, trauma, and (most commonly) medications, among other causes, and may present with hyponatremia; treatment

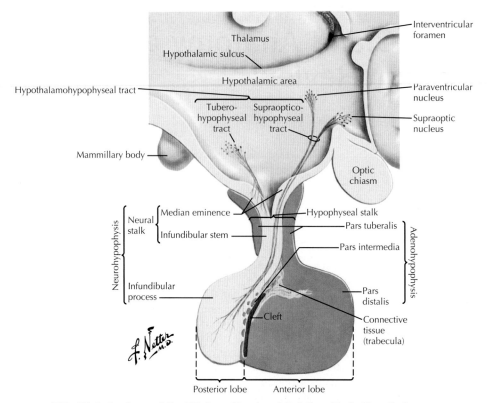

FIG. 80.1 Anatomy of the Pituitary Gland and Relationship to Hypothalamus.

involves treating/removing underlying causes and fluid restriction (see Chapter 27 for further details).

Patients with DI present with massive polyuria that can lead to dehydration and hypernatremia if affected patients are unable to access water or lose their thirst mechanism. There are two forms: central or hypothalamic and nephrogenic. In central DI, there is a deficiency in secretion of ADH due to damage and improper functioning of the posterior pituitary. ADH analogues, such as desmopressin, can treat central DI. In nephrogenic DI, the kidney is unable to respond to ADH, usually through damage to the nephrons or genetic disease encoding mutated ADH receptors or aquaporins. Treatment involves a low-salt, low-protein diet, diuretics (to induce mild volume depletion and thus increase sodium and water resorption earlier in the nephron), and NSAIDs to decrease synthesis of prostaglandins, which ordinarily antagonize ADH.

Anterior Pituitary (Fig. 80.3)
Adrenocorticotropic hormone
Adrenocorticotropic hormone (ACTH) is secreted from corticotroph cells in the anterior pituitary in response to **corticotropin-releasing hormone (CRH)** from the hypothalamus, which is stimulated by stress. ACTH then acts upon the adrenal glands to stimulate secretion of glucocorticoids, primarily **cortisol**. In addition to its systemic effects, cortisol creates a negative feedback loop on the hypothalamus, inhibiting CRH secretion. ACTH is synthesized as pro-opiomelanocortin (POMC), a large precursor protein, which includes several other peptides (e.g., melanocyte-stimulating hormone [MSH], which controls melanin pigmentation).

The most common disease related to ACTH oversecretion is Cushing syndrome, of which most cases are caused by **Cushing disease,** in which a hyperfunctioning pituitary adenoma overproduces ACTH. This leads to hypercortisolism and its attendant symptoms (see Chapter 77 for further details).

Thyroid-stimulating hormone
Thyroid-stimulating hormone (TSH), or **thyrotropin,** is secreted by thyrotroph cells in the anterior pituitary gland in response to thyroid-releasing hormone (TRH) from the hypothalamus. TSH is a glycoprotein composed of two subunits (α and β), which are noncovalently bonded to

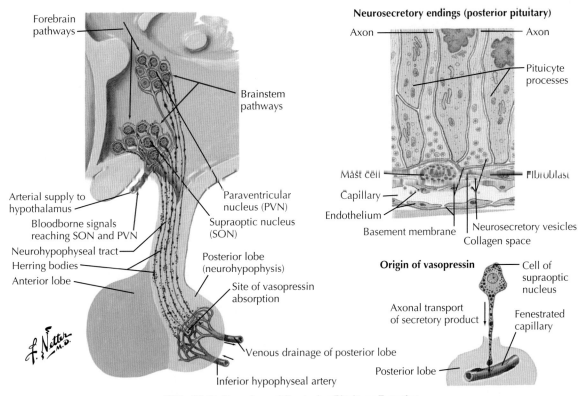

Neurosecretory endings (posterior pituitary)

Origin of vasopressin

FIG. 80.2 **Overview of Posterior Pituitary Function.**

each other and only have activity when bonded together. TSH binds to receptors in the thyroid gland to stimulate production of thyroxine (T_4) and triiodothyronine (T_3), forms of thyroid hormone that regulate multiple metabolic pathways. TSH also promotes extrathyroidal conversion of T_4 to T_3, while T_4 and T_3 inhibit both TSH and TRH secretion. Disruptions in TSH levels can cause either hyperthyroidism or hypothyroidism (see Chapter 71 for further details).

Prolactin

Prolactin is a single-chain protein hormone secreted as a prohormone by lactotroph cells in the anterior pituitary and by the pregnant uterus. It targets the mammary gland and stimulates development and milk production. Prolactin also decreases the levels of **estrogen** and **testosterone**. In contrast to other anterior pituitary hormones, the hypothalamus tonically suppresses prolactin secretion via dopamine inhibition. Prolactin is only secreted once this dopamine inhibition is released, although nipple stimulation and other hormones such as TSH can also stimulate prolactin. **Hyperprolactinemia** is a common disorder that can cause amenorrhea (lack of menstrual cycles) and galactorrhea (excessive/spontaneous milk secretion) in women, and hypogonadism and gynecomastia (breast enlargement) in men (see Chapter 81 for further details).

Growth hormone

Growth hormone (GH), or **somatotropin,** is a protein composed of about 190 amino acids that is synthesized by somatotroph cells of the anterior pituitary. It serves to regulate growth and metabolism directly through binding to GH receptors on fat cells and indirectly through stimulation of secretion of insulin-like growth factor-1 (IGF1) in the liver. IGF1 stimulates growth of muscle, bone, and cartilage, as well as regulates protein, fat, and carbohydrate metabolism. The synthesis and secretion of GH is stimulated by the secretion of growth hormone–releasing hormone (GHRH) from the hypothalamus as well as **ghrelin,** a peptide hormone synthesized in the stomach. **Somatostatin,** a peptide produced in the hypothalamus, inhibits GH release in response to GHRH stimulation. In addition, IGF1 inhibits both GH and GHRH secretion in a negative feedback loop, and GH itself inhibits GHRH secretion. This complex system

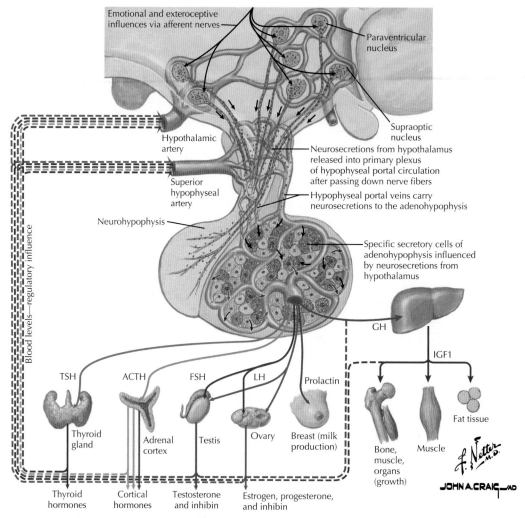

Emotional and exteroceptive
influences via afferent nerves

Paraventricular
nucleus

Hypothalamic
artery

Supraoptic
nucleus

Neurosecretions from hypothalamus
released into primary plexus
of hypophyseal portal circulation
after passing down nerve fibers

Superior
hypophyseal
artery

Hypophyseal portal veins carry
neurosecretions to the adenohypophysis

Neurohypophysis

Specific secretory cells of
adenohypophysis influenced
by neurosecretions from
hypothalamus

Blood levels—regulatory influence

GH

IGF1

TSH   ACTH   FSH   LH   Prolactin

Fat tissue

Thyroid
gland

Adrenal
cortex

Testis   Ovary   Breast (milk
production)

Bone,
muscle,
organs
(growth)

Muscle

Thyroid
hormones

Cortical
hormones

Testosterone
and inhibin

Estrogen, progesterone,
and inhibin

JOHN A. CRAIG—AD

FIG. 80.3 Overview of Anterior Pituitary Function. *ACTH*, Adrenocorticotropic hormone; *FSH*, follicle-stimulating hormone; *GH*, growth hormone; *IGF1*, insulin-like growth factor-1; *LH*, luteinizing hormone; *TSH*, thyroid-stimulating hormone.

leads to a pulsatile pattern of GH release with low basal concentrations of GH that peak during sleep.

Deficiencies in GH or defects in its binding receptor can lead to growth retardation and **dwarfism.** Excessive secretion of GH can result in either giantism in children or **acromegaly** in adults (Fig. 80.4). Recombinant GH is available to treat children with pathologically short stature.

Follicle-stimulating hormone and luteinizing hormone

Follicle-stimulating hormone (FSH) and **luteinizing hormone (LH),** commonly known as **gonadotropins,**

are essential reproductive hormones that stimulate the gonads—testes in males and ovaries in females. They consist of large glycoproteins composed of the same α-subunit as TSH but with different β-subunits. FSH stimulates ovarian follicle maturation in preparation for ovulation in women and supports sperm production and Sertoli cell function in men. In men, LH binds to receptors on Leydig cells that stimulate the synthesis and secretion of testosterone. In women, LH binds to the theca cells of the ovary to stimulate secretion of testosterone, which is then converted to estrogen by neighboring granulosa cells. In women, LH also serves an important function in stimulating ovulation with an

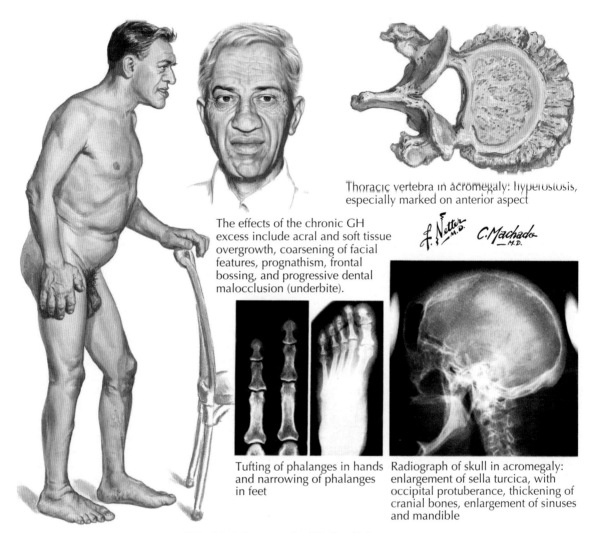

Thoracic vertebra in acromegaly: hyperostosis, especially marked on anterior aspect

The effects of the chronic GH excess include acral and soft tissue overgrowth, coarsening of facial features, prognathism, frontal bossing, and progressive dental malocclusion (underbite).

Tufting of phalanges in hands and narrowing of phalanges in feet

Radiograph of skull in acromegaly: enlargement of sella turcica, with occipital protuberance, thickening of cranial bones, enlargement of sinuses and mandible

FIG. 80.4 **Acromegaly.** *GH*, Growth hormone.

LH surge, which results in release of an egg from a follicle and formation of the **corpus luteum,** an important source of **progesterone** and **estradiol** necessary to maintain a healthy pregnancy.

Secretion of FSH and LH is regulated through **gonadotropin-releasing hormone (GnRH),** which is a peptide synthesized and secreted in the hypothalamus. GnRH binds to receptors on gonadotroph cells in the anterior pituitary to stimulate release of FSH/LH. Synthesis of FSH/LH is also regulated through a

negative feedback loop by sex steroids (testosterone, estrogen, and progesterone), which results in pulsatile secretion of FSH/LH, leading to the cyclic pattern of menstruation. Hormonal contraceptives, which often contain a combination of estrogen and progesterone, utilize this negative feedback loop to suppress the LH surge and ovulation. Diminished LH/FSH secretion manifests as decreased sperm production in men and oligomenorrhea/amenorrhea in women.

CHAPTER 81

Pituitary Masses

PAULA ROY-BURMAN

INTRODUCTION

Pituitary tumors represent 10% to 15% of all intracranial neoplasms. Approximately 90% of these masses are benign **adenomas** arising from the anterior pituitary, which will be the focus of this section.

Pituitary adenomas are classified by two characteristics: size and cell origin. Masses ≥10 mm are known as **macroadenomas,** and those <10 mm are **microadenomas.** The anterior pituitary is comprised of five major cell types—lactotroph, gonadotroph, corticotroph, somatotroph, and thyrotroph—from which adenomas arise. Pituitary adenomas may go unrecognized for many years until one of the following things occur: development of a neurological complaint (such as headache or visual deficit), development of a hormonal disturbance (such as amenorrhea or galactorrhea), or discovery of an incidental sellar mass on MRI **(pituitary incidentaloma).**

It is important to note that the differential of sellar masses is broad, and other diagnoses may present under similar conditions. Pituitary hyperplasia, of which lactotroph hyperplasia during pregnancy is the most common, may present as a sellar mass mimicking an adenoma. **Hypophysitis,** or inflammation of the pituitary, causes pituitary enlargement associated with a severe headache. Remnants of Rathke pouch can form a cyst (Rathke cleft cyst), which is the most common etiology of an incidentaloma. When sufficiently large, cysts can cause headache, visual impairment, and hormonal abnormalities. Benign tumors, such as craniopharyngiomas and meningiomas, also cause headache and visual impairment, particularly when arising from the perisellar region. Less common, but notable, causes of pituitary masses include primary malignancy (e.g., ectopic pinealoma, pituicytoma, and lymphoma), metastases (e.g., breast and lung cancer most commonly), arteriovenous fistula of the cavernous sinus, and pituitary abscess.

PATHOPHYSIOLOGY

Clinical syndromes related to pituitary adenomas are categorized into downstream endocrine effects and local tumor effects.

Each anterior pituitary cell type releases hormones that feed into the **hypothalamic-pituitary-adrenal axis** (see Chapter 80 for further details). Impaired feedback inhibition is the root of the hormonal effects of corticotroph, somatotroph, and thyrotroph tumors.

- Corticotroph adenomas secrete **adrenocorticotropic hormone (ACTH),** which causes adrenal production of cortisol. Negative feedback by cortisol is ineffective, and the unopposed ACTH causes signs and symptoms of hypercortisolism. This is known as **Cushing disease** (whereas Cushing syndrome is hypercortisolism due to causes other than corticotroph adenoma).
- Somatotroph adenomas hypersecrete **growth hormone (GH).** Downstream production of insulin-like growth factor-1 (IGF1) by the liver fails to inhibit tumor secretion of GH. A wide range of clinical effects owed to excess IGF1 and GH are observed, resulting in **acromegaly.**
- In the same vein, thyrotroph adenomas secrete thyroid-stimulating hormone (TSH) resistant to feedback inhibition by thyroxine (T_4) and triiodothyronine (T_3). In addition to causing signs and symptoms of hyperthyroidism, up to one-fourth of thyrotroph adenomas will cosecrete clinically significant amounts of GH or prolactin and cause additional symptomatology.

Gonadotroph adenomas and lactotroph adenomas **(prolactinomas)** deviate slightly from the general mechanism described earlier. Gonadotroph tumors are very inefficient hormone producers and are almost exclusively clinically silent. Prolactinomas, conversely, tend to be very efficient. High levels of prolactin exert influence on gonadotrophs by inhibiting hypothalamic gonadotropin-releasing hormone (GnRH). Without follicle-stimulating hormone (FSH) and luteinizing hormone (LH) to activate gonad production of estrogen, progesterone, and testosterone, **hypogonadotropic hypogonadism** results.

Macroadenomas can exert local tumor mass effects, which can result in neurological symptoms and/or hormone deficiencies. Headaches, sometimes associated with nausea and vomiting, are caused by tumor

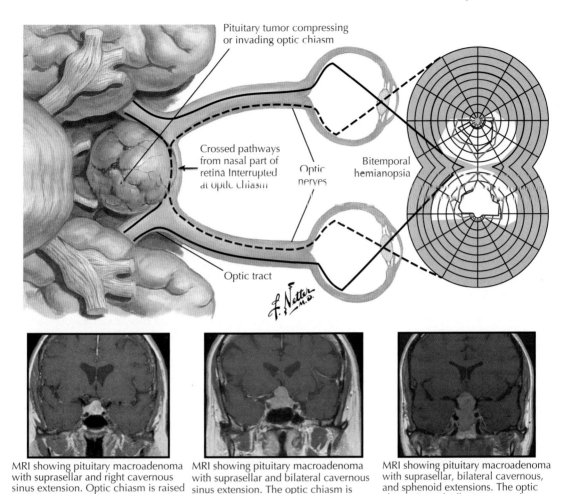

Pituitary tumor compressing or invading optic chiasm

Crossed pathways from nasal part of retina Interrupted at optic chiasm

Optic nerves

Bitemporal hemianopsia

Optic tract

f. Netter.
M.D.

MRI showing pituitary macroadenoma with suprasellar and right cavernous sinus extension. Optic chiasm is raised slightly, but visual fields are normal.

MRI showing pituitary macroadenoma with suprasellar and bilateral cavernous sinus extension. The optic chiasm is compressed, causing bitemporal superior quadrant vision loss.

MRI showing pituitary macroadenoma with suprasellar, bilateral cavernous, and sphenoid extensions. The optic chiasm is markedly compressed, causing complete bitemporal hemianopsia.

FIG. 81.1 Effect of Pituitary Masses on Visual Fields.

invasion into bone or expansion into the diaphragma sellae. Suprasellar extension of the tumor causes visual disturbance. **Bitemporal hemianopsia** (loss of vision in the lateral halves of the right and left visual fields) results from tumor compression of the optic chiasm (Fig. 81.1). Tumor compression of the hypothalamic-pituitary stalk, termed **stalk effect,** leads to hormone deficiencies, most commonly GH and FSH/LH. Though GH deficiency has no clinical consequence in adults, FSH/LH deficiency causes hypogonadotropic hypogonadism. Furthermore, stalk compression impairs upstream inhibition of lactotrophs by dopamine, causing a mild-moderate elevation of prolactin in nonprolactin-secreting adenomas.

RISK FACTORS

Pituitary adenomas are associated with several genetic conditions. **Multiple endocrine neoplasia type 1 (MEN1)** is an autosomal dominant syndrome characterized by pituitary, parathyroid, and pancreatic islet cell tumors. **Familial isolated pituitary adenoma (FIPA)** is an autosomal dominant condition, which occurs in families with variable penetrance. Sporadic cases may result from pituitary tumor transforming gene (PTTG) overexpression or, in some somatotroph adenomas, Gsα-activating mutations.

PRESENTATION, EVALUATION, AND DIAGNOSIS

Though a majority of adenomas cause hormone abnormalities, neurological symptoms more commonly prompt patients to seek care. Visual impairment is typified by bitemporal hemianopsia, but may also present as diplopia or diminished visual acuity. Symptoms are insidious in onset, and headaches do not have a stereotyped description. However, a severe headache of sudden onset and concomitant diplopia should raise suspicion of **pituitary apoplexy** (acute hemorrhage or infarct of the pituitary), which is often associated with an adenoma (Fig. 81.2).

Prolactinomas and tumors causing stalk effect present with **hypogonadotropic hypogonadism,** which manifests in several ways. In men, direct questioning may reveal decreased libido, impotence, and infertility; examination may find gynecomastia. In premenopausal women, the most common complaint is oligomenorrhea (or amenorrhea) and infertility. Unless there are neurological symptoms, the diagnosis in postmenopausal women may be missed as they are already hypogonadal. Patients may note fatigue and lethargy, which, though nonspecific, reflect hypopituitarism. With prolactinomas, premenopausal women and men (rarely) may present with galactorrhea.

Corticotroph, somatotroph, and thyrotroph tumors present with signs and symptoms of hypercortisolism, acromegaly, and thyrotoxicosis, respectively. Hypercortisolism is associated with myriad findings, including centripetal obesity, moon facies, dorsal fat pad, facial plethora, hirsutism, easy bruisability, purple striae, hypertension, insulin resistance, and fractures. Acromegaly is typified by enlarged hands/feet, macrognathia, macroglossia, deepening of the voice, and visceral organ enlargement. The changes in acromegaly are insidious; the mean diagnosis is 12 years, usually when the tumor is large enough to exert local mass effects. Although these tumors are exceedingly rare, patients with thyrotroph adenomas can present with diffuse goiters in addition to symptoms of heat intolerance, palpitations, tremor, diarrhea, and diaphoresis.

The general workup for a pituitary adenoma includes cross-sectional imaging and screening for hormonal abnormalities. MRI with contrast is the imaging modality of choice. Hormonal screening includes serum prolactin, IGF1 (which represents an integrative index of GH secretion), 8 a.m. serum or 24-hour urine cortisol (to account for the diurnal variation in serum cortisol), TSH, and free T_4. Screening for hypogonadism includes FSH and LH in addition to testosterone (in men) and estrogen (in women).

Diagnosis varies by adenoma type but is generally made in the presence of consistent MRI findings and hormone abnormalities. Prolactin levels >500 ng/mL and >250 ng/mL are diagnostic and suggestive of prolactinoma, respectively. A prolactin level between 20 and 200 ng/mL in the presence of a mass may represent a nonlactotroph adenoma or other sellar mass (Fig. 81.3).

Corticotroph adenomas are challenging to diagnose, as most cases present with a microadenoma or no adenoma seen on imaging. If 24-hour urine cortisol is elevated, and morning ACTH is at the upper limits of normal or elevated, a corticotroph adenoma may be suspected and further workup needed. Elevated IGF1 indicates acromegaly; equivocal results can be further evaluated with a GH level checked after an oral glucose load, which should be suppressed in normal patients. Elevated T_4 and T_3 levels in the presence of inappropriately normal or elevated TSH can be diagnostic of a thyrotroph tumor. Unless the serum levels of the α-subunit common to LH and FSH are elevated, the diagnosis of gonadotroph adenomas is usually made postoperatively on pathology evaluation of the adenoma.

TREATMENT

Management of pituitary adenomas is dictated by tumor size and cell type and involves medical and surgical therapies.

With the exception of prolactinomas, **transsphenoidal surgery** is the treatment of choice for all symptomatic adenomas. Some corticotroph microadenomas lack an image correlate on MRI and are diagnosed solely by hormone levels. In this case, **inferior petrosal sinus sampling** is performed to localize the high ACTH to the pituitary gland; if this test is positive for a central-to-peripheral gradient for ACTH, 80% to 90% of the pituitary gland is removed in hopes of resecting the microadenoma. Thyrotroph adenomas are pretreated with somatostatin analogs to achieve euthyroidism and reduce the tumor burden. Patients with acromegaly from somatotroph tumors may require treatment with somatostatin analogues following surgical resection, with serial IGF1 levels used to guide therapy. Perioperative management with steroids should be considered in any patient with a large adenoma since nonadenomatous tissue may be accidentally removed during resection.

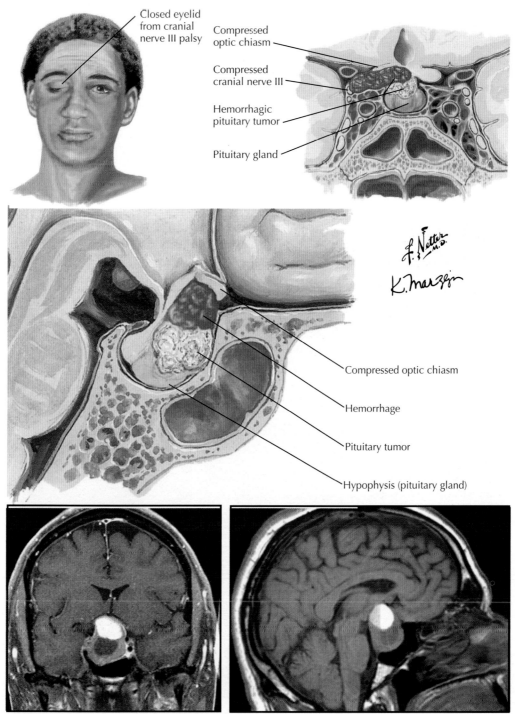

MRI showing pituitary tumor apoplexy. Coronal image *(left)* shows the partially cystic pituitary tumor in the sella with the hemorrhagic component extending above the sella. Sagittal image *(right)* shows fluid-fluid level within the area of recent hemorrhage.

Images reprinted with permission from Young WF: *The Netter collection of medical illustrations, vol 2: endocrine system,* Philadelphia, 2011, Elsevier.

FIG. 81.2 **Pituitary Apoplexy.**

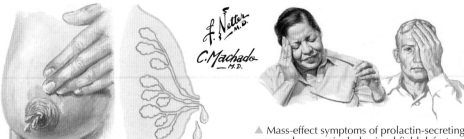

▲ In premenopausal women, hyperprolactinemia causes bilateral spontaneous galactorrhea.

▲ Mass-effect symptoms of prolactin-secreting macroadenomas include visual field defects with suprasellar extension, cranial nerve palsies with lateral (cavernous sinus) extension (e.g., diplopia, ptosis), headaches, and varying degrees of hypopituitarism.

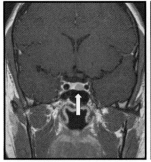 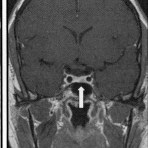

◀ Serial head MRI scans (coronal views) from a patient with a 9-mm prolactin-secreting pituitary microadenoma (*arrows*). At the time of diagnosis (image on *left*), the serum prolactin concentration was 280 ng/mL. The image on the *right* was obtained 6 months after normalizing the serum prolactin concentration with a dopamine agonist. The size of the prolactinoma decreased more than 50% (image on *right*).

▶ Head MRI (coronal view on *left* and sagittal view on *right*) from a patient with a 6.5-cm prolactin-secreting pituitary macroadenoma. There are scattered cystlike areas within the mass, the largest in the right inferior frontal region deforms the frontal horn, resulting in mild midline shift to the left. The mass wraps around the superior and lateral margins of the cavernous sinuses. The patient presented with visual field defects and secondary hypogonadism. Baseline serum prolactin concentration was 6100 ng/mL.

▶ Head MRI (coronal view on *left* and sagittal view on *right*) from the same patient 6 months after normalizing the serum prolactin concentration with a dopamine agonist. Dramatic shrinkage on the MRI is evident. Visual field defects resolved, and pituitary function returned to normal.

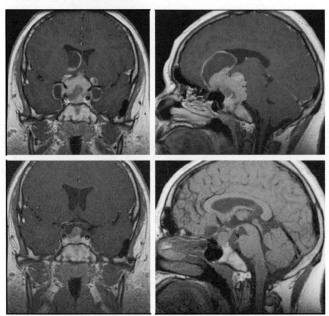

FIG. 81.3 **Prolactinoma.**

First-line treatment for prolactinomas is medical therapy with dopamine agonists. Cabergoline is preferred given its favorable side effect profile and dosing schedule. Bromocriptine is an alternative agent but is associated with more gastrointestinal side effects and is dosed more frequently. If the tumor is resistant to or the patient is unable to tolerate dopamine agonist therapy, surgery may be indicated.

After surgery, patients are followed with serial MRIs and hormone levels to monitor for tumor recurrence and hormonal deficiencies that may have occurred as an unintended side effect from surgery. Should the tumor recur, a patient may be offered repeat surgery, medical therapy, or radiation therapy.

CHAPTER 82

Respiratory System Anatomy Review

BINA CHOI

THORACIC CAVITY

The lungs sit in the thoracic cavity, which is defined by the thoracic ribcage peripherally and superiorly, and the **diaphragm** inferiorly. The ribs are connected by three sets of intercostal muscles from peripheral to central: external, internal, and innermost intercostals.

Muscles comprising the thoracic cavity aid in respiration, and the diaphragm is the primary muscle of respiration. During **inspiration,** the diaphragm contracts inferiorly, and the external intercostals contract to expand the ribcage peripherally and superiorly, thus increasing the volume of, and creating negative pressure within, the thoracic cavity. The negative pressure created induces air entry from the atmosphere into the lungs, expanding them. Expiration is mostly a passive process, but the internal and innermost intercostal muscles may contract to contribute. During exercise, the body recruits additional muscles to meet increased oxygen demand. The scalene muscles (anterior, middle, and posterior) and sternocleidomastoids contract during inspiration to further raise the ribcage, while the rectus abdominis, obliques, and transverse abdominis contribute to expiration.

The thoracic cavity and lung surfaces are lined by serosa called **pleura.** The lungs are lined externally by the **visceral pleura,** which is continuous with the **parietal pleura** that lines the inside of the chest wall. The pleural cavity, which is the potential space between the two pleurae, is normally thin and filled with about 20 mL of pleural fluid, which acts as a lubricant between the lungs and chest wall during respiration. This potential space can expand and be filled in various disease states causing a pleural effusion, or become inflamed leading to pleuritis (pleurisy).

The lungs remain stable within the thoracic cavity via attachments to the hilum, which runs from the mediastinum and carries blood vessels, lymphatics, and the airways, as well as the pulmonary ligament.

The pulmonary ligament is not a true ligament, but a downward extension of the parietal pleura from the hilum that fuses with the visceral pleura and helps anchor the lower lung into position.

LUNGS

The lungs comprise the left and right lung, each of which has four surfaces. The anterior and posterior surfaces are convex and contact the internal thoracic ribcage. The inferior surface is concave and contacts the underlying diaphragm. The medial surface contacts the mediastinum and has the imprints of the heart and descending aorta. The medial surface contains the hilum, which contains the structures that lead to and from the lungs: **pulmonary arteries, pulmonary veins,** bronchi, and lymphatics (Fig. 82.1).

Each lung is further separated into lobes. The right lung has three lobes: upper, middle, and lower. The horizontal fissure separates the upper and middle lobes anteriorly to the hilum. The right oblique fissure separates the lower lobe from the middle lobe anteriorly, and from the upper lobe posteriorly and cranially to the hilum. The left lung has two lobes: upper and lower, which are separated by the oblique fissure, and a lingula, located in the anterior and caudal aspect of the superior lobe.

NOSE, OROPHARYNX, AND LARYNX

During inspiration, air flows from the surrounding atmosphere through the nares and into the nasal cavity. The air is warmed and humidified by the four connecting **paranasal sinuses** on each side of the face: frontal, maxillary, ethmoid, and sphenoid. The paranasal sinuses are lined with columnar epithelial cells projecting cilia that trap dust particles. Air then travels to the back of the throat, termed the nasopharynx. Air can also enter the lungs through the mouth into the oral cavity, then

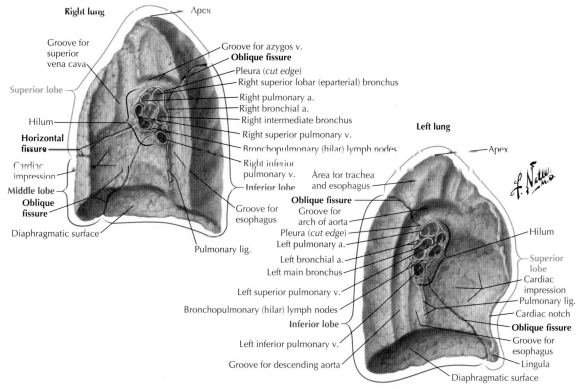

FIG. 82.1 Gross Anatomy of the Lungs. *a.*, Artery; *v.*, vein.

travel into the oropharynx. The nasopharynx and oropharynx are separated by the soft palate and the uvula, and together make up the pharynx. From the pharynx, air moves into the laryngopharynx (or hypopharynx), and finally the **larynx,** or the voicebox.

The larynx is separated from the rest of the upper airways by the epiglottis, which closes the entrance to the larynx during swallowing to prevent aspiration. The vocal cords reside in the larynx and are composed of twin mucous membrane folds that open, close, and vibrate to allow for phonation. Air continues from the larynx into the trachea.

CONDUCTING AIRWAYS

The **trachea** divides into two bronchi, left and right, that respectively lead to the left and right lungs. The **carina** is the dividing point from trachea to bronchi, and each bronchus further divides, on average a total of 23 times, into bronchioles. These bronchioles divide further, into terminal bronchioles, followed by transitional bronchioles, and finally respiratory bronchioles, which terminate in alveolar sacs **(alveolus/alveoli).**

The trachea, bronchi, terminal, and transitional bronchioles make up the **conducting airways.** The purpose of the conducting airways is to conduct air from the environment into the body, and carbon dioxide from the body back out to the environment. The conducting airways do not participate in gas exchange and thus make up the anatomical dead space (~150 mL). The conducting airways are made of an inner epithelial layer, a medial basement membrane layer, and cartilage rings, which provide rigid, structural support for the conducting airways. The inner epithelium is composed of ciliated, pseudostratified columnar epithelium, as well as goblet cells that secrete mucus. Mucus traps dust that enters the airway, and the cilia push the mucus to larger and larger airways, up to the bronchi, trachea, and pharynx, where it is swallowed. This action is called the **mucociliary escalator.**

The basement membrane layer contains smooth muscle cells that are controlled by the sympathetic and parasympathetic nerves that open and constrict the airways, respectively. These nerves play an important role in disease processes such as asthma and chronic obstructive pulmonary disease (COPD).

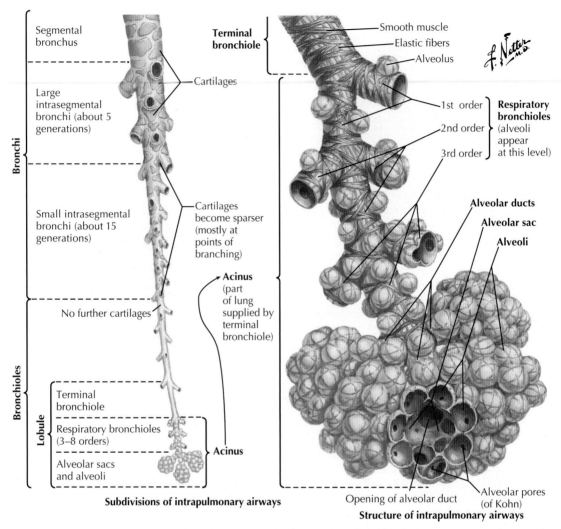

Subdivisions of intrapulmonary airways

Structure of intrapulmonary airways

FIG. 82.2 **Structure of the Bronchioles and Alveoli.**

ACINAR AIRWAYS

The respiratory bronchioles, alveolar ducts, and sacs make up the **acinar airways** (Fig. 82.2). The purpose of the respiratory bronchioles is to conduct gas exchange. Thus the cartilage rings disappear and the cell layers become thinner. Club (originally Clara) cells appear in the smaller bronchioles, and they secrete glycosaminoglycans to protect the respiratory lining and regenerate goblet cells.

Once the air enters the alveoli, it must travel through a thin layer of tissue to enter the bloodstream. The tissue is composed of three layers: epithelial layer of the alveoli, interstitial layer, and endothelial layer of the pulmonary capillaries (Fig. 82.3).

The epithelial layer is comprised of two primary types of cells:

- Type I squamous cells that allow for diffusion of gas from the alveolar space into the pulmonary capillaries. They are squamous cells, flat to facilitate gas exchange, and notable for their small nuclei and thin cytoplasmic projections that allow for diffusion of gas. These cells make up the majority of the surface area of alveoli but do not have the ability to divide by mitosis.
- Type II cuboidal secretory cells that produce **surfactant,** which lines the inside of the alveoli and decreases surface tension during alveoli collapse. With

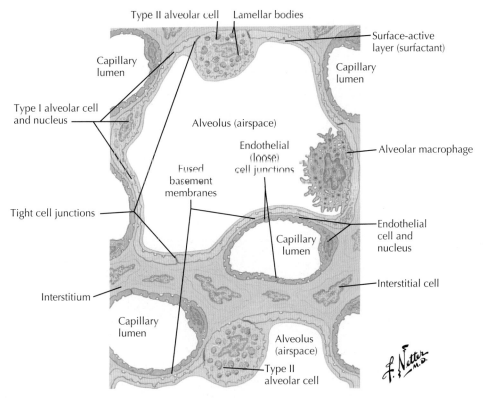

FIG. 82.3 **Structure of Pulmonary Alveoli and Capillaries.**

normal respiration, the difference in thoracic pressure between inspiration and expiration is large enough to completely collapse the alveoli. Thus surfactant coats the inside lining of alveoli and decreases the surface tension required to open the alveoli during inspiration. Surfactant also contributes to innate immunity and prevents interstitial fluid from entering the alveoli. Type II cells also have the capability to divide by mitosis and thus regenerate type I cells in response to damage.

The interstitial layer is made of connective tissue, and it contains fibroblasts, histiocytes, and mast cells.

The endothelial cells of the capillaries are similar to type I cells in that they also have small nuclei and thin cytoplasmic projections to promote diffusion of gas. Notably, the cell junctions are somewhat leaky and allow fluid and solutes to pass between the blood and the interstitial layer. The endothelial cells also contribute to the production of proteins (e.g., angiotensin) and lipids (e.g., prostaglandins).

PULMONARY VASCULATURE

Blood flows from the right ventricle to the pulmonary arteries, which divide into pulmonary arterioles, and later, capillaries made of the endothelial cells (described earlier). The capillaries form a dense network, which surrounds the alveoli for diffusion-mediated gas exchange. Gas exchange happens easily with passive diffusion of oxygen, as the walls of the alveoli are 0.2 to 0.3 μm thick and encompass 50 to 100 m^2 of surface area, and the walls of the capillaries are <0.3 μm thick. The newly oxygenated blood then travels to the pulmonary veins into the left atrium (Fig. 82.4).

RESPIRATORY CONTROL

The reticular formation of the medulla, along with the apneustic and pneumotaxic centers of the pons, controls respiration. The cortex can override this automatic control, as evidenced by a person's ability to hold his or her breath or hyperventilate if he or she so chooses. The

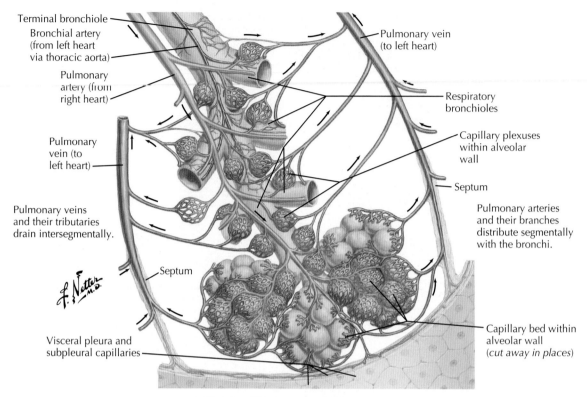

Terminal bronchiole

Bronchial artery (from left heart via thoracic aorta)

Pulmonary artery (from right heart)

Pulmonary vein (to left heart)

Pulmonary veins and their tributaries drain intersegmentally.

Septum

Visceral pleura and subpleural capillaries

Pulmonary vein (to left heart)

Respiratory bronchioles

Capillary plexuses within alveolar wall

Septum

Pulmonary arteries and their branches distribute segmentally with the bronchi.

Capillary bed within alveolar wall (*cut away in places*)

FIG. 82.4 The Pulmonary Vasculature.

rate and pattern of breathing are affected by the limbic system and hypothalamus in emotional states, but more importantly by chemoreceptors. Central chemoreceptors are located in the medulla and respond to changes in H^+ and $PaCO_2$ concentration in the blood. For example,

a rise in $PaCO_2$ leads to a respiratory acidosis, which is sensed by the chemoreceptors. These receptors then trigger an increase in respiratory rate to increase ventilation, or exhalation of CO_2, thus decreasing $PaCO_2$ and returning blood pH to normal.

CHAPTER 83

Respiratory System Physiology Review

WILLIAM C. MCMANIGLE

INTRODUCTION

The primary purpose of respiration is to maintain appropriate levels of oxygen and carbon dioxide within the body. This is accomplished via a coordinated series of integrated functions performed within a specialized anatomical framework. This chapter will focus on respiratory physiology, including pulmonary mechanics, **ventilation, diffusion,** and **perfusion.**

PULMONARY MECHANICS

To effectively exchange oxygen and carbon dioxide, the human body must be able to inspire and expire air. For air to be inspired, pressure external to the lung (atmospheric pressure) must exceed pressure internal to the lung (intrapleural pressure), drawing air internally. For air to be expired, the opposite must be true, driving air externally. The muscles of respiration are primarily responsible for altering the dimensions of the lung, and thus the lung's total volume and, by extension, the intrapleural pressure. Of note, contraction and relaxation of these muscles can be either active or passive. One additional key consideration of pulmonary mechanics is the ability of the lung tissue itself to expand and recoil. Lung **compliance** can be calculated by determining volume change per pressure change within the lung tissue. Certain disease states can cause pathologically increased compliance, such as severe emphysema. Other disease states can cause pathologically decreased compliance, such as fibrotic lung disease. Related to compliance is **elasticity,** defined as the ability for the lung to return to its prior dimensions after inhalation. It is essential for the lung to be able to expand and recoil effectively with each breath. Both compliance and elasticity depend on the presence of functional elastic tissues within the lung, as well as on **surfactant,** a liquid substance synthesized

in the lung that lines the alveoli and affects surface tension.

VENTILATION

Ventilation is defined as the movement of air from the external environment to the **alveolus–pulmonary capillary interface,** where gas exchange occurs. A healthy individual's brain triggers passive breaths and has the ability to initiate active, purposeful breaths. The volume of air moved with a passive breath (either inspired or expired) is termed the tidal volume (TV). The volume of air capable of being moved with a full, forced inspiration, starting at passive end expiration, is termed the inspiratory capacity (IC). Subtracting TV from IC determines the inspiratory reserve volume (IRV). The volume of air capable of being moved with a full, forced expiration, starting at passive end expiration, is termed expiratory reserve volume (ERV), and the air remaining in the airways by the end of expiration is the residual volume (RV). RV, in other words, is the volume of air that cannot be actively expired. Addition of IC and ERV is termed the vital capacity (VC), or the total volume of air able to be moved starting at full, forced expiration to full, forced inspiration. Addition of the VC and RV is termed the total lung capacity (TLC). In addition to lung volumes, another important aspect of a patient's ability to ventilate is termed the **minute ventilation,** defined as the volume of air entering and exiting the airways per minute. There are specific maneuvers that can be performed to measure these values in the clinical setting, including spirometry, body plethysmography, and dilutional techniques. Proper ventilation requires a concerted effort involving the nervous system, the chest wall and associated musculature (including the diaphragm), and the airways. Carbon dioxide and oxygen present in the alveolus are measured as partial pressures, denoted $PaCO_2$ and PaO_2, respectively (see Chapter 46 for further details).

DIFFUSION

The principle of diffusion states that a molecule moves passively from a region of higher concentration to a region of lower concentration. This principle holds true for oxygen and carbon dioxide at the alveolus–pulmonary capillary interface. External air (and thus the gas within alveoli at end inspiration) has a higher concentration of oxygen and a lower concentration of carbon dioxide compared to deoxygenated mixed venous blood of a healthy individual. Applying the principle of diffusion, oxygen moves from the alveolus (higher $[O_2]$), across the alveolus–pulmonary capillary interface, to the mixed venous blood of the pulmonary capillaries (lower $[O_2]$). Conversely, carbon dioxide moves from the mixed venous blood (higher $[CO_2]$), across the alveolus–pulmonary capillary interface, to the alveolus (lower $[CO_2]$), ultimately expired via ventilation. This ensures the cycle through which oxygen, the necessary reactant of aerobic metabolism, is made continually available to cells supplied by the systemic circulation, and through which carbon dioxide can be continually removed from those same tissues. In certain circumstances, despite appropriate ventilation and perfusion, abnormal diffusion can lead to inadequate gas exchange.

PERFUSION

Perfusion is defined as the movement of blood from the systemic circulation to the alveolus–pulmonary capillary interface. Perfusion, necessary to facilitate gas exchange, relies on a functioning heart to circulate blood and a sufficient amount of hemoglobin-rich red blood cells (Fig. 83.1).

Deoxygenated blood travels from peripheral tissues through the venous vasculature, ultimately reaching the inferior or superior vena cava before emptying into the right atrium. From there, deoxygenated blood travels through the right ventricle to the pulmonary arteries, which, like the systemic vasculature, give rise to pulmonary arterioles and eventually capillaries. As in systemic circulation, the pulmonary arteries are responsible for modulating the blood pressure within the pulmonary circuit. The alveolus–pulmonary capillary interface is the site of gas exchange; both oxygen and carbon dioxide diffuse down their respective concentration gradients as blood traverses the capillaries. Assuming appropriate ventilation and diffusion, newly oxygenated blood travels from the efferent pulmonary capillaries through the pulmonary veins to the left side of the heart, moving through the left atrium, left ventricle, and aorta to the systemic arterial vasculature and systemic capillaries. At this interface, the intravascular blood is oxygen-rich and carbon dioxide–poor relative to surrounding tissues. Oxygen is transferred from oxygen-rich blood to oxygen-poor tissue, and carbon dioxide is transferred from carbon dioxide–rich tissue to carbon dioxide–poor blood, and the circulatory cycle then begins again. The level of carbon dioxide and oxygen dissolved in blood is represented as a partial pressure in the arterial system, denoted $PaCO_2$ and PaO_2.

A balance between ventilation (V) and perfusion (Q) is necessary to allow adequate gas exchange, and the ratio of the two is termed V/Q matching. Ideally, in a healthy individual, the amount of blood circulating through the alveolus every minute is an adequate volume to ensure appropriate oxygen and carbon dioxide exchange. The body adjusts blood flow to different areas of the lung in an attempt to optimize V/Q matching, as needed. In pathological states, V/Q ratio can become dysfunctional and lead to inappropriate levels of oxygen and/or carbon dioxide in the body. Consider an individual with a right lung that suddenly receives no ventilation, such as if the right mainstem bronchus became blocked by a foreign object, mucous plug, or cancerous growth. To optimize perfusion, blood vessels supplying the right lung should constrict, minimizing blood flow to the alveoli incapable of effectively exchanging oxygen and carbon dioxide. If blood flow to the left and right lung did not compensate, half of the blood passing through the lungs back to the systemic circulation would be deoxygenated. Alternatively, a large pulmonary embolus blocked perfusion to the left lung, while blood continued to flow to the right lung, no blood passing through the pulmonary vasculature would be oxygenated. Thus V/Q matching is a crucial component of appropriate gas exchange and depends on numerous factors, including adequate cardiac function, appropriate blood pressure control within the systemic and pulmonary circulation, and appropriate distribution of blood flow within the lungs (Fig. 83.2).

Of note, perfect V/Q matching is not present at every alveolus-pulmonary capillary interface because the lungs are oriented vertically within the body and thus impacted by gravity. The apex of the lung sees more ventilation than perfusion and has a higher V/Q ratio, while the base of the lung has more perfusion than ventilation, constituting a lower V/Q ratio. Taken as a whole, the typical V/Q ratio is 0.8.

A. Conditions with low ventilation-perfusion ratio

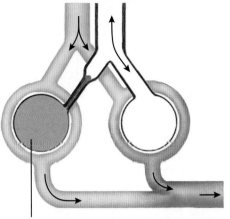

No ventilation, normal perfusion

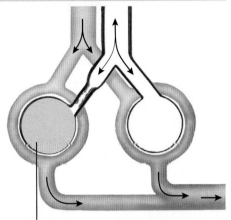

Hypoventilation, normal perfusion

B. Conditions with high ventilation-perfusion ratio

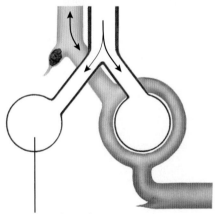

Normal ventilation,
no perfusion (physiological dead space)

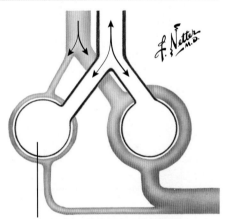

Normal ventilation, hypoperfusion

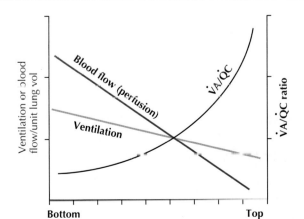

Both ventilation and blood flow
are gravity dependent and
decrease from bottom to top of
lung. Gradient of blood flow is
steeper than that of ventilation,
so ventilation-perfusion ratio
increases up lung.

FIG. 83.1 **Ventilation-Perfusion (VA/QC) Relationships.**

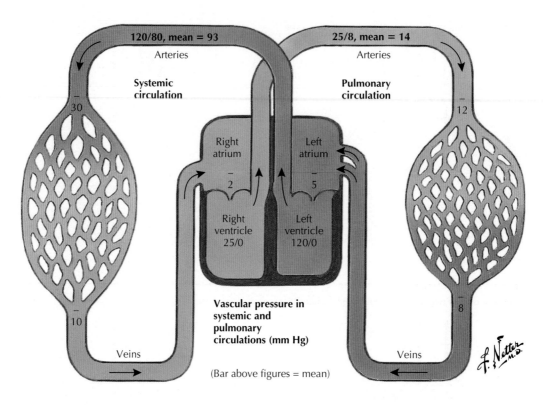

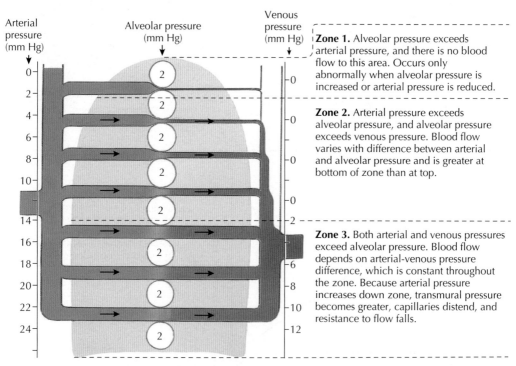

FIG. 83.2 Vascular Pressure in Systemic and Pulmonary Circulations (mm Hg)—Distribution of Pulmonary Blood Flow.

ACID-BASE REGULATION

Apart from gas exchange, the lungs are also one of the organs primarily responsible for acid-base regulation in the body. In the human body, the major contributors to acid-base balance in a clinical sense are bicarbonate (HCO_3^-), regulated by the kidneys, and carbon dioxide (CO_2), regulated by the lungs. While the kidneys can take days to adjust the level of bicarbonate within the body through differences in excretion and resorption, the concentration of carbon dioxide can be altered relatively quickly by respiration. Hyperventilation, which increases minute ventilation, decreases levels of carbon dioxide in the body and thus increases pH. Hypoventilation, which decreases minute ventilation, increases levels of carbon dioxide in the body and thus decreases pH. Respiratory regulation is more fully covered in Chapter 31.

CHAPTER 84

Asthma

JESSE TUCKER

INTRODUCTION

Asthma is a complex chronic disorder of the airways characterized by variable and recurring symptoms, **airflow obstruction,** bronchial hyperresponsiveness, smooth muscle proliferation, and underlying inflammation. Asthma is a common disease, the prevalence of which has increased globally over several decades and is now recognized as a major cause of disability, medical expense, and preventable death. In the United States, the prevalence and severity of asthma are highest in certain vulnerable populations, including children, those living below the poverty line, and specific minority groups (Puerto Ricans and black, non-Hispanic Americans). African Americans are more likely than Caucasians to be hospitalized and have a higher rate of mortality due to asthma.

For years, asthma management focused primarily on allergic mechanisms, but more recent investigations have demonstrated that asthma is quite heterogeneous, with various pathophysiological mechanisms, contributing risk factors, and molecular/clinical phenotypes.

PATHOPHYSIOLOGY

Asthma is characterized by episodic airway obstruction, lung hyperinflation, and airflow limitation resulting from multiple cellular and molecular processes (Figs. 84.1 and 84.2). **Type 2 immune responses** in the lower airway are the primary immunological abnormality in the disease and are mediated by T-helper type 2 (Th2) CD4+ cells and **immunoglobulin E (IgE).** Type 2 immune responses drive a cascade of downstream events, including IgE-mediated hypersensitivity, activation of airway epithelial cells, chemoattraction of effector cells (mast cells, eosinophils, and basophils), and remodeling of the epithelium and subepithelial matrix. The **eosinophil** is the most characteristic cell that accumulates in asthma and allergic inflammation; its presence is often related to disease severity. **Mast cells** are also increased in number in asthmatic airways and may be found in close association with airway smooth muscle cells. In addition to producing bronchoconstrictive mediators (e.g., histamine, prostaglandins, and leukotrienes), mast cells

also store and release tumor necrosis factor-α (TNFα), which is important in the recruitment and activation of inflammatory cells and in altered function of airway smooth muscle.

RISK FACTORS

Asthma results from complex interactions between multiple environmental, host, and genetic influences. The strongest risk factor for asthma is a family history of **atopy,** defined as having IgE antibodies to specific allergens, which is a prerequisite for developing allergic disease. In adults, the odds of having asthma increase with the number of positive skin tests to common allergens. Because much allergic asthma is associated with sensitivity to indoor allergens (including house dust mite, dog and cat dander, and cockroach allergens), increased allergen exposure in infancy and early childhood is implicated as a driver of rising asthma prevalence. Other environmental exposures, including occupational exposures (e.g., fires, mixing cleaning agents, industrial spills, nursing and commercial cleaning occupations), are associated with increased risk of new-onset asthma. Although it is accepted that air pollution can exacerbate preexisting asthma, it has been difficult to demonstrate that it can contribute to the onset of asthma.

Severe viral infections early in life, particularly respiratory syncytial virus (RSV) and certain strains of rhinovirus, are associated with the development of asthma in childhood and potential persistence to adulthood. Although typical bacterial infections are not thought to cause asthma, two causes of atypical pneumonia, *Chlamydia pneumoniae* and *Mycoplasma pneumoniae,* have been implicated in the development of chronic wheezing illnesses.

PRESENTATION, EVALUATION, AND DIAGNOSIS

Most patients with asthma have periods of normal, symptom-free breathing disrupted by dyspnea, cough, and/or **wheezing.** Dyspnea and wheezing, often

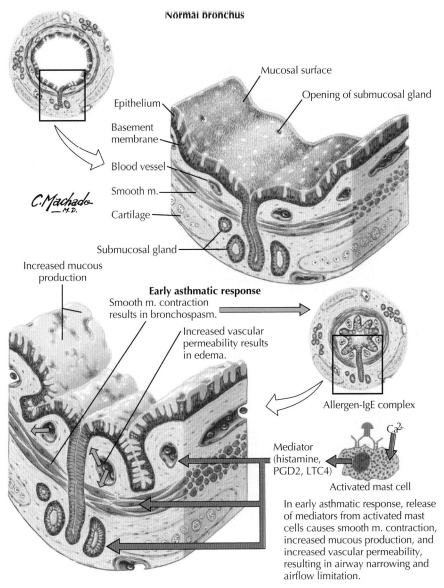

Normal bronchus

Mucosal surface

Opening of submucosal gland

Epithelium

Basement membrane

Blood vessel

Smooth m.

Cartilage

Submucosal gland

C. Machado M.D.

Increased mucous production

Early asthmatic response

Smooth m. contraction results in bronchospasm.

Increased vascular permeability results in edema.

Allergen-IgE complex

Mediator (histamine, PGD2, LTC4)

Ca^{2+}

Activated mast cell

In early asthmatic response, release of mediators from activated mast cells causes smooth m. contraction, increased mucous production, and increased vascular permeability, resulting in airway narrowing and airflow limitation.

FIG. 84.1 **Airway Pathophysiology in Asthma.** *IgE,* Immunoglobulin E; *LTC,* leukotriene; *m.,* muscle; *PGD,* prostaglandin.

accompanied by a prolonged expiratory phase, manifest during an exacerbation and can be triggered by infection, cold air, exercise, or environmental exposures. Cough may be accompanied by sputum production and can worsen at night or with activity. In addition, some patients describe bandlike chest tightness during an exacerbation. Aside from these symptoms, patients with asthma often have signs of allergic conditions (eczema, hives, atopic dermatitis) and evidence of upper respiratory tract inflammation and obstruction with inflamed nasal passages and/or nasal polyps. A number of different diseases can mimic asthma, including rhinosinusitis, vocal cord dysfunction, chronic obstructive pulmonary disease (COPD), cystic fibrosis, bronchiectasis, congestive heart failure, sleep apnea, pneumonia, allergic bronchopulmonary aspergillosis or mycosis (ABPA or ABPM), aspirin sensitivity as a part of Samter triad, and sarcoidosis.

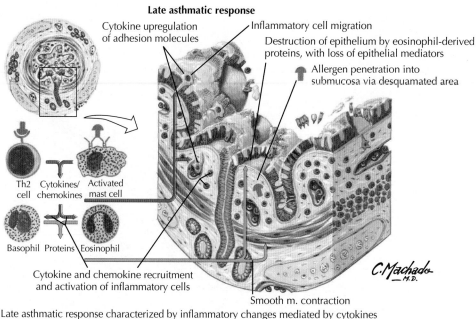

Late asthmatic response

Cytokine upregulation of adhesion molecules

Inflammatory cell migration

Destruction of epithelium by eosinophil-derived proteins, with loss of epithelial mediators

Allergen penetration into submucosa via desquamated area

Th2 cell

Cytokines/ chemokines

Activated mast cell

Basophil Proteins Eosinophil

Cytokine and chemokine recruitment and activation of inflammatory cells

Smooth m. contraction

Late asthmatic response characterized by inflammatory changes mediated by cytokines and chemokines, and epithelial destruction mediated by eosinophils and basophils

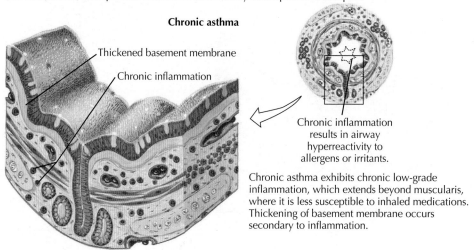

Chronic asthma

Thickened basement membrane

Chronic inflammation

Chronic inflammation results in airway hyperreactivity to allergens or irritants.

Chronic asthma exhibits chronic low-grade inflammation, which extends beyond muscularis, where it is less susceptible to inhaled medications. Thickening of basement membrane occurs secondary to inflammation.

FIG. 84.2 **Airway Pathophysiology in Asthma (Continued).** *m.*, Muscle; *Th*, T helper.

Clinical testing for asthma begins with pulmonary function testing. Diagnosis is most supported by an **obstructive** pattern on spirometry that improves after bronchodilator therapy, defined as an increase in the forced expiratory volume in 1 second (FEV1) >12% and 200 mL after two to four puffs of a short-acting bronchodilator. With mild obstructive disease, the ratio of the FEV1 to forced vital capacity (FVC) may be normal at baseline, with the only abnormality being a decrease in airflow at the middle range of lung volume (FEV 25%–75%). In cases in which the spirometry is normal, the diagnosis can be made by showing responsiveness to methacholine challenge; this is considered positive when the challenge causes a decline in the FEV1 of 20% from baseline (see Chapter 46 for details).

No blood tests are available that can determine the presence or absence of asthma or gauge its severity, but a complete blood count (CBC) with differential to screen

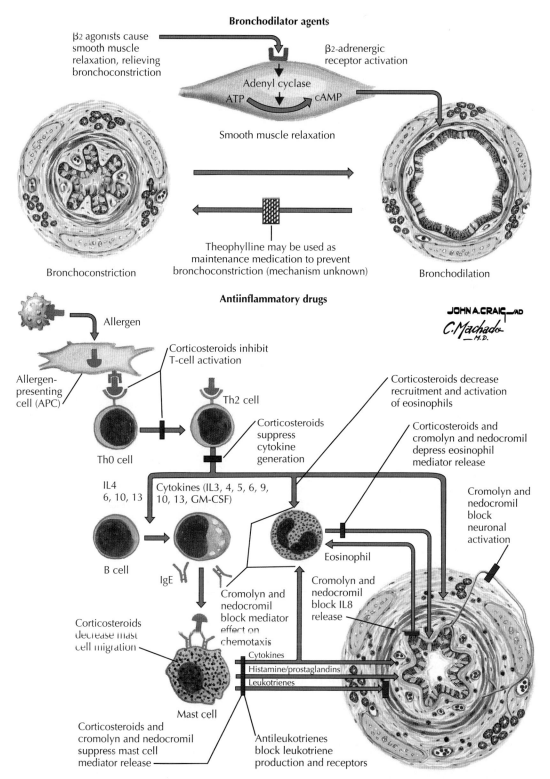

Bronchodilator agents

β2 agonists cause smooth muscle relaxation, relieving bronchoconstriction

β2-adrenergic receptor activation

Adenyl cyclase
ATP → cAMP

Smooth muscle relaxation

Theophylline may be used as maintenance medication to prevent bronchoconstriction (mechanism unknown)

Bronchoconstriction

Bronchodilation

Antiinflammatory drugs

JOHN A. CRAIG—MD
C. Machado—M.D.

Allergen

Corticosteroids inhibit T-cell activation

Allergen-presenting cell (APC)

Th0 cell

Th2 cell

Corticosteroids suppress cytokine generation

Corticosteroids decrease recruitment and activation of eosinophils

Corticosteroids and cromolyn and nedocromil depress eosinophil mediator release

IL4 6, 10, 13

Cytokines (IL3, 4, 5, 6, 9, 10, 13, GM-CSF)

Cromolyn and nedocromil block neuronal activation

B cell

IgE

Eosinophil

Cromolyn and nedocromil block IL8 release

Cromolyn and nedocromil block mediator effect on chemotaxis

Corticosteroids decrease mast cell migration

Cytokines
Histamine/prostaglandins
Leukotrienes

Mast cell

Corticosteroids and cromolyn and nedocromil suppress mast cell mediator release

Antileukotrienes block leukotriene production and receptors

FIG. 84.3 **Mechanisms of Asthma Medications.** *ATP,* Adenosine triphosphate; *cAMP,* cyclic adenosine monophosphate; *GM-CSF,* granulocyte-macrophage colony-stimulating factor; *IgE,* immunoglobulin E; *IL,* interleukin; *Th,* T helper.

for eosinophilia or significant anemia may be helpful. Allergy tests are generally not useful for the diagnosis of asthma, but they can be helpful to confirm sensitivity to suspected allergic triggers of respiratory symptoms. Measurement of total serum IgE levels is indicated in patients with moderate-to-severe persistent asthma when considering treatment with anti-IgE monoclonal antibody (omalizumab) or when allergic bronchopulmonary aspergillosis is suspected.

In the absence of comorbid illness or acute exacerbation, the chest x-ray is often normal in patients with asthma. Chest radiography may be useful in adults over age 40 with new-onset, moderate-to-severe asthma to exclude the occasional alternative diagnosis (e.g., the mediastinal mass with tracheal compression, heart failure, or Churg-Strauss syndrome). Cross-sectional imaging (high-resolution CT) is performed when abnormalities seen on conventional chest radiography need clarification or when other processes are suspected, such as bronchiectasis, bronchiolitis obliterans, tracheomalacia, or anatomical anomalies compromising central airways.

TREATMENT

Medical management of asthma involves chronic symptom control and developing an **asthma action plan** for acute exacerbations (Fig. 84.3). Current guidelines recommend adjusting therapy in a stepwise fashion to reduce daily symptoms and risk of exacerbations while minimizing the use of medications. Generally, such a plan includes the daily use of an antiinflammatory disease-modifying medication such as a low-dose **inhaled corticosteroid (ICS)** for long-term control and an as-needed short-acting **bronchodilator** such as albuterol for quick relief of episodic symptoms. Short-acting β-agonists (SABAs), including albuterol and levalbuterol, are the cornerstone of quick-relief therapy for episodic symptoms using a metered dose inhaler (MDI), as well as for rapid treatment of exacerbations in the emergency or inpatient setting using a nebulized solution.

ICS medications are the primary therapy for disease maintenance because they reduce asthmatic symptoms, improve lung function, and decrease airway inflammation. As a result, these medications are considered to be first-line therapy for all patients requiring more than twice-weekly SABA use. Systemic corticosteroids continue to be a cornerstone of the management of acute exacerbations, but are associated with a variety of undesirable side effects and thus generally have little role in long-term therapy. Long-acting β-agonists (LABAs) for long-term symptom management have modest effects on improving asthma control and reducing severe exacerbations, but patients must be counseled that LABAs do not serve as rescue inhalers. Additionally, it is critical to prescribe LABAs only with concomitant ICS and to warn patients about the potential dangers of LABA monotherapy. Additional therapies useful during acute asthma exacerbations, especially refractory cases, include intravenous (IV) magnesium sulfate and inhaled heliox (a mixture of 70% helium and 30% oxygen) delivered with albuterol to improve turbulent flow of oxygen. Noninvasive ventilation has not been studied as well as in patients with COPD or heart failure, but a trial of noninvasive ventilation may be warranted in patients who are not responding to medical treatment but do not need intubation. Indications for intubation include decreased respiratory rate/effort, altered mental status, and progressive hypercapnia or hypoxemia.

Leukotriene modifiers (LTMs) act on the leukotriene pathway, which mediates bronchoconstriction, mucous hypersecretion, and mucosal edema in airway smooth muscle. LTMs have a modest bronchodilator effect and may improve asthma symptoms and exacerbation rates but are generally less effective than ICS. LTMs generally serve as adjuncts to ICS therapy, but they can be used as monotherapy in exercise-induced asthma and in patients with relatively mild asthma symptoms that do not require therapy with ICS.

Omalizumab is a monoclonal antibody that is approved for patients with moderate-to-severe persistent allergic asthma with demonstrable sensitivity to an aero-antigen and incomplete control on existing maintenance therapy. Omalizumab targets the receptor-binding portion of IgE, preventing it from interacting with immune cells to cause degranulation. High cost, the requirement for monitoring during treatment, and the need for careful selection of patients likely to benefit have limited its use. Future therapeutic targets include interleukin-5 (IL5), which mediates eosinophil hematopoiesis, and IL13, which promotes IgE production in B cells, smooth muscle contraction, and the generation of eosinophil chemoattractants.

CHAPTER 85

Chronic Obstructive Pulmonary Disease

MICHAEL MURN

INTRODUCTION

Chronic obstructive pulmonary disease (COPD) is a progressive disease defined by airflow limitation. The mechanism by which this occurs is thought to be an inflammatory response out of proportion to noxious stimuli, which impact both the small airways and parenchyma of the lung. Consistent irritation causes chronic irreversible changes, which, in turn, greatly impact quality of life.

The most significant cause of COPD is smoking exposure in a dose-dependent nature. Other environmental inhalation exposures coupled with genetic factors such as **α1-antitrypsin deficiency** play a much smaller role but are important to consider.

While COPD causes chronic airflow limitation and symptoms, **acute exacerbation of COPD (AECOPD)** is defined by sudden worsening of cough and sputum production unable to be managed with the baseline outpatient medical regimen. Upper respiratory infections are the most likely acute irritant, with bacterial causes almost twice as likely as their viral counterparts. The gold standard for diagnosis and severity classification in stable COPD is the **pulmonary function test** (PFT).

COPD impacts an estimated 30 million Americans. Despite being a chronic condition, it remains the fourth leading cause of death in the United States. Worldwide, however, COPD is one of the leading causes of deaths and thus should be well understood by all clinicians regardless of field of practice or country of origin.

PATHOPHYSIOLOGY

COPD is the result of irreversible large or small airway obstruction triggered by an inciting agent that causes an inflammatory response persisting longer than would be predicted by duration of exposure. Many recurrent exposures lead to chronic inflammation and eventual airway fibrosis, reducing airway caliber and thus airflow rate (Fig. 85.1). These changes can lead to limited gas exchange and airway obstruction.

Mechanistically, obstruction of airflow occurs with the breakdown of lung parenchyma providing less elastic recoil to keep airways patent (Fig. 85.2). With

reduction of airway radius, as predicted by **Poiseuille's law**, resistance increases by a factor of 4, greatly decreasing flow rate. Eventually, elasticity is so reduced that airway collapse occurs, creating air trapping and lung expansion as the entirety of each subsequent breath cannot be fully expelled. Ongoing hyperinflation flattens the diaphragm, and in seeking to regain mechanical advantage and expel trapped air, as predicted by Laplace's law, the body recruits accessory muscles in the neck, thorax, and abdomen to generate exceedingly higher amounts of tension to reopen the airways.

As lung parenchyma breaks down, total surface area of air exchange is limited. As to be expected, this is a heterogeneous process across the lung surface resulting in significant ventilation-perfusion (V/Q) mismatch.

RISK FACTORS

By far and away the best studied risk factor is smoking. While found to be a dose-dependent response, the causal relationship has a significant genetic and environmental component leading to wide variability in individuals. For example, increased age and the male sex have been identified as independent risk factors. Inhalation of airway irritants can be a risk factor in the absence of smoking, such as indoor cookstove and smoked wood.

The interplay of individual genes with the development and progression of COPD is under continued investigation. The most well-studied genetic risk factor is α1-antitrypsin deficiency; this protease protects tissues from enzymes such as elastase, and when deficient, elastase activity is unchecked and leads to degradation of lung parenchyma. This genetic abnormality should be considered in anyone developing COPD before age 50 years. Other risk factors that should be clinically considered, but of which a link has not definitively been proven, are occupational and environmental exposures such as gold and coal dusts, and airway hyperresponsiveness such as asthma.

AECOPD risk factors include age, prior COPD exacerbations, certain comorbidities (including heart failure and diabetes mellitus), lower respiratory infections, medication nonadherence, and gastroesophageal reflux disease (GERD).

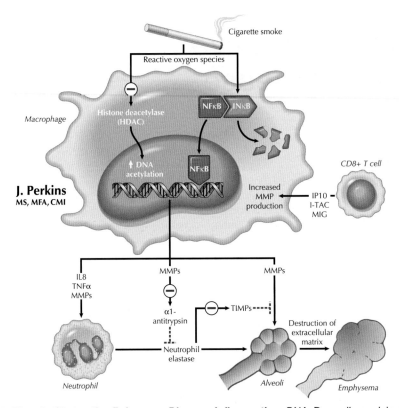

FIG. 85.1 Chronic Obstructive Pulmonary Disease: Inflammation. *DNA,* Deoxyribonucleic acid; *IL,* interleukin; *INκB,* inhibitor of nuclear factor kappa-light-chain enhancer of activated B cells; *IP,* interferon γ-induced protein; *I-TAC,* interferon-inducible T-cell α-chemoattractant; *MIG,* monokine induced by gamma interferon; *MMP,* matrix metalloproteinases; *NFκB,* nuclear factor κ-light-chain enhancer of activated B cells; *TIMPs,* tissue inhibitors of metalloproteinases; *TNFα,* tumor necrosis factor-α.

PRESENTATION, EVALUATION, AND DIAGNOSIS

It is crucial to establish a baseline of symptoms for continuity of care as treatment is driven by symptomatic changes characterized by subjective reports of dyspnea and cough. Important information to elicit includes baseline functional status, such as current exercise capacity and ability to complete activities of daily living. Physicians should inquire about cough quality, duration, and sputum production, as well as any recent changes. Previous respiratory-related hospitalizations are the best predictor of the likelihood for future hospitalizations and should always be investigated. Finally, clinicians should discuss the current treatment regimen, including level of adherence and questions about regimen, as many AECOPD events stem from lack of adherence or incorrect inhaler technique.

A patient's general appearance can be variable based on severity of disease, ranging from normal appearance to generalized wasting, tripod positioning, and cyanotic extremities. On pulmonary exam, expect to hear wheezes,

crackles, and a prolonged expiratory phase indicative of reduced air movement and trapping (see Chapter 24 for details).

The gold standard for COPD evaluation is the PFT with a telltale obstructive picture in both forced expiratory volume in 1 second (FEV1) and FEV1 to forced vital capacity (FVC) ratio (see Chapter 46 for further details). PFTs are utilized as one of the major classification criteria in the **Global Initiative for Chronic Obstructive Lung Disease (GOLD) criteria.** The diagnostic threshold is an FEV1:FVC ratio <0.70. Disease severity is classified by the FEV1 percent predicted. Typically, COPD is termed mild at >80%, moderate between 50% and 80%, severe between 30% and 50%, and very severe at <30%. While useful in the outpatient clinic setting, PFTs are not recommended in the setting of an acute exacerbation. As previously noted, physicians should consider testing for α1-antitrypsin is patients who develop COPD prior to age 50.

Diagnosis of AECOPD entails a good history demonstrating increased dyspnea, cough, or a change in

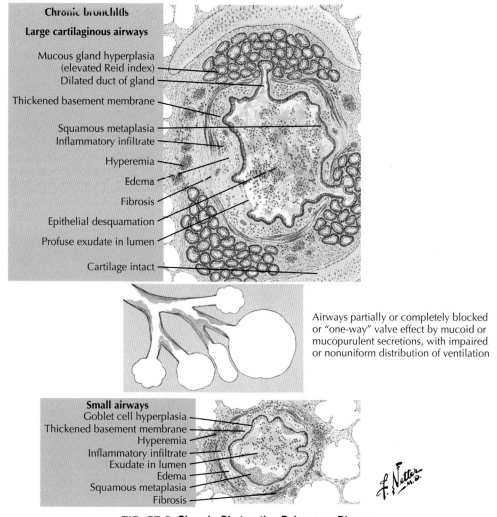

Chronic bronchitis

Large cartilaginous airways

Mucous gland hyperplasia (elevated Reid index)
Dilated duct of gland
Thickened basement membrane
Squamous metaplasia
Inflammatory infiltrate
Hyperemia
Edema
Fibrosis
Epithelial desquamation
Profuse exudate in lumen
Cartilage intact

Airways partially or completely blocked or "one-way" valve effect by mucoid or mucopurulent secretions, with impaired or nonuniform distribution of ventilation

Small airways
Goblet cell hyperplasia
Thickened basement membrane
Hyperemia
Inflammatory infiltrate
Exudate in lumen
Edema
Squamous metaplasia
Fibrosis

FIG. 85.2 **Chronic Obstructive Pulmonary Disease.**

amount and character of sputum. Chest radiography demonstrates hyperinflated lungs and can reveal potential exacerbation triggers or help rule out alternative causes of shortness of breath, including acute decompensated heart failure, pneumothorax, or pleural effusions (Fig. 85.3). Arterial blood gases can determine the degree of hypercarbia present and demonstrate the effectiveness of compensatory mechanisms such as tachypnea and the need for respiratory support.

TREATMENT

Treatment of COPD should be broken down into the acute and chronic/stable settings. Only three interventions have demonstrated decreased mortality rates: smoking cessation, oxygen therapy in those with

resting O_2 saturation <88%, and **lung volume reduction surgery** in a small subtype of patients with upper lobe–predominant emphysema.

The primary medication categories used in COPD treatment are **β_2 agonists, anticholinergics,** and **corticosteroids.** These medications seek to reduce chronic inflammation, which leads to progressive airway destruction, and increase the caliber of airways to allow for better airflow. Choice of a specific type should be based around local availability, individual symptomatic response, and financial considerations. Additionally, while no direct mortality benefit has been shown, yearly flu vaccination and pulmonary rehabilitation are recommended in COPD patients.

Acute exacerbations should be treated with frequent nebulized short-acting β_2 agonists (i.e., albuterol)

Upper lobe

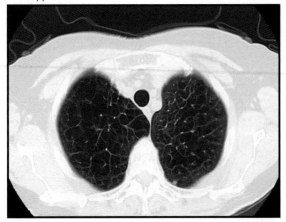

Middle lobe

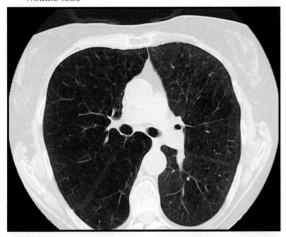

Lower lobe

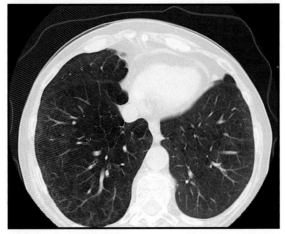

FIG. 85.3 High-Resolution CT Scan of Lungs in Chronic Obstructive Pulmonary Disease. CT scans show severe panacinar emphysema of the upper *(above and middle)* and lower *(below)* lobes of the lung.

and anticholinergics (i.e., ipratropium), systemic corticosteroids, and supplemental oxygen to maintain peripheral oxygen saturation (SpO_2) >88%. The use of antibiotics should be considered in those who are having a moderate to severe exacerbation with choice dictated by local resistance patterns. Common selections include doxycycline or azithromycin for uncomplicated cases or amoxicillin-clavulanate or levofloxacin for complicated cases; patients with risk factors for *Pseudomonas aeruginosa* should receive antibiotics with activity against this organism. Patients with declining respiratory status should be considered for **noninvasive positive pressure ventilation** or, if respiratory compromise is imminent, endotracheal intubation and mechanical ventilation.

Stable COPD treatment is based around the GOLD criteria, with medications added on to the treatment plan of less severe classifications. The goal of these treatment modalities is symptomatic management and to reduce severity and frequency of exacerbations. In GOLD stages 1 and 2, short-acting β_2 agonists (albuterol, terbutaline) or anticholinergics should be selected to start and be used on an as-needed basis. As symptoms become more consistent, physicians can add a long-acting anticholinergic (tiotropium, umeclidinium, aclidinium) and/or long-acting β_2 agonist (salmeterol, formoterol, oldanterol). Once FEV1 decreases <50% (GOLD stages 3 and 4) an inhaled corticosteroid should be added.

Therapy can be further refined by classifying a patient's COPD by severity of symptoms (minimal vs. more determined by the COPD Assessment Test) and risk of exacerbation (low vs. high), termed GOLD "ABCD." Group "A" (minimal symptoms, low risk of exacerbation) therapy begins with as-needed short-acting bronchodilators. Group "B" (more symptoms, low exacerbation risk) utilizes either a long-acting B2 agonist or anticholinergic, while Group "C" (minimal symptoms, high exacerbation risk) recommends initial therapy with a long-acting anticholinergic. Group "D" (more symptoms, high risk) should begin with a long-acting anticholinergic, combination long-acting therapy, or a long-acting B2 agonist with an inhaled corticosteroid. Further exacerbations on therapy may necessitate additional medications as described above.

In recurrent exacerbations, we may consider advanced therapies such as **roflumilast**. It is a selective phosphodiesterase type 4 inhibitor that may help to reduce exacerbations. Pulmonary rehabilitation helps COPD patients to reduce their symptoms and prevent exacerbations. Lung volume reduction surgery is an option to consider in severe air trapping, upper lobe–predominant emphysema, and FEV1 <30% predicted with poor exercise tolerability as this procedure will prolong life.

CHAPTER 86

Cystic Fibrosis

ANNE M. MATHEWS

INTRODUCTION

Cystic fibrosis (CF) is a multiorgan disease affecting the lungs, digestive system (including the liver), sweat glands, and reproductive tract. Patients with CF have abnormal transport of chloride and sodium across secretory epithelia, resulting in thickened, viscous secretions in the bronchi, biliary tract, pancreas, intestines, and reproductive system (Fig. 86.1). Although the disease is systemic, progressive lung disease continues to be the major cause of morbidity and mortality. Therefore this chapter will focus on highlighting the pathophysiology, presentation, evaluation, and diagnosis of CF-related sinus and pulmonary complications.

CF is the most common life-shortening autosomal recessive disease among Caucasians. It has been reported to occur with a frequency of 1 in 2500 to 3000 live births. In recent years, due to a better understanding of the genetic underpinnings leading to CF, it has been more frequently recognized in minority populations, and approximately 7% of CF is diagnosed in adulthood. According to the Cystic Fibrosis Foundation 2014 Registry Report of CF centers from the United States, Canada, and Europe, the median survival was about 40 years. Females seem to have a higher morbidity and mortality than males, and this has been demonstrated across many populations. It has been hypothesized that the underlying mechanism is due to the proinflammatory effects of estrogens.

The progression of CF can occur over a highly variable time course, ranging from months to decades after birth. Individuals eventually develop chronic infection of the respiratory tract with a characteristic array of bacterial flora. Chronic bacterial infection within the airways occurs in most CF patients, and the prevalence of each bacterial type varies with patient age. Ultimately, chronic respiratory infection and airway obstruction result in progressive respiratory insufficiency and eventual **respiratory failure.**

GENETICS AND PATHOPHYSIOLOGY

The pathogenesis of organ dysfunction observed in CF has been studied in humans and animal models (specifically CF transmembrane conductance regulator [CFTR] knockout mice) but remains poorly understood. CF is caused by mutations in a single large gene on chromosome 7 that encodes the **CFTR protein** (Fig. 86.2). CFTR functions as a regulated chloride channel, which may also in turn regulate the activity of other chloride and sodium channels at the cell surface. There have been over 2000 mutations characterized and divided into five classes, which range from no synthesis or reduced synthesis to blunted processing, regulation, and conductance. The net result of genetic mutations is alteration in airway secretions, which become thick and difficult to clear. In addition to thickened secretions, there are alterations in airway pH and defects in mucociliary transport that play a role in disease progression.

The viscous secretions and chronic inflammation result in characteristic chronic airway obstruction. The physical and chemical abnormalities of the CF airway secretions result in chronic infections with unique bacterial pathogens, particularly *Pseudomonas* species but also include *Haemophilus influenzae, Staphylococcus aureus,* and *Burkholderia cepacia* complex species. Other commonly seen organisms in CF include *Stenotrophomonas maltophilia, Alcaligenes xylosoxidans,* and *Klebsiella* species. Additionally, nontuberculous mycobacteria and fungal species such as *Aspergillus* contribute to clinical disease in some CF patients.

Once infection occurs, there is massive infiltration of inflammatory cells, particularly neutrophils, into the lung tissue. However, the neutrophils are unable to control the bacteria and subsequently release elastase, which overwhelms the antiproteases of the lung and contributes to tissue destruction. Furthermore, large amounts of deoxyribonucleic acid (DNA) and cytosol matrix proteins

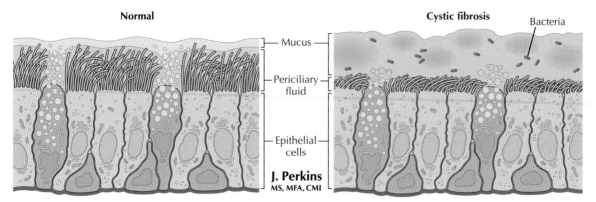

Normal **Cystic fibrosis** Bacteria

Mucus
Periciliary fluid
Epithelial cells

J. Perkins
MS, MFA, CMI

Abnormal electrolyte transport at the airway epithelium leads to a net absorption of sodium and water from the periciliary liquid (PCL) layer and airway mucus. The smaller PCL volume leads to trapping of cilia in tenacious mucus, impairing effective mucous clearance.

FIG. 86.1 **Abnormal Electrolyte Transport.**

are released by degranulating neutrophils, contributing to increased viscosity of airway mucus.

Chronic inflammation leads to damage of the airways that, through airway remodeling and fibrosis, ultimately advance to irreversible **bronchiectasis** and progressive respiratory failure. Often lung parenchyma becomes severely congested with grossly purulent secretions, both in and around dilated airways (Fig. 86.3). Airway epithelium is hyperplastic with areas of erosion and squamous metaplasia. There is also submucosal gland hypertrophy and hyperplasia of airway smooth muscle. Plugs of mucoid material and inflammatory cells are often present in the airway lumen and contribute to air trapping. Late-stage disease can manifest, as well as hypoxemia, hypercapnia, and development of pulmonary hypertension.

PRESENTATION, EVALUATION, AND DIAGNOSIS

The usual presenting symptoms and signs include persistent pulmonary infection, pancreatic insufficiency, and elevated sweat chloride levels. However, many patients demonstrate mild or atypical symptoms, and clinicians should remain alert to the possibility of CF even when only a few of the usual features are present. Classic CF is diagnosed in patients with more than one organ system involvement and a positive diagnostic test, usually a sweat chloride test. Nonclassic CF characterizes patients with mild disease limited to one organ system or indeterminate diagnostic testing.

Pulmonary function testing (PFT) plays a key role in determining prognosis and evaluating the efficacy of therapies. Early signs on PFT include increased

reserve volume when compared to total lung volumes. Subsequent changes demonstrate an obstructive pattern and include a decline in forced expiratory volume in 1 second (FEV1) and FEV1/forced vital capacity (FVC) and increased total lung capacity due to hyperinflation (see Chapter 46 for further details). PFT can also be used to evaluate acute exacerbations.

TREATMENT

A variety of modalities for the treatment of CF-associated lung disease have been studied and shown to be effective. These include mechanical airway clearance, antimicrobials, bronchodilators, supplemental oxygen, mucolytics, and other novel treatments.

Antibiotics have not been well validated, but standard practice has been to use two antipseudomonal antibiotics in addition to therapies targeted at culture-proven microbiota in acute exacerbations. There has been considerable variation in duration of therapy, and no validated studies have definitively outlined the duration of therapy. While oral antibiotics may be appropriate in mild exacerbations with known culture data, inhaled antibiotics are not considered alternatives and instead function as adjuncts and maintenance therapy. Inhaled therapies, such as tobramycin, aztreonam, and colistin, can improve lung function, improve quality of life, and reduce exacerbations when used for maintenance therapy. Intermittent oral azithromycin can also be implemented. There is no evidence supporting chronic antistaphylococcal or antipseudomonal therapy.

Other chronic therapies commonly used include bronchodilators, although these should be utilized only

CFTR mutation classes

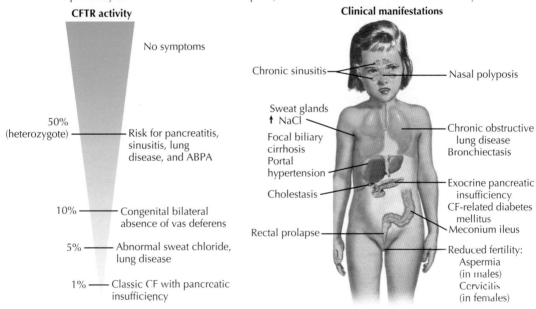

Class I Absent protein synthesis due to defective transcription; **Class II** Defective protein maturation and degradation; **Class III** Defective regulation; **Class IV** Defective chloride conductance; **Class V** Reduced protein synthesis due to reduced transcription; **Class VI** Defective chloride channel stability

CFTR activity

No symptoms

50%
(heterozygote) — Risk for pancreatitis, sinusitis, lung disease, and ABPA

10% — Congenital bilateral absence of vas deferens

5% — Abnormal sweat chloride, lung disease

1% — Classic CF with pancreatic insufficiency

Clinical manifestations

Chronic sinusitis

Nasal polyposis

Sweat glands ↑ NaCl

Focal biliary cirrhosis
Portal hypertension

Cholestasis

Rectal prolapse

Chronic obstructive lung disease
Bronchiectasis

Exocrine pancreatic insufficiency
CF-related diabetes mellitus
Meconium ileus

Reduced fertility:
Aspermia (in males)
Cervicitis (in females)

Pathogenesis

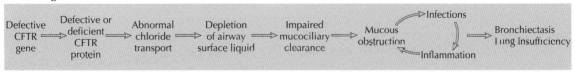

Defective CFTR gene ⟹ Defective or deficient CFTR protein ⟹ Abnormal chloride transport ⟹ Depletion of airway surface liquid ⟹ Impaired mucociliary clearance ⟹ Mucous obstruction ⟹ Infections / Inflammation ⟹ Bronchiectasis Lung insufficiency

FIG. 86.2 **Pathophysiology and Clinical Manifestations of Cystic Fibrosis** *(CF). ABPA,* Allergic bronchopulmonary aspergillosis; *CFTR,* CF transmembrane conductance regulator.

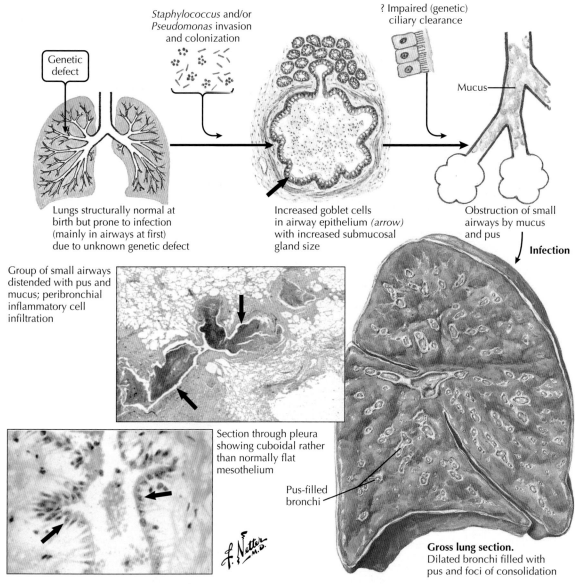

Genetic defect

Staphylococcus and/or *Pseudomonas* invasion and colonization

? Impaired (genetic) ciliary clearance

Mucus

Lungs structurally normal at birth but prone to infection (mainly in airways at first) due to unknown genetic defect

Increased goblet cells in airway epithelium *(arrow)* with increased submucosal gland size

Obstruction of small airways by mucus and pus

Infection

Group of small airways distended with pus and mucus; peribronchial inflammatory cell infiltration

Section through pleura showing cuboidal rather than normally flat mesothelium

Pus-filled bronchi

Gross lung section. Dilated bronchi filled with pus and foci of consolidation

FIG. 86.3 **Pathogenesis of Cystic Fibrosis.**

if there is evidence of airway hyperreactivity. Inhaled glucocorticoids also have insufficient evidence, and systemic glucocorticoids for maintenance therapy are not indicated. High-dose NSAIDs have been validated as chronic therapy in children. Mucous clearance agents have a favorable safety profile and include dornase, hypertonic saline, chest physiotherapy, and flutter devices. These are utilized to improve airway clearance and reduce frequency and duration of exacerbations. All patients should be

vaccinated with PCV12 and PPSV23 pneumococcal vaccines, as well as annual influenza vaccination.

Novel therapies targeting specific genetic mutations have been implemented over the past decade. Ivacaftor, approved in 2012, increases ion flow through the malfunctioning ion gate. This drug was later combined with lumacaftor, a drug aimed at increasing cell surface density of CFTR channels, to offer therapies to patients with cell surface localization mutations.

Bilateral **lung transplant** remains an option for end-stage CF patients, and their survival is better than lung transplant survival in other diseases; on average they survive 8.3 years.

OTHER ORGAN INVOLVEMENT AND CONSIDERATIONS

CF is a multiorgan chronic disease, and the CFTR channel plays key roles in other organ systems. The GI tract is commonly affected, and patients with CF can develop bowel obstruction, focal cirrhosis, and cholelithiasis. CF is one of the leading indications of liver transplantation in children, and liver failure results from thickening of secretions in bile ducts. **Pancreatic insufficiency** contributes significantly to morbidity, as it leads to fat malabsorption and loss of fat-soluble vitamins, as well as CF-related diabetes. Sinus disease leads to chronic rhinosinusitis and nasal polyposis. CF patients may also have difficulty with fertility due to congenital bilateral absence of the vas deferens in men and thickened cervical mucus in women.

CHAPTER 87

Sleep Apnea

KARTIK N. RAJAGOPALAN • DIANNE M. AUGELLI

INTRODUCTION

Sleep apnea, or sleep-disordered breathing (SDB), is a disease that results in the disruption of normal breathing during sleep and encompasses both central sleep apnea (CSA) and obstructive sleep apnea (OSA). CSA occurs in the absence of any structural airway hindrance and is caused by dysregulation of the brain's respiratory control center. CSA can be primary (idiopathic) or caused by injury to the central nervous system, including toxins, or associated with conditions such as congestive heart failure, atrial fibrillation, or renal failure. Treatment of CSA involves addressing underlying diseases as well as therapy with positive pressure ventilation. This chapter, however, will focus primarily on OSA, which results from the collapse of the upper airway during sleep and accounts for the vast majority of SDB.

As the incidence of **obesity** has increased, the incidence of OSA has increased as well, with certain studies estimating that it affects 2% to 4% of the adult population. The prevalence of OSA also increases with age and with male gender.

RISK FACTORS AND PATHOPHYSIOLOGY

OSA results from an **unstable upper airway,** as the neurological impulses that maintain its tone are reduced during sleep and are overcome by risk factors that promote collapse. When the reduced tone of the upper airway is combined with the increased extraluminal pressure, airflow is obstructed. Efforts to breathe against a transiently obstructed airway lead to snoring and variable intrathoracic pressures, and apneic events self-terminate with neuromuscular impulses, which restore airway patency (Fig. 87.1).

Apneic episodes result in hypoxemia and hypercapnia, changes that are sensed by the carotid chemoreceptors, which then signal to various oxygen-sensitive and carbon dioxide–sensitive neurons in the brain and cause sympathetic excitation. This contributes to numerous microarousals, and repeated surges from the sympathetic autonomic nervous system lead to one of the most common consequences of OSA: daytime **hypertension,** which is found in approximately half of all individuals with OSA. In fact, individuals with OSA have elevated levels of angiotensin II and aldosterone as a result of increased sympathetic activity.

During apneic or hypopneic events, sharp decreases in intrathoracic pressure cause pooling of blood in the pulmonary circulation, leading to decreased left ventricular preload and resultant stroke volume. Decreased stroke volume in turn leads to reflexive systemic vasoconstriction, increasing cardiac afterload. These transient increases in afterload and the hypertension that results from OSA contribute to the systolic and diastolic cardiac dysfunction that is seen in these patients. Furthermore, the combination of increased **sympathetic vasoconstriction** leading to decreased coronary perfusion and increased left ventricular afterload results in myocardial ischemia and arrhythmias, including bradyarrhythmias and atrial fibrillation/flutter. Increased hypoxia during sleep, secondary to airway obstruction, causes **pulmonary vasoconstriction,** which serves to remodel and increase the pulmonary vascular pressures leading to right ventricular dysfunction.

The most common risk factor for OSA is obesity due to the propensity for increased pharyngeal fat deposits that increase extraluminal pressure and collapsibility of the upper airway. Individuals with truncal obesity also have increased extrathoracic pressure, which can reduce chest compliance and thus the generation of negative intrathoracic pressure. Other important contributors are craniofacial abnormalities, such as a small mandible, or retroposition of the maxilla that leads to a narrowed airway.

PRESENTATION, EVALUATION, AND DIAGNOSIS

The most common symptom of OSA is excessive **daytime sleepiness.** This may be present despite reportedly adequate amounts of sleep. Other symptoms include nocturia, morning headaches, decreased concentration,

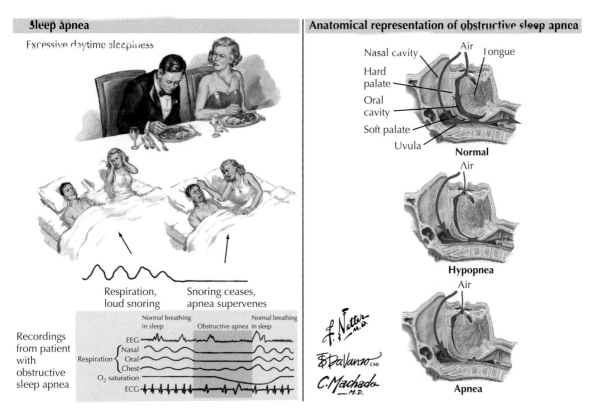

Sleep apnea

Excessive daytime sleepiness

Respiration, loud snoring

Snoring ceases, apnea supervenes

Recordings from patient with obstructive sleep apnea

Normal breathing in sleep — Obstructive apnea — Normal breathing in sleep

EEG
Respiration { Nasal / Oral / Chest }
O₂ saturation
ECG

Anatomical representation of obstructive sleep apnea

Nasal cavity — Air — Tongue
Hard palate
Oral cavity
Soft palate
Uvula

Normal

Air

Hypopnea

Air

Apnea

FIG. 87.1 **Obstructive Sleep Apnea.** *ECG*, Electrocardiogram; *EEG*, electroencephalogram.

memory loss, decreased libido, and irritability. Very importantly, if the patient has a sleep partner, this individual can be questioned about whether the patient snores, makes gasping/choking sounds during sleep, or potentially stops breathing for short periods (see Fig. 87.1). Patients may have undiagnosed OSA at the time of physician encounter and already suffer from sequelae; testing should be considered in those with congestive heart failure without other clear cause, treatment refractory hypertension, atrial fibrillation, or pulmonary hypertension. Of note, patients who live at high altitudes may present with episodes of apnea and compensatory hyperventilation; this is called high-altitude breathing and is a known subset of CSA.

Patients with suspected OSA should undergo **polysomnography (PSG)**, more commonly known as a sleep study, which is required for the diagnosis of OSA. PSG has traditionally occurred in a sleep laboratory with technical support, but portable units are now available for home testing. While monitoring fewer clinical parameters, home sleep testing can be safely utilized in patients without known cardiopulmonary disease and moderate to high probability of OSA. Various physiological parameters

are monitored during a sleep study and include airflow, oxygen saturation, and respiratory effort. During PSG, a patient's **apnea/hypopnea index (AHI)**, which is the number of obstructed airway episodes that occur per hour, can be ascertained. The severity of OSA is graded by the AHI: mild for 5 to 15 events, moderate for 15 to 29 events, and severe for >30 events per hour. While an AHI of 5 or greater confirms a diagnosis of OSA, the diagnosis of OSA syndrome is clinically defined by an AHI of 5 or greater and comorbidities such as hypersomnia, hypertension, mood disorder, cognitive dysfunction, coronary artery disease, stroke, congestive heart failure, atrial fibrillation, or type 2 diabetes. Alternatively, it can be defined by an AHI of 15 or greater in the absence of any symptoms.

TREATMENT

Positive airway pressure (PAP) is the standard of care and the most efficacious treatment for OSA. PAP seeks to overcome the extraluminal forces leading to airway collapse and includes several different modes: continuous PAP (CPAP), bilevel PAP (BiPAP), or autotitrating PAP (APAP). These modes can be delivered through nasal

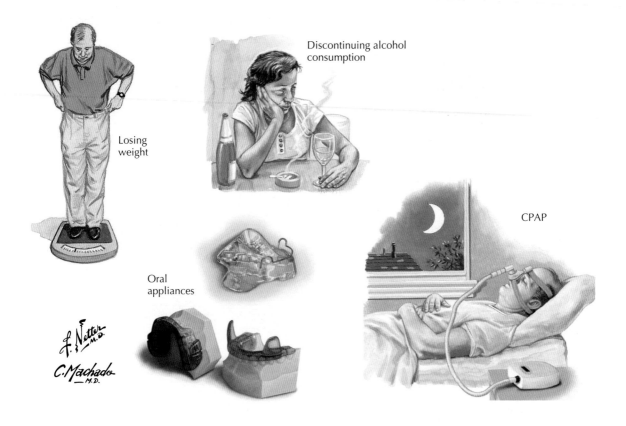

Losing weight

Discontinuing alcohol consumption

CPAP

Oral appliances

FIG. 87.2 **Treatment for Obstructive Sleep Apnea.** *CPAP,* Continuous positive airway pressure.

or oronasal user interfaces. CPAP is generally used first, with BiPAP being second-line treatment in patients who are intolerant of CPAP due to having difficulties exhaling against high pressures and for patients with hypoventilatory disorders, such as obesity hypoventilation and neuromuscular disorders. Additionally, due to changes in airway tone during sleep, the pressure required to splint it open at different points of the night can vary. APAP devices, which can titrate the positive pressure based on apneic/hypopneic events of the patient, can also be used if an in-lab titration is not available. After institution of PAP, compliance, resolution of sleepiness, and patient and bed-partner satisfaction must be addressed at subsequent visits.

In addition to PAP, patients must institute **behavioral modifications** to improve sleep hygiene. Obese patients should be started on a weight-loss program, and all patients should be counseled to avoid caffeine, nicotine, and alcohol before bed and use the bed exclusively for sleep. Oral appliances to reposition the mandible or

tongue to increase the caliber of the airway can be used in mild to moderate OSA and is an option in moderate and severe OSA patients who are intolerant or fail PAP therapy (Fig. 87.2).

Surgical therapies are also an option in OSA and are indicated for patients who fail other noninvasive therapies. These surgeries may involve reconstruction of the upper airway or mandibular/maxillary advancement. Newer options, such as hypoglossal nerve stimulators, may also be appropriate for those who fail traditional therapies. Bariatric surgery is uncommon in regular cases of OSA but can be an adjunct to PAP; it should be considered in patients who have a body mass index (BMI) ≥40, or ≥35 with comorbidities, and who are unable to reduce their own weight. There is a paucity of pharmacological therapies that can be used to treat OSA, though nasal corticosteroids can be helpful in patients who suffer from rhinitis. Oxygen therapy alone is not helpful in treating OSA and might prolong apneas, thus increasing hypercapnia during sleep.

CHAPTER 88

Diffuse Parenchymal Lung Disease

MARY ELIZABETH CARD

INTRODUCTION

Diffuse parenchymal lung disease (DPLD), or **interstitial lung disease (ILD)**, refers to a heterogeneous group of >100 distinct lung disorders that cause varying degrees of inflammation and fibrosis in the lung parenchyma. The airspace, peripheral airways, and blood vessels may also be affected. Diagnosis is made largely on the basis of the patient's clinical history and radiographic studies, including chest radiograph and high-resolution CT scan (HRCT); however, diagnosis occasionally requires histopathological testing (Figs. 88.1 and 88.2). Generally speaking, the natural history of DPLD ranges from complete recovery in patients with predominantly inflammatory parenchymal disease to death in patients with end-stage fibrosis. Management should target stabilization and prevention of progression. It is usually individualized based on the patient's specific DPLD diagnosis, respiratory status, comorbidities, and personal approach to medical care.

PATHOPHYSIOLOGY AND RISK FACTORS

DPLD refers to a wide spectrum of lung diseases, each with its own unique pathophysiology. Risk factors for the development of DPLD include (1) exposure to noxious environmental and/or occupational stimuli, (2) genetic predisposition, (3) comorbid disease such as collagen vascular diseases, (4) infectious organisms, and (5) genomics-based aberrant repair responses that ultimately lead to sustained inflammation and remodeling of the lung parenchyma.

CLASSIFICATION

Diagnosing DPLD is challenging because it requires the synthesis of clinical, radiographical, and sometimes pathohistological data (Table 88.1). Broadly speaking, DPLD can be divided into lung disease from known versus unknown causes. The known causes include pneumoconiosis (e.g., asbestos, silica, hard metals, coal dust), connective tissue disorder–associated DPLD (CTD-associated DPLD), and hypersensitivity pneumonitis (e.g., birds, hay, fungi, *Mycobacteria*).

The classification system of the unknown (idiopathic) causes of DLPD is complicated and has undergone multiple revisions. The most recent and widely accepted consensus guidelines published in 2013 classify **idiopathic interstitial pneumonias (IIPs)** into three major groups: major IIPs, rare IIPs, and unclassifiable IIPs. Major IIPs include chronic fibrosing lung diseases, such as **idiopathic pulmonary fibrosis (IPF)** and **nonspecific interstitial pneumonia (NSIP)**; smoking-related lung diseases, such as respiratory bronchiolitis with ILD (RB-ILD) and desquamative interstitial pneumonia (DIP); and acute and subacute IIPs, such as **acute interstitial pneumonia (AIP)** and **cryptogenic organizing pneumonia (COP)**. Rare IIPs include idiopathic lymphoid interstitial pneumonia (LIP) and idiopathic pleuroparenchymal fibroelastosis (PPFE). Finally, unclassifiable IIPs include DPLD that are either diseases with inadequate clinical, radiological, or pathological data to make a firm diagnosis, either due to discrepencies among available data or presentations with multiple disease patterns present.

PRESENTATION, EVALUATION, AND DIAGNOSIS

Different forms of DPLD may require vastly different treatment and management strategies, typically with a dynamic integrated approach using multidisciplinary discussion (MDD) comprised of a clinician, a radiologist, and (when appropriate) a pathologist.

A detailed medical history is the most important tool for diagnosing DPLD. Typically, patients with DPLD present similarly with exertional dyspnea and a dry cough, with symptoms evolving over months to years, although there are exceptions to this rule, such as AIP, acute eosinophilic pneumonia, acute hypersensitivity pneumonitis, diffuse alveolar hemorrhage, COP drug reactions, and acute exacerbations. In the case of acute DPLD, the clinician's suspicion for DPLD may be raised if the patient's symptoms fail to improve after antibiotics

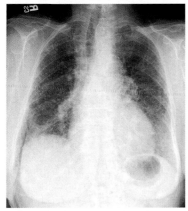

PA chest film shows extensive pulmonary fibrosis with typical honeycomb pattern.

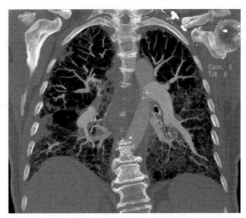

Coronal reconstruction of chest from CTA shows extensive interstitial thickening, cystic changes, and honeycombing bilaterally with cystic changes involving more the upper than lower lungs. Confluent pleural thickening is seen laterally on the right.

FIG 88.1 **Severe Pulmonary Fibrosis.** *CTA,* CT angiogram; *PA,* posteroanterior.

or diuretics. Other nonspecific systemic complaints, such as night sweats, fever, fatigue, unintentional weight loss, ophthalmological complaints, gastrointestinal symptoms, and musculoskeletal concerns, can assist in diagnosis and may suggest an etiology. Thorough medication histories are necessary, and patients should also be questioned about a broad variety of environmental/occupational exposures, including inorganic toxins, molds, pets (birds), and cigarette smoking.

Although most DPLD are not heritable, some forms of the disease are associated with particular genetic abnormalities, and patients with particular genetic variants do seem to be at higher risk of developing DPLD, particularly IPF, **sarcoidosis,** and chronic beryllium syndrome.

Physical exam findings vary depending on the specific type of DPLD. For example, most patients with pulmonary fibrosis will have fine, inspiratory, ripping-like crackles, and digital clubbing, whereas patients without fibrosis will sound normal on lung auscultation. Non-pulmonary exam findings include erythema nodosum, skin tightening or ulcerations of the digits, or sicca symptoms, all of which may suggest a CTD-associated DPLD. If CTD-associated DPLD is suspected, the patient should have confirmatory serological testing done (e.g., antinuclear and antiextractable nuclear antibody testing).

Chest radiography will generally show diffuse, bilateral pulmonary infiltrates. Pulmonary function testing (PFT) demonstrates a restrictive ventilatory defect as a result of decreased lung compliance as well as a decreased diffusion capacity due to the presence of fibrotic and/or inflammatory cells in the lung interstitium. HRCT

is more sensitive and specific than a chest radiograph and has an extremely high negative predictive value. Some forms of DPLD, such as IPF, have characteristic HRCT findings such that further testing is not required to make a diagnosis. If, however, HRCT is nondiagnostic, additional histopathological evaluation should be pursued via bronchoscopy with bronchoalveolar (BAL) analysis and/or transbronchial lung biopsy. Additional tests such as microbiologic testing, special stains and cell marking testing, and malignant cell cytology can be sent depending on the clinician's clinical suspicion. If the BAL cellular analysis in conjunction with the patient's history, physical exam, and chest imaging is still not diagnostic for a specific DPLD diagnosis, then the practitioner should proceed to surgical lung biopsy, which may be performed via video-assisted thoracoscopic surgery (VATS) or open biopsy.

TREATMENT AND PROGNOSIS

Management and prognosis of DPLD depends on the specific diagnosis. In general, management consists of one or a combination of the following: supportive therapy, treatment of the patients' underlying comorbidities, immunosuppressive therapy, antifibrotic drugs, lung transplant, and palliative care. In the case of DPLD due to a particular exposure, that exposure must be eliminated.

There are a variety of objective measures the clinician may use to monitor for disease progression, including PFT, diffusion capacity of the lung for carbon monoxide (DLCO), the 6-minute walk test (6MWT), oxyhemoglobin

Nonspecific interstitial pneumonia

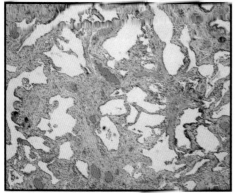

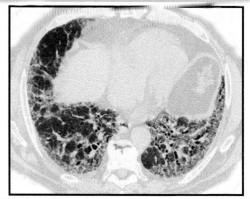

The fibrotic NSIP pattern is present showing the alveolar walls to be uniformly thickened by dense fibrosis. The architecture of the lung is relatively preserved, and the dense fibrosis is approximately of the same age. Fibroblastic foci are absent. Fibrotic NSIP can be difficult to reliably distinguish from UIP.

HRCT shows bilateral symmetric ground-glass opacities with traction bronchiectasis and volume loss. Honeycombing is absent.

Respiratory bronchiolitis-associated ILD **Lymphoid interstitial pneumonitis**

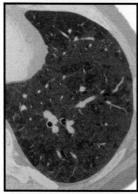

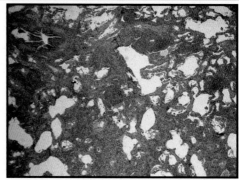

HRCT shows patchy areas of ground-glass opacities and a few poorly defined nodular opacities.

A diffuse lymphoid infiltrate with several reactive follicles extends through the pulmonary interstitium. A mixture of lymphocytes and plasma cells is present in the interstitium.

FIG. 88.2 Idiopathic Interstitial Pneumonias. *HRCT,* High-resolution CT; *ILD,* interstitial lung disease; *NSIP,* nonspecific interstitial pneumonia; *UIP,* usual interstitial pneumonia.

saturation change, and serial chest radiograph. Of note, obtaining serial HRCT as a means for monitoring for disease progression is not currently recommended due to lack of validation and the radiation risk it poses to the patient.

Patients should be assessed for the need of supplemental oxygen, with the goal SpO_2 >90% at rest and on exertion. Referral to pulmonary rehabilitation can be helpful to patients by teaching them breathing techniques, as a form of social support and to help identify comorbidities, such as anxiety and depression, so that patients can be referred to the appropriate specialists. Gastroesophageal reflux disease (GERD) control, as well

as postnasal drip and secretions, may prevent disease worsening.

In addition, patients' comorbidities should be treated. These include coronary artery disease (CAD), for which patients with IPF are at increased risk (from management options); lung nodules, which tend to arise at the junction of diseased and normal lung parenchyma; GERD, which some believe leads to the development of DPLD; secondary pulmonary hypertension; and metabolic bone disease.

Some forms of DPLD, such as COP, eosinophilic pneumonia, sarcoidosis, and NSIP respond quite well

Text continued on p. 380

TABLE 88.1
Classification and Characteristics of Specific Diffuse Parenchymal Lung Diseases (DPLDs)

Clinical Diagnosis	Clinical History	Physical Exam	Histological Pattern	Radiographical Findings	Bronchoalveolar Lavage (BAL) Cell Analysis
KNOWN DPLD, PNEUMOCONIOSIS					
Chronic beryllium disease (CBD)	Exposure history			Hilar LAD; nodules along bronchovascular bundles	Consistent cell pattern; positive lymphocyte proliferation test
Asbestosis	Exposure history Gradual onset of dyspnea			Irregular linear opacities with thickened interlobular septae that predominate in dorsal, subpleural areas; pleural plaques	Infection, hemorrhage, malignancy excluded
Silicosis	Exposure history Gradual onset of dyspnea			Dense, well-circumscribed nodules in upper-lung and middle-lung zones	Silica-laden macrophages; infection, hemorrhage, malignancy excluded
KNOWN DPLD, CTD-ASSOCIATED DPLD					
CTD • Rheumatoid arthritis (RA) • Systemic sclerosis (SSc) • Systemic lupus erythematosus (SLE) • Polymyositis/dermatomyositis (PM/DM) • Primary Sjögren syndrome • Mixed connective tissue disease • Undifferentiated connective tissue disease (UCTD)	Rapid onset, worsening Pleurisy (SLE, RA) Eye symptoms Rash GERD, dysphagia (scleroderma) Raynaud phenomenon Arthralgias, arthritis Morning stiffness Sicca symptoms (Sjögren) Myalgias, muscle weakness Young, female	Pleural rub on pulmonary auscultation (RA, SLE) Erythema nodosum Telangiectasia (scleroderma) Calcinosis (scleroderma, PM/DM) Subcutaneous nodules (RA) Skin tightening, ulcerations over the digits (scleroderma) Scleritis (SLE) Keratoconjunctivitis sicca HSM Synovitis, arthritis Pericardial rub (SLE) Raynaud phenomenon Keratoconjunctivitis sicca (Sjögren) Enlarged salivary glands (Sjögren) Heliotrope rash (PM/DM) Gottron papules (PM/DM) Mechanic's hands (PM/DM) Muscle weakness, myositis (PM/DM)		GGOs Pleural effusions Pericardial effusion Pericardial thickening Esophageal dilatation NSIP pattern on HRCT	Infection, hemorrhage, malignancy excluded

KNOWN DPLD, HYPERSENSITIVITY

Condition	Clinical	Exam/Auscultation	Pattern	Imaging	BAL
Hypersensitivity (HP)	• Acute or chronic presentation with exposure history. Note, however, that up to 30% of patients with histological HP have no exposure history[a]	Squeaks on pulmonary auscultation		Acute: bilateral GGOs and poorly defined centrilobular nodules. Chronic: reticular fibrotic pattern +/- honeycomb change, and traction bronchiectasis +/- GGOs. Upper-lobe distribution	>15% lymphocytes (>50% lends even more support); exclude infection, hemorrhage, malignancy
Eosinophilic pneumonia (EP)	• Diffuse CXR infiltrates • Rapid response to steroids			Bilateral peripheral subpleural airspace consolidation	>1% eosinophils (>25% eosinophils virtually diagnostic for acute/chronic EP)
Drug reaction	• Rapid onset, worsening • Drug exposure			Can appear similar to various ILD	>15% lymphocytes; hemorrhage; infection and malignancy excluded

IDIOPATHIC, MAJOR, FIBROSING CONDITIONS

Condition	Clinical	Exam/Auscultation	Pattern	Imaging	BAL
Idiopathic pulmonary fibrosis (IPF)	• Age >70 • Male • Subacute/chronic onset of dyspnea • Nonproductive cough	• Bibasilar Ripping-like crackles on pulmonary auscultation • Prominent P2 • Digital clubbing	UIP	Reticulation, traction, and bronchiectasis are common. Distribution is predominantly peripheral, subpleural, and basilar, may be asymmetric and patchy. Very little or no GGOs	>3% neutrophils

Continued

TABLE 88.1
Classification and Characteristics of Specific Diffuse Parenchymal Lung Diseases (DPLDs)—cont'd

Clinical Diagnosis	Clinical History	Physical Exam	Histological Pattern	Radiographical Findings	Bronchoalveolar Lavage (BAL) Cell Analysis
Nonspecific interstitial pneumonia (NSIP)	• Age 40–50, may also occur in children • Male = female • Subacute onset of dyspnea, cough, fatigue, weight loss	• Basilar crackles	NSIP	Bilateral GGOs, irregular reticular opacities with traction bronchiectasis and bronchiolectasis. Distribution is predominantly peripheral, subpleural, basilar and symmetric, and homogenous. Fibrosis is predominantly basilar, often symmetric. Honeycombing uncommon	Typical BAL profile; hemorrhage, infection, and malignancy excluded
IDIOPATHIC, MAJOR, SMOKING RELATED					
Respiratory bronchiolitis with ILD (RB-ILD)	• Age 30–40 • Male > female • Smokers • Mild, nondisabling symptoms; however, some experience significant dyspnea and hypoxemia		Respiratory bronchiolitis (RB)	Bronchial wall thickening and GGOs. Distribution is diffuse. Mild, upper lung-predominant centrilobular ground-glass nodularity is common	Increased, heavily pigmented alveolar macrophages and absence of lymphocytosis; hemorrhage, infection, and malignancy excluded

Disease	Clinical features	Histologic pattern	Imaging findings	BAL/Biopsy
Pulmonary Langerhans cell histiocytosis of lung (PLCH)	• Subacute onset of dyspnea • History of pneumothorax		Cysts and centrilobular nodules that can cavitate; most prominent in mid-lung to upper-lung zones	CD1a-positive cells >5%; infection, hemorrhage, malignancy excluded
Desquamative interstitial pneumonia (DIP)	• Age 30–40 • Male > female • Smoking history • Weeks–months of dyspnea and dry cough that may progress to respiratory failure	DIP	GGOs that span several pulmonary lobules, typically in the lower and peripheral lung distribution. Multiple-clustered cysts within areas of GGOs Desquamative interstitial pneumonia	Increased, heavily pigmented alveolar macrophages. Typical BAL profile; hemorrhage, infection, and malignancy excluded
IDIOPATHIC, MAJOR, ACUTE/SUBACUTE				
Acute interstitial pneumonia (AIP)	• Age 50 • Male = female • Acute, viral-like prodrome followed by rapidly progressive hypoxemia • Diffuse crackles and consolidation	Diffuse alveolar damage (DAD)	Early, exudative: diffuse alveolar damage. Patchy consolidation and GGOs. Consolidation is greater in dependent lung. Later, organizing: distortion of bronchovascular bundles and traction bronchiectasis	Prominent neutrophils; infection and hemorrhage excluded

Continued

TABLE 88.1
Classification and Characteristics of Specific Diffuse Parenchymal Lung Diseases (DPLDs)—cont'd

Clinical Diagnosis	Clinical History	Physical Exam	Histological Pattern	Radiographical Findings	Bronchoalveolar Lavage (BAL) Cell Analysis
Cryptogenic organizing pneumonia (COP)	• Age 55 • Male = female • Subacute onset (median, <3 months) of cough, dyspnea, weight loss, chills, intermittent fever, myalgias following viral URI-like symptoms		Organizing pneumonia (OP) (patchy process characterized by organizing pneumonia involving alveolar ducts and alveoli with or without bronchiolar intraluminal polyps)	Patchy, migratory consolidation. Distribution is predominantly in a subpleural, peribronchial or bandlike pattern; often basilar and peripheral but can be anywhere; often bilateral. Consolidation with wispy borders and GGOs, transient bronchial dilation and distortion of lung architecture. Atoll/reverse halo sign (a central region of GGO with a surrounding rim of consolidation) and perilobular thickening can be suggestive	>15% lymphocytes (>25% lends even more support)
IDIOPATHIC, RARE					
Lymphocytic interstitial pneumonia (LIP)	• Female • Age 40 • Gradually worsening cough and dyspnea ≥3 years • Presents with symptoms consistent with the underlying systemic/autoimmune disorder	• Crackles • Lymphadenopathy	LIP	Lower-lung predominant perilymphatic cysts, typically adjacent to the peribronchovascular bundles. Patchy bilateral GGOs. Subpleural and perilymphatic nodularity	>15% lymphocytes; hemorrhage, infection, and malignancy excluded

Disease	Clinical features / History	Radiographic / HRCT findings	BAL findings
Idiopathic pleuroparenchymal fibroelastosis (PPFE)	Age 50-60; Recurrent infections; Pneumothorax	Subpleural consolidation with traction bronchiectasis, architectural distortion and upper-lobe volume loss	
Lymphangioleiomyomatosis (LAM)	Hemoptysis; Female; Subacute onset of dyspnea; History of pneumothorax	Randomly distributed, thin-walled cysts throughout lungs surrounded by normal parenchyma	Infection, hemorrhage, malignancy excluded
Diffuse alveolar hemorrhage (DAH)	Rapid onset, worsening; Hemoptysis; Collagen vascular disease (especially lupus erythematosus)	Patchy or diffuse areas of GGOs	Progressive increase in RBCs with sequential BAL aliquots excluding infection, malignancy
IDIOPATHIC, OTHER			
Sarcoidosis	Eye symptoms; Rash; Arthralgias, arthritis; Bilateral hilar LAD; Uveitis; Enlarged salivary glands; Lymphadenopathy; HSM; Muscle weakness, myositis; Synovitis; Prominent P2 (if end stage); Pericardial rub	Hilar/ mediastinal adenopathy. Nodules along bronchovascular bundles in mid-lung/ upper-lung fields	>15% lymphocytes (≥25% lends even more support). CD4/CD8 ratio >3.5 increases specificity
Pulmonary alveolar proteinosis (PAP)	Subacute onset of dyspnea	Alveolar filling pattern	Milky fluid with positive PAS-staining and amorphous debris; hemorrhage, infection, malignancy excluded

BAL, Bronchoalveolar; CTD, connective tissue disorder; CXR, chest x-ray; GERD, gastroesophageal reflux disease; GGO, ground glass opacity; HRCT, high-resolution CT; HSM, hepatosplenomegaly; ILD, interstitial lung disease; LAD, lymphadenopathy; PAS, periodic acid–Schiff; RBC, red blood cell; UIP, usual interstitial pneumonia; URI, upper respiratory infection.

[a]Data from Travis W, Costabe U, Hansell D, et al: An Official American Thoracic Society/European Respiratory Society Statement: Update of the International Multidisciplinary Classification of the Idiopathic Interstitial Pneumonias, Am J Respir Crit Care Med 188:733–748, 2013.

to immunosuppressive treatment with steroids. Other DPLD, such as CTD-associated DPLD, may require a prolonged course of steroids, in which case one should consider adding a steroid-sparing medication such as azathioprine or mycophenolate mofetil to the treatment regimen. More severe forms of DPLD may require more aggressive immunosuppression with cytotoxic drugs such as cyclophosphamide. There exist few effective treatment options for patients with fibrotic lung disease. Two drugs that have shown potential benefit are pirfenidone, an antifibrotic small molecule drug, and nintedanib, a multikinase inhibitor that targets multiple growth factor receptors. These drugs have shown modest benefit at delaying symptoms, but given their side effects, guidelines suggest shared decision making regarding their use.

In patients with fibrotic lung disease, lung transplant may ultimately be required, and the International Society for Heart and Lung Transplantation (ISHLT) has guidelines for transplant listing. If transplant is not an option, palliative services, including hospice, may be appropriate. An emerging area of research is aimed at identifying biomarkers that may be used to help diagnose, manage, and/or prognosticate DPLD. To date, the biomarkers that have been identified have not been validated in any large-scale, independent studies.

CHAPTER 89

Pulmonary Embolism

EMILIA A. HERMANN

INTRODUCTION

A **pulmonary embolus** (PE) is an obstruction of the pulmonary artery or distal arteriole, most commonly by a thrombus. In >95% of cases, emboli originate as **deep venous thrombosis** (DVT) in the lower extremities; however, thrombi may also originate in the upper extremities or right side of the heart. PEs are common, with an estimated incidence of 70 per 100,000 population; however, the actual figures are likely to be substantially higher because clinically silent PE can develop in up to 40% to 50% of patients with DVT. Acute PE-related mortality approaches 30% if untreated, whereas the mortality rate of diagnosed and treated PE is approximately 8%. The clinical presentation of PE is varied, and diagnosis requires a high degree of clinical suspicion. Diagnostic work-up and treatment are determined by the patient's initial clinical presentation and hemodynamic stability.

PATHOPHYSIOLOGY

Thrombus classically forms when Virchow triad is present: stasis of blood flow, hypercoagulability, and endothelial injury. A PE occurs when thrombus originating in the venous system of the legs dislodges, travels through the venous vasculature and right side of the heart, and obstructs a branch of the pulmonary artery. Pulmonary arterial occlusion results in an increase in pulmonary artery pressure and vasospasm distal to the clot. In addition, alveolar collapse and atelectasis occur in the lung distal to the obstruction. Because the lung has dual circulation with both pulmonary and bronchial arteries, infarction is not common but can occur, especially with large occlusive clots. Although PEs are most commonly caused by thrombosis, nonthrombotic occlusion of the pulmonary artery or arterioles may also occur with embolism of air, fat, amniotic fluid, or foreign bodies.

RISK FACTORS

Risk factors for PE include circumstances that increase the likelihood of DVT formation, including immobility (i.e., long car or plane rides, convalescence during hospitalization/after surgery), congenital or acquired prothrombotic disorders, trauma, or malignancy (Fig. 89.1). Prior PE/DVT is also a risk factor for PE.

PRESENTATION AND EVALUATION

Patients with acute PE may have a range of presentations from largely asymptomatic to cardiogenic shock. Classically, patients with PE are described as having sudden-onset shortness of breath or increased dyspnea with mild exertion (Fig. 89.2). Patients also may complain of pleuritic chest pain, cough, orthopnea, and (rarely) hemoptysis.

Because a PE increases pulmonary vascular resistance, and therefore increases resistance against the right ventricle, patients will often present with tachycardia. PE also causes hypoxemia due to a mismatch of ventilation and perfusion with disruption of pulmonary arterial blood flow, leading to inefficient excretion of carbon dioxide and reduced uptake of oxygen. This produces tachypnea, another common vital sign abnormality in patients presenting with PE. Importantly, because of the dead space created by a portion of the lung that is ventilated but not perfused, hypoxemia in patients with PE may persist despite the administration of supplemental oxygen.

Physical exam findings for PE are nonspecific. Hemodynamically significant PE may present with signs of cardiogenic shock (cool extremities, altered mental status), or right-sided cardiac strain (jugular venous distension, new tricuspid murmur, or accentuated second heart sound). Patients with hemodynamically stable PE may present more subtly with nonspecific abnormalities in lung auscultation, such as crackles or scattered wheezing. A history or presence of asymmetric leg swelling or calf pain with dorsiflexion of the foot (Homan sign) suggests the presence of DVT.

Routine laboratory findings and initial screening tests are not diagnostic for PE but may raise or lower clinical suspicion. The most common test used is a **D-dimer**, which measures fibrin degradation products

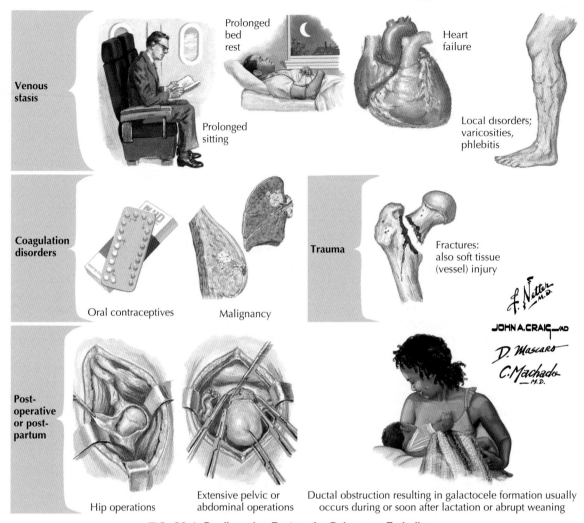

Venous stasis

Prolonged bed rest

Prolonged sitting

Heart failure

Local disorders; varicosities, phlebitis

Coagulation disorders

Oral contraceptives

Malignancy

Trauma

Fractures: also soft tissue (vessel) injury

Post-operative or post-partum

Hip operations

Extensive pelvic or abdominal operations

Ductal obstruction resulting in galactocele formation usually occurs during or soon after lactation or abrupt weaning

FIG. 89.1 Predisposing Factors for Pulmonary Embolism.

and is elevated with DVT/PE. Its primary use, however, is as a test to rule out thromboembolism given its high sensitivity. Common abnormalities seen on arterial blood gas include hypoxemia, respiratory alkalosis, and an increased alveolar to arterial (A-a) oxygen gradient, though a normal A-a gradient is not sensitive enough to rule out a PE. Cardiac biomarkers such as pro-BNP and troponin may also be elevated in patients with hemodynamically significant PE and right ventricular (RV) strain.

The classic electrocardiogram (ECG) pattern of S1Q3T3—deep S wave in lead 1, Q wave in III, and inverted T wave in III—is rare and may occur in only 10% of patients with acute PE. More commonly, ECG findings in patients with PE include sinus tachycardia as well as evidence of RV strain, including complete or incomplete right bundle branch block (RBBB), T-wave inversions in leads V_1 to V_4 or the inferior leads (II, III, and aVF), right axis deviation, P pulmonale (peaked P wave in lead II >2.5 mm in height), and a dominant R wave in V_1 (Fig. 89.3).

Chest radiographs are nonspecific in patients with PE but may show atelectasis or a pleural effusion. Less commonly, direct evidence of a PE may be seen, including an abrupt cutoff of a proximal pulmonary vessel (Westermark sign), enlarged pulmonary arteries at the hilum (Fleischner sign), or wedge-shaped opacity at the pleura (Hampton hump).

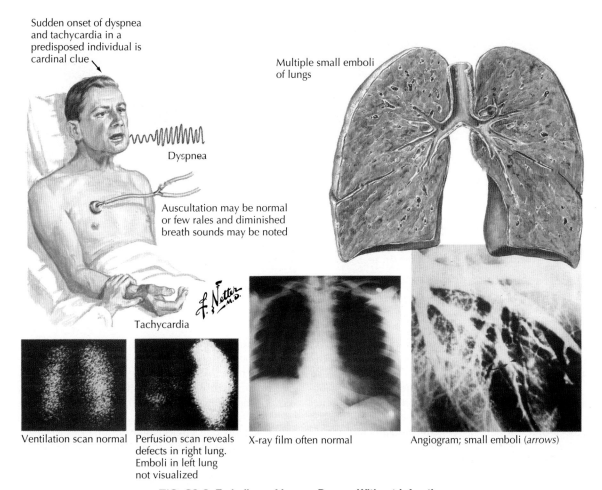

Sudden onset of dyspnea and tachycardia in a predisposed individual is cardinal clue

Dyspnea

Auscultation may be normal or few rales and diminished breath sounds may be noted

Tachycardia

Multiple small emboli of lungs

Ventilation scan normal

Perfusion scan reveals defects in right lung. Emboli in left lung not visualized

X-ray film often normal

Angiogram; small emboli (*arrows*)

FIG. 89.2 **Embolism of Lesser Degree Without Infarction.**

DIAGNOSIS AND TREATMENT

Diagnostic workup and treatment of patients with suspected PE are based on the hemodynamic stability of the patient. Treatment algorithms have historically classified PEs as massive, submassive, or nonmassive based on hemodynamic stability and evidence of RV strain.

In hemodynamically stable patients, diagnosis of PE should follow a stepwise approach starting with a clinical probability assessment based on a patient's clinical presentation and underlying risk factors. Clinical decision aids, such as **Wells criteria** or the Geneva score, may be used to classify patients into categories of pretest probability for PE, which then informs the choice of diagnostic testing and interpretation of test results.

In stable patients with low or intermediate clinical probability of PE, an enzyme-linked immunosorbent assay (ELISA)–based D-dimer assay has a high negative predictive value. Patients with low clinical probability of PE and negative D-dimer assay have an estimated 3-month risk of PE of ~0.15% and do not need to undergo further workup. Importantly, the specificity of an elevated D-dimer is reduced by other medical conditions, such as active malignancy, kidney function, and/or pregnancy. Age-adjusted D-dimer with clinical scores are very helpful to exclude PE in elderly.

Patients with a high clinical probability of PE and/or positive D-dimer testing should undergo CT pulmonary angiography (CTPA), which is the imaging study with the best sensitivity and specificity for PE. Other imaging modalities, such as ventilation-perfusion (V/Q) scanning, may be performed where CTPA is unavailable or contraindicated (such as in renal failure); however, V/Q

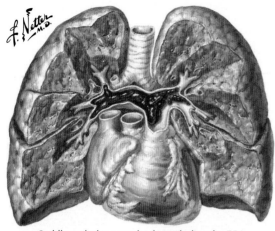

X-ray film showing dense shadow of the RPA with increased luminescence of peripheral lung fields

Saddle embolus completely occluding the RPA and partially obstructing main and left arteries

Sinus tachycardia is the most common electrocardiographic finding in acute pulmonary embolism. This ECG also demonstrates the "classic," though rare, S1Q3T3, and right-axis deviation.

FIG. 89.3 **Massive Embolization.** *ECG*, Electrocardiogram; *RPA*, right pulmonary artery.

scans have a lower positive predictive value than CTPA and are diagnostic in only 50% to 70% of patients with suspected PE.

In hemodynamically unstable patients, management should initially be focused on stabilizing the patient with supplemental oxygenation, intravenous (IV) fluids, and vasopressor support (usually norepinephrine) if necessary. CTPA is also the preferred imaging modality to confirm PE in hemodynamically unstable patients. However, if CTPA is not available immediately, or if the patient is too unstable for transport, assessment for RV dysfunction using transthoracic echocardiography or assessment for evidence of emboli in the main pulmonary arteries using transesophageal echocardiography should be performed to confirm PE diagnosis.

Once diagnosed with PE, patients should be stratified for risk of adverse outcome based on evidence of myocardial dysfunction to guide disposition and treatment decisions. RV dysfunction can be assessed either via laboratory evaluation with cardiac markers (B-type natriuretic peptide [BNP]/pro-BNP, troponin) or via echocardiography. CTPA may suggest RV strain with septal bowing/flattening or RV enlargement by calculating the RV to left ventricular (LV) ratio.

Hemodynamically unstable patients with PE should undergo immediate IV thrombolysis. Contraindications to thrombolytic therapy include uncontrolled hypertension, recent major surgery or trauma, and intracranial disease, which raises the probability of fatal intracranial hemorrhage. In patients for whom thrombolysis is contraindicated or

unsuccessful, surgical or catheter-directed embolectomy should be considered. Surgical embolectomy is most effective for proximal emboli, especially when there are clots-in-transit (visualized intracardiac emboli by echocardiography or CTPA), with patent foramen ovale (PFO). Risk of a cerebrovascular accident increases in these patients, and surgical intervention in a specialized center is recommended. Catheter-directed thrombolysis, such as ultrasound-assisted technique, has progressed greatly over the last few years. It can function close to systemic thrombolysis in certain cases.

Hemodynamically stable patients with evidence of RV dysfunction should be admitted for monitoring in the intensive care unit or a stepdown bed with cardiac monitoring. They should receive systemic anticoagulation. Patients with a large clot burden, high oxygen requirement, significant tachycardia, or evidence of severe RV strain/dysfunction should be considered for catheter-based thrombolysis therapies on a case-by-case basis. Determination of that is highly valuable with the presence of PE response team (PERT) consultants.

Hemodynamically stable patients without evidence of RV strain may be considered for outpatient anticoagulation. The simplified Pulmonary Embolism Severity Index (sPESI) is a tool that has been developed to help clinicians determine the safety of outpatient management of patients with stable, low-risk PE in the right clinical and social context.

Options for systemic anticoagulation include low molecular weight heparin, fondaparinux, IV unfractionated heparin, warfarin, or direct oral anticoagulants. Patient factors, such as obesity, malignancy, prior heparin-induced toxicity, renal failure, and pregnancy, must be considered when choosing the most appropriate agent. Absolute contraindications for anticoagulation include recent surgery, hemorrhagic stroke, or active bleeding. In these patients, alternative treatments include vena cava filter placement.

Duration of treatment depends on whether the diagnosed PE was provoked—developed due to a clear precipitating risk factor—or unprovoked. If provoked with transient risk factors, patients should be anticoagulated for a minimum 3 months. Select patients should be considered for indefinite anticoagulation, including patients with unprovoked PE, patients with recurrent PE, and patients with persistent PE risk factors.

CHAPTER 90

Pulmonary Hypertension

ASHLEY L. SPANN

INTRODUCTION

Pulmonary hypertension (PH) is the existence of sustained elevations in blood pressure within the pulmonary arteries. PH is defined by a mean pulmonary arterial pressure >25 mm Hg, with higher pressures corresponding to increased severity. There are several processes that can lead to this; as such, the clinical presentation of PH can be quite variable. Patients with PH are grouped according to cause of PH, which guides potential management options.

PATHOPHYSIOLOGY

Blood supply to the lungs involves two different circulatory pathways. The bronchial circulation is a high-pressure, low-flow system responsible for maintaining pulmonary function by providing well-oxygenated blood directly to the vessels feeding the conducting airways. The pulmonary circulation, on the other hand, is a low-pressure, high-flow system that supplies venous blood from the right ventricle to the alveolar capillaries for gas exchange, later emptying into the left atrium (Fig. 90.1).

The pulmonary circulation consists of precapillary pulmonary arterial vessels, the pulmonary capillary bed, and postcapillary pulmonary veins. The pressure within the main pulmonary artery is a function of right ventricular cardiac output, pulmonary vascular resistance, and postcapillary pressure; conditions that increase the latter two can lead to pulmonary hypertension. While increased pressure due to increased right ventricular output is offset by vasodilation of the pulmonary vascular bed, decreased left ventricular cardiac output can increase postcapillary pressures, leading to pulmonary hypertension. The pulmonary vascular tree undergoes modifications to accommodate chronically elevated pulmonary pressures, such as hypertrophy in the pulmonary muscular and elastic arteries. The right ventricle can hypertrophy to increase contractility and systolic force to overcome increased pressures, but as the pulmonary system is traditionally a low-pressure system, the ventricle tends to dilate in response to pulmonary hypertension, resulting in right ventricular failure and clinical manifestations of pulmonary hypertension.

EPIDEMIOLOGY

Given the variety of conditions that lead to the pathophysiological changes that contribute to pulmonary hypertension, the disease can occur at any age. PH is classified into World Health Organization (WHO) groups based on the cause of PH (Fig. 90.2):
- Group 1: Pulmonary arterial hypertension (PAH)
- Group 2: PH due to left heart disease
- Group 3: PH due to chronic hypoxemia or lung disease
- Group 4: PH due to chronic thromboembolism (CTEPH)
- Group 5: PH from unclear or multifactorial causes

Group 1 includes connective tissue diseases (most commonly systemic sclerosis), which are significant risk factors for development of PAH. HIV can lead to pulmonary arteriopathies causing PAH. Drugs that have been previously linked to PAH include appetite suppressants (fen-phen, dexfenfluramine) and selective serotonin reuptake inhibitor (SSRI) use in pregnancy. Cardiac etiologies include left ventricular systolic and diastolic dysfunction, heart failure with a preserved ejection fraction, and left-sided valvulopathy. Pulmonary diseases such as chronic obstructive pulmonary disease (COPD) and interstitial lung disease (ILD), including idiopathic and secondary to connective tissue disease, are risk factors, as are systemic diseases, including sarcoidosis, sickle cell disease, and glycogen storage diseases.

PRESENTATION, EVALUATION, AND DIAGNOSIS

The evaluation of potential PH should start with a focused history and physical exam. The most common complaints include exertional dyspnea or reductions in exercise tolerance and fatigue that precedes more advanced complaints of syncope, lower extremity edema, and abdominal distention due to right ventricular failure.

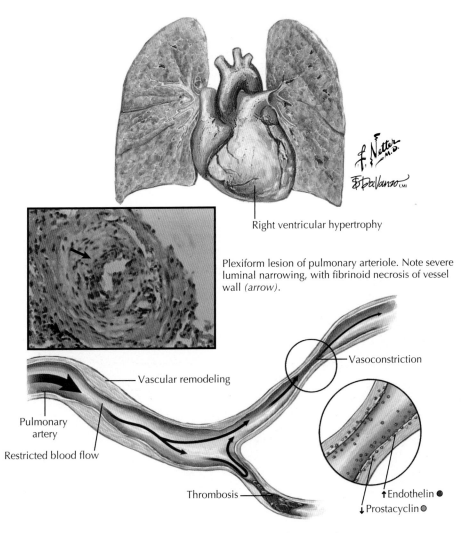

Right ventricular hypertrophy

Plexiform lesion of pulmonary arteriole. Note severe luminal narrowing, with fibrinoid necrosis of vessel wall (arrow).

Vasoconstriction

Vascular remodeling

Pulmonary artery

Restricted blood flow

Thrombosis

↑Endothelin ●
↓Prostacyclin ○

FIG. 90.1 **Pathology of Pulmonary Hypertension.**

Physical exam can reveal elevated jugular venous pressure, and a right ventricular heave can be best felt along the left parasternal border. Auscultation can reveal an accentuated pulmonic component of S2, a tricuspid regurgitation murmur, and an S4 heart sound. In advanced pulmonary hypertension, clinical findings of right ventricular failure manifest (e.g., S3 heart sound, hepatomegaly, ascites, peripheral edema, hypotension, and decreased peripheral pulses).

Echocardiography is the most appropriate initial screening study when pulmonary hypertension is suspected. Doppler ultrasound on echocardiography can estimate the **right ventricular systolic pressure (RVSP)**, which functions as a surrogate for the systolic pulmonary

artery pressure. Echocardiography also reveals morphological consequences of PH, including right ventricular function/hypertrophy/dilation, tricuspid regurgitation, right atrial enlargement, and interventricular septal flattening, as well as the status of the left ventricle, mitral valves, and aortic valves. If the RVSP on echocardiogram is elevated and/or other parameters exist for suspecting PH, **right heart catheterization** is indicated to diagnose PH and evaluate for left-sided cardiac disease with the **pulmonary capillary wedge pressure (PCWP)**. Patients can undergo simultaneous immediate evaluation of therapeutic response to vasodilator therapies to determine the appropriateness of starting them in these patients.

1. Pulmonary arterial hypertension (PAH)

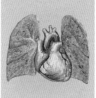

- Idiopathic pulmonary arterial hypertension
- Heritable
- Drug and toxin induced
- Persistent PH of newborn
- Associated with:
  - connective tissue disease
  - HIV infection
  - portal hypertension
  - coronary heart disease
  - schistosomiasis
  - chronic hemolytic anemia

1A. Pulmonary venoocclusive disease and pulmonary capillary hemangiomatosis

2. Pulmonary hypertension due to left heart disease

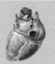

- Systolic dysfunction
- Diastolic dysfunction
- Valvular disease

3. Pulmonary hypertension due to lung diseases and/or hypoxia

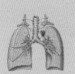

- Chronic obstructive pulmonary disease
- Interstitial lung disease
- Other pulmonary diseases with mixed restrictive and obstructive pattern
- Sleep-disordered breathing
- Alveolar hypoventilation disorders
- Developmental abnormalities

4. Pulmonary hypertension due to chronic thrombotic and/or embolic disease

- Chronic thromboembolic pulmonary hypertension

5. Pulmonary hypertension with unclear multifactorial mechanisms

- Hematological disorders
- Systemic disorders
- Metabolic disorders
- Others

Modified from Simonneau G, Gatzoulis MA, Adatia I, et al: Updated clinical classification of pulmonary hypertension, *J Am Coll Cardiol* 62:D34–D41, 2013.

FIG. 90.2 World Health Organization Classification System of Pulmonary Hypertension.

Other testing includes a chest radiograph, electrocardiogram (ECG), and laboratory studies (Fig. 90.3). A chest radiograph can show prominent pulmonary vessels and right ventricular enlargement, and an ECG may have evidence of right ventricular hypertrophy with strain and right axis deviation. In addition to basic chemistries (including assessment of liver function to look for portopulmonary hypertension), patients should be tested for HIV and undergo antinuclear antibody (ANA) screening for connective tissue diseases. Patients with a history of thromboembolism can undergo a ventilation-perfusion (V/Q) scan, and pulmonary function tests (PFTs) can elucidate the presence of pulmonary disease.

Patients with established PH should undergo exercise testing, most commonly with the **6-minute walk test** (6MWT). This simple test involves continuous pulse oximetry while measuring how far a patient can walk in 6 minutes; serial measurements can be used to evaluate exercise tolerance over time, as well as potential response to therapeutics. Longer distances on 6MWT are associated with longer survival.

TREATMENT

Therapies should be directed toward symptomatic relief of dyspnea and improving exercise tolerance,

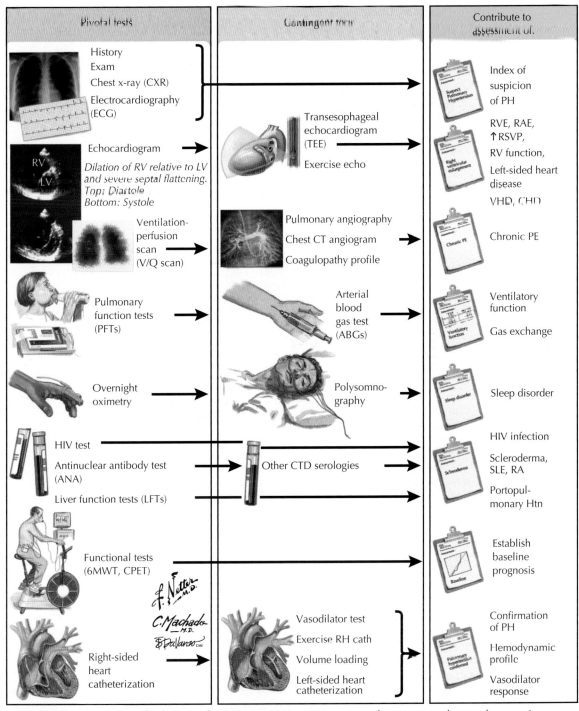

Pivotal tests	Contingent tests	Contribute to assessment of:

Pivotal tests:

History
Exam
Chest x-ray (CXR)
Electrocardiography (ECG)

Echocardiogram

Dilation of RV relative to LV and severe septal flattening. Top: Diastole Bottom: Systole

RV
LV

Ventilation-perfusion scan (V/Q scan)

Pulmonary function tests (PFTs)

Overnight oximetry

HIV test

Antinuclear antibody test (ANA)

Liver function tests (LFTs)

Functional tests (6MWT, CPET)

Right-sided heart catheterization

Contingent tests:

Transesophageal echocardiogram (TEE)

Exercise echo

Pulmonary angiography
Chest CT angiogram
Coagulopathy profile

Arterial blood gas test (ABGs)

Polysomno-graphy

Other CTD serologies

Vasodilator test
Exercise RH cath
Volume loading
Left-sided heart catheterization

Contribute to assessment of:

Index of suspicion of PH

RVE, RAE, ↑RSVP, RV function, Left-sided heart disease
VHD, CHD

Chronic PE

Ventilatory function
Gas exchange

Sleep disorder

HIV infection
Scleroderma, SLE, RA
Portopul-monary Htn

Establish baseline prognosis

Confirmation of PH
Hemodynamic profile
Vasodilator response

J. Netter M.D.
C. Machado M.D.
B. Dallanzo CMI

McLaughlin VV, Archer SL, Badesch DB, et al: ACCF/AHA 2009 expert consensus document on pulmonary hypertension a report of the American College of Cardiology Foundation Task Force on Expert Consensus Documents and the American Heart Association developed in collaboration with the American College of Chest Physicians; American Thoracic Society, Inc.; and the Pulmonary Hypertension Association, *J Am Coll Cardiol* 53:1573–1619, 2009.

FIG. 90.3 **Diagnosis of Pulmonary Hypertension.** *CHD,* Coronary heart disease; *CPET,* cardiopulmonary exercise testing; *CTD,* connective tissue disease; *Htn,* hypertension; *LV,* left ventricle; *PF,* pulmonary embolism; *PH,* pulmonary hypertension; *RA,* rheumatoid arthritis; *RAE,* right atrial enlargement; *RH,* right heart; *RVSP,* right ventricular systolic pressure; *RV,* right ventricle; *RVE,* right ventricular enlargement; *SLE,* systemic lupus erythematosus; *VHD,* valvular heart disease.

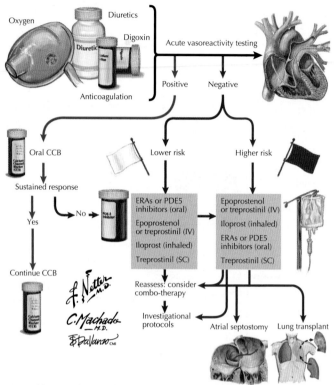

McLaughlin VV, Archer SL, Badesch DB, et al: ACCF/AHA 2009 expert consensus document on pulmonary hypertension a report of the American College of Cardiology Foundation Task Force on Expert Consensus Documents and the American Heart Association developed in collaboration with the American College of Chest Physicians; American Thoracic Society, Inc.; and the Pulmonary Hypertension Association, *J Am Coll Cardiol* 53:1573–1619, 2009.

FIG. 90.4 **Therapy for Pulmonary Hypertension.** *CCB,* Calcium channel blocker; *ERAs,* endothelin receptor antagonists; *IV,* intravenous; *PDE5,* phosphodiesterase type 5 inhibitor; *SC,* subcutaneous.

right ventricular function, and overall hemodynamics. Patients are stratified by WHO classification (Fig. 90.4):

- Class I: Minimal symptoms, no targeted pharmacological management needed
- Class II: Slight limitation in physical activity
- Class III: Marked limitation in physical activity but comfortable at rest
- Class IV: Inability to carry out physical activity with symptoms at rest and/or presence of syncope

In general, all patients with pulmonary hypertension should receive nonpharmacological therapies consisting of **pulmonary rehabilitation,** dietary counseling, and exercise training. All patients should receive influenza and pneumococcal vaccinations, and all female patients with PH should be advised to avoid pregnancy. Patients with pulmonary hypertension due to a systemic disease should receive primary therapeutic interventions for that disease in the hopes of relieving PH symptoms.

Supportive therapies that are beneficial in all PH patients include diuretic therapy for fluid retention and oxygen supplementation to decrease hypoxic vasoconstriction (particularly in WHO group 3 PH). Digoxin may be used in patients with group 2 PH, and anticoagulation with potential pulmonary endarterectomy is indicated in patients with group 4 CTEPH.

Patients with class II to IV disease are candidates for pharmacological therapies and should undergo right heart catheterization prior to beginning therapy. In those patients who are responsive to vasodilator therapy, calcium channel blockers (e.g., long-acting diltiazem, amlodipine, nifedipine) are beneficial. Verapamil should be avoided due to its negative inotropic effects. Prostacyclin pathway agonists promote dilation of the pulmonary arteries and are most commonly given via continuous intravenous infusion (epoprostenol, treprostinil), subcutaneously (treprostinil), inhaled (iloprost and treprostinil), or oral (treprostinil and selexipag, a prostacyclin receptor agonist). Nitric oxide (NO)–promoting therapies include phosphodiesterase type V inhibitors (sildenafil, tadalafil) and soluble guanylate cyclase stimulators such as riociguat (stimulate NO production and inhibit its metabolism), which increase vasodilation as well. Endothelin receptor antagonists (bosentan, ambrisentan, and macitentan) work to decrease the smooth muscle constrictive effects on the pulmonary circulation. These therapies are often used in combination.

Surgical management of pulmonary hypertension includes pulmonary endarterectomy for WHO group 4 disease and, in severely symptomatic patients, balloon atrial septostomy, which is typically a palliative measure to decrease right-sided pressures in the heart and as a bridge to lung transplantation. Bilateral lung or heart-lung transplantation is the procedure of choice for definitive management of pulmonary hypertension and is indicated in patients with disease refractory to medical therapies, rapidly progressive disease, or WHO class III/IV disease.

CHAPTER 91

Acute Respiratory Distress Syndrome

NEELIMA NAVULURI

INTRODUCTION

Acute respiratory distress syndrome (ARDS) is a clinical syndrome characterized by acute, diffuse, inflammatory lung injury that interferes with effective gas exchange. The pathological hallmarks include **diffuse alveolar damage (DAD)**, leaky vasculature, higher lung weight, and reduced aeration. ARDS is more common in adults than children, remains underrecognized by clinicians, and carries a mortality rate as high as 40% in the United States. Survivors are at risk for long-term decreased functional capacity, psychiatric illness, and less desirable quality of life.

PATHOPHYSIOLOGY

Etiologies of ARDS include direct and indirect injuries. Direct causes include pneumonia, aspiration of gastric contents, inhalational injury, pulmonary contusion, vasculitis, and drowning. Indirect injuries usually occur from generalized inflammatory states. These include nonpulmonary sepsis, major trauma, pancreatitis, severe burns, noncardiogenic shock, drug overdose, multiple transfusions, and transfusion-associated acute lung injury.

These various insults initiate a process of inflammation, cytokine release, and free radical production that damages pulmonary endothelial and alveolar cells, thereby increasing the permeability of pulmonary capillaries (Fig. 91.1). This results in accumulation of exudative fluid in the alveolar space and the formation of hyaline membranes—or the acute phase of DAD.

In a later phase, the pulmonary edema resolves but the lungs remain noncompliant and unable to perform effective gas exchange due to cellular proliferation, collagen deposition, and lack of surfactant. Ultimately, this damage may progress to a fibrotic state. The extensive parenchymal destruction and consequent hypoxia-induced pulmonary vasoconstriction can also lead to pulmonary hypertension and right-sided heart failure.

The supportive treatment for ARDS may paradoxically perpetuate the vicious cycle of lung injury. Excess of positive-pressure ventilation can lead to barotrauma and volutrauma, further increasing inflammation and edema, while high levels of supplemental oxygen may lead to additional oxygen free radical formation.

PRESENTATION, DIAGNOSIS, AND EVALUATION

The initial presentation varies according to the precipitating event. All patients have acute-onset dyspnea, hypoxemia, and diffuse crackles on lung auscultation. Depending on the severity of the lung injury, patients may present with signs of severe respiratory distress, including tachypnea, tachycardia, diaphoresis, and use of the accessory muscles of respiration (Fig. 91.2).

Patients with suspected ARDS should undergo a comprehensive workup that includes chest imaging (x-ray or CT scan), arterial blood gas testing, and an assessment of cardiac function. Per the standard **Berlin definition**, ARDS can be diagnosed when respiratory failure:
- Occurs within 1 week of a known clinical insult or onset of respiratory symptoms (with most patients identified in the first 72 hours)
- Features bilateral opacities consistent with pulmonary edema on chest radiograph or CT scan
- Is not fully explained by cardiac failure or volume overload

Prior definitions of ARDS required pulmonary artery wedge pressures to exclude cardiogenic pulmonary edema, but given the declining use of pulmonary artery catheters, noninvasive assessments (e.g., physical examination, brain natriuretic peptide, echocardiography) are recommended.

The severity of ARDS is determined using the ratio of the partial pressure of arterial oxygen (PaO_2) to the fraction of inspired oxygen (FiO_2), so long as patients are receiving at least 5 cm H_2O of continuous positive airway pressure. Mild ARDS is defined as a **PaO_2/FiO_2 ratio** of 200 to 300, moderate 100 to 200, and severe <100. The mortality increases from 35% among those with mild ARDS to 46% among those with severe ARDS.

Pulmonary arteries and veins

Structure of intrapulmonary airways

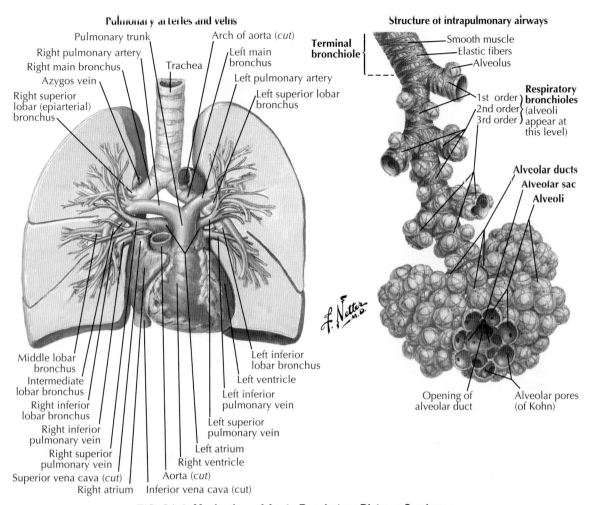

FIG. 91.1 **Mechanism of Acute Respiratory Distress Syndrome.**

TREATMENT

Most patients with ARDS require sedation, intubation, and mechanical ventilation. Patients should be placed in an intensive care unit with careful monitoring of their hemodynamics, gas exchange, and acid-base status (see Chapter 47 for details).

The pivotal ARDS Network (ARDSNet) randomized clinical trial established optimal ventilation strategies in patients with ARDS. The major finding was that the use of **low tidal volumes** (i.e., 6 mL/kg of ideal body weight vs. the traditional 10–15 mL/kg), with a target plateau pressure ≤30 cm H_2O, decreased overall mortality. The protocol recommends that the initial ventilator settings include tidal volumes of 8 mL/kg, and that the tidal volume be lowered by 1 mL/kg every 2 hours to a goal

of 6 mL/kg. If the plateau pressure remains ≥30 cm H_2O, the tidal volume can be further lowered to a minimum 4 mL/kg.

The use of low tidal volumes may result in hypoventilation and respiratory acidosis. Respiratory acidosis in this setting may be termed **permissive hypercapnia,** as the risks of acidosis may be outweighed by both lung protection and, indeed, the hypercapnic acidosis itself. These benefits include increased oxygen delivery from increased cardiac output, potentiation of hypoxic vasoconstriction facilitating better ventilation-perfusion (V/Q) matching, and rightward shift of the oxygen-hemoglobin dissociation curve. If the pH is <7.30, the protocol recommends increasing the respiratory rate to a maximum of 35 to maximize minute ventilation. If the

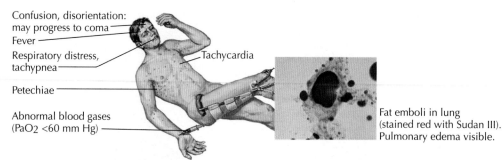

Confusion, disorientation: may progress to coma

Fever

Respiratory distress, tachypnea

Tachycardia

Petechiae

Abnormal blood gases (PaO_2 <60 mm Hg)

Fat emboli in lung (stained red with Sudan III). Pulmonary edema visible.

Criteria for diagnosis of adult respiratory distress syndrome (ARDS) include development of respiratory symptoms within 1 week of a clinical insult, bilateral diffuse infiltrates on the chest radiograph in the absence of pneumonia, and absence of cardiogenic pulmonary edema. In this example of ARDS due to a fat embolism, associated findings of petechiae and confusion merge into systemic inflammatory response syndrome (SIRS).

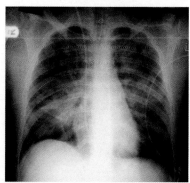

Chest radiograph in a patient with adult respiratory distress syndrome due to extrathoracic trauma. Bilateral airspace opacity is seen. Reprinted with permission from Adam A, Dixon AK, Grainger RG, et al: *Grainger & Allison's diagnostic radiology,* ed 5, Philadelphia, 2007, Elsevier.

FIG. 91.2 Adult Respiratory Distress Syndrome.

TABLE 91.1
FiO₂ and PEEP Settings for Oxygenation in ARDS

FiO$_2$	0.3	0.4	0.5	0.6	0.7	0.8	0.9	1.0
Lower PEEP (cm H$_2$O), higher FiO$_2$	5	5–8	8–10	10	10–14	14	14–18	18–24
Higher PEEP (cm H$_2$O), lower FiO$_2$	5–14	14–16	16–20	20	20	20–22	22	24

ARDS, Acute respiratory distress syndrome; *FiO$_2$,* fraction of inspired oxygen; *PEEP,* positive end-expiratory pressure.
Data derived from ARDSnet: *NIH NHLBI ARDS clinical network mechanical ventilation protocol summary.* http://www.ardsnet.org/files/ventilator_protocol_2008-07.pdf. (Accessed 13 January 2020).

pH remains <7.15 despite these measures, the protocol recommends increasing tidal volumes, even if the plateau pressure begins to exceed 30 cm H_2O.

The protocol also provides guidance for determining appropriate combinations of **positive end-expiratory pressure (PEEP)** and FiO_2; the goal should be a PaO_2 of 55 to 80 mm Hg or peripheral oxygen saturation of 88% to 95% (Table 91.1).

Additional therapies that benefit patients with severe or refractory ARDS include **neuromuscular blockade** and **prone positioning.** Both interventions were studied in patients with early ARDS and PaO_2/FiO_2 <150 who

failed to improve with low tidal volume ventilation and were deeply sedated.

Patients who still fail to improve despite these measures may be candidates for salvage therapy with high-frequency oscillatory ventilation or (increasingly) **extracorporeal membrane oxygenation (ECMO).** In ECMO, blood is drained from the vena cava or right atrium, circulated using a mechanical pump through an oxygenator and heat exchanger, and returned to the body through a catheter in a major vein (i.e., venovenous [VV] ECMO) or artery (venoarterial [VA] ECMO). ECMO therefore bypasses the lungs and, in a VA circuit, the heart.

The oxygenator fully saturates hemoglobin with oxygen and removes carbon dioxide (CO_2), with the degree of CO_2 removal dependent on the flow rate (sweep) of the countercurrent gas. Given the complexity and potential morbidity associated with ECMO, it should not be used for the initial treatment of ARDS or outside of experienced centers.

The pharmacological options for treatment of ARDS are limited. The use of surfactant therapy has been studied in children with ARDS, but there is no evidence of benefit among adults. The use of corticosteroids to reduce lung inflammation is controversial. The use of inhaled nitric oxide to improve the perfusion of oxygenated lung is under active investigation.

CHAPTER 92

Urinary System Anatomy Review

PEROLA LAMBA

GROSS ANATOMY

The kidneys are bean-shaped organs approximately the size of a fist, weighing about 150 g each in adults. They are located in the retroperitoneal space just under the ribcage, one on each side of the vertebral column, along the borders of the psoas muscles. The right kidney is positioned lower than the left kidney due to its relationship to the liver.

The kidneys are physically supported by perirenal fat, the renal vascular pedicle, abdominal muscles, and the abdominal viscera. They have a rounded, outer convex surface and an inner concave surface with a cleft known as the hilum, which is penetrated by blood vessels, nerves, and the **ureter.**

The capsule is the outermost surface of the kidney, comprised of thin connective tissue. The kidneys are macroscopically divided into the **renal cortex** and the **renal medulla.** The working mass of the kidney consists of tubules and blood vessels, which are present in both the cortex and medulla, and are surrounded and supported by the interstitium.

The cortex is the outer region of the kidney under the capsule, and the medulla is the central region of the kidney. Portions of the cortex project toward the renal pelvis in structures known as columns of Bertin. The cortex contains the **renal corpuscles** and randomly intertwined tubules and blood vessels, whereas the medulla contains pyramids with tubules and blood vessels that are more organized in a parallel arrangement. The pyramids are arranged radially around the hilum. The tip of the pyramid is called a papilla and projects into the **minor calyx,** which collects the urine formed in the tubules. Several minor calices converge to form a **major calyx,** and the major calyces join to form the renal pelvis, which narrows into the ureter (Fig. 92.1).

The ureter drains urine from the kidney and transports it to the **bladder.** The ureters course for ~30 cm, following a smooth S curve and entering obliquely on the posteroinferior surface of the bladder. The bladder is a hollow, muscular viscus, which serves as the reservoir for urine, with a capacity of 400 to 500 mL. Its walls are composed mainly of the detrusor muscles, which contract to expel urine through the urethra. The bladder lies in the pelvis, behind the pubic symphysis when empty, and rising above when full. The inner surface of the calices, renal pelvis, ureters, bladder, and urethra is composed of **transitional cell epithelium,** allowing these organs to stretch and accommodate different volumes of urine.

THE NEPHRON

The **nephron** is the functional unit of the kidney, controlling volume and composition of blood, including acid-base status and electrolyte levels, and facilitating the removal of water, toxins, and by-products of metabolism. Each kidney contains ~1 million nephrons. Each nephron consists of the renal corpuscle and the renal tubule, which merge with tubules of other nephrons to form **collecting ducts,** which merge with other collecting ducts in the renal papilla to form calyxes and eventually the ureter.

The renal corpuscle is a spherical structure composed of **Bowman capsule,** a hollow sphere composed of epithelial cells. Blood from the afferent arteriole enters the **glomerulus,** a compact tuft of interconnected capillary loops. Bowman capsule surrounds the glomerulus, with the afferent (entry) and efferent (exit) arterioles penetrating at the vascular pole. The blood from the glomerulus is ultrafiltered across the basement membranes of the capillaries into the empty space within Bowman capsule, referred to as Bowman space (Fig. 92.2).

The renal tubule leads out of the Bowman capsule opposite the vascular pole, draining the contents of the capsule. The tubule is lined with epithelial cells, which possess multiple channels and exchange proteins to facilitate reabsorption and secretion of electrolytes and

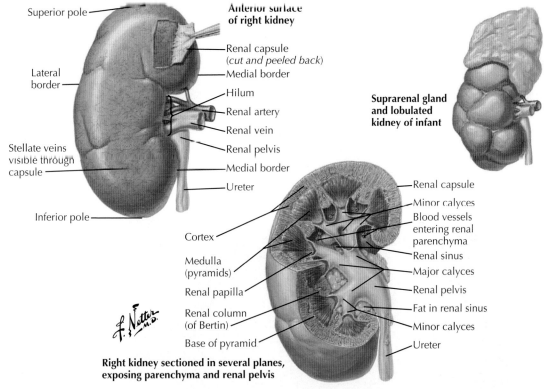

Superior pole

Anterior surface
of right kidney

Renal capsule
(*cut and peeled back*)

Medial border

Lateral
border

Hilum

Renal artery

Renal vein

Renal pelvis

Stellate veins
visible through
capsule

Medial border

Ureter

Inferior pole

**Suprarenal gland
and lobulated
kidney of infant**

Renal capsule

Minor calyces

Blood vessels
entering renal
parenchyma

Renal sinus

Cortex

Major calyces

Medulla
(pyramids)

Renal pelvis

Renal papilla

Fat in renal sinus

Renal column
(of Bertin)

Minor calyces

Base of pyramid

Ureter

f. Netter
M.D.

**Right kidney sectioned in several planes,
exposing parenchyma and renal pelvis**

FIG. 92.1 **Gross Structure of the Kidney.**

other compounds, depending on the body's physiological state (see Chapter 93 for further details).

The first segment of the renal tubule is the proximal tubule, which contains a coiled segment, the **proximal convoluted tubule,** followed by a shorter, straight segment, the **proximal straight tubule.** The proximal convoluted tubule has a brush border consisting of microvilli for major reabsorptive function. The proximal tubule is contained primarily within the cortex and outer medulla.

The next segment is the **descending limb of the loop of Henle,** which penetrates down to varying depths in the medulla, where it abruptly reverses at a hairpin turn and becomes the **ascending portion of the loop of Henle.** The ascending portion of the loop of Henle initially has a thin portion (the ascending thin limb) followed by a portion where the epithelium thickens (the ascending thick limb). The ascending thick limb rises out of the medulla into the cortex, in close proximity to the vascular pole of the Bowman capsule. This region of the tubule

contains specialized cells called the **macula densa.** The region is collectively referred to as the **juxtaglomerular apparatus,** which plays an important role in regulating nephron flow and systemic blood pressure.

This is followed by the **distal convoluted tubule,** which leads to the connecting tubule, which merges with collecting tubules from several other nephrons to form the cortical collecting duct. The cortical collecting ducts run downward to enter the medulla, merging to form larger ducts, eventually emptying into the calyx of the renal pelvis, which is continuous with the ureter (Fig. 92.3).

VASCULATURE

The renal arteries arise from the abdominal aorta at the L1/L2 level immediately inferior to the superior mesenteric artery. The right renal artery is longer and passes posterior to the inferior vena cava. Near the hilum, each artery divides into five segmental arteries, which

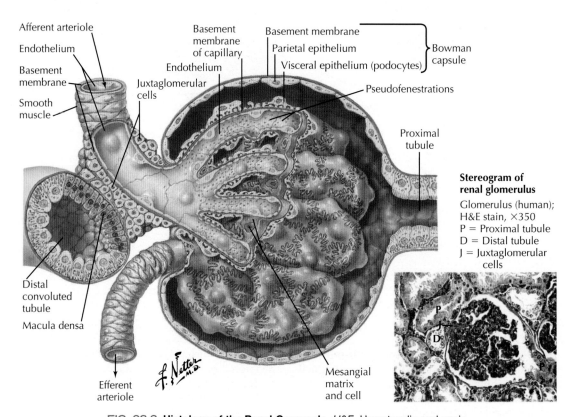

Afferent arteriole

Endothelium

Basement membrane

Smooth muscle

Juxtaglomerular cells

Basement membrane of capillary

Endothelium

Basement membrane

Parietal epithelium

Visceral epithelium (podocytes)

Bowman capsule

Pseudofenestrations

Proximal tubule

Distal convoluted tubule

Macula densa

Efferent arteriole

Mesangial matrix and cell

Stereogram of renal glomerulus

Glomerulus (human); H&E stain, ×350
P = Proximal tubule
D = Distal tubule
J = Juxtaglomerular cells

FIG. 92.2 Histology of the Renal Corpuscle. *H&E,* Hematoxylin and eosin.

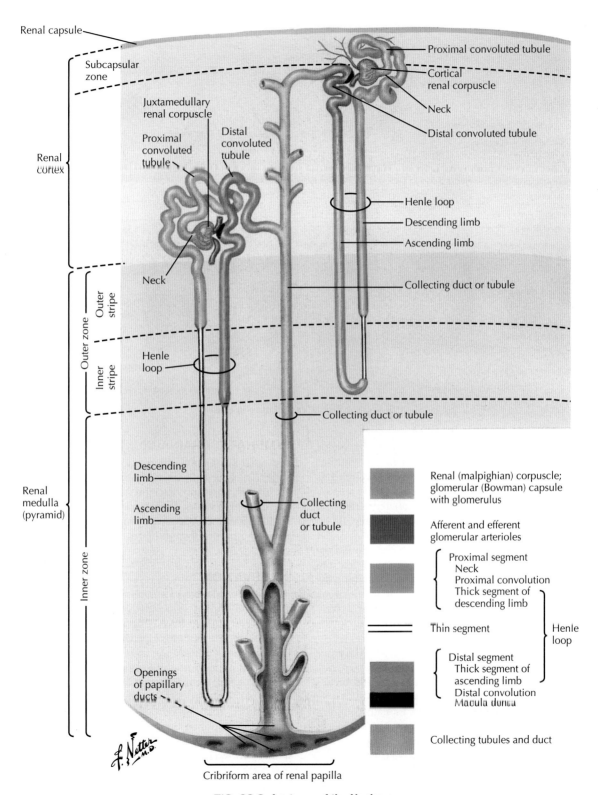

FIG. 92.3 **Anatomy of the Nephron.**

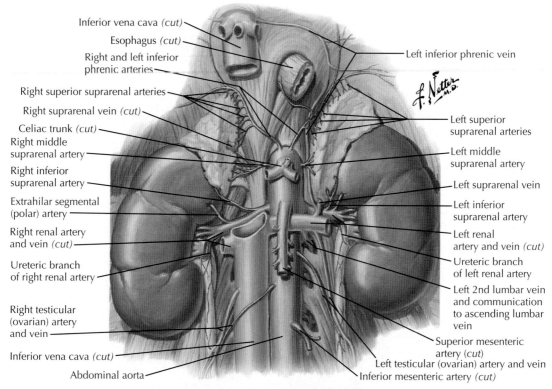

Inferior vena cava *(cut)*
Esophagus *(cut)*
Right and left inferior phrenic arteries
Right superior suprarenal arteries
Right suprarenal vein *(cut)*
Celiac trunk *(cut)*
Right middle suprarenal artery
Right inferior suprarenal artery
Extrahilar segmental (polar) artery
Right renal artery and vein *(cut)*
Ureteric branch of right renal artery
Right testicular (ovarian) artery and vein
Inferior vena cava *(cut)*
Abdominal aorta

Left inferior phrenic vein
Left superior suprarenal arteries
Left middle suprarenal artery
Left suprarenal vein
Left inferior suprarenal artery
Left renal artery and vein *(cut)*
Ureteric branch of left renal artery
Left 2nd lumbar vein and communication to ascending lumbar vein
Superior mesenteric artery *(cut)*
Left testicular (ovarian) artery and vein
Inferior mesenteric artery *(cut)*

FIG. 92.4 **Renal Vasculature in Situ.**

supply the different renal segments, and further divide into interlobar arteries, which travel in the columns of Bertin and arch along the base of the pyramids as arcuate arteries and then divide as interlobular arteries.

The smallest arteries divide into afferent arterioles, which deliver blood to the glomerular capillaries. Blood leaves the glomerular capillaries into efferent arterioles and then to peritubular capillaries, which surround the nephron (vasa recta). The peritubular capillaries flow into small veins, which unite in a variable fashion to form the renal vein. The renal veins drain into the inferior vena cava. The renal veins lie anterior to the renal arteries, and the longer left renal vein passes anterior to the aorta (Fig. 92.4).

The arterial supply to the ureters arises from three main sources: the renal artery, testicular/ovarian arteries, and abdominal aorta. The venous drainage of the ureters goes into the renal and testicular/ovarian veins. Accessory renal veins are common and may occasionally compress the ureter, resulting in hydronephrosis. The bladder is supplied by branches of the internal iliac arteries and drained by tributaries of the internal iliac veins.

LYMPHATIC DRAINAGE

The renal lymphatics drain into the lumbar lymph nodes. The lymphatic vessels from the ureter drain into the lumbar, common iliac, internal lymph nodes, and external lymph nodes. The lymphatic drainage from the bladder goes into vesical, external iliac, internal iliac, and common iliac lymph nodes.

INNERVATION

The kidneys and ureters are innervated by the renal nerve plexus and consist of sympathetic, parasympathetic, and visceral afferent fibers. This plexus is supplied by fibers from the abdominopelvic splanchnic nerves. The abdominal parts of the ureters are also innervated by the abdominal aortic and superior hypogastric plexuses. The sympathetic fibers to the bladder are supplied by the pelvic plexus (T11–L3 spinal cord levels); parasympathetic fibers, which are motor to the detrusor muscle, are supplied by the pelvic splanchnic nerves and the inferior hypogastric plexuses, arising from sacral spinal cord levels.

CHAPTER 93

Urinary System Physiology Review

FANGFEI ZHENG

INTRODUCTION

The kidney performs several key homeostatic functions, including the excretion of water and electrolytes, regulation of acid-base balance, and control of blood pressure through the retention or excretion of fluids and release of vasoactive hormones. The kidney also contributes to the activation of vitamin D and the regulation of erythropoiesis.

The functional unit of the kidney is the nephron (Fig. 93.1), which includes the glomerulus and renal tubule. The tubule itself is divided into a proximal portion, the loop of Henle, and a distal portion, which joins with other tubules to form collecting ducts that drain into the renal pelvis (see Chapter 92 for details).

GLOMERULAR FILTRATION

The first step of urine production is the filtration of plasma through the glomerular capillaries, which allows the passage of molecules of certain sizes and charges while blocking others (e.g., albumin, red blood cells). The **glomerular filtration rate (GFR)** is the amount of blood that is filtered per unit of time and serves as a quantitative measure for renal function.

The GFR can be estimated based on the plasma and urine concentration of substances that are freely filtered across the glomerular capillaries, then neither absorbed, metabolized, or secreted in the tubules. Although the ideal such substance is **inulin**, which is sometimes used for precise GFR measurement (as opposed to estimation) in the laboratory setting, the substance most widely assessed in clinical practice is **creatinine,** which is freely filtered at the glomerulus and is neither metabolized nor absorbed in the tubules. Creatinine is, however, secreted into the proximal tubule in increasing amounts as GFR falls, and formulas based on it can thus overestimate the true GFR. Creatinine is produced during the metabolism of creatine, and so the calculation of GFR has to be adjusted for muscle mass or its surrogates (e.g., age, gender); several equations help with this approximation (Table 93.1).

Renal artery pressure, which corresponds to the systemic arterial pressure, is the primary determinant of GFR. When the mean arterial pressure falls, activation of the **renin-angiotensin-aldosterone system (RAAS)** increases tone in the efferent arterioles, increasing pressure in the glomerular capillaries and thereby the filtration fraction (see later for details).

THE TUBULAR SYSTEM

The renal tubules reabsorb most of the filtered plasma and electrolytes back into the peritubular capillaries, using ion channels, exchangers, cotransporters, and adenosine triphosphate (ATP) pumps. These mechanisms are subject to numerous regulatory controls to preserve homeostasis. For example, the urine osmolality can range from 50 to 1200 mOsm/L depending on serum osmolality, intravascular volume status, and release of regulatory hormones such as **antidiuretic hormone (ADH).**

Most sodium reabsorption occurs in the proximal tubule (Fig. 93.2). By the end of this segment, two-thirds of the filtered sodium has been reabsorbed on Na-H exchangers and various cotransporters, which couple its reabsorption with that of glucose, amino acids, organic acids, and phosphate. The H^+ that is secreted in exchange for Na^+ is combined in the tubular lumen with filtered bicarbonate by carbonic anhydrase into carbonic acid, H_2CO_3. This then dissociates into CO_2 and H_2O, both of which are passively reabsorbed. Once in the tubular cell, CO_2 and H_2O are again combined by carbonic anhydrase into H_2CO_3. A proton dissociates (and is secreted in exchange for another Na^+ ion), and HCO_3 is cotransported with Cl^- into the peritubular capillaries. In this manner, virtually all filtered bicarbonate is reabsorbed.

The reabsorption of sodium establishes an osmotic gradient that promotes the paracellular reabsorption of water. The passive diffusion of water occurring in proportion to the reabsorption of solutes causes the filtrate at the end of proximal tubule to remain isosmotic with plasma. The proximal tubule also secretes numerous substances into the urine, such as organic anions, drugs (e.g., furosemide), and a small quantity of creatinine.

The isosmotic filtrate leaving the proximal tubule enters the loop of Henle and passes through the renal medulla. The descending limb is highly permeable to water, which is reabsorbed through the aquaporin-1 transporter. In contrast, the thick ascending loop is impermeable to

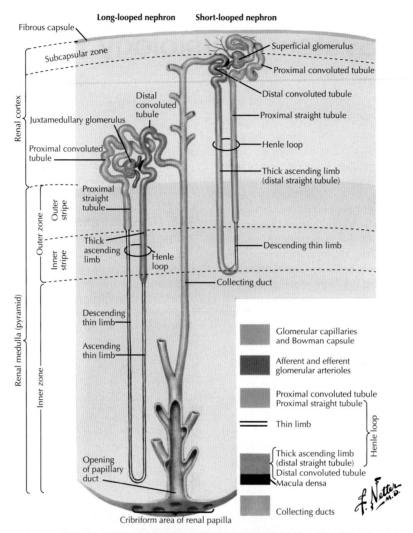

FIG. 93.1 **Anatomy of the Nephron and Collecting Tubule.**

TABLE 93.1
Glomerular Filtration Rate (GFR) Estimating Equations

GFR Estimating Equation	Date of Publication	GFR in mL/min/1.73 m²
Cockcroft-Gault[a]	1973	$[(140 - \text{age}) \times \text{weight}]/(72 \times \text{Scr}) \times 0.85$ (if female)
MDRD (four variable)[b]	1999	$175 \times \text{SerumCr}^{-1.154} \times \text{Age}^{-0.203} \times 1.212$ (if patient is black) $\times$ 0.742 (if female)
CKD-EPI[c]	2009	$141 \times \min(\text{Scr}/\kappa,1)^{\alpha} \times \max(\text{Scr}/\kappa,1)^{-1.209} \times 0.993^{\text{Age}} \times 1.018$ (if female) $\times 1.159$ (if black) Where Scr is serum creatinine (mg/dL), κ is 0.7 for females and 0.9 for males, α is −0.329 for females and −0.411 for males, min indicates the minimum of Scr/κ or 1, and max indicates the maximum of Scr/κ or 1.

[a]*Cockcroft-Gault:* Cockcroft DW, Gault MH: Prediction of creatinine clearance from serum creatinine, *Nephron* 16(1):31–41, 1976.
[b]*MDRD:* Levey AS, Bosch JP, Lewis JB, et al: A more accurate method to estimate glomerular filtration rate from serum creatinine: a new prediction equation. Modification of Diet in Renal Disease Study Group, *Ann Intern Med* 130(6):461–470, 1999.
[c]*CKD-EPI:* Levey AS, Stevens LA, Schmid CH, et al: A new equation to estimate glomerular filtration rate, *Ann Intern Med* 150(9):604–612, 2009.

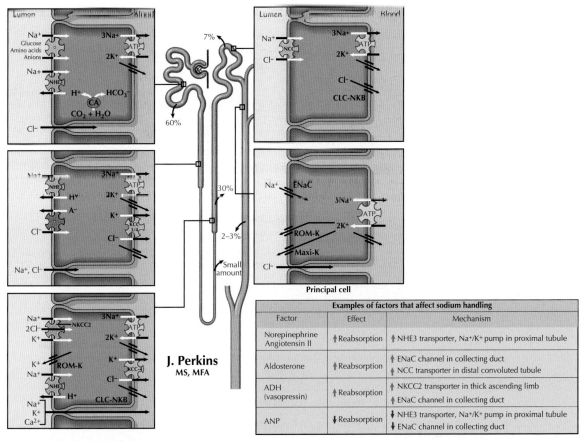

FIG. 93.2　Nephron Sites of Sodium Reabsorption. *ADH*, Antidiuretic hormone; *ANP*, atrial natriuretic peptide; *ATP*, adenosine triphosphate.

water but actively transports Na$^+$, K$^+$, and Cl$^-$ into the interstitium on Na$^+$-K$^+$-2Cl$^-$ (NKCC2) cotransporters; for this reason, the thick ascending limb is also referred to as the "diluting segment." Solute reabsorption in the thick ascending limb creates a hyperosmotic interstitium that drives the earlier reabsorption of water through the descending limb; interstitial fluid then equilibrates with blood flow through the vasa recta, which carries the reabsorbed water and solutes away. At this point, the descending limb tubular fluid is hyperosmotic (due to water reabsorption) compared to the thick ascending limb fluid (hypoosmotic due to solute reabsorption). New filtrate flows from the proximal convoluted tubule, pushing tubular fluid along the loop of Henle, and the hypoosmotic fluid in the thick ascending limb empties into the distal convoluted tubule and collecting duct. This repetitive process maximizes solute reabsorption and minimizes water loss and is termed the **countercurrent multiplication system.**

Although only one-tenth of the filtrate volume reaches the collecting tubule, this segment determines the urine osmolality and is also critical to potassium homeostasis

and acid-base regulation. ADH is released in response to increased serum osmolality or volume depletion; it binds to the vasopressin-2 receptor, triggering the insertion of aquaporin-2 receptors into the luminal membrane and thereby rendering this segment permeable to water.

The direction of water flow in the collecting tubule depends on the concentration gradient between the tubular lumen and the interstitium. At the beginning of the collecting tubule, the interstitium has a higher osmotic concentration than filtrate, and thus water is reabsorbed. As a result, however, the filtrate becomes more concentrated. The further the filtrate moves along the collecting tubule, the more concentrated it becomes. For further water reabsorption to occur, the interstitial space must continue to rise in concentration as well, always staying ahead of the tubular lumen to maintain a concentration gradient that favors water reabsorption (rather than secretion). Such a gradient is established by the passive diffusion of urea into the inner medullary region, as well as the reabsorption of ions on NKCC2 cotransporters in the thick ascending

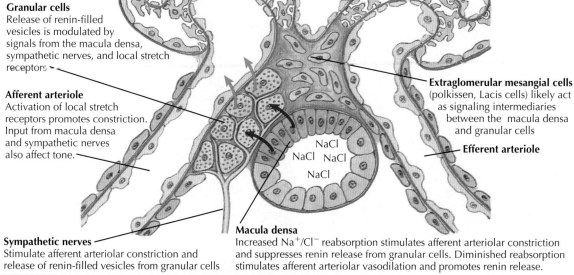

Granular cells
Release of renin-filled vesicles is modulated by signals from the macula densa, sympathetic nerves, and local stretch receptors

Afferent arteriole
Activation of local stretch receptors promotes constriction. Input from macula densa and sympathetic nerves also affect tone.

Extraglomerular mesangial cells (polkissen, Lacis cells) likely act as signaling intermediaries between the macula densa and granular cells

Efferent arteriole

NaCl
NaCl   NaCl
NaCl

Sympathetic nerves
Stimulate afferent arteriolar constriction and release of renin-filled vesicles from granular cells

Macula densa
Increased Na^+/Cl^- reabsorption stimulates afferent arteriolar constriction and suppresses renin release from granular cells. Diminished reabsorption stimulates afferent arteriolar vasodilation and promotes renin release.

Stimulus	Effect
Increased tubular flow	Afferent arteriolar constriction. Suppression of renin release
Decreased tubular flow	Afferent arteriolar dilation. Activation of renin release
Afferent arteriole stretching	Afferent arteriolar constriction. Suppression of renin release
Sympathetic tone	Afferent arteriolar constriction. Activation of renin release

FIG. 93.3 Renin-Angiotensin-Aldosterone System.

limb. The urine-concentrating ability of the kidney is impaired by loop diuretics, which inhibit the NKCC2 cotransporters; thus loop diuretics may be used in the treatment of hyponatremia (see Chapter 27 for details).

JUXTAGLOMERULAR APPARATUS AND THE RENIN-ANGIOTENSIN-ALDOSTERONE SYSTEM

The **juxtaglomerular apparatus (JGA),** located in a portion of the thick ascending limb adjacent to the glomerulus, is the kidney's primary means of sensing and responding to circulating volume (Fig. 93.3). A specialized portion of the thick ascending limb, known as the **macula densa,** is the sensing limb of the JGA.

In response to a reduction in sodium chloride delivery and urine flow, which may occur in the setting of volume depletion, the macula densa promotes the release of **renin** from nearby granular cells. Activation of the sympathetic nervous system, which also occurs in response to volume depletion, can similarly trigger renin release. Renin activates an enzymatic cascade that increases the serum levels of angiotensin II and aldosterone. Angiotensin II causes systemic vasoconstriction, constricts efferent

arterioles (thereby increasing glomerular hydrostatic pressure and filtration fraction), and increases sodium reabsorption in the proximal tubule. **Aldosterone** further increases sodium reabsorption in the distal nephron. The net effect is volume retention and an increase in blood pressure. Although the sympathetic nervous system promotes constriction of the afferent arterioles, the effect is mitigated by the sensing of decreased flow at the macula densa, which leads to afferent arteriolar vasodilation.

In contrast, in response to increased sodium chloride delivery and urine flow, the macula densa (along with stretch receptors in the afferent arteriole) promotes afferent arteriolar vasoconstriction (to bring urine flow back down to normal) and suppresses renin release (to decrease volume retention).

It is important to note that effective circulating volume is not equivalent to total body volume. Under certain edematous disease states (e.g., congestive heart failure, cirrhosis), extensive third spacing of fluids results in chronic stimulation of the RAAS; however, the retained volume does not remain in the vascular space and instead causes worsened edema and volume overload. The RAAS is also stimulated in renovascular disease (i.e., renal artery stenosis), which can lead to volume-mediated hypertension.

CHAPTER 94

Acute Tubular Necrosis

DIVYANSHU MALHOTRA

INTRODUCTION

Acute kidney injury (AKI) (see Chapter 30) is an important cause of morbidity and mortality worldwide. The two leading causes overall are prerenal azotemia and acute tubular necrosis (ATN), which together account for 65% to 75% of cases. ATN accounts for almost three-quarters of causes of intrinsic kidney injury and is common among hospitalized patients. It is thus essential to adapt universal preventative strategies and to be able to recognize this entity early on, given the lack of effective therapies.

PATHOPHYSIOLOGY

Historically, the two main types of ATN have been ischemic and nephrotoxic, the incidences of which are nearly equal. Recently it has been recognized that severe inflammation in general, and sepsis in particular, can result in ATN from direct tubular toxicity from cytokines, irrespective of blood pressure and renal perfusion. In many instances, ATN results from multiple insults acting together.

In ATN, the injury is to the tubular epithelial cell (Fig. 94.1) and occurs through a variety of mechanisms, as described later. Even though glomeruli are generally spared, filtration falls because of tubuloglomerular feedback (Fig. 94.2). The impaired reabsorption of solutes (secondary to tubular epithelial cell injury) leads to increased delivery of sodium and chloride to the macula densa, resulting in the release of adenosine, which causes intense vasoconstriction of the afferent arterioles. The damaged nephron thereby halts incoming filtrate to prevent massive losses of sodium and a corresponding systemic volume collapse when ATN is severe.

Two other mechanisms contribute to the decrease in filtration. First, there is backleak of filtered material into the peritubular capillaries between the injured and no longer adherent epithelial cells. Second, obstruction of tubular flow (from sloughed cells, crystals, etc.) causes increased hydrostatic pressure in Bowman capsule.

Ischemic Acute Tubular Necrosis

Ischemic ATN occurs in the setting of prolonged, severe renal hypoperfusion and occurs on a spectrum with **prerenal azotemia.** In prerenal azotemia, some nephrons (based on their location and proximity to blood supply) become ischemic, but a sufficient majority are spared any structural injury. Thus when perfusion is restored, filtration returns essentially to baseline. In ischemic ATN, a sufficient number of nephrons are damaged such that filtration does not improve with improved renal perfusion. There are multiple phases of ischemic ATN, including impairment of perfusion (specific to ischemic ATN), initiation of injury, extension of injury, maintenance, and repair.

Ischemic ATN is most commonly seen in the setting of surgery (especially cardiac surgery and abdominal aortic aneurysm repair), sepsis, acute pancreatitis, and severe volume depletion. There is a complex interplay of pathophysiological mechanisms, which include increased sympathetic tone, an imbalance between vasoconstrictors and vasodilators (including increased endothelin and decreased nitric oxide), endothelial injury with disruption of perfusion and decreased tissue oxygenation, generation of reactive oxygen species, tubular shredding and obstruction, backleak of filtrate through injured tubular epithelium, and recruitment of inflammatory mediators, with reperfusion causing further tubular cell injury.

Toxic Acute Tubular Necrosis

Nephrotoxic ATN can occur in response to a variety of toxins, which are further categorized as endogenous or exogenous (Box 94.1). Tubular injury can result from a variety of direct toxic effects, changes in intrarenal hemodynamics, or a combination.

Endogenous toxins

Myoglobin and hemoglobin promote the generation of reactive oxygen species and decrease renal perfusion by inhibiting the synthesis of nitric oxide. Substances such as uric acid and calcium oxalate can crystallize

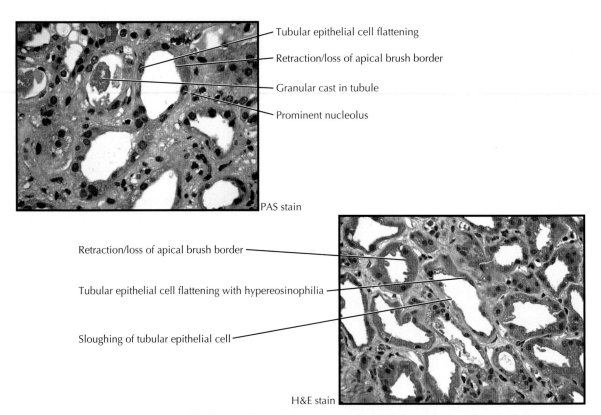

FIG. 94.1 **Histopathologic Findings of Acute Tubular Necrosis.** *H&E,* Hematoxylin and eosin; *PAS,* periodic acid–Schiff.

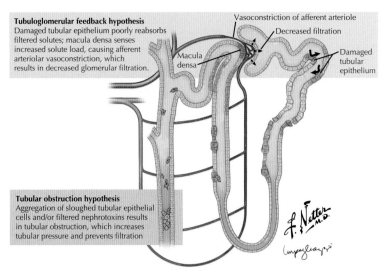

FIG. 94.2 **Mechanisms of Decreased Filtration in Acute Tubular Necrosis.**

BOX 94.1
Common Causes of Acute Tubular Necrosis

- Severe renal ischemia
- Hemorrhage
- Circulatory collapse
- Sepsis
- Toxic exposures
  - Exogenous toxins
    Radiocontrast agents
    Antibiotics (e.g., aminoglycosides)
    Antivirals (e.g., cidofovir)
    Antifungals (amphotericin B)
    Calcineurin inhibitors
    Ethylene glycol
    Toluene
  - Endogenous toxins
    Myoglobin
    Hemoglobin
    Oxalate
    Uric acid
    Myeloma light chains

in the renal tubules, causing injury and obstruction; risk factors include tumor lysis syndrome (which causes elevated levels of uric acid) and bariatric surgery (which causes increased oxalate reabsorption). Substances such as myeloma light chains can form obstructive casts that impede tubular flow and cause direct tubular toxicity.

Exogenous toxins

A variety of therapeutic drugs have direct nephrotoxic effects. Aminoglycosides frequently cause proximal tubular injury via mitochondrial damage, typically after ~1 week of treatment. In high doses, vancomycin has also been associated with tubular injury. Amphotericin B destroys cellular membranes through sterol interactions; lysosomal preparations are somewhat less nephrotoxic. The antiviral agents cidofovir and tenofovir disrupt mitochondrial and other cellular functions, while acyclovir, indinavir, and atazanavir (as well as ciprofloxacin) cause crystal formation and tubular obstruction/injury. Numerous chemotherapeutic agents have been associated with tubular injury, the most common being platinum-based drugs, ifosfamide, imatinib, and mithramycin. Iodinated contrast causes both vasoconstrictive effects and direct tubular damage (see Chapter 42 for further details). Osmolar agents (e.g., sucrose, dextran, mannitol, Hetastarch) cause osmotic nephropathy, with tubular

swelling, cellular disruption, and occlusion of tubular lumens.

PRESENTATION, EVALUATION, AND DIAGNOSIS

Depending on the degree and duration of tubular injury, the initial presentation can range from an asymptomatic rise in serum creatinine concentration to a fulminant oligoanuric picture with life-threatening electrolyte and acid-base disturbances. As described in Chapter 30, the differential diagnosis includes prerenal AKI, acute interstitial nephritis, acute glomerulonephritis, and urinary obstruction. ATN should be suspected in those with no evidence of volume depletion based on history, exam, and laboratory assessment (i.e., functional excretion of sodium >2%, urine sodium >20 mEq/L, urine osmolality <350 mOsm/L); a urine microscopy with coarse muddy-brown granular casts (composed of sloughed and degraded tubular epithelial cells) and/or free tubular epithelial cells; and a recent episode of sustained hypotension, extreme inflammation, or exposure to a known nephrotoxin.

TREATMENT AND PREVENTION

The **prevention of ATN** among hospitalized patients is essential for reducing the risk of mortality and improving outcomes. It is important to avoid exogenous nephrotoxins when possible and, when exposure is necessary, to closely monitor renal function and ensure that any exposure stops if injury occurs.

The treatment of ATN is **supportive,** as no therapy has been shown to be beneficial once ATN has occurred. Diuretics are often given in the setting of volume overload in an attempt to convert oliguric to nonoliguric ATN; however, although this may improve patient symptoms, it has not been shown to decrease the duration of ATN or risk of death. Multiple medications have been assessed for the prevention or amelioration of ATN. While several of these have proved successful in animal studies, clinical trials of agents such as low-dose dopamine, fenoldopam (a dopamine agonist), vasopressin, and N-acetylcysteine have all produced disappointing results. The reason for the discrepancy is likely a combination of the heterogeneous pathways of cellular apoptosis in clinical ATN, as well as a delay in treatment owing to the lag between a rise in creatinine concentration and the actual structural injury.

Renal replacement therapy (RRT) should be offered if complications of renal failure have occurred, including refractory volume overload, severe acidosis, or life-threatening electrolyte abnormalities (usually hyperkalemia). There has been no conclusive evidence regarding the appropriate timing of RRT initiation in the absence of such complications.

The outcomes for ATN are variable. Poor prognostic factors include advanced age, poor nutritional status, male sex, oliguria, need for mechanical ventilation, liver failure, myocardial infarction (MI), and overall severity of illness. The in-hospital mortality rate is ~50% in such settings and can be even higher in postoperative or septic patients.

CHAPTER 95

Glomerulonephritis

BRYAN M. TUCKER

INTRODUCTION

Glomerulonephritis (GN) refers to glomerular inflammation, which may occur secondary to many different disease processes. The various causes of GN are generally grouped into three categories, which reflect shared pathogenesis features and microscopy findings: immune complex mediated, **antineutrophil cytoplasmic antibody (ANCA)** associated, and **antiglomerular basement membrane (anti-GBM)** antibody associated.

PATHOGENESIS

Immune complex GN occurs when immune complexes are captured in the glomerular capillaries, causing activation of complement, recruitment of neutrophils, and elaboration of cytotoxins. These immune complexes can reflect the presence of a systemic immune disorder (i.e., lupus nephritis) or of antibodies targeting antigens that are bound to glomerular capillaries (i.e., postinfectious GN).

ANCA-associated GNs occur when antineutrophil cytoplasmic antibodies directly activate neutrophils, causing a vasculitis that can affect the glomerular capillaries either alone or as part of a systemic disorder. Finally, anti-GBM antibodies bind directly to the GBM and trigger an inflammatory response. In some cases, anti-GBM antibodies also bind the pulmonary capillaries, causing diffuse alveolar hemorrhage (Goodpasture syndrome) (Box 95.1).

PRESENTATION

The clinical presentation of GN can range from asymptomatic **hematuria** to varying degrees of the **nephritic syndrome** (acute kidney injury [AKI], **hypertension, edema, proteinuria,** and hematuria). The term rapidly progressive GN (RPGN) is applied whenever a GN causes a sudden, significant loss of renal function, irrespective of the pathogenesis.

In general, milder presentations are seen with immune complex GNs (in particular IgA nephropathy), while RPGN is more common with ANCA-associated or anti-GBM antibody–associated GNs; however, any acute GN can have a severe or fulminant course.

Unlike other causes of hematuria, acute GN is associated with **dysmorphic red blood cells** (RBCs) and/or RBC casts on urine microscopy (Fig. 95.1). These findings are highly specific for glomerular bleeding because RBCs become dysmorphic upon passing through the damaged GBM, while RBC casts are created in the thick ascending limb. Although the presence of dysmorphic RBCs and RBC casts is essentially diagnostic of GN, their absence does not rule it out.

DIAGNOSIS

All patients presenting with the nephritic syndrome should undergo a thorough evaluation. Proteinuria should be quantified. Complement levels should be measured, as they are depressed in all of the immune complex GNs (except for IgA nephropathy) but are normal in pauciimmune GN and anti-GBM disease.

The different causes of GN are distinguished based on history, clinical findings, serological tests, and (in most cases) renal biopsy findings (Fig. 95.2).

Light microscopy often demonstrates endocapillary hypercellularity, which is occlusion of the capillaries by proliferation of endothelial and mesangial cells as well as infiltration of neutrophils. Meanwhile, a defining feature of RPGN, irrespective of the specific disease process, is extracapillary proliferation, which occurs when inflammation is so intense that neutrophils rupture the glomerular capillaries and accumulate along the rim of Bowman space, where they resemble crescents.

The pattern observed on immunofluorescent staining of glomeruli for antibodies and/or complement proteins offers insights into the underlying process (Fig. 95.3).

A pattern of patchy, granular staining for antibodies and complement proteins suggests immune complex GN. In these diseases, a pattern of continuous, linear staining for antibodies and complement proteins along the capillary walls suggests direct binding of antibodies

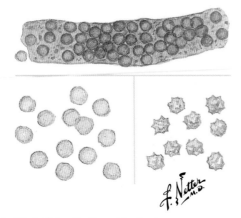

FIG. 95.1 **Urine Sediment in Acute Glomerulonephritis.** Red blood cell casts *(top)*, red blood cells *(bottom left)*, and dysmorphic red blood cells *(bottom right)* may be seen.

BOX 95.1
Types of Glomerulonephritis (GN)

- Immune complex GNs
  - IgA nephropathy
  - Henoch-Schönlein purpura
  - Postinfectious (poststreptococcal) GN
  - Membranoproliferative GN
  - Lupus nephritis
- ANCA-associated GNs
  - Granulomatosis with polyangiitis (Wegener syndrome)
  - Microscopic polyangiitis
  - Churg-Strauss disease
- Anti-GBM antibody–associated GN
  - Goodpasture syndrome

ANCA, Antineutrophil cytoplasmic antibody; *GBM,* glomerular basement membrane; *IgA,* immunoglobulin A.

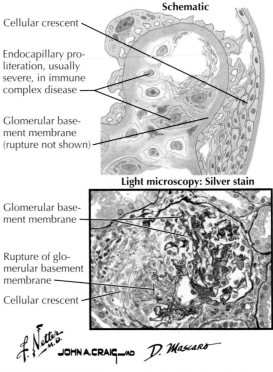

FIG. 95.2 **Light Microscopy in Rapidly Progressive Glomerulonephritis.**

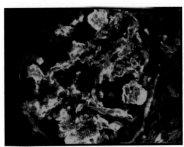

Granular staining for IgG, consistent
with immune complex disease

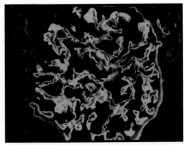

Linear staining for IgG, consistent
with anti-GBM disease

FIG. 95.3 **Immunofluorescence in Glomerulonephritis (GN).** Patchy staining typical of immune complex GN *(top)* and linear staining typical of anti-glomerular basement membrane *(anti-GBM)* disease *(bottom)*. IgG, Immunoglobulin G.

to the GBM and is therefore characteristic of anti-GBM disease.

A general lack of staining for antibodies or complement proteins (i.e., pauciimmune staining) suggests the presence of circulating ANCAs, which are thought to directly activate neutrophils in the glomerular capillaries. The ensuing inflammation often leads to RPGN, and it may be either isolated or part of a systemic vasculitis. ANCAs can be subdivided into those with predominantly cytoplasmic (c-ANCA) or perinuclear (p-ANCA) staining. c-ANCAs are often associated with granulomatosis with polyangiitis (Wegener granulomatosis). p-ANCAs are often associated with Churg-Strauss syndrome and microscopic polyangiitis. Wegener granulomatosis and microscopic polyangiitis often feature pulmonary hemorrhage, whereas Churg-Strauss syndrome often features asthma and eosinophilia.

TREATMENT

The treatment for acute GN depends on the cause but generally involves suppression of the immune response; one exception is postinfectious GN, in which treatment centers on eradicating any residual infection.

CHAPTER 96

Acute Tubulointerstitial Nephritis

DENNIS G. MOLEDINA

INTRODUCTION

Acute tubulointerstitial nephritis (AIN) is a major cause of acute kidney injury (AKI) that occurs most often in response to medication exposure and less often as a result of autoimmune disorders or **infection**. The loss of renal function results from the presence of inflammatory cells in the interstitial space, resulting in edema and injury to the renal tubules. Up to 2% to 3% of all kidney biopsies have evidence of AIN; in patients with AKI, the proportion increases to 13% to 20%.

PATHOPHYSIOLOGY AND RISK FACTORS

The major causes of AIN are medications, autoimmune disorders, and infections (Fig. 96.1).

Medications are implicated in >70% causes of AIN in the developed world. The kidneys are particularly sensitive to drug hypersensitivity, and kidneys are often affected in the absence of systemic manifestations. The most commonly implicated drug classes are antibiotics, proton-pump inhibitors (PPIs), and NSAIDs. PPIs have become a common cause of AIN due to their widespread use, and multiple recent studies have demonstrated increased risk of AIN, AKI, and chronic kidney disease (CKD) in individuals who take PPIs. Immune checkpoint inhibitors, including cytotoxic T-cell antigen-4 (CTLA4) and programmed cell death-1 or its ligand (PD1/PD-L1), restore T-cell activity against tumor cells and have revolutionized cancer treatment; however, they have also been associated with various immune phenomena, such as AIN. There are numerous case reports of patients who were previously tolerant to drugs known to cause AIN but then became intolerant due to immune checkpoint inhibition therapy.

Systemic autoimmune disorders are the second most common cause of AIN in the developed world. Autoimmune AIN is more common among younger individuals and is uncommon in the elderly. The major causes are sarcoidosis and Sjögren syndrome. AIN may also occur as part of the **tubulointerstitial nephritis and uveitis (TINU) syndrome;** thus younger patients with

AIN of unclear etiology should be monitored for uveitis. **Immunoglobulin G4 (IgG4)**–related kidney disease is one of several disorders that are characterized by elevated serum levels of IgG4 subclass antibodies, tissue deposition of IgG4, and involvement of various organ systems (including salivary glands, pancreas, retroperitoneum, and kidneys). Systemic lupus erythematosus (SLE) and antineutrophil cytoplasmic antibody (ANCA)–associated vasculitis can also cause isolated AIN but are more commonly associated with glomerulonephritis.

Infections are an uncommon cause of AIN in the developed world and account for <5% of cases.

Through a variety of mechanisms, the abovementioned exposures trigger an infiltrate of lymphocytes (and, in some cases, eosinophils) into the renal interstitium (Fig. 96.2). The resulting edema increases intratubular pressure and can interfere with normal renal filtration function. Moreover, lymphoctytes can cross from the interstitium into the tubular wall and then lumen, a phenomenon known as **tubulitis**. The passage of lymphocytes into the tubules results in the presence of white blood cells (WBCs) and WBC casts in the urine. The ensuing injury to tubules may also result in renal tubular cells and granular casts in the urine. Ongoing, unchecked interstitial inflammation can progress to interstitial fibrosis, which is irreversible and leads to CKD.

PRESENTATION, EVALUATION, AND DIAGNOSIS

Most patients with drug-associated AIN are asymptomatic. Signs of a systemic allergic reaction, such as fever and urticaria, are more likely to be present with β-lactam–associated AIN but are characteristically absent in PPI-associated or NSAID-associated AIN. The classic clinical triad of fever, rash, and eosinophilia is observed in <10% of patients with drug-induced AIN.

The time from drug initiation to the diagnosis of AIN is usually a few days for antibiotics and weeks to months for PPIs and NSAIDs. Patients with systemic diseases associated with AIN (e.g., sarcoidosis, syndrome, IgG4)

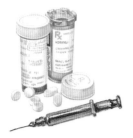

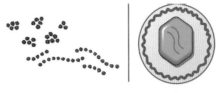

Medications (major cause)

- Antibiotics
  (esp. β-lactam,
  fluoroquinolones,
  vancomycin,
  rifampin)
- NSAIDs
- Sulfonamides
- Proton-pump inhibitors
- Immune checkpoint inhibitors
- Diuretics
- Mesalamine

Infections
*Streptoccocus, Escherichia coli, Mycobacterium
tuberculosis, Legionella, Leptospira,*
cytomegalovirus, Epstein-Barr virus, adenovirus

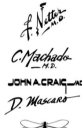

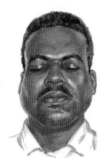

Autoimmune diseases
- Sarcoidosis
- Sjögren syndrome
- Tubulointerstitial nephritis and
  uveitis (TINU) syndrome
- IgG4-related kidney disease
- Systemic lupus erythematosus
- ANCA-associated vasculitis

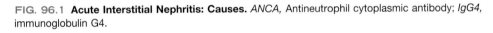

FIG. 96.1 **Acute Interstitial Nephritis: Causes.** *ANCA,* Antineutrophil cytoplasmic antibody; *IgG4,* immunoglobulin G4.

often have known histories of these diseases. In TINU syndrome, patients may present with uveitis, manifest as painful red eyes and photophobia.

Although patients always undergo evaluation for AIN on the basis of an elevation in serum creatinine concentration, up to half of patients with biopsy-proven AIN do not meet criteria for AKI and instead have a much more insidious decline in renal function over the course of months. Such changes may be indistinguishable from progressive CKD and can lead to a delay in the recognition of AIN.

In up to 20% of patients, the urinary sediment appears normal. In most cases, however, some abnormality can be detected. The presence of pyuria or WBC casts in the absence of infection is highly suggestive of AIN. Likewise, patients can have low-grade (tubular) proteinuria. (One exception is NSAID-associated AIN, which can present with nephrotic-range proteinuria if there is concomitant glomerular disease.) **Urine eosinophil** testing is neither sensitive nor specific, and the common causes of AIN

have significantly changed since the original studies on the significance of urine eosinophils. Significant serum eosinophilia suggests AIN but does not confirm the diagnosis. A small percentage of individuals may present with gross hematuria.

Renal imaging, generally with ultrasonography, is helpful to rule out other causes of renal disease. Patients with AIN may have increased kidney size and echogenicity, although this finding is nonspecific. Patients with IgG4-associated AIN may have retroperitoneal fibrosis, which can result in ureteral obstruction.

Overall, AIN is challenging to diagnose as there is no pathognomonic clinical feature, the renal function decline is slowly progressive, and there is no definitive noninvasive test. The gold standard for diagnosis remains a kidney biopsy. Thus it is necessary to maintain a high index of suspicion and consider biopsy in cases of nonresolving or progressive AKI, or in patients with preexisting CKD and a sudden acceleration in loss of renal function.

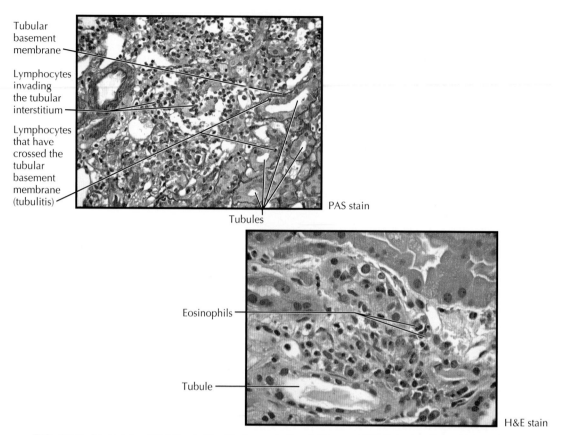

Tubular basement membrane

Lymphocytes invading the tubular interstitium

Lymphocytes that have crossed the tubular basement membrane (tubulitis)

Tubules

PAS stain

Eosinophils

Tubule

H&E stain

FIG. 96.2 **Acute Interstitial Nephritis: Findings on Renal Biopsy.** *H&E,* Hematoxylin and eosin; *PAS,* periodic acid–Schiff.

TREATMENT

The mainstay of AIN management is identification of the offending agent and prompt discontinuation. As drug-associated AIN is often a class effect, switching to another agent in the same class is not recommended. Given the underlying mechanism of AIN, immunosuppressive therapy is an attractive treatment option; however, there have been no randomized controlled trials of their efficacy, and the existing evidence is derived from retrospective, small, single-center studies. These limitations notwithstanding, a short course (<4 weeks) of glucocorticoid therapy should be considered in those with potential for renal recovery (indicated by minimal interstitial fibrosis) and no contraindication to glucocorticoids. Delays in diagnosis, more prolonged exposure to the offending medication, and delay in the initiation of glucocorticoids are all associated with incomplete recovery and risk of CKD.

CHAPTER 97

Nephrotic Syndrome

ROBERT DIEP

INTRODUCTION

The nephrotic syndrome occurs when individuals develop **glomerular** disease associated with heavy (or nephrotic-range) **proteinuria,** defined as >3.5 g/24 hours, along with **hypoalbuminemia** (<3 g/dL), peripheral edema, and hyperlipidemia.

Nephrotic syndrome can occur either as a primary phenomenon or secondary to a systemic disease. The major primary renal diseases that cause nephrotic syndrome include **minimal change disease, focal segmental glomerulosclerosis,** and **membranous nephropathy.** Of note, these same conditions can also occur secondary to other insults; for example, minimal change disease has been associated with hematological malignancies, while membranous nephropathy may be the first manifestation of a solid tumor.

The major secondary causes of nephrotic syndrome include diabetes mellitus **(diabetic nephropathy),** systemic lupus erythematosus (lupus nephritis), amyloidosis, multiple myeloma, and HIV infection (HIV-associated nephropathy). Finally, some of the **glomerulonephritides** can cause sufficient proteinuria to cause nephrotic syndrome; the major causes include immunoglobulin A (IgA) nephropathy and membranoproliferative glomerulonephritis (see Chapter 95 for further details).

PATHOPHYSIOLOGY

The glomerular capillaries selectively filter molecules based on their charge and size. In normal individuals, albumin is absent or nearly absent from the glomerular ultrafiltrate due to both its large molecular weight and negative charge; the small amount that passes through the glomerular capillaries is reabsorbed in the proximal tubules. In the diseases responsible for the nephrotic syndrome, disruption of the normal glomerular barrier leads to a significant loss of protein and lipids into urine (Fig. 97.1).

The mechanisms for such disruption are diverse. Minimal change disease, for example, features idiopathic effacement of podocyte foot processes, which are essential components of the filtration barrier. Membranous nephropathy, in contrast, features immune complex–mediated injury to and loss of podocytes.

When proteinuria becomes advanced, patients become hypoalbuminemic, reducing intravascular oncotic pressure and leading to the third spacing of fluids. The resulting intravascular volume depletion results in renal hypoperfusion, leading to increased sodium and water retention and progressive worsening of edema. Historically, the associated hyperlipidemia was thought to be a by-product of increased hepatic synthetic activity in an attempt to create more albumin. More recent data suggest that a more significant mechanism may be reduced lipid metabolism through alterations in lipoprotein lipase activity.

While albumin is the principal protein that is spilled in the urine in nephrotic syndrome, other plasma proteins are lost as well, including transferrin, clotting factors (in particular, proteins C and S), immunoglobulins, and hormone-carrier proteins. Advanced nephrotic syndrome can therefore also be complicated by hypercoagulability (with particular risk of renal vein thrombosis,), immunodeficiency, and even vitamin deficiencies (such as vitamin D from loss of vitamin D–binding protein).

RISK FACTORS

The numerous potential causes of nephrotic syndrome each have their own risk factors. In the general population, the most common cause of nephrotic syndrome is diabetes mellitus. The most common primary cause of nephrotic syndrome, however, is focal segmental glomerulosclerosis, a condition that can be either idiopathic or related to conditions such as obesity, intravenous drug use, sickle cell disease, and anabolic steroid use. Also very common in adults is membranous nephropathy, which can be either idiopathic or secondary and associated with hematological and solid malignancies, drugs (gold, penicillamine, NSAIDs, antitumor necrosis factor [anti-TNF] agents), and chronic infections (hepatitis B virus [HBV] or syphilis). Hepatitis C virus (HCV) can

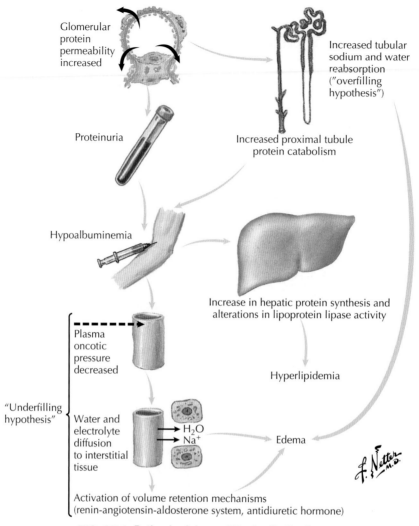

FIG. 97.1 **Pathophysiology of Nephrotic Syndrome.**

lead to membranoproliferative glomerulonephritis or, much more rarely, to membranous nephropathy. HIV can result in nephrotic syndrome through the development of HIV-associated nephropathy (HIVAN). Among children, minimal change disease is by far the most common cause of nephrotic syndrome; in adults, NSAIDs are the most common cause of secondary minimal change disease.

PRESENTATION, EVALUATION, AND DIAGNOSIS

Nephrotic syndrome should be considered in any patient with edema and/or a positive urine dipstick for proteinuria (Fig. 97.2). One characteristic, but somewhat infrequent, complaint is facial edema that is worst when first arising in the morning, after sleeping in a prone position. Unlike patients with heart failure, those with nephrotic syndrome do not experience significant orthopnea, so sleeping in a prone position is not necessarily uncomfortable but does cause dependent edema. Some patients may also describe their urine as frothy or soapy, owing to the large amounts of lipoproteins.

The history should investigate recent exposures to medications and assess all known and potential systemic illnesses. Older adults should be asked about malignancy screening and risk factors. The physical examination

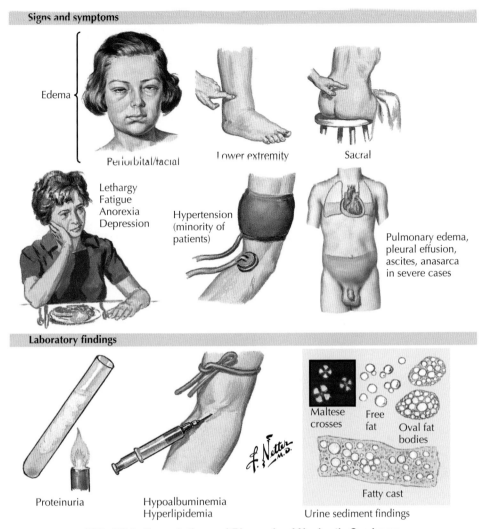

FIG. 97.2 Presentation and Diagnosis of Nephrotic Syndrome.

is most notable for edema, which, in extreme cases, may be frank anasarca. Patients may also have findings consistent with pleural effusions, thromboembolism, or dyslipidemia (i.e., eruptive xanthomata or xanthelasmata). Additional findings may depend on the underlying diseases (e.g., retinopathy in a patient with diabetic nephropathy).

Microscopic inspection of the urine sediment may reveal fatty casts due to lipiduria, with a Maltese cross pattern evident under polarized light. The urinalysis is usually acellular but can run the gamut to very active if the proteinuria is secondary to a glomerulonephritis. A 24-hour urine collection provides the most accurate quantitation and can distinguish between albumin and

nonalbumin proteinuria; however, a protein-to-creatinine ratio (mg/mg) on a random urine specimen is often an adequate substitute, as the ratio correlates closely with daily protein excretion.

Additional laboratory tests can be sent to assess for systemic inflammation and specific diseases in the context of other signs and symptoms, including C-reactive protein, hemoglobin A1c, antinuclear antibody (ANA), anti–double-stranded DNA antibody, complement levels, serum free light-chain concentrations, serum and urine protein electrophoresis and immunofixation, rapid plasma reagin (RPR), HIV serologies, hepatitis B and C serologies, and cryoglobulins. The presence of antiphospholipase-A2-receptor (PLA2R) autoantibodies is quite specific to the diagnosis of idiopathic membranous nephropathy (though only ~70% sensitive), and the titer also follows disease activity and progression. Testing for PLA2R autoantibodies is currently performed in only a limited number of laboratories but is available for clinical use.

A renal ultrasound can provide useful information regarding the chronicity of a disease and can establish the safety of biopsy. Enlarged kidneys are characteristic of diabetes, HIV, and infiltrative disease (e.g., amyloidosis). Renal biopsy is generally safe unless the kidneys appear shrunken and atrophic, in which case the bleeding risk becomes high and the potential yield low. A biopsy is almost always required to establish the diagnosis and guide therapy; the only exception is nephrotic syndrome in children, which is presumed to be minimal change disease and evaluated further only if it is refractory to empiric treatment with steroids.

TREATMENT

The treatment must address both the underlying cause of nephrotic syndrome and its manifestations. The mainstays of symptom management include high-dose ACE inhibitors and angiotensin II receptor blockers (ARBs) to reduce and reverse proteinuria by lowering intraglomerular pressure; spironolactone can act as an effective adjuvant to these, but patients much be closely monitored for hyperkalemia. High-dose diuretics can be used to reduce edema and statins to reverse hyperlipidemia. Patients should adapt a low-sodium diet (<2 g/day) and restrict their fluid intake (<2 L/day). There is not strong evidence to support prophylactic anticoagulation, but many clinicians do so if a patient's serum albumin is consistently <1.5 g/dL. If anticoagulation is required but contraindicated, an inferior vena cava (IVC) filter should be placed superior to the renal vein, given its risk of thrombosis.

CHAPTER 98

Polycystic Kidney Disease

MARYAM GONDAL

INTRODUCTION

Polycystic kidney disease (PKD) is an inherited disorder characterized by the formation of renal cysts that cause progressive growth and eventual dysfunction of the kidneys (Fig. 98.1). There are two distinct PKD syndromes, distinguished by their inheritance patterns. **Autosomal dominant PKD (ADPKD)** is more common and features slow but progressive enlargement of the kidneys, with renal failure occurring in the fifth to sixth decade. ADPKD affects approximately 1 in 800 to 1000 individuals and accounts for 2.5% of all cases of end-stage renal disease (ESRD). **Autosomal recessive PKD (ARPKD)** typically presents at a younger age and frequently is associated with dysgenesis of the biliary ductal plate, resulting in hepatic fibrosis. The incidence is estimated as 1 in 20,000 live births.

PATHOPHYSIOLOGY

In both ADPKD and ARPKD, a defect in cilia-mediated signaling is the primary abnormality that leads to cyst formation. The primary cilium is a hairlike organelle present on the surface of most cells in the body, including the nephron, where it projects from the apical surface of the renal epithelium into the tubule lumen. Disruption of the signaling pathways within the primary cilium, including intracellular calcium, Hedgehog signaling, and cyclic adenosine monophosphate (cAMP), may trigger cystogenesis and cyst expansion in PKD.

ADPKD has been associated with mutations in the gene *PKD1* or *PKD2*; these encode the proteins polycystin-1 and polycystin-2, which have important roles in cilia formation. *PKD1* is located on the short arm of chromosome 16 and *PKD2* is on the long arm of chromosome 4. *PKD1* accounts for ~80% of cases and is typically associated with an earlier age at onset. Meanwhile ARPKD is associated with mutations of the polycystic kidney and hepatic disease-1 gene *(PKHD1)*, which is located on the short arm of chromosome 6 and encodes the protein fibrocystin.

PRESENTATION, EVALUATION, AND DIAGNOSIS

Most patients with ADPKD present in the fourth or fifth decade of life with flank pain or hematuria, which reflects spontaneous cyst rupture. Hypertension is another common manifestation, occurring in about two of three patients. This is secondary to cyst expansion, which results in compression of renal vessels, in turn causing intrarenal ischemia and activation of the renin-angiotensin-aldosterone system (RAAS). Other signs include early satiety, abdominal fullness/bloating, shortness of breath, and lower back discomfort—all resulting from the mass effect of the enlarged kidneys on adjacent organs (Fig. 98.2). Nephrolithiasis is also common, due to urinary stasis, and it occurs in 20% to 30% of patients. Extrarenal manifestations include intracranial **aneurysms,** as well as hepatic, pancreatic, thyroid, and seminal vesicle cysts. Of ADPKD patients, 40% have concomitant intracranial aneurysms identified.

ARPKD has a more heterogeneous clinical presentation. Most diagnoses occur either in utero or during the perinatal period. The typical findings include oligohydramnios, large echogenic kidneys, pulmonary hypoplasia, facial defects, spine deformities, and abnormal extremities. Some patients have milder renal abnormalities and present later in childhood, usually with complications of hepatic fibrosis and biliary disease, such as portal hypertension or cholangitis.

All patients with suspected ADPKD must have a thorough evaluation of family history, especially for the purposes of future counseling. Ultrasonography is an appropriate initial test to assess the kidneys and readily reveals multiple, large cysts. Standard criteria dictate that for the diagnosis of ADPKD, patients between 15 and 39 years of age must have at least three unilateral or bilateral cysts; those between 40 and 59 years of age must have at least two cysts in each kidney; those >60 years of age must have at least four cysts in each kidney. MRI, either with or without gadolinium contrast, is the gold standard for assessing changes in kidney volume over time. As

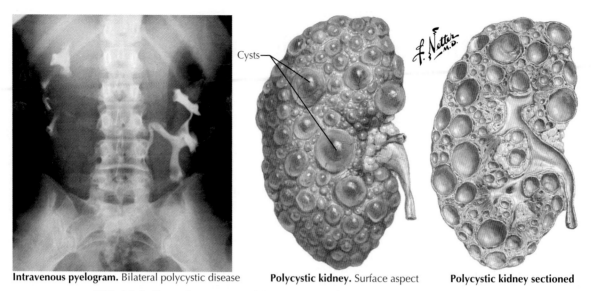

Cysts

Intravenous pyelogram. Bilateral polycystic disease   Polycystic kidney. Surface aspect   Polycystic kidney sectioned

FIG. 98.1   **Gross Appearance of Autosomal Dominant Polycystic Kidney Disease.**

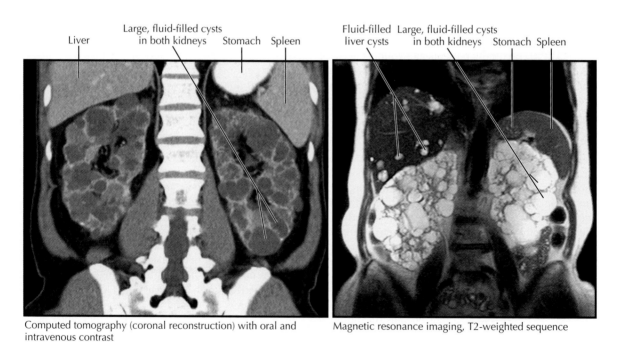

Liver   Large, fluid-filled cysts in both kidneys   Stomach   Spleen

Fluid-filled liver cysts   Large, fluid-filled cysts in both kidneys   Stomach   Spleen

Computed tomography (coronal reconstruction) with oral and intravenous contrast

Magnetic resonance imaging, T2-weighted sequence

(Note that these images depict different patients.)

FIG. 98.2   **Radiographic Findings of Autosomal Dominant Polycystic Kidney Disease.**

cyst expansion leads to the symptoms and pathology of PKD, serial measurements of kidney volume (increasing over time) are negatively correlated with and reflect a decline in glomerular filtration rate (GFR).

TREATMENT

Although there is no cure for ADPKD, several interventions can slow the progression of the disease. Hypertension control is essential, as patients with persistently elevated blood pressure have an earlier progression to ESRD and experience more cardiovascular complications than normotensive patients. RAAS inhibitors, such as ACE or angiotensin receptor blockers (ARBs), are generally preferred. A reduction in sodium intake (<2–4 g/day) and protein, as well as daily exercise, are associated with blood pressure control, which leads to better outcomes. Cyst growth is stimulated by antidiuretic hormone (ADH), and thus patients with ADPKD should have aggressive water intake to suppress ADH production.

Abdominal pain may respond to analgesics, although NSAIDs should be avoided. NSAIDs reduce synthesis of prostaglandins, which play a critical role in preservation of renal blood flow in patients with chronic kidney disease, heart failure, cirrhosis, older age, or volume depletion via dilating the afferent arteriole. Reduced prostaglandin synthesis therefore reduces GFR and can lead to acute kidney injury. Cyst decortication may alleviate cases of severe, refractory pain. Renal replacement therapy is appropriate for patients with ESRD. Novel therapies, including mTOR inhibitors, octreotide, and (most promisingly) vasopressin receptor antagonists, are under investigation and appear to be promising in managing this condition, especially in slowing cyst expansion and potentially preserving renal function.

Patients with ARPKD generally require multiple, concerted interventions starting at a very young age. Growth retardation is common and may mandate supplemental nutrition with gastrostomy or nasogastric tube feedings. Renal replacement therapy and eventual renal transplantation often are indicated. Depending on the extent of hepatic fibrosis and associated complications, patients do occasionally end up requiring liver transplant.

CHAPTER 99

Nephrolithiasis

MARINA MUTTER

INTRODUCTION

Nephrolithiasis refers to the formation of stones in the upper urinary tract, which are also known as renal calculi or **kidney stones.** Renal calculi are common, occurring in ~10% of men and 7% of women during their lifetime. About 75% to 80% of all stones are calcium based **(calcium oxalate or calcium phosphate).** The remaining types include struvite (magnesium-ammonium-phosphate) stones (15%), uric acid stones (5%), and cysteine stones (1%). It is important to note, however, that stones are frequently of mixed composition, and management decisions must take this into account.

The passage of calculi from the kidney through the ureter is painful and is a common reason for both primary care and emergency department (ED) visits. The treatment depends on the size of the calculus and the clinical condition of the patient. Preventive strategies are also important to reduce the risk of recurrence.

PATHOPHYSIOLOGY AND RISK FACTORS

Renal stones occur when urine becomes **supersaturated** with stone-forming constituents, which can result from increased excretion of those compounds and/or a decrease in fluid content of the urine. In addition, the presence of inhibitors of crystallization, such as citrate, can help prevent the formation of calcium-based or uric acid kidney stones. Microscopic crystals act as nidi for stone formation, upon which subsequent crystals can anchor and grow (Fig. 99.1).

The concentration and composition of urine determine the likelihood of calculus formation and the type of kidney stone formed. For calcium oxalate stones, the primary risk factors include low urinary volume, excess renal calcium excretion (from primary hyperparathyroidism, vitamin D excess), excess oxalate excretion (from inflammatory bowel disease [IBD], dietary excess, decreased dietary calcium), and/or a low renal citrate excretion (e.g., from renal tubular acidosis [RTA], other acidosis, chronic bowel disease). Risk factors for uric acid stones include a urinary pH <5.5 and elevated serum

uric acid. Struvite stones are usually caused by infections with urease-producing organisms, and cysteine stones occur in individuals with cystinuria, an inborn error of metabolism.

CLINICAL MANIFESTATIONS

Renal calculi require weeks to months of growth before they become large enough to cause symptoms. Some patients may be incidentally diagnosed during this period, but most renal calculi are not detected until pain occurs (Fig. 99.2).

The severity of the pain can vary from mild discomfort to severe, disabling pain that requires intravenous medications. The pain itself is typically paroxysmal and colicky, resulting from ureteral spasm as the calculus migrates from the renal pelvis toward the bladder. The pain is often located in the ipsilateral **flank** but can radiate depending on its location. For example, stones in the upper ureter can cause pain in the abdomen, while stones in the lower ureter can cause pain in the genitals.

Most patients also have gross or microscopic **hematuria.** Less common symptoms include nausea, vomiting, dysuria, and urinary urgency.

DIAGNOSIS

Urinalysis usually reveals hematuria and, in some cases, a variable amount of pyuria. The imaging modality of choice is a **noncontrast CT scan of the abdomen and pelvis,** which can detect both calculi and evidence of any associated complications, such as urinary obstruction or superinfection. If a CT scan cannot be performed, an ultrasound is another acceptable imaging modality, though it is less sensitive to smaller calculi and those located in the ureter. A study in 2014 compared ultrasound to CT for the diagnosis of nephrolithiasis and found no differences in diagnostic accuracy or serious adverse events between the two modalities, but lower radiation dose in the ultrasound group. However, a

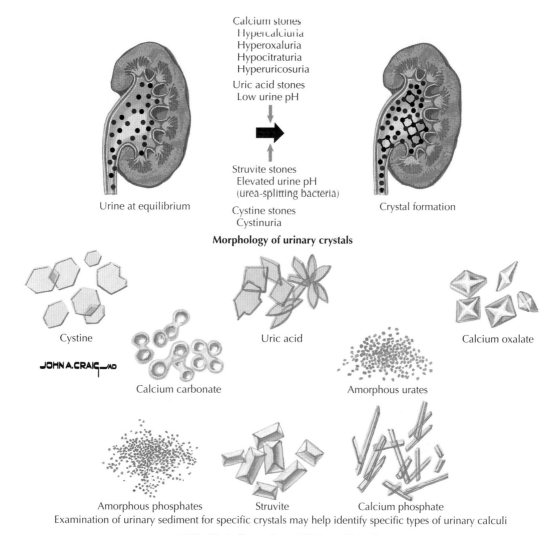

Calcium stones
    Hypercalciuria
    Hyperoxaluria
    Hypocitraturia
    Hyperuricosuria
Uric acid stones
    Low urine pH

Struvite stones
    Elevated urine pH
    (urea-splitting bacteria)
Cystine stones
    Cystinuria

Urine at equilibrium

Crystal formation

Morphology of urinary crystals

Cystine

JOHN A. CRAIG—AD

Calcium carbonate

Uric acid

Amorphous urates

Calcium oxalate

Amorphous phosphates

Struvite

Calcium phosphate

Examination of urinary sediment for specific crystals may help identify specific types of urinary calculi

FIG. 99.1 **Formation of Urinary Calculi.**

noncontrast CT scan of the abdomen remains the imaging modality of choice for the diagnosis of nephrolithiasis as it can identify other culprit abdominal pathologies in the differential diagnosis.

MANAGEMENT

The management of renal calculi depends on the clinical condition of the patient and the calculus size. Many patients can be managed with a combination of analgesics and hydration. Most stones <5 mm in diameter can reach the bladder without intervention, and patients can be managed at home, with instructions to strain their urine. A kidney stone collected by the straining of

urine can later be used for stone analysis. α-Adrenergic agonists, such as tamsulosin, can also facilitate passage of stones <10 mm by dilating the bladder neck. Passage can also be aided by vigorous hydration and smooth muscle relaxation with calcium channel blockers.

Calculi >10 mm in diameter are unlikely to pass without a urological intervention. Calculi between 5 and 10 mm often receive a trial of conservative management first, though up to half ultimately require intervention. If complications are already present (such as acute renal failure, urosepsis, anuria, or unrelenting pain, nausea, and vomiting), more urgent intervention is required.

For urgent removal of renal calculi and decompression of the collecting system, standard procedures include

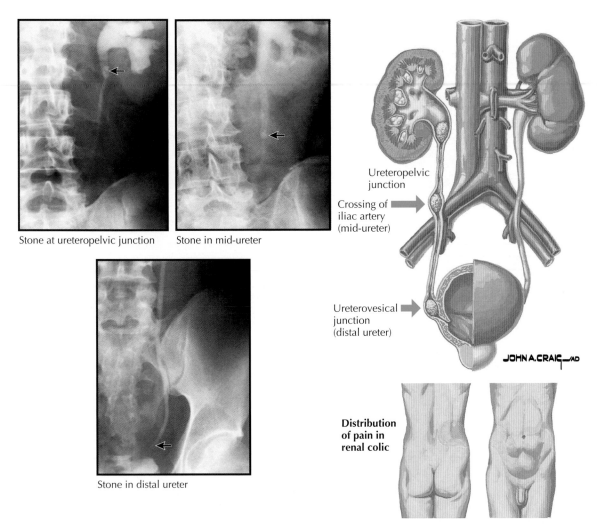

Stone at ureteropelvic junction

Stone in mid-ureter

Ureteropelvic junction

Crossing of iliac artery (mid-ureter)

Ureterovesical junction (distal ureter)

JOHN A.CRAIG᷄AD

Stone in distal ureter

Distribution of pain in renal colic

FIG. 99.2 **Major Sites of Renal Stone Impaction.**

a nephrostomy tube or insertion of a ureteral stent. A **nephrostomy tube** is a tube inserted through the skin into the renal pelvis, with a nephrostomy bag as collection for the urine. This diverts urine into the tube instead of down the ureter and into the bladder. A **ureteral stent** is a thin tube inserted into the ureter to allow drainage of urine around the stone. In less urgent settings, **extracorporeal shockwave lithotripsy (ESWL)** may be performed to fragment calculi and facilitate their passage. In ESWL, shockwaves are produced and transmitted directly to the renal calculi, with concentration and release of energy at the stone surface and subsequent fragmentation of the stone (Fig. 99.3).

More than half of patients with symptomatic renal calculi will experience a recurrent event within 10 years.

Thus if there is no obvious explanation for a calculus (e.g., dehydration) or the patient has experienced multiple episodes, a workup to determine the etiology and composition of the calculi is appropriate. Laboratory testing should include a urinalysis and serum chemistries (blood urea nitrogen [BUN], creatinine, uric acid, calcium, phosphate, chloride, bicarbonate, parathyroid hormone [PTH]). On the urinalysis, note should be made of the pH, as alkaline urine promotes the formation of calcium phosphate and struvite stones, while an acidic environment promotes uric acid and cysteine stones. The urinalysis may also reveal crystals that indicate the type of stone (calcium oxalate, uric acid, cysteine, etc.). The initial workup may suggest the cause for the stone, such as elevated PTH/calcium (Ca)

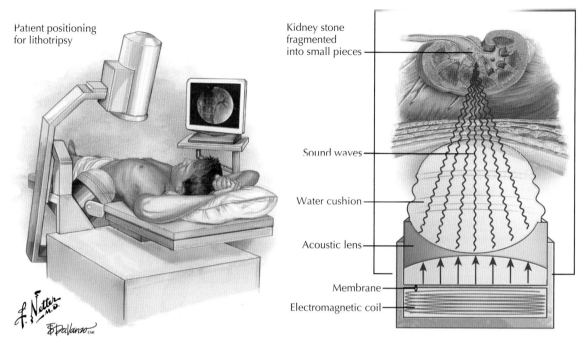

Patient positioning for lithotripsy

Kidney stone fragmented into small pieces

Sound waves

Water cushion

Acoustic lens

Membrane

Electromagnetic coil

FIG. 99.3 **Extracorporeal Shockwave Lithotripsy.**

in primary hyperparathyroidism, elevated uric acid in uric acid stones, or metabolic acidosis/RTA that may contribute to stones.

Based on clinical suspicion, a 24-hour urine collection for certain electrolytes may be indicated. In a 24-hour collection, levels of calcium, phosphate, sodium, oxalate, citrate, uric acid, magnesium, and cysteine are measured, in addition to urinary volume. High levels of any of the abovementioned components promote stone formation, with the exception of citrate, when low levels promote calcium-based stone formation. In addition, if a kidney stone or stone fragment is available, stone composition analysis should be performed.

PREVENTION

Urine dilution reduces the risk of any type of stone formation; therefore patients should be encouraged to drink at least 2 to 3 L water per day. Further prevention of renal calculi depends on the specific composition of the stone. For calcium oxalate stones, treatment of the underlying cause is important; for idiopathic hypercalciuria, a thiazide diuretic is often prescribed to lower urinary calcium excretion. A low oxalate diet should be pursued for hyperoxaluria, and citrate supplementation can be prescribed for hypocitraturia. Somewhat paradoxically, patients with calcium oxalate stones should eat dairy with most meals as the calcium binds oxalate in the intestines and prevents its absorption. However, use of calcium supplements increases stone risk. For primary hyperparathyroidism, surgery is indicated in the presence of nephrolithiasis (see Chapter 74 for further details). Alkalinization of the urine and increased fluid intake are helpful for both uric acid and cysteine stones, whereas antibiotics are indicated for struvite stones.

CHAPTER 100

Chronic Kidney Disease

CAROL TRAYNOR

INTRODUCTION

Chronic kidney disease (CKD) affects >20 million people in the United States; it is defined as ≥3 months of reduced kidney function or kidney damage (abnormal urinalysis, imaging, or biopsy studies). CKD is classified into different stages based on **estimated glomerular filtration rate (eGFR)** and degree of albuminuria (Table 100.1).

In 2015, >660,000 Americans had stage 5 CKD **(end-stage renal disease [ESRD])**; one-third had a functioning transplant, while the remainder require ongoing dialysis. The annual incidence of ESRD has stabilized due to better treatment of hypertension and the use of ACE inhibitors, which delay the progression of renal dysfunction. The life expectancy for patients with CKD is significantly reduced compared to age-matched, gender-matched, and race-matched controls.

ETIOLOGY AND PATHOGENESIS

Diabetes mellitus (DM) and hypertension account for more than two-thirds of all CKD cases in the United States. Additional causes include focal segmental glomerulosclerosis, glomerulonephritis, HIV-associated nephropathy, polycystic kidney disease (PKD), and chronic obstructive or reflux nephropathy. Regardless of the underlying disease, the remaining nephrons initially compensate by increasing their filtration rate to maintain GFR. These changes ultimately become maladaptive, however, as these nephrons experience intraglomerular hypertension, afferent arteriolar vasodilation, and an increase in profibrotic cytokines (driven in part by increased angiotensin II) that together promote glomerular sclerosis, tubulointerstitial fibrosis, and further nephron loss.

ASSESSMENT OF RENAL FUNCTION

GFR is the best overall index of kidney function in health and disease; however, GFR is not directly measured in clinical practice and is instead estimated from equations based on serum creatinine (Table 100.2). Of note, eGFR is inaccurate in the setting of acute kidney injury, since kidney function (and therefore creatinine concentration) is not in steady state.

PRESENTATION

The presentation of CKD depends on the underlying cause and stage. Many patients with long-standing DM or hypertension, for example, have CKD detected on screening. In contrast, patients with autosomal dominant PKD (ADPKD) may present with abdominal masses and hypertension (see Chapter 98). Some patients present with nonspecific symptoms, such as fatigue and anorexia, due to progressive anemia and azotemia. In the most severe cases, patients may present with **uremia,** a constellation of symptoms related to the accumulation of toxins normally cleared by the kidneys (Fig. 100.1).

COMPLICATIONS AND MANAGEMENT

Patients with CKD are typically asymptomatic until the disease becomes advanced. Thus it is important to screen for CKD and its complications in high-risk patients, such as those with DM or hypertension. The initial treatment of CKD should focus on the underlying disease. General recommendations include discontinuation of tobacco products (to reduce cardiovascular risk and potentially slow the progression of CKD) and avoidance of nephrotoxins (e.g., NSAIDs and iodinated contrast media).

Hypertension

Hypertension occurs in >80% of patients as both a cause and consequence of CKD. The treatment of hypertension can slow the progression of CKD and reduce the risk of cardiovascular complications. A common blood pressure goal is <130/80, and renin-angiotensin system (RAS) inhibitors (either ACE inhibitors or angiotensin receptor blockers) are preferred, particularly in patients with proteinuria. The initiation of RAS inhibition requires monitoring for hyperkalemia and acute kidney injury. A rise of creatinine within 30% of the baseline value is

TABLE 100.1
Chronic Kidney Disease Stages

GFR Stage	Description	eGFR (mL/min/1.73 m²)
1	Kidney damage with normal or increased GFR	>90
2	Mildly decreased	60–89
3a	Mildly to moderately decreased	45–59
3b	Moderately to severely decreased	30–44
4	Severely decreased	15–29
5	Kidney failure	<15
Albuminuria Stage	**Description**	**Albumin Excretion Rate (mg/day)**
A1	Normal to mildly increased	<30
A2	Moderately increased	30–300
A3	Severely increased	>300

eGFR, Estimated glomerular filtration rate; GFR, glomerular filtration rate.
Modified from Levey AS, de Jong PE, Coresh J, et al: The definition, classification, and prognosis of chronic kidney disease: a KDIGO Controversies Conference report, Kidney Int 80(1), 2011.

TABLE 100.2
GFR Estimating Equations

Method	Equation
CKD-EPI equation	GFR (mL/min/1.73 m²) = 141 × min(SCr/κ, 1)^α × max(SCr/κ, 1)$^{-1.209}$ × 0.993^{Age} *(1.018 if female)*(1.159 if black) SCr is serum creatinine (in mg/dL) κ is 0.7 for females and 0.9 for males α is −0.329 for females and −0.411 for males min is the minimum of SCr/κ or 1 max is the maximum of SCr/κ or 1
Four-variable MDRD equation	GFR (mL/min/1.73 m²) = 175 × (SCr)$^{-1.154}$ × (Age)$^{-0.203}$ × (0.742 if female) × (1.212 if black) SCr is serum creatinine (in mg/dL)

CKD-EPI, Chronic Kidney Disease Epidemiology Collaboration; GFR, glomerular filtration rate; MDRD, Modification of Diet in Renal Disease.

acceptable, since it is typically not indicative of actual structural kidney injury but rather a reduction in filtration fraction due to efferent arteriole dilatation. Many patients need at least two antihypertensives, and the additional agents can be based on specific indications (e.g., a diuretic may be given for edema or a β-blocker for ischemic heart disease).

Anemia

Many patients with more advanced CKD develop normochromic, normocytic **anemia**. The major causes are decreased renal erythropoietin production and iron deficiency (due to increased levels of hepcidin, which impairs oral absorption and inhibits mobilization of iron from the reticuloendothelial system). It is important, however, to screen patients for other causes of anemia, checking red cell indices, iron studies, vitamin B$_{12}$ level, folate level, reticulocyte count, and platelet count (see Chapter 32 for details). Available therapies for anemia of CKD include iron supplementation and **erythrocyte-stimulating agents (ESAs).** Iron should be supplemented when the transferrin saturation is <30% and ferritin concentration is ~<500 ng/mL. As oral iron supplements may not be reliably absorbed, intravenous iron is more appropriate. Patients with hemoglobin levels persistently <10 g/dL despite adequate iron stores may require treatment with ESAs (such as epoetin alfa or darbepoetin). The goal is to maintain hemoglobin in the range of 10 to 11.5 g/dL, as higher hemoglobin targets are associated with increased cardiovascular events.

Bone Disease

Renal phosphorous excretion declines along with eGFR. In addition, gastrointestinal (GI) calcium absorption decreases owing to low levels of 1,25-dihydroxyvitamin D (the active form of vitamin D produced by the kidney). The resulting hyperphosphatemia, hypocalcemia, and decreased 1,25-dihydroxyvitamin D levels produce **secondary hyperparathyroidism.** The rise in parathyroid

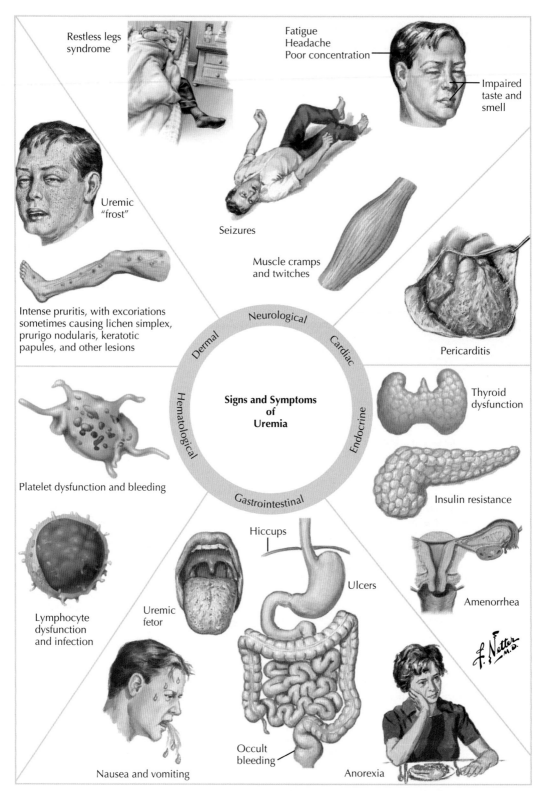

Restless legs syndrome

Fatigue
Headache
Poor concentration

Impaired taste and smell

Uremic "frost"

Seizures

Muscle cramps and twitches

Pericarditis

Intense pruritis, with excoriations sometimes causing lichen simplex, prurigo nodularis, keratotic papules, and other lesions

Dermal

Neurological

Cardiac

Hematological

Endocrine

Signs and Symptoms of Uremia

Thyroid dysfunction

Platelet dysfunction and bleeding

Gastrointestinal

Insulin resistance

Hiccups

Ulcers

Lymphocyte dysfunction and infection

Uremic fetor

Amenorrhea

Occult bleeding

Nausea and vomiting

Anorexia

FIG. 100.1 **Uremia.**

hormone (PTH) initially serves to maintain serum calcium and serum phosphorous within normal ranges, albeit at the expense of increased bone turnover. Uncontrolled secondary hyperparathyroidism can lead to osteitis fibrosa cystica, a form of bone disease characterized by high bone turnover and fibrosis (see Chapter 74).

The treatment for secondary hyperparathyroidism includes dietary phosphate restriction, oral phosphate binders, and active vitamin D analogs such as calcitriol. Cinacalcet is a calcimimetic that is used in refractory cases; it acts on the calcium-sensing receptor in the parathyroid glands to lower serum PTH levels, thereby decreasing serum phosphorus concentrations.

Acidosis

Metabolic acidosis is a common complication of CKD. As the GFR declines below 40 to 50, the reduced nephron mass is unable to excrete acid at normal rates or create new bicarbonate via ammoniagenesis. The ensuing chronic metabolic acidosis causes muscle catabolism, increased systemic inflammation, impaired myocardial contractility, and increased mortality. It is also associated with a higher risk of progressive renal dysfunction. Patients with metabolic acidosis should be treated with alkali therapy, such as sodium bicarbonate, to maintain bicarbonate in the normal range.

Hyperkalemia

Hyperkalemia becomes more common as CKD progresses and renal excretion is unable to match oral intake. Preventative measures include a low potassium diet and avoidance of medications that can increase serum potassium, such as NSAIDs (which inhibit renal prostaglandin synthesis and impair angiotensin II–induced aldosterone secretion, thereby decreasing urinary potassium excretion). The use of loop diuretics and treatment of metabolic acidosis also lower serum potassium levels. Dialysis may be required if hyperkalemia becomes refractory to medical management.

Volume Overload

Overt signs of volume overload, such as peripheral and pulmonary edema, occur more commonly with advanced CKD. Even in the earlier stages of CKD, however, the ability to handle a salt load is impaired, and increased salt intake with concomitant heart failure can lead to volume overload. Patients with CKD and volume overload are typically treated with sodium restriction (<2 g/day) and a loop diuretic.

Cardiovascular Disease

Cardiovascular disease is the leading cause of death in patients with CKD. Although patients with CKD have an increased prevalence of traditional risk factors (e.g., diabetes, hypertension, hyperlipidemia), CKD itself is an independent risk factor, as it is associated with left ventricular hypertrophy (due to hypertension and anemia), vascular calcification (driven primarily by abnormalities in calcium and phosphate), and chronic inflammation.

Preparation and Timing of Renal Replacement Therapy

All patients with CKD should be counseled regarding the different **renal replacement therapy (RRT)** modalities (including the possible need for vascular access surgery) and potential for renal transplantation (see Chapter 54 for details).

RRT is generally indicated when patients experience volume overload refractory to diuretics, metabolic disturbances (such as hyperkalemia or metabolic acidosis) that cannot be corrected with medications, or uremic signs such as pericarditis and encephalopathy. Among asymptomatic patients with progressive CKD, there is no specific threshold eGFR for the initiation of dialysis; however, RRT initiation should be considered when eGFR is <10 mL/min/1.73 m^2 due to the risk of life-threatening complications.

Patients opting for hemodialysis should be referred for arteriovenous fistula (AVF) creation when dialysis is likely to become necessary within 1 year, as fistula maturation can take several months. Native AVFs are associated with the lowest mortality risk compared to other forms of vascular access (such as tunneled dialysis catheters) and have good long-term patency rates. Venipuncture of peripheral veins can render them unsuitable for AVF placement; therefore patients and health care providers should be instructed to avoid venipuncture above the level of the hands, particularly in the nondominant extremity, to preserve potential access sites. Patients opting for peritoneal dialysis (PD) should have a PD catheter inserted 3 to 4 weeks before the anticipated need for dialysis.

Kidney transplantation is the treatment of choice for most patients with ESRD. Timely referral of patients with progressive CKD facilitates early identification of potential living donors and enables preemptive transplantation, which improves patient and graft survival.

CHAPTER 101

Osteoarthritis

JOHN I. O'REILLY

INTRODUCTION

Osteoarthritis (OA) is the most common joint disease. It can affect either one or multiple joints and occurs most commonly in weight-bearing joints such as the spine, knee, and hips, as well as the small joints of the hands. OA had been classically thought of as a wear-and-tear disease due to aging, leading to erosion of the articular cartilage, but the pathology is now understood to be more complex. Proinflammatory molecules lead to involvement of the whole joint, including the overlying capsule, the synovial fluid, and underlying subchondral bone.

OA is best thought of as a related group of underlying causes leading to common radiological, pathological, and clinical findings. It can be classified as **primary** or **secondary;** secondary disease is due to a known inciting factor such as trauma, surgery, hip dysplasia, or an inflammatory arthritis such as rheumatoid arthritis. Primary OA is idiopathic, but it is related to genetic risk factors as well as age and obesity.

OA is one of the leading causes of morbidity across the world. Prevalence varies markedly depending of the definition used, since more than half of patients with radiographical findings of OA will not yet have symptoms. Prevalence also increases dramatically with age, with OA of the hand being particularly common, and is seen in over 50% of patients age ≥65 years.

PATHOPHYSIOLOGY

The articular cartilage is an avascular, aneural matrix composed of chondrocytes and a meshwork of collagen and proteoglycans. The proteoglycans have hydrophilic side chains, which trap water and provide the lubrication necessary for joint function. Classically, OA has been considered noninflammatory since there are minimal leukocytes in the synovial fluid. However, it is now understood that there is innate immune system activation in OA leading to cytokine and chemokine activation.

Initially, chondrocytes undergo injury in areas of maximal stress, causing them to proliferate and release inflammatory mediators. The mediators degrade and remodel the matrix, exposing the underlying bone. In addition, vascular growth factors released lead to new blood vessel and nerve development, causing inflammation and pain. The underlying bone becomes the new articular surface, resulting in joint space narrowing. Mechanical stress on this surface leads to growth and hardening of the bone, manifested as subchondral sclerosis. Local areas of bony overgrowth from this stress are called **osteophytes,** or bone spurs. Small pieces of cartilage and bone eventually break off, forming the loose bodies seen on imaging. Another radiographical finding in advanced OA is **bone cysts,** which develop in areas of localized bone necrosis and subsequent reabsorption (Fig. 101.1).

RISK FACTORS

The strongest risk factor for OA is age; the prevalence increases significantly over the age of 50. Other risk factors include obesity, female gender, congenital hip dysplasia, previous trauma, or an occupation requiring manual labor. Physical exercise is protective against OA before joint disease develops, but may worsen symptoms in joints that are already affected. Twin studies have shown a strong genetic correlation for OA as well.

PRESENTATION, EVALUATION, AND DIAGNOSIS

A patient with OA in an affected joint typically presents with pain and stiffness, and has decreased range of motion and crepitus on exam. Pain is often the initial complaint that brings patients into their provider. The pain is deep and aching, developing over a number of months to years. It becomes progressively worse during

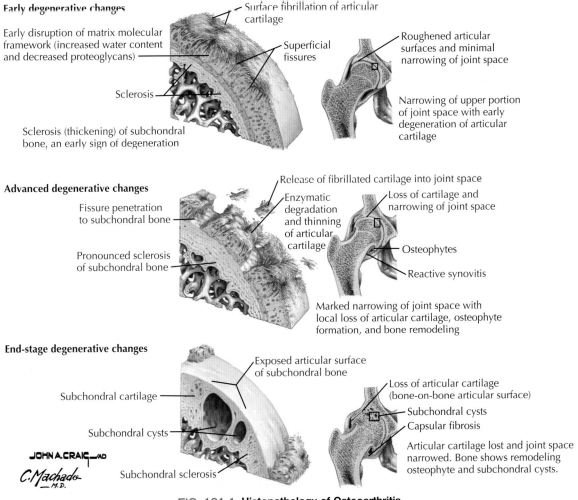

Early degenerative changes

Early disruption of matrix molecular framework (increased water content and decreased proteoglycans)

Sclerosis

Sclerosis (thickening) of subchondral bone, an early sign of degeneration

Surface fibrillation of articular cartilage

Superficial fissures

Roughened articular surfaces and minimal narrowing of joint space

Narrowing of upper portion of joint space with early degeneration of articular cartilage

Advanced degenerative changes

Fissure penetration to subchondral bone

Pronounced sclerosis of subchondral bone

Release of fibrillated cartilage into joint space

Enzymatic degradation and thinning of articular cartilage

Loss of cartilage and narrowing of joint space

Osteophytes

Reactive synovitis

Marked narrowing of joint space with local loss of articular cartilage, osteophyte formation, and bone remodeling

End-stage degenerative changes

Subchondral cartilage

Subchondral cysts

JOHN A.CRAIG—MD
C.Machado—M.D.

Subchondral sclerosis

Exposed articular surface of subchondral bone

Loss of articular cartilage (bone-on-bone articular surface)

Subchondral cysts

Capsular fibrosis

Articular cartilage lost and joint space narrowed. Bone shows remodeling osteophyte and subchondral cysts.

FIG. 101.1 **Histopathology of Osteoarthritis.**

the day due to physical overuse. Pain that presents acutely or is stabbing in nature suggests another diagnosis.

The stiffness is classically present in the morning but resolves in <30 minutes with activity; this brief stiffness is known as **gelling.** Stiffness that is present for >1 hour in the morning is more consistent with rheumatoid arthritis or another inflammatory joint disease. The joint may have bony swelling and joint line tenderness, and often it will become bulky and deformed in severe disease. As OA progresses, the patient may become immobile and develop muscle wasting, leading to sensation that the joint is giving out, although no joint instability is present on exam (Fig. 101.2). No joint warmth or erythema should be present in OA, although effusions may occur.

OA most often affects a single joint. It is often bilateral when found in weight-bearing joints, although one side

may predominate. Less often, it is found in the ankles, elbows, and shoulders; this suggests a pattern of repetitive occupational overuse in the patient. Hand OA is a special case, as it is typically bilateral and preferentially affects the distal and proximal interphalangeal joints. **Heberden and Bouchard nodes** are osteophytes that may appear on the distal interphalangeal (DIP) and proximal interphalangeal (PIP) joints, respectively. Metacarpophalangeal (MCP) involvement, along with boutonnière and swan neck deformities, are more characteristic of rheumatoid arthritis.

OA is a clinical diagnosis, and further workup is often unnecessary. If the diagnosis is uncertain, plain radiographs can provide additional supporting evidence. Occasionally MRI is used to detect early pathological changes not seen on plain imaging. Laboratory testing

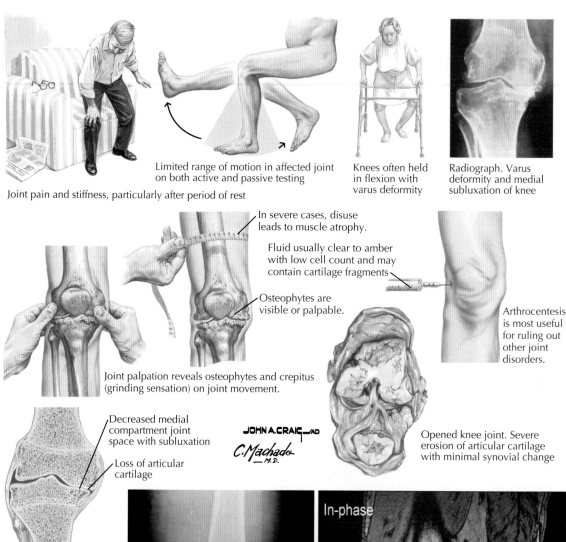

Joint pain and stiffness, particularly after period of rest

Limited range of motion in affected joint on both active and passive testing

Knees often held in flexion with varus deformity

Radiograph. Varus deformity and medial subluxation of knee

In severe cases, disuse leads to muscle atrophy.

Fluid usually clear to amber with low cell count and may contain cartilage fragments

Osteophytes are visible or palpable.

Arthrocentesis is most useful for ruling out other joint disorders.

Joint palpation reveals osteophytes and crepitus (grinding sensation) on joint movement.

Decreased medial compartment joint space with subluxation

Loss of articular cartilage

JOHN A. CRAIG—AD

C. Machado—M.D.

Opened knee joint. Severe erosion of articular cartilage with minimal synovial change

Knee with osteoarthritis exhibits varus deformity, medial subluxation, loss of articular cartilage, and osteophyte formation

Semiflexed AP view *(left)* and MRI *(right)* of left knee. In addition to joint space narrowing (cartilage loss) and osteophyte formation seen on routine x-ray, MRI provides scoring of a number of additional features such as subarticular bone marrow edema, synovitis, and meniscal integrity.
Courtesy Dr. Steven B. Abramson

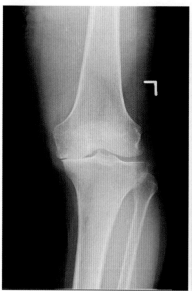

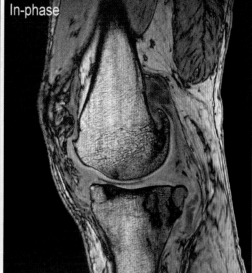

In-phase

FIG. 101.2 **Clinical Findings in Osteoarthritis.** *AP,* Anteroposterior.

and arthrocentesis are performed solely to rule out other causes of joint disease.

TREATMENT

The core interventions for all patients with OA are education, weight loss, and physical exercise. Even small amounts of weight loss can lead to noticeable improvements in symptoms of OA. Physical exercise should aim to improve muscle strength around the affected joints. There are currently no medications that have been proven to slow the progression of OA. Pain should be initially treated with acetaminophen or topical NSAIDs. Oral NSAIDs and opioids should be avoided due to their considerable side effects, especially in patients with renal, cardiovascular, and gastrointestinal comorbidities in the case of NSAIDs. Glucosamine and chondroitin are over-the-counter supplements, but they have not been shown to be beneficial. If pain persists, intraarticular steroid injections may provide short-term relief. Hyaluronic acid injections may also help alleviate symptoms but are expensive for patients.

If the patient has persistent severe pain or functional limitations despite these measures, surgery is an option. The most common joint replacement surgeries are for the knee and hip, but shoulder and elbow replacements also have excellent clinical outcomes. Arthroscopy has no role in OA unless ligament damage is also present.

CHAPTER 102

Rheumatoid Arthritis

ISABELLE AMIGUES

INTRODUCTION

Rheumatoid arthritis (RA) is a chronic inflammatory disease that principally affects the joints, causing symmetric pain, stiffness, swelling, and limitation in the motion and function of multiple joints. Although joints are the principal body parts affected by RA, inflammation can develop in other organs as well. If left untreated, or if it is unresponsive to therapy, inflammation and joint destruction lead to deformity, loss of physical function, and significant disability in addition to increased risk of mortality.

An estimated 1.3 million Americans with no clear racial predilection have RA. Average age of onset is 50 years, and it generally affects women twice as often as men.

PATHOPHYSIOLOGY AND RISK FACTORS

RA is best characterized as an immune-mediated inflammatory disease. Inflammatory **synovitis** is the initial lesion that is also responsible for joint destruction (Fig. 102.1). This synovitis is due to multiple mechanisms, including the cellular immune activation of T lymphocytes. Plasma cells produce antibodies (e.g., **rheumatoid factor [RF], anticitrullinated protein antibodies [ACPA]**) that participate in the production of immune complexes but are not required for the development of erosive RA. In addition to activated T lymphocytes, macrophages also migrate to the diseased synovium early in the disease and produce inflammatory cytokines and chemokines such as tumor necrosis factor (TNF), interleukin-1 (IL1), and IL6. The systemic and joint manifestations are thought to be the consequence of the release of these inflammatory mediators.

At the joint level, the inflamed hyperplastic synovial tissue called pannus develops many villous folds and releases inflammatory mediators that lead to excess synovial fluid production, as well as cartilage and bone destruction via the production and activation of matrix metalloproteinases and osteoclasts, respectively.

RA typically occurs in women between the ages of 40 and 60. Cigarette smoking is the most significant behavioral risk factor for the development of the disease and is especially associated in patients with autoantibodies for RA (RF or **anticyclic citrullinated protein [anti-CCP]**) or with a family history of autoimmune disease. Being overweight or obese has also been associated with an increased risk of developing RA.

PRESENTATION, EVALUATION, AND DIAGNOSIS

It is now widely accepted that a therapeutic window of opportunity exists for patients early in the course of RA when the disease is most amenable to treatment. Thus a patient with suspected RA should be rapidly evaluated, including a detailed history, physical exam, blood work, and joint x-ray to confirm the diagnosis so that appropriate treatment can be started to prevent further damage.

The typical manifestation of RA is that of a chronic (>6 weeks), fixed, symmetric inflammatory polyarthritis affecting the small joints of the wrists and hands with involvement of the metacarpophalangeal (MCP) and proximal interphalangeal (PIP), but not the distal interphalangeal, joints. The feet are also very often affected, particularly the metatarsophalangeal (MTP) joints. However, early RA may occasionally present as monoarthritis or oligoarthritis or in a palindromic manner, in which symptoms, including pain and joint swelling, appear and disappear.

The symptoms are usually insidious. The inflammatory nature of the arthritis is evidenced by the report of morning stiffness that lasts >30 minutes, swelling, and tender joints that respond at least partially to antiinflammatory medications. It is recommended that general practitioners do not delay the referral of these patients to rheumatologists when they have one or more of the following symptoms: positive hand and foot squeeze test (at the MCP and MTP joints), one or more swollen

Joint pathology

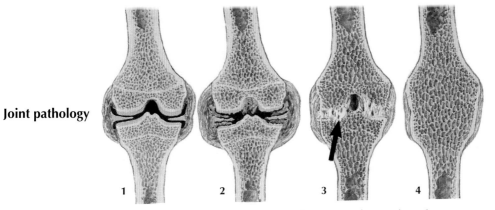

Progressive stages in joint pathology. 1. Acute inflammation of synovial membrane (synovitis) and beginning proliferative changes. 2. Progression of inflammation with pannus formation; beginning destruction of cartilage and mild osteoporosis. 3. Subsidence of inflammation; fibrous ankylosis *(arrow)*. 4. Bony ankylosis; advanced osteoporosis.

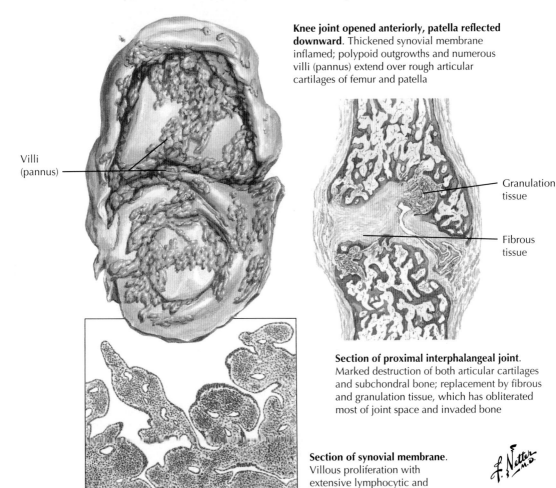

Knee joint opened anteriorly, patella reflected downward. Thickened synovial membrane inflamed; polypoid outgrowths and numerous villi (pannus) extend over rough articular cartilages of femur and patella

Villi (pannus)

Granulation tissue

Fibrous tissue

Section of proximal interphalangeal joint. Marked destruction of both articular cartilages and subchondral bone; replacement by fibrous and granulation tissue, which has obliterated most of joint space and invaded bone

Section of synovial membrane. Villous proliferation with extensive lymphocytic and plasma cells

FIG. 102.1 **Joint Pathology in Rheumatoid Arthritis.**

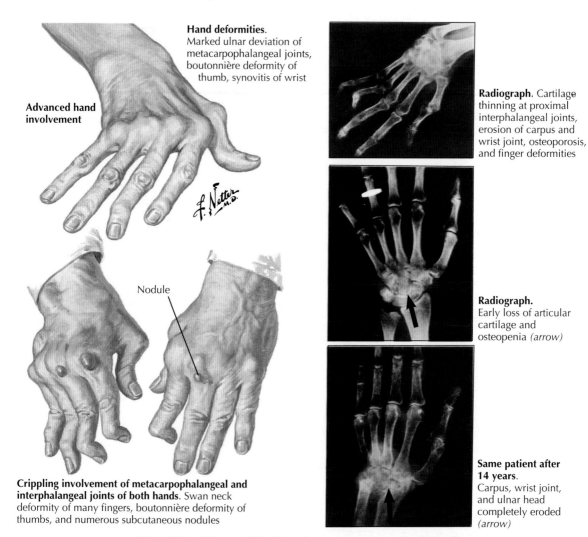

Hand deformities. Marked ulnar deviation of metacarpophalangeal joints, boutonnière deformity of thumb, synovitis of wrist

Advanced hand involvement

Radiograph. Cartilage thinning at proximal interphalangeal joints, erosion of carpus and wrist joint, osteoporosis, and finger deformities

Nodule

Radiograph. Early loss of articular cartilage and osteopenia *(arrow)*

Same patient after 14 years. Carpus, wrist joint, and ulnar head completely eroded *(arrow)*

Crippling involvement of metacarpophalangeal and interphalangeal joints of both hands. Swan neck deformity of many fingers, boutonnière deformity of thumbs, and numerous subcutaneous nodules

FIG. 102.2 **Advanced Hand Involvement in Rheumatoid Arthritis.**

joints, or morning stiffness that lasts ≥30 minutes. When RA has been progressing for months or years, there may also be joint deformities and restriction in the range of motion (Fig. 102.2). The examiner should also carefully look for extraarticular manifestations of RA (Fig. 102.3), which may require a higher level of immunosuppression.

Once suspected, laboratory tests may also confirm the inflammatory nature of the disease with elevation of the C-reactive protein (CRP) and erythrocyte sedimentation rate (ESR) and the presence of anemia of chronic inflammation on a complete blood count. A comprehensive metabolic panel as well as hepatitis B and C serology are needed as a baseline and to rule out any contraindication to using **disease-modifying antirheumatic drugs (DMARDs).**

In excluding other etiologies such as infection or crystalline arthritis, **arthrocentesis** should be performed to evaluate the synovial fluid for bacteria, crystal evaluation, and cell count. The synovial fluid of patients with RA is inflammatory (with cell counts usually of 2000 to 50,000) and is sterile and without crystals. X-rays are often normal in early RA but are important to assess for erosion, subluxations, and deformities. Hand and foot x-rays are often the earliest to show signs of joint damage and are useful as a baseline.

The evaluation of **autoantibodies** is useful for both diagnosis and prognosis. About 60% of patients are positive for RF. The specificity and sensitivity of this test is about 75%. ACPA can be found in up to 40% seronegative for RF and are much more specific for RA

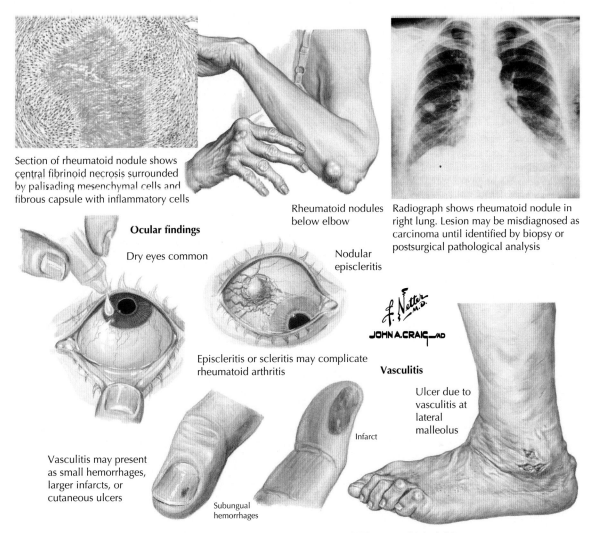

Section of rheumatoid nodule shows central fibrinoid necrosis surrounded by palisading mesenchymal cells and fibrous capsule with inflammatory cells

Rheumatoid nodules below elbow

Radiograph shows rheumatoid nodule in right lung. Lesion may be misdiagnosed as carcinoma until identified by biopsy or postsurgical pathological analysis

Ocular findings

Dry eyes common

Nodular episcleritis

Episcleritis or scleritis may complicate rheumatoid arthritis

Vasculitis

Ulcer due to vasculitis at lateral malleolus

Infarct

Vasculitis may present as small hemorrhages, larger infarcts, or cutaneous ulcers

Subungual hemorrhages

FIG. 102.3 **Extraarticular Manifestations of Rheumatoid Arthritis.**

(95%). Their presence is also associated with a higher risk of developing erosion. Antinuclear antibodies (ANA) also can be present (15%–20%), and are at times associated with anti-SSA and anti-SSB, which can be suggestive of a diagnosis of secondary Sjögren syndrome. The natural history and presence of erosion help in confirming the RA diagnosis.

TREATMENT

In the last decade, we have significantly increased our knowledge of the underlying pathophysiology of RA, and many treatment options have been developed.

Treating patients appropriately as early as possible is key to preventing further damage.

The mainstay of treatment in RA consists of control of inflammation with DMARDs to prevent damage to the joints and the other organs. A treat-to-target strategy is the most accepted treatment approach for patients with RA, the goal being to reach the target of remission or low disease activity and thus to obtain the best outcome for patient.

The American College of Rheumatology has created guidelines for the treatment of RA. In patients with a new diagnosis of RA and in whom the disease activity is low or moderate, methotrexate monotherapy with folic acid supplementation is usually recommended unless contraindicated (namely for chronic liver or pulmonary diseases). Other nonbiological DMARDs (leflunomide, hydroxychloroquine, sulfasalazine) can be used as alternatives. In patients with persistent disease activity despite 3 months of an appropriate dose of methotrexate (up to 25 mg weekly), the addition of two more DMARDs to achieve triple therapy (methotrexate, hydroxychloroquine, sulfazalazine) or the addition of a biological agent (generally a **TNF inhibitor** such as etanercept, infliximab, or adalimumab) to the nonbiological DMARD is recommended. Small doses of prednisone (5–15 mg daily) can be used for a limited period of time at the beginning of the disease or during flares of the disease.

Prior to starting any biological agent, patients should be evaluated for latent tuberculosis using a **purified protein derivative (PPD)** or **interferon-γ release assay (IGRA)** and, if it is positive, should be treated (the biological can safely be started after a month of treatment). In addition to the recommended vaccinations for the general population, including the yearly influenza vaccine, it is recommended to vaccinate against pneumococcus and herpes zoster. These vaccinations are particularly important before the use of a biological agent, as the risk of severe infection is heightened on these agents. Once started, live vaccinations are contraindicated in patients on biologicals.

Patients should be followed regularly, usually every 3 to 4 months once the disease is under control, to evaluate their tolerance to treatment (complete blood count, comprehensive metabolic panel) and to evaluate their response to treatment. Therapy should be adjusted if disease control is not adequate.

CHAPTER 103

Septic Arthritis and Bursitis

PRANAY SINHA

INTRODUCTION

Septic arthritis is a critical diagnosis to consider among patients presenting with monoarticular pain and swelling. If left untreated, the infection can rapidly damage cartilage in the affected joint and injure the subchondral bone. Many patients go on to develop permanent arthritis, joint instability, or deformity. The mortality ranges from 7% to 15% but can be as high as 30% to 50% in patients with polyarticular involvement (seen in ~10%–20% of cases) or additional comorbidities. To prevent adverse outcomes, rapid evaluation of the synovial fluid, initiation of antibiotics, and evacuation of the joint effusion is necessary. Septic bursitis is a distinct and less severe entity that can mimic septic arthritis. This chapter will cover infections within native joints, not prosthetic joint infections seen following joint replacement.

PATHOPHYSIOLOGY

Pathogens enter the joint space hematogenously, by direct inoculation, or through contiguous spread from an adjacent focus of infection. Bacteria adhere to adhesive proteins on the synovial membrane and begin replicating, while the host immune system responds by initiating an inflammatory cascade. Leukocytes invade the joint space and release inflammatory cytokines, leading to purulent synovial fluid and the symptoms described later.

Bacterial enzymes damage cartilage and decrease the viscosity, and hence the lubricative property, of the synovial fluid. The body's inflammatory response, however, causes much of the damage to the joint. The inflammatory response corrodes cartilage, inhibits cartilage proliferation, and damages subchondral bone. The inflammatory exudate also increases the intraarticular pressure and decreases blood flow to the joint, causing ischemic damage to the synovium. Thus a combination of inflammation, friction, and vascular compromise can rapidly damage intraarticular cartilage within days if left untreated (Fig. 103.1).

Septic bursitis usually follows the trauma of a superficial bursa. Deeper bursae can be affected through hematogenous seeding, but this is rare. The degree of inflammation in infected bursae is significantly lower than that in infected joints.

RISK FACTORS

Hematogenous seeding occurs in patients with bacteremia, endocarditis, or intravenous (IV) drug use. Direct inoculation of pathogens occurs through trauma, bites, joint injections, and joint surgery. Contiguous spread can occur from nearby bones or soft tissue infections. Sexual activity increases risk for gonococcal arthritis. Immunosuppression due to diabetes mellitus, HIV disease, complement deficiency, or use of immunosuppressive medications has been linked to septic arthritis. Abnormal joint architecture due to preexisting rheumatoid arthritis (RA) and osteoarthritis also increases the risk of infection.

PRESENTATION, EVALUATION, AND DIAGNOSIS

Septic arthritis can be acute or chronic. A large majority of cases are monoarticular, but ~10% to 20% of cases are oligoarticular. The knee is the most common site of infection followed by the hip. Other commonly affected joints include shoulders, wrists, and elbows. Septic bursitis is largely seen in the olecranon bursa and the prepatellar bursa.

Moderate to severe pain around the joint, decreased range of motion, and **joint effusion** are common symptoms of septic arthritis (Fig. 103.2). Patients with infected knees and hips may be unable to bear weight on the affected leg due to pain. Fever is common, but not always present. Acute septic arthritis from a bacterial process presents with symptoms over days to 1 to 2 weeks. Chronic septic arthritis from tuberculosis (TB) or nonbacterial organisms tends to be more indolent and presents insidiously over longer periods with a lower intensity of symptoms. The impairment of range of motion and pain is typically lower in septic bursitis. In elbow bursitis, flexion of the elbow increases bursal

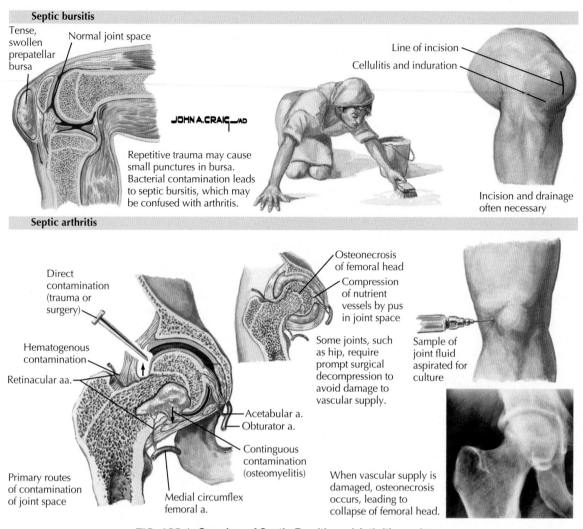

FIG. 103.1 **Overview of Septic Bursitis and Arthritis.** *a.,* Artery.

pressure and is more painful. Extension increases synovial pressures and exacerbates pain in septic arthritis of the elbow. Severe cases of bursitis can be difficult to distinguish clinically from septic arthritis.

Staphylococcus aureus is the most common cause of septic arthritis, followed by *Streptococcus* species, which often produce polyarticular infections. Gram-negative infections are more common in neonates, the elderly, the immunocompromised, and IV drug users. Overall, gram-negative septic arthritis represents 5% to 20% of cases. The incidence of gonococcal arthritis has decreased in recent years.

Peripheral leukocyte count, erythrocyte sedimentation rate, and C-reactive protein levels may be elevated in

patients with septic arthritis and bursitis, but these are not specific markers. Synovial fluid or bursal fluid Gram stain, culture, cell count, and crystal analysis are necessary for diagnosis. Fungi and mycobacterial cultures should also be collected for patients with chronic arthritis or bursitis, although if suspicion is high, synovial biopsy should be considered as it is far more sensitive.

Bacterial arthritis typically causes a synovial leukocyte count >50,000 cells/µL with a neutrophilic predominance, but lower levels of leukocytosis do not preclude this diagnosis. Mycobacterial and fungal infections, in particular, produce leukocyte counts <50,000 cells/µL in the synovial fluid without neutrophilic predominance. Conversely, crystal arthropathies can also produce synovial leukocyte counts >50,000 cells/μL. In septic bursitis, the aspirated fluid usually has >1000 cells/μL, but the cell count is significantly lower than that in septic arthritis. Synovial fluid cultures are positive in ~90% of patients with nongonococcal bacterial arthritis.

Blood cultures have a high yield and should be drawn before initiation of antimicrobial therapy. If there is a contiguous wound, it should be cultured as well. If gonococcal arthritis is suspected, mucosal cultures and nucleic acid amplification testing for *Neisseria gonorrhoeae* should be obtained on specimens taken from mouth, rectum, and genitals (see Chapter 121 for further details).

Patients with risk factors for tick bites or those living in endemic regions should be tested for Lyme disease via serology.

Plain film radiography of the affected joints should be performed to establish a baseline (Fig. 103.3). Foreign bodies, periarticular osteoporosis, loss of joint space, and subchondral bone destruction can be assessed through plain radiography. CT and MRI have higher sensitivities for adjacent osteomyelitis and are also used to assess for infection in deep bursae.

The differential diagnosis for septic arthritis and bursitis is large. Viral arthritides due to parvovirus B19, Chikungunya virus, rubella, hepatitis B virus, hepatitis C virus, and various α-viruses can present acutely, but they do not generate purulent synovial fluid like bacteria or fungi. Crystal arthritides, such as gout and pseudogout, can mimic septic arthritis and bursitis, and they are diagnosed through microscopic visualization of crystals in the synovial fluid. Occasionally, patients can present with concomitant crystal and septic arthritis. Inflammatory conditions such as reactive arthritis, RA, systemic lupus erythematosus, Still disease, and systemic vasculitides also produce polyarticular arthritis.

TREATMENT

Timely joint drainage coupled with early and appropriate antibiotics can decrease the morbidity and mortality of septic arthritis. Evacuation of pus from the affected joints should be done emergently. This can be done

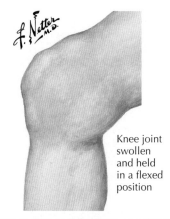

Knee joint swollen and held in a flexed position

FIG. 103.2 **Physical Findings of a Septic Knee.**

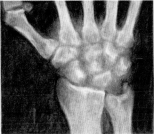

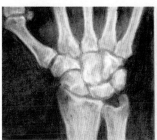

Rapid progression of wrist involvement within 4 weeks, from almost normal *(left)* to advanced destruction of articular cartilages and severe osteoporosis *(right)*

Biopsy specimen of synovial membrane shows infiltration with polymorphonuclear cells, lymphocytes, and mononuclear cells, and tissue proliferation with neovascularization

FIG. 103.3 **Radiography and Biopsy of Septic Arthritis.**

with needle aspiration, **arthroscopy,** or arthrotomy. The evacuated fluid is sent for culture and Gram stain, which help guide antibiotic therapy.

Deep joints such as hips require emergent arthrotomy to prevent necrotic damage of the femoral head. Arthroscopy is usually preferred for drainage of knees and shoulders. Any septic arthritis should be managed with orthopedic guidance.

Antibiotics should be initiated rapidly after cultures are collected and should be adjusted based on culture data at the earliest. Bactericidal agents are necessary in septic arthritis and should be delivered intravenously. Duration of therapy depends on the causative pathogen.

S. aureus should be covered empirically; vancomycin is widely used for methicillin-resistant *S. aureus* (MRSA) coverage. If the incidence of MRSA is <10%, nafcillin or cefazolin can be considered. Patients with immunocompromising conditions, such as diabetes or RA, are at risk for gram-negative infection and should receive coverage with a third-generation cephalosporin. Ongoing or historic infections with extended-spectrum β-lactamase–producing organisms should prompt use of carbapenems for gram-negative coverage. IV drug use or concern for pseudomonal infections should prompt consideration of antipseudomonal antibiotics (e.g., ceftazidime, piperacillin-tazobactam).

Lyme arthritis is treated with doxycycline, while gonococcal arthritis is treated with ceftriaxone. Tuberculous arthritis is treated with the same protocol as pulmonary TB. Treatment for fungal arthritis is targeted toward the causative organism.

Septic bursitis should be treated with daily aspiration of the bursa until the aspirate becomes sterile as well as antibiotics. Bursa fluid cultures determine antibiotic therapy. A course of 14 to 21 days is usually appropriate. In severe cases, bursectomy may be necessary.

CHAPTER 104

Gout

PAULINE B. YI

INTRODUCTION

Gout is a type of **inflammatory arthropathy** that affects >8 million Americans and results from the precipitation of **monosodium urate crystals** in joints. It is often associated with **hyperuricemia** and conditions such as insulin resistance, hypertension, and chronic kidney disease (CKD). The diagnosis is typically confirmed upon visualization of monosodium urate crystals in synovial fluid. Patients with multiple, recurrent episodes may develop chronic tophaceous gout.

Pseudogout, or calcium pyrophosphate dihydrate (CPPD) disease, is another type of inflammatory arthropathy that is often confused with gout. It results from the formation of CPPD crystals in the cartilage. These crystals are released from the joint into the synovial fluid and can cause a similar presentation of an acute gout flare. The rhomboid crystals present as positively birefringent under polarized light. The most common site of CPPD is the knee and the most common setting is that of osteoarthritis. Other, less common causes of CPPD are hypothyroidism, hyperparathyroidism, hypomagnesemia, hypercalcemia, and/or hemochromatosis. For acute pseudogout, treatment includes NSAIDS, colchicine, intraarticular steroids, and/or systemic corticosteroids.

PATHOPHYSIOLOGY

Uric acid is the final product of purine metabolism and in physiological conditions exists as urate. **Xanthine oxidase** is the terminal enzyme in uric acid synthesis; however, humans lack the uricase enzyme that converts urate into the more soluble allantoin (Fig. 104.1). When urate concentration in serum increases, and remains increased over a period of time, it is deposited in the joint. Crystallization of monosodium urate crystals can then trigger an immune response. Cytokines and neutrophils flood the area, propagating the immune response; this inflammatory activation is responsible for the symptoms of acute gout.

Urate is cleared by the kidneys, where it freely enters the glomerular filtrate and is then both secreted and reabsorbed in the proximal tubules. The most common risk factor for gout is underexcretion of urate by the kidneys. Although high levels of uric acid are needed for crystal precipitation and deposition, hyperuricemia by itself affects up to 20% of the adult population and may be asymptomatic. Measuring serum uric acid concentration therefore is not a useful screening tool for gout in the absence of typical signs and symptoms.

PRESENTATION

Gout is diagnosed clinically with the sudden development of arthritis with classical features of swelling and redness. A classic presentation is **podagra,** in which the first metatarsophalangeal joint becomes painful, red, and swollen over 12 to 24 hours. First episodes are typically monoarticular, whereas recurrent episodes with progressively more urate burden deposited in the joints can be either monoarticular or polyarticular. Signs of systemic inflammation are common, including fever, leukocytosis, and elevated **inflammatory markers** (Fig. 104.2). Soft tissue inflammation can occur and often is confused with cellulitis. Of note, serum urate levels can be low during acute episodes, as a gout attack can be triggered by anything that acutely raises or lowers serum uric acid levels. Because of this variability, the serum urate level should be assessed after acute episodes. Purine-rich foods such as alcohol, red meat, shellfish, and foods with high fructose content increase the risk of gout flares. A number of drugs, including diuretics such as furosemide and thiazides, low-dose aspirin, and cyclosporine, also increase uric acid.

Poorly controlled gout and recurrent flares put patients at risk for chronic gouty arthropathy. A **tophus** (or tophi, if multiple) is a collection of monosodium crystals in a matrix of lipids and glycoproteins and may form in chronically affected joints. Tophaceous gout can lead to

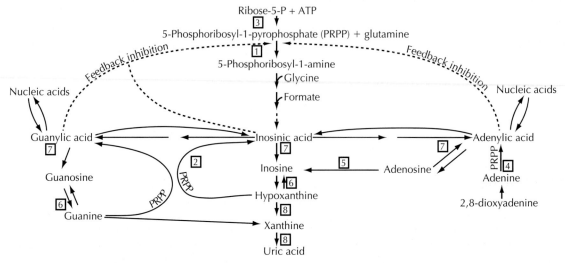

FIG. 104.1 **Purine Elimination Biochemical Pathway.** *ATP*, Adenosine triphosphate.

bony erosions and disfiguring joint damage, as well as skin ulcerations and infections (Fig. 104.3).

DIAGNOSIS

Gout should be suspected in any acute monoarticular joint swelling and clinically can be confused with septic arthritis. Diagnosing gout requires **arthrocentesis** of the affected joint with synovial fluid analysis. The synovial fluid can be examined with microscopy; identification of needle-shaped monosodium crystals with negative birefringence on polarized light microscopy clinches the diagnosis of gout. Extracellular crystals are more noted in chronic gout, whereas intracellular crystals are seen more typically in acute episodes. The synovial fluid is inflammatory, characterized by 2000 to 50,000 nucleated cells/µL with a neutrophilic (polymorphonuclear [PMN]) predominance. Gram stain and cultures are warranted to exclude infection.

Gout can also be diagnosed clinically using the American College of Rheumatology (ACR) classification criteria for gout (Box 104.1). Radiographs can be used to identify classic gouty erosions such as punched-out lesions, described as overhanging edges where bones have been affected by tophaceous deposits.

TREATMENT

Acute gout attacks should be treated within the first 24 hours of symptom onset. Treatment selection depends on a patient's comorbidities and ability to take oral medications. NSAIDs such as naproxen and indomethacin are useful for mild to moderate or monoarticular episodes, but their use may be limited by renal, cardiovascular, and gastrointestinal comorbidities. Colchicine also may be used if given early enough, and some patients can use colchicine to abort gout episodes at the earliest symptoms. Glucocorticoids remain an effective option for counteracting the inflammatory response typical of gout.

For monoarticular attacks, intraarticular steroid injections can be quickly effective at relieving symptoms, though physicians must be wary of possible septic arthritis (either on its own or concurrent with gouty arthritis). Oral glucocorticoids are helpful if patients have polyarticular gout or cannot readily receive an intraarticular injection. Interleukin-1 (IL-1) has been identified as a major cytokine for acute gout flares. IL-1 inhibitors such as anakinra, canakinumab, or rilonacept are being studied as potential agents in both treatments of ongoing flares and prophylaxis to prevent acute flares during initiation of urate-lowering therapies.

Following resolution of an acute gout attack, patients should be considered for urate-lowering therapy. The ACR specifies that urate-lowering therapies should be initiated in the following patients:

- Those with more than two acute gout attacks within a 1-year period
- Clinical or radiographical signs of chronic gout arthropathy
- Presence of tophi
- Stage II or higher CKD
- History of urate kidney stones

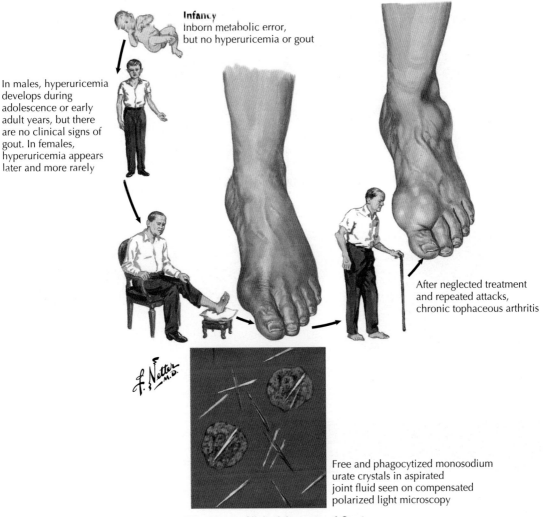

Infancy
Inborn metabolic error, but no hyperuricemia or gout

In males, hyperuricemia develops during adolescence or early adult years, but there are no clinical signs of gout. In females, hyperuricemia appears later and more rarely

After neglected treatment and repeated attacks, chronic tophaceous arthritis

Free and phagocytized monosodium urate crystals in aspirated joint fluid seen on compensated polarized light microscopy

FIG. 104.2 **Clinical Aspects of Gout.**

Urate-lowering therapy is usually started after the resolution of an episode. Target serum urate is <6 mg/dL in patients without tophi and <5 mg/dL in patients with tophi. Urate-lowering therapy usually acts by either decreasing the creation of uric acid like in xanthine oxidase inhibitors or facilitating its excretion in the urine.

In patients with moderate or severe CKD, allopurinol, a xanthine oxidase inhibitor, is the first-line drug of choice. It lowers the production of uric acid. Allopurinol should be avoided in patients with an increased likelihood of HLA-B5801 positivity because of increased risk of cutaneous adverse reactions. High-risk populations such as Han Chinese, Thai, and Koreans with CKD should also be monitored carefully while on allopurinol, Febuxostat,

another xanthine oxidase inhibitor, is also an alternative for patients who do not reach the target uric acid goal on maximal doses of allopurinol, patients who have a higher risk of adverse effects, or patients with creatinine clearance as low as 15 mL/min.

Probenecid is a uricosuric agent that blocks renal acid reabsorption. It can be used as adjunct therapy in patients who do not have limitations to uricosuric treatment such as a CKD or uric acid overproduction. Monotherapy with probenecid can be considered to treat gout, but in the United States it is not considered first-line therapy as the majority of patients underexcrete uric acid. Probenecid increases the risk of kidney stones and is therefore contraindicated in patients who have a history

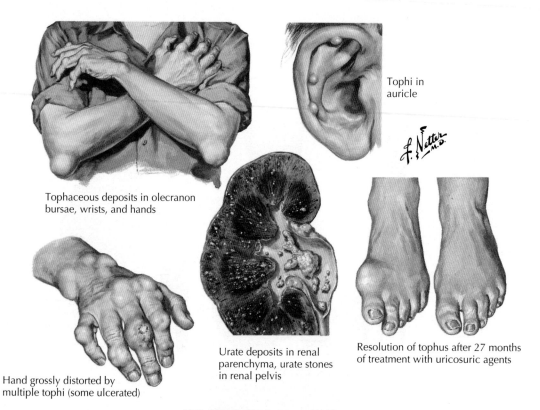

Tophi in
auricle

Tophaceous deposits in olecranon
bursae, wrists, and hands

Hand grossly distorted by
multiple tophi (some ulcerated)

Urate deposits in renal
parenchyma, urate stones
in renal pelvis

Resolution of tophus after 27 months
of treatment with uricosuric agents

FIG. 104.3 **Tophaceous Gout.**

BOX 104.1
American College of Rheumatology Criteria for Acute Arthritis in Primary Gout

Must meet six of the following findings, even in the absence of crystal identification:

• More than one episode of acute arthritis
• Maximum inflammation within 1 day
• Monoarthritis episode
• First metatarsophalangeal joint painful or swollen
• Unilateral first metatarsophalangeal joint episode
• Unilateral tarsal joint episode
• Presence of tophi
• Hyperuricemia
• Asymmetric joint swelling on examination
• Subcortical cysts without erosions on radiograph
• Monosodium urate monohydrate microcrystals in joint fluid
• Negative joint fluid culture during episode

Reused with permission from Wallace SL, Robinson H, Masi AT, et al: Preliminary criteria for the classification of the acute arthritis of primary gout, *Arthritis Rheum* 20(3):895–900, 1977.

of urate nephrolithiasis. Other uricosuric agents, such as losartan or fenofibrate, may be useful in patients with hypertension or hyperlipidemia already on allopurinol.

For patients with advanced gout refractory to treatment or with significant tophaceous disease, pegloticase or rasburicase can be used. **Uricase** is the enzyme that converts urate into allantoin, a more soluble purine degradation product. Due to accumulated mutations, however, this enzyme is not active in humans. Pegloticase is a pegylated urase that has been shown to be effective in 40% of patients who have not responded to conventional urate-lowering therapy. This drug must be monitored carefully when administered because of the high risk of anaphylaxis. Treatment with this drug should also be discontinued if the urate levels start to increase, which can signify antibodies to the drug that develop in a large majority of the patients receiving it. High titers of the antibodies were associated with decreased effectiveness of the drug and higher risks of adverse infusion reactions. Other urate-lowering medications should not be used while on pegloticase as they may mask early increases in serum urate levels, which need to be monitored very closely. Rasburicase is nonpegylated uricase used in the prevention of acute uric acid nephropathy in tumor lysis syndrome, and has not been studied closely as an agent in the treatment of gout.

As changes in the serum uric acid level can lead to gout attacks, colchicine or NSAIDs can be coadministered during initiation of urate-lowering therapy as prophylaxis.

The ACR recommends that prophylaxis medications be continued 3 months after achieving serum target without tophi or 6 months with the presence of tophi. Patients on urate-lowering therapies should continue medications through the acute episode as changes in serum urate can worsen a gout flare.

CHAPTER 105

Spondyloarthridities

AMIT LAKHANPAL

INTRODUCTION

Spondyloarthridities (SpA) are characterized by inflammatory joint-related symptoms, classically involving the sacroiliac (SI) joints, the spine, as well as tendon-insertion sites (enthesis arthritis) and certain extraarticular manifestations. Generally there are no associated serological tests aside from elevation in inflammatory markers. In Caucasian populations, they are frequently associated with the class I gene **HLA-B27**. Their variable and nonspecific presentation often delays diagnosis until well after the onset of symptoms. Overall prevalence of SpA ranges from 0.1% to 1.4%, correlated with the baseline incidence of the HLA-B27 allele. In the United States, the prevalence is ~1%, with the most commonly observed being **ankylosing spondyloarthropathy (AS)** and **psoriatic arthritis (PsA)**. Novel treatments have improved our ability to limit the progression of these diseases.

CLASSIFICATION

Although diagnosis of the SpA is clinical, a variety of classification schemes have been used for screening and research purposes. The most widely used is the Assessment of SpondyloArthritis International Society (ASAS) classification based on clinical, imaging, and lab data. A variety of sensitivity and specificity data for the system have been reported in the literature, both generally in the 70% to 80% range, by comparing criteria fulfillment with expert clinical diagnoses.

Based on the specific manifestations, SpA can be one of these recognized disease entities:
- AS
- PsA
- **Enteropathic SpA (EnA)**
- **Reactive arthritis (ReA)**
- **Undifferentiated SpA (uSpA)**

PATHOPHYSIOLOGY

The pathophysiology of SpA is incompletely understood and likely varies among clinical entities. A combination of genetic predisposition and environmental factors plays a role in disease pathogenesis. Whatever the upstream molecular mechanisms, disease in the spine progresses from inflammation to syndesmophyte and results in erosion and destruction in the joints.

The HLA complex, the human form of the major histocompatibility complex (MHC), presents peptide fragments, including pathological antigens, to the adaptive immune system. Approximately one-fifth of the heritability of SpA is related to variation in the HLA region. HLA-B alleles, governing part of the MHC1 complex, which generally presents intracellular contents to cytotoxic T cells, have been associated with SpA. Most prominently, HLA-B27 is associated with all SpA and most strongly AS. However, despite the much higher frequency of HLA-B27 in SpA patients than in controls, <5% of HLA-B27 individuals develop disease, making it useful to establish a diagnosis but not as a screening test.

The mechanism by which specific HLA alleles affect pathogenesis in SpA remains unclear. Early theories posited that those alleles present bacterial peptides structurally similar to self-antigens, stimulating an antiself T-cell response. However, T-cell–negative animal models can still develop disease. Alternatively, certain HLA allele products may be more prone to misfolding and accumulation leading to interleukin-23 (IL-23) release.

Genome-wide association studies have also obtained a number of non-HLA associations, including several members of the IL-23/Th17 axis—this may hint at a molecular mechanism of disease, as IL-23 induces IL-17 production, which itself activates synoviocytes, chondrocytes, and osteoclasts. Variation in NOD2 has been linked specifically to intestinal involvement in SpA patients.

Given the frequency of bowel-related symptoms and the influence of enteric infection in SpA, the **gut microbiome** is an area of considerable interest. Microbial metabolites may directly prime the host immune system to generate pathological responses or alter intestinal permeability to microbial antigens that might activate an immunological response. The fecal microbiomes of PsA

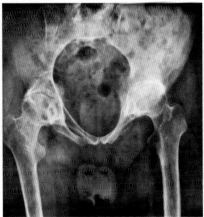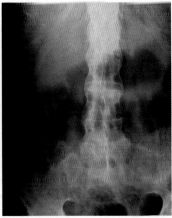

Radiograph shows complete bony ankylosis of both sacroiliac joints in late stage of disease

"Bamboo spine." Bony ankylosis of joints of lumbar spine. Ossification exaggerates bulges of intervertebral disks

FIG. 105.1 **Plain Radiography of Ankylosing Spondyloarthropathy.**

and AS patients are distinct from healthy controls, and while differences in the gut immune profiles of animal models make direct translation to humans difficult, the prospect of modulating the microbiome to treat disease remains an area of interest.

PRESENTATION, EVALUATION, AND DIAGNOSIS

Symptoms often manifest in younger patients, and history should extend to the juvenile years. The male-to-female ratio, previously thought skewed toward males, is closer to 1:1, but some sex-based differences remain. Male patients tend to be younger with less disease activity and more often axial disease. Female patients tend to be older with more severe disease, and display more frequent manifestations of dactylitis and enthesitis with a higher number of affected joints overall.

Clinical features include some combination of inflammatory back pain, dactylitis, asymmetric oligoarthritis, and enthesitis. Nonmusculoskeletal complaints commonly involve the eyes, skin, and bowel. Crucial in any SpA is determining whether the pain is inflammatory in nature, guided by five criteria:

- Onset before age 40
- Insidious onset with over several months' duration
- Pain at night with improvement after awakening
- Improvement with exercise
- No improvement with rest

Ankylosing Spondyloarthropathy (AS)

AS is the most common spondyloarthritis. Its cardinal manifestation is inflammatory lower back pain, often reported as pain in the buttocks alternating between each side, which can be mistaken for other etiologies given the typical age of onset between age 15 and 40 years. One-quarter of cases can have pain in the hips or shoulders, with the upper extremities otherwise almost always spared. Examination maneuvers to quantify axial mobility can be used to monitor disease in established cases, but baseline population variation is too wide to serve as a useful diagnostic criterion. Workup includes radiographical assessment of the SI joint and spine to look for **sacroiliitis** (Fig. 105.1), although the disease may be advanced by the time findings are apparent on plain radiography, giving rise to the concept of non-radiographic AS; MRI of the SI joints may be of help in suspected cases, but may also lead to false positive results. Laboratory testing is of limited utility, except to exclude other entities, to assess inflammatory markers, and to check for the presence of HLA-B27.

Nonaxial manifestations are common in AS, particularly acute **anterior uveitis** (30%–40%), psoriasis (10%), and inflammatory bowel disease (IBD, 5%–10%). Anterior uveitis manifests as abrupt unilateral circumlimbal hyperemia, pain, and visual changes. Attacks may occur repeatedly without predilection for one eye over the other and are the one aspect of AS that is responsive to steroid treatment. Psoriatic skin lesions may indicate

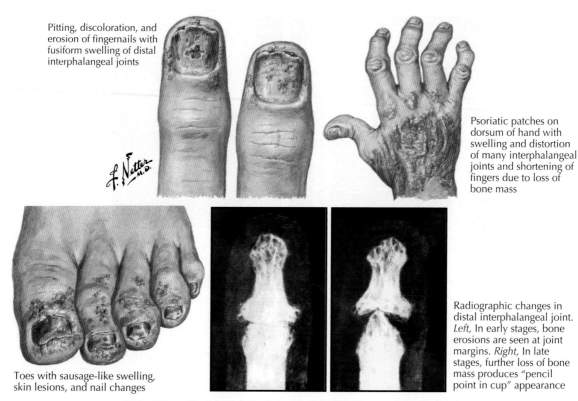

Pitting, discoloration, and erosion of fingernails with fusiform swelling of distal interphalangeal joints

Psoriatic patches on dorsum of hand with swelling and distortion of many interphalangeal joints and shortening of fingers due to loss of bone mass

Radiographic changes in distal interphalangeal joint. *Left,* In early stages, bone erosions are seen at joint margins. *Right,* In late stages, further loss of bone mass produces "pencil point in cup" appearance

Toes with sausage-like swelling, skin lesions, and nail changes

FIG. 105.2 Clinical and Radiographic Findings in Psoriatic Arthritis.

PsA but can occur with AS. Similarly, patients with AS have a higher incidence of bowel inflammation than controls, but clinically apparent IBD should prompt consideration of enteropathic SpA.

Psoriatic Arthritis (PsA)

Patients with personal or family history of psoriasis and either oligoarthritis or distal polyarthritis should raise suspicion of PsA. Although the diagnosis is difficult and generally requires consultation with a rheumatologist, the CASPAR classification criteria, which include the features described in this section, can aid in early recognition of potential disease. History should include questions on smoking, trauma, and infection history. Retrospective studies have noted PsA in ~30% of patients with psoriasis, of whom ~10% also developed axial disease. Physical examination should take careful note of the patient's nails, with 90% of PsA demonstrating either pitting across multiple nails or onycholysis. The other examination finding commonly associated with PsA is dactylitis, or swelling and erythema of the entire finger, present in half of PsA patients. Enthesitis is more common than

true arthritis. Imaging of affected joints may reveal periarticular erosions or new bone formation, bearing a characteristic pencil-in-cup appearance (Fig. 105.2). Laboratory findings are limited, though elevated acute phase reactants may portend a more severe course.

Enteropathic SpA (EnA)

Manifestations of SpA coincident with chronic bloody diarrhea, abdominal pain, and weight loss should prompt concern for EnA. The symptomatic profiles tend to fall into two categories: (1) an oligoarticular, asymmetric large-joint arthritis where the articular symptoms correlate with the IBD severity, or (2) a polyarticular small-joint arthritis that is less correlated with IBD symptoms (see Chapter 134).

Reactive Arthritis (ReA)

ReA should be suspected in a patient with recent infection with an intracellular organism who develops either articular or extraarticular features of SpA, especially dactylitis in the feet. Classically, the disease is a triad of lower extremity asymmetric oligoarthritis/enthesitis,

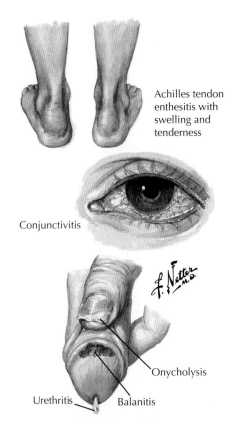

Achilles tendon enthesitis with swelling and tenderness

Conjunctivitis

Onycholysis

Urethritis   Balanitis

FIG. 105.3 **The Classic Triad of Reactive Arthritis.**

conjunctivitis, and urethritis, although all three rarely occur together (Fig. 105.3). Infections classically associated with ReA are urogenital (e.g., *Chlamydia*) or enteric (e.g., *Salmonella, Shigella, Yersinia, Campylobacter*). Arthritic symptoms generally occur in the 1 to 6 weeks after the acute infectious process, and actively inflamed joints may require arthrocentesis to rule out septic arthritis.

Undifferentiated SpA (uSpA)

Patients who present with SpA symptoms but do not fall into any of the established diagnoses are classified as uSpA. Data regarding the progression from uSpA to the defined forms are limited, although there is often enough symptomatic burden in uSpA to warrant its treatment.

MANAGEMENT

Physical therapy and exercise, to the extent that is tolerable, is common to the management of all SpA. As with most inflammatory diseases, pharmacological treatment for SpA centers on downregulating the inflammatory response with agents including NSAIDs, steroids, disease-modifying antirheumatic drugs (DMARDs), and specific biological agents. **Tumor necrosis factor (TNF) inhibitors** have been extremely effective in ~60% of cases resistant to NSAID treatment in AS, and include infliximab, etanercept, adalimumab, golimumab, and certolizumab. More recently, treatments targeting the IL-17/IL-23 axis either directly (secukinumab, ustekinumab) or indirectly (tofacitinib) have shown promise as well.

For peripheral joint symptoms of SpA, first-line treatment with NSAIDs is often effective. Glucocorticoid therapy can bring relief to joint symptoms but should be avoided in patients with psoriasis as it can trigger severe rebound flares when tapered. Intraarticular glucocorticoid injections may improve symptoms if the number of affected joints is low. Other DMARDs, such as sulfasalazine, methotrexate, or leflunomide, generally should be attempted before biological agents. TNF inhibitors are commonly used, although after discontinuation there is a high rate of relapse within months. Axial disease is managed similarly, although therapy generally progresses from NSAID to biological in light of less effective results with steroids or DMARDs.

In ReA, resolution of acute symptoms can be hastened by NSAID treatment but may evolve into a chronic condition requiring treatment with DMARD or biological. For ReA induced by gastrointestinal (GI) infection, sulfasalazine is preferred. Methotrexate and etanercept are effective for persistent joint issues in chronic disease.

In EnA, NSAID and COX-2 inhibitors should be used with caution given the risk of worsened bowel disease. Among DMARDs sulfasalazine is preferred, but if resistant, TNF inhibitors with the exception of etanercept can be effective.

CHAPTER 106

Systemic Lupus Erythematosus

ALEXANDRA C. PEREL-WINKLER

INTRODUCTION

Systemic lupus erythematosus (SLE) is a chronic autoimmune disease characterized by the production of autoantibodies and multiorgan involvement. Lupus symptoms can be variable, and its presentation exists on a continuum; some patients have mild involvement of skin and joints, while others may have severe, life-threatening organ involvement. Patients with SLE are at higher risk of other illnesses, including coronary artery disease, malignancy infections, and the **antiphospholipid syndrome (APLS)** (see Chapter 145 for details). This disease most commonly affects young women of childbearing age and is more severe in Asian, African American, and Hispanic populations.

Patients with SLE usually present between the ages of 15 and 45 years. The reported prevalence of SLE is 20 to 150 cases per 100,000. Women have a higher incidence, with a female-to-male ratio of 10 to 15 : 1 before the age of 55. After menopause, this ratio narrows to 3 : 1. There is evidence that genetics plays a role in the development of SLE. Identical twin studies have shown a 25% to 50% chance of an identical twin developing SLE and only a 2% to 5% risk for a nonidentical twin. First-degree relatives have an increased chance of developing SLE (sixfold) as well as non-SLE autoimmune disease (fourfold).

PATHOPHYSIOLOGY

The exact underlying pathophysiology of SLE remains unknown, but both genetic and environmental factors play a role. Defective immune regulatory mechanisms, such as poor clearance of apoptotic cells, loss of immune tolerance, complement deficiencies, increased T-cell activation, and defective B-cell suppression lead to B-cell hyperactivity and the production of pathogenic autoantibodies. These autoantibodies can lead to the formation of immune complexes, leading to tissue damage.

RISK FACTORS

Risk factors for SLE include both fixed (nonmodifiable) and modifiable risk factors. Fixed risk factors include genetic predisposition, such as possessing MHC-DR2 and 3 alleles or C1q deficiency, being of African American, Asian, or Hispanic origin, and female sex. Modifiable risk factors include ultraviolet (UV) light exposure, exogenous estrogen use, smoking, and certain drugs that may exacerbate disease, including thiazides, sulfa drugs, and NSAIDs.

PRESENTATION, EVALUATION, AND DIAGNOSIS

Due to its multisystem involvement and variable presentation, SLE can be challenging to diagnose and treat. The Systemic Lupus International Collaborating Clinics **(SLICC)** criteria for classification lists common clinical and immunological findings in patients with SLE and can be used as a guideline for the diagnosis of SLE (Table 106.1). A person who satisfies four or more criteria (including at least one clinical and one immunological criterion) is considered to have SLE (97% sensitivity, 84% specificity) for the purposes of clinical studies.

Antibody testing is recommended as part of the diagnostic workup for SLE. See Table 106.2 for a list of SLE-related antibodies and their associations. It is important to note that patients who have biopsy-proven **lupus nephritis** in the presence of a positive antinuclear antibody (ANA) or anti–double-stranded DNA (dsDNA) antibody also fulfill criteria for a diagnosis of SLE.

The classic lupus rash is called a **malar rash,** also known as a butterfly rash. This rash involves the cheeks and nasal bridge and (importantly) spares the nasolabial folds. It is usually pink, and the skin may appear slightly raised. Photosensitivity is common, defined as erythema or irritation of the skin after exposure to UV light. Discoid rashes affect the face, scalp, and ears and are light pink, expanding outward but leaving a central scar, which may be hypopigmented or hyperpigmented. These rashes can be biopsied to assist in diagnosis (Fig. 106.1).

Arthralgia is joint pain in the absence of swelling and synovitis but can be associated with increased severity in the morning, while arthritis is joint pain with objective findings of warmth, swelling, effusion,

TABLE 106.1

Systemic Lupus International Collaborating Clinics Classification Criteria for SLE (2012)

Clinical Criteria	Description
1. Acute cutaneous lupus (+++)	Malar (nondiscoid), photosensitive, maculopapular; may be bullous or toxic epidermal necrolysis
2. Chronic cutaneous lupus (+)	Discoid lupus (scarring), lupus panniculitis/profundus
3. Alopecia (++)	Nonscarring; diffuse hair thinning, broken hairs
4. Oral or nasal ulcers (++)	Nonpainful; palate, buccal cavity, tongue, nares
5. Inflammatory arthritis (synovitis) (+++)	Two or more peripheral joints with tenderness, swelling, effusion, warmth, boggy synovium on palpation or morning stiffness >30 min
6. Serositis (++)	Pleuritis, pericarditis
7. Renal disease (++)	Persistent proteinuria ≥0.5 g/day or RBC casts
8. Neurological disease (++)	CNS: seizure, psychosis, cranial nerve defects, encephalitis, coma, myelitis, brain fog PNS: mononeuritis multiplex
9. Hemolytic anemia (+)	Positive direct Coombs test
10. Leukopenia (++)	Leukopenia <4000 cells/μL *or* Lymphopenia <1000 cells/μL at least once
11. Thrombocytopenia (++)	Platelets <100,000 cells/μL
Immunological Criteria	
1. ANA (+++)	Positive test (usually 1:320 or higher)
2. Anti-dsDNA (++)	Positive
3. Anti-Sm (++)	Positive
4. Antiphospholipid antibody positive (++)	One of the following: positive lupus anticoagulant test, anticardiolipin antibody (medium-high titer), B2-glycoprotein antibody, or falsely positive RPR
5. Low complement (+++)	Low C3, C4, or CH50
6. Direct Coombs test (+)	In the absence of hemolytic anemia

+, Uncommon; *++,* common; *+++,* very common; *ANA,* antinuclear antibody; *CNS,* central nervous system; *dsDNA,* double-stranded deoxyribonucleic acid; *PNS,* peripheral nervous system; *RBC,* red blood cell; *RPR,* rapid plasma reagin; *SLE,* systemic lupus erythematosus.
Reused with permission from Petri M, Orbai AM, Alarcon GS, et al: Derivation and validation of the Systemic Lupus International Collaborating Clinics classification criteria for systemic lupus erythematosus, *Arthritis Rheum* 64(8):2677–2686, 2012.

and/or synovitis on exam. Lupus patients do not develop erosive arthritis but can have a reversible deformity called Jaccoud arthropathy that appears similar to the swan neck deformity and is caused by joint capsule and ligamental laxity, not bony destruction.

Patients with anemia should be evaluated for hemolytic anemia. Patients will often have positive Coombs tests without hemolytic anemia, so other markers of hemolysis (e.g., lactate dehydrogenase, haptoglobin, and bilirubin) are useful. Negative tests for hemolysis make anemia from chronic inflammation more likely. Leukopenia correlates with increased disease activity, and while lymphopenia is more common than neutropenia, both rarely fall to the point of increased infectious risk.

Lupus nephritis (LN) is one of the most common and serious manifestations of lupus. Patients with active lupus nephritis may present with findings consistent with the nephrotic syndrome, but some patients may be asymptomatic. Therefore all patients with SLE should have their renal function and urine screened every 3 months for increasing creatinine, proteinuria, and cellular casts. Biopsy should be considered for urine protein/urine creatinine ratios >1, >0.5 with hematuria or cellular casts, or rising creatinine without alternative cause (Fig. 106.2).

TABLE 106.2
Lupus Antibody Targets and Their Associations

Antibody Target	Association
dsDNA	High specificity for SLE Can correlate with disease activity
Smith	High specificity for SLE
Histone	Drug-induced lupus, SLE
Ro/SSA	Neonatal lupus, photosensitivity, Sjögren syndrome, subacute cutaneous lupus
La/SSB	Neonatal lupus, Sjögren syndrome
Ribosomal P protein	High specificity for SLE, psychiatric disease
Phospholipid antibodies	Thrombosis, recurrent abortion/fetal loss, thrombocytopenia
U1-RNP	Mixed connective tissue disease/overlap syndrome

SLE, Systemic lupus erythematosus.

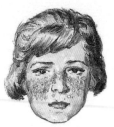

Malar rash

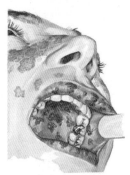

Painless oral ulcers

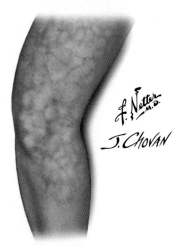

Livedo reticularis

FIG. 106.1 Skin and Mucous Membrane Manifestations of Systemic Lupus Erythematosus.

Central nervous system (CNS) involvement can be diffuse or focal. Encephalopathy can range from mild cognitive dysfunction to confusion and coma. The cerebrospinal fluid (CSF) often has elevated cells and may have increased immunoglobulin G (IgG) and oligoclonal bands (markers of autoantibody production in the CSF) in diffuse disease. Focal disease, such as strokes and transient ischemic attacks, are often noted in the setting of concomitant APLS.

Pericarditis is the most common cardiac manifestation (up to 40%–50% of patients) and is often asymptomatic and noted on echocardiogram. Libman-Sacks endocarditis is the buildup of inflammatory material on valves, and although noninfectious, it does put patients at risk for subacute bacterial endocarditis. Premature coronary artery disease (not explained by typical risk factors), myocardial infarction, and congestive heart failure are the leading causes of mortality in lupus patients.

The most concerning pulmonary sequela is diffuse alveolar hemorrhage, usually noted in patients with poorly controlled, highly active disease. Pleuritis is more common and usually bilateral (infection should be ruled out if unilateral). Interstitial lung disease is rare, and pulmonary embolism can occur most commonly with concomitant APLS. Gastrointestinal (GI) involvement is uncommon and can include esophageal dysmotility, serositis, and (more rarely) mesenteric vasculitis, protein-losing enteropathy, and autoimmune hepatitis.

TREATMENT

Modifiable risk factors should be addressed with medication changes and lifestyle changes, including starting an exercise program and avoiding smoking and exogenous estrogen. All lupus patients should avoid direct sunlight and wear UVA and UVB protection (SPF ≥30). Patients

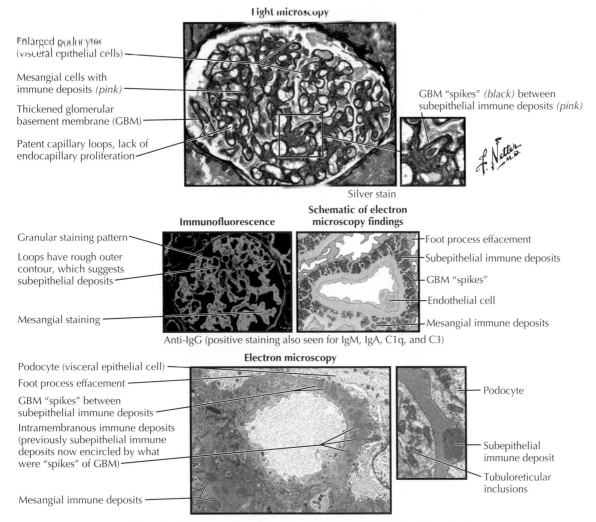

Light microscopy

Enlarged podocytes (visceral epithelial cells)

Mesangial cells with immune deposits *(pink)*

Thickened glomerular basement membrane (GBM)

Patent capillary loops, lack of endocapillary proliferation

GBM "spikes" *(black)* between subepithelial immune deposits *(pink)*

Silver stain

Immunofluorescence

Schematic of electron microscopy findings

Granular staining pattern

Loops have rough outer contour, which suggests subepithelial deposits

Mesangial staining

Foot process effacement

Subepithelial immune deposits

GBM "spikes"

Endothelial cell

Mesangial immune deposits

Anti-IgG (positive staining also seen for IgM, IgA, C1q, and C3)

Electron microscopy

Podocyte (visceral epithelial cell)

Foot process effacement

GBM "spikes" between subepithelial immune deposits

Intramembranous immune deposits (previously subepithelial immune deposits now encircled by what were "spikes" of GBM)

Mesangial immune deposits

Podocyte

Subepithelial immune deposit

Tubuloreticular inclusions

FIG. 106.2 **Lupus Nephritis: Renal Histopathology (Class V Lesions).**

should receive appropriate immunizations prior to starting immunosuppressive therapies.

Immunosuppressants constitute the core of SLE therapy, and the choice of particular therapies depends on clinical manifestations. **Hydroxychloroquine** (HCQ) is the only medication with evidence for mortality and morbidity benefit, and all patients should be on it unless contraindicated. HCQ is often used as monotherapy for mild skin disease, cytopenias, and arthralgias.

Topical steroids are useful for active skin disease, but oral steroids may be necessary for more serious skin flares. Steroid-sparing therapies include HCQ and dapsone. Serious chronic skin disease can be treated with azathioprine, mycophenolate mofetil, or tacrolimus (topical or oral). Belimumab is a monoclonal antibody against a B-cell survival factor (BAFF) and has shown efficacy but takes 4 to 6 months for effect. Discoid lesions may be treated with thalidomide and cyclosporine; rituximab is not useful. Joint disease that does not respond to HCQ may require additional medications such as methotrexate; azathioprine, abatacept, belimumab, and rituximab are other options. Tumor necrosis factor (TNF) inhibitors are not recommended in lupus due to risk of flare.

Lupus nephritis treatment involves induction with high-dose methylprednisolone and a steroid-sparing agent (often cyclophosphamide or mycophenolate mofetil), followed by steroid-sparing maintenance therapy. Adjunct therapy includes HCQ, ACE inhibitor of angiotensin receptor blocker (ARB) for proteinuria, blood pressure control (goal ≤130/80), and statins for low-density lipoprotein (LDL) >100 mg/dL.

Other moderate to severe SLE manifestations can be treated with azathioprine, mycophenolate mofetil, cyclophosphamide, and antibody therapy (including rituximab and belimumab). Patients presenting with acute moderate to severe symptoms usually receive glucocorticoids (e.g., methylprednisolone, prednisone) while steroid-sparing therapies are considered.

CHAPTER 107

Systemic Sclerosis

JAE HEE YUN

INTRODUCTION

Systemic sclerosis (SSc) is a rare autoimmune connective tissue disease characterized by **vasculopathy** and **fibrosis**. Most patients can be classified as having **limited** cutaneous SSc (lcSSc) or **diffuse cutaneous SSc** (dcSSc) (Table 107.1). Patients with lcSSc typically experience **Raynaud phenomenon** and have skin thickening limited to the face and distal extremities **(sclerodactyly).** They also frequently have one or more other symptoms of **CREST syndrome:** cutaneous calcification, Raynaud, esophageal dysmotility, sclerodactyly, and telangiectasias. Late in the course, pulmonary hypertension or pulmonary fibrosis are common causes of significant morbidity and mortality. **Anticentromere** antibodies are common but not terribly sensitive or specific.

The dcSSc is characterized by much more **diffuse skin involvement** and early-onset internal organ involvement, including interstitial lung disease (ILD), sclerodermal renal disease, diffuse gastrointestinal involvement, and myocardial disease. Patients typically have Raynaud phenomenon sometimes leading to digital ischemia and digital loss. **Anti-Scl-70** antibodies are associated with dcSSc, but are neither sensitive nor entirely specific.

PATHOPHYSIOLOGY

The pathogenesis of SSc is complex and incompletely understood. At a molecular level, it involves both vascular factors and inappropriate innate and adaptive immune activation, leading to vascular damage and excessive synthesis of extracellular matrix resulting in increased amount of collagen depositions and fibrosis. The activated fibrogenic fibroblasts are likely the main mediators facilitating the fibrotic pathology in SSc, but the factors that initially trigger inappropriate activation are not completely understood.

RISK FACTORS

SSc most commonly affects women, with a female-to-male ratio of 4:1, and diagnosis occurs between the ages of 30 and 60 years. African American women are more likely to be diagnosed and seem to have more severe symptoms than Caucasian women. The risk of SSc in first-degree relatives of individuals with SSc is significantly increased.

Interestingly, Choctaw Native Americans have a disease prevalence 20 times higher than the general population. Studies on this population and others demonstrate genetic risk loci in the major histocompatibility complex (MHC) genes as well as in other areas of the genome. Environmental exposures in some situations also seem to have an etiological role. Clusters of SSc or SSc-like diseases have been related to exposure to vinyl chloride, rapeseed oil, L-tryptophan, and chemotherapy drugs, such as bleomycin. Other studies demonstrate that occupational silica exposure in men is associated with a significantly increased risk of SSc.

PRESENTATION, EVALUATION, AND DIAGNOSIS

SSc is a multisystem disease that can affect various organ systems due to vasculopathy and progressive fibrosis. It should be suspected in patients who present with skin thickening, puffy fingers, Raynaud phenomenon, and gastroesophageal reflux disease (GERD) (Fig. 107.1). Clinical presentation of SSc varies according to different types of sclerosis as well as early versus late phase. As dcSSc has a more rapidly progressive course, unlike lcSSc, an early phase is considered <3 years for dcSSc while <10 years for lcSSc.

The lcSSc manifests with skin thickening limited to the neck, face, or distal parts of upper and lower extremities. Patients often have a long-standing Raynaud phenomenon, GERD, and may have calcinosis (skin calcifications), telangiectasia, and sclerodactyly (digital edema).

The presence of anti-Scl-70 antibody is associated with a high risk of progressive ILD, and the presence of anticentromere antibody is associated with a high risk for pulmonary arterial hypertension (PAH). However,

TABLE 107.1
Symptoms of Limited and Diffuse Cutaneous Systemic Sclerosis

	Limited Cutaneous Systemic Sclerosis	Diffuse Cutaneous Systemic Sclerosis
Constitutional	None	Fatigue, weight loss during early phase, possible weight gain during late phase Weight gain
Vascular	Raynaud, telangiectasia, with digital ulceration during late phase	Raynaud, telangiectasia, with digital ulceration during late phase
Cutaneous	Slow progression of sclerosis, involving face, distal extremities, sparing trunk	Rapid progression of sclerosis involving proximal arms, trunk, face; stable or regression during late phase
Pulmonary	No involvement during early phase, lung fibrosis and PAH during late phase	Interstitial pulmonary fibrosis developed during early phase, with progression during late phase
Cardiac	No involvement during early phase, secondary right ventricular failure from PAH during late phase	Myocarditis, pericardial effusion mostly in early phase
Gastrointestinal	Dysphagia, GERD during early phase with progression of dysmotility and fecal incontinence during late phase	Dysphagia, GERD during early phase with progression of dysmotility and fecal incontinence during late phase
Renal	No involvement during early phase, rarely renal crisis during late phase	Renal crisis typically during first 5 years
Musculoskeletal	Occasional joint stiffness during early phase, mild flexion contractures during late phase	Arthralgia, stiffness, myalgia, muscle weakness, tendon friction rubs during early phase, flexion contracture and deformities during late phase

GERD, Gastroesophageal reflux disease; *PAH*, pulmonary arterial hypertension.

renal crisis is rare in lcSSc. Patients with lcSSc often do not present until 5 to 10 years after symptom onset.

The dcSSc manifests skin thickening proximal to elbows or knees; it often involves the trunk but spares the face and neck. Unlike lcSSc, patients with dcSSc usually present acutely with Raynaud phenomenon, puffy hands, arthritis, and rapidly progressive skin thickening.

All patients with dcSSc are at high risk of progressive ILD, especially within 5 years of disease onset and are at risk for PAH. Patients are also much more likely to develop scleroderma renal crisis (SRC).

SRC is an early complication of dcSSc and occurs in 5% to 20% of patients. Risk factors include a rapid progression of skin thickening, a presence of anti–ribonucleic acid (anti-RNA) polymerase III antibody, and glucocorticoid use. It is characterized by acute onset of renal failure and abrupt onset of moderate to severe hypertension. Patients can have proteinuria in the range of 500 mg to 1 g due to hypertension, but glomerulonephritis with an active urine sediment is not a feature of SRC. Microangiopathic hemolytic anemia and thrombocytopenia can also be seen.

In examining patients whose presentation is concerning for SSc, physicians should pay particular attention to extremity findings, including nonpitting edema of hands, digital ulcerations, and nailfold capillary changes, as well as cutaneous skin thickening in hands/feet/face/trunk, perioral skin tightening with decreased oral aperture, and calcinosis of hands/elbows/knees.

In addition to routine laboratory studies and urinalysis, physicians should check renal function, anticyclic citrullinated peptide (anti-CCP), and lupus serologies (double-stranded deoxyribonucleic acid [dsDNA], anti-Smith, C3, C4, and RNP antibody) to narrow the diagnosis. The following labs have clinical significance in the diagnosis and progression of SSc:

- Antinuclear antibody (ANA): positive in >90% patient with SSc
- Anti-Scl-70: associated with a higher risk of severe ILD
- Anticentromere antibody: usually associated with lcSSc, 5% in dcSSc
- Anti-RNA polymerase III antibody: associated with dcSSc, rapidly progressive skin involvement and SRC

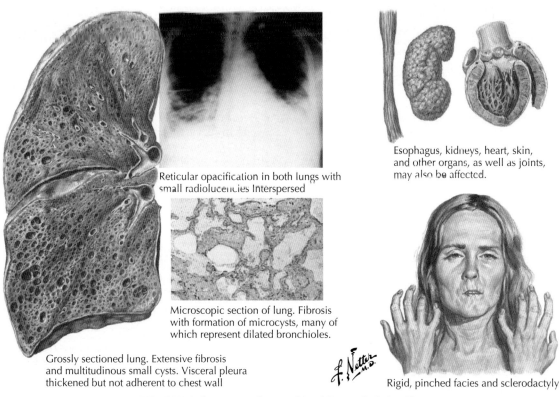

Reticular opacification in both lungs with small radiolucencies Interspersed

Esophagus, kidneys, heart, skin, and other organs, as well as joints, may also be affected.

Microscopic section of lung. Fibrosis with formation of microcysts, many of which represent dilated bronchioles.

Grossly sectioned lung. Extensive fibrosis and multitudinous small cysts. Visceral pleura thickened but not adherent to chest wall

Rigid, pinched facies and sclerodactyly

FIG. 107.1 **Symptoms Suggestive of Systemic Sclerosis.**

All patients with suspected SSc should be monitored for any evidence of SRC and receive high-resolution chest CT, pulmonary function tests, and Doppler echocardiography to investigate ILD and PAH.

The 2013 American College of Rheumatology/European League Against Rheumatism (ACR/EULAR) classification criteria (Table 107.2) are useful to diagnose SSc (sensitivity 91%, specificity 92%). While containing common diagnostic features of SSc, some patients with the disease may not fulfill the criteria. Therefore it should be used as an initial guidance, and the ultimate diagnosis should be established from a clinical suspicion based on individual presentation. Patients with a total of score of ≥9 are classified as having definitive SSc.

TREATMENT

There is no treatment for underlying disease mechanisms of SSc, but there are therapies that can help manage specific disease manifestations. Initial treatment for Raynaud phenomenon involves keeping the hands and body warm to improve distal blood flow; smoking cessation is required. Calcium channel blockers, excluding verapamil, are the first choice to increase vasodilation, and angiotensin II receptor blockers and topical nitroglycerin ointment may be effective, as well. Digital sympathectomy and hyperbaric oxygen treatment can promote digital ulcer healing. Treatment of calcinosis is less successful with limited data supporting methotrexate, infliximab, or rituximab. Surgical resection is considered as a last resort.

H2 blockers and proton-pump inhibitors (PPIs) are the first line of therapy for esophageal dysmotility, and endoscopic injection of botulinum toxin into pyloric sphincter can also be used for resistant cases of GERD.

Promotility agents such as metoclopramide, domperidone, and erythromycin are useful for small bowel dysmotility, and cisapride or injectable octreotide can also be tried in refractory cases.

Antibiotics may be useful for diarrhea from small intestine bacterial overgrowth, but persistent symptoms should prompt a malabsorption workup. For fecal incontinence due to anorectal neuropathy, biofeedback, sacral nerve stimulations, and, lastly, surgical repair can be considered.

TABLE 107.2
ACR/EULAR Criteria for the Diagnosis of Systemic Sclerosis[a]

Items	Subitems	Score[b]
Skin thickening of the fingers of both hands extending proximal to the metacarpophalangeal joints *(sufficient criterion)*		9
Skin thickening of the fingers *(only count the higher score)*	Puffy fingers	2
	Sclerodactyly of the fingers (distal to the metacarpophalangeal joints but proximal to the proximal interphalangeal joints)	4
Fingertip lesions *(only count the higher score)*	Digital tip ulcers	2
	Fingertip pitting scars	3
Telangiectasia		2
Abnormal nailfold capillaries		2
Pulmonary arterial hypertension and/or interstitial lung disease *(maximum score is 2)*	Pulmonary arterial hypertension	2
	Interstitial lung disease	2
Raynaud phenomenon		3
SSc-related autoantibodies *(maximum score is 3)*	Anticentromere	3
	Antitopoisomerase 1 (Anti-Scl-70)	
	Anti-RNA polymerase III	

[a]These criteria are applicable to any patient considered for inclusion in an SSc study. The criteria are not applicable to patients with skin thickening sparing the fingers or to patients who have a scleroderma-like disorder that better explains their manifestations (e.g., nephrogenic sclerosing fibrosis, generalized morphea, eosinophilic fasciitis, scleredema diabeticorum, scleromyxedema, erythromyalgia, porphyria, lichen sclerosis, graft-versus-host disease, diabetic cheiroarthropathy).
[b]The total score is determined by adding the maximum weight (score) in each category. Patients with a total score of 9 are classified as having definite SSc.
ACR/EULAR, American College of Rheumatology/European League Against Rheumatism; *RNA,* ribonucleic acid; *SSc,* systemic sclerosis.
Reused with permission from Van den Hoogen F, Khanna D, Fransen J, et al: 2013 classification criteria for systemic sclerosis, *Arthritis Rheum* 65(11):2737–2747, 2013.

For symptomatic ILD, mycophenolate mofetil or cyclophosphamide is the first line of therapy. For patients who cannot tolerate either agent, azathioprine can be the alternative therapy. For refractory disease, rituximab can be considered as well as lung transplantation or stem cell transplant. Patients may develop PAH and should receive calcium channel blockers, diuretics for fluid/volume control, and supplemental oxygen as needed. Patients can also be on PAH-specific therapies (see Chapter 90).

Patients who present with acute increase in serum creatinine or renal failure in the setting of moderate to severe hypertension should be hospitalized immediately for SRC and started on a short-acting ACE inhibitor. The goal is to decrease systolic pressure by 20 mm Hg within the first 24 hours. If refractory to maximum dose of ACE inhibitor, patients should also be on calcium channel blockers and/or angiotensin receptor blockers. Complete blood count (CBC), basic metabolic panel (BMP), haptoglobin, and serum lactate dehydrogenase should be checked daily to monitor kidney function and intravascular hemolysis. Approximately 20% to 50% of patients with SRC may initially require dialysis. However, most of them recover renal function and discontinue dialysis after an appropriate ACE inhibitor therapy.

CHAPTER 108

Polymyositis and Dermatomyositis

ELIZABETH MATHEW

INTRODUCTION

The term **inflammatory myositis** includes a heterogeneous group of chronic systemic autoimmune diseases, including **dermatomyositis** (DM), **polymyositis** (PM), and **inclusion body myositis** (IBM). DM and PM, with a prevalence of about 21.5 per 100,000, are the most common. Though they share common clinical features of gradually progressing proximal muscle weakness, along with biochemical, electrophysiological, and histological evidence of muscle inflammation, DM and PM differ with regard to genetics and immunological mechanisms, and typical skin manifestations in the former. The recognition of myositis-specific autoantibodies has allowed better clinical characterization, identification of risks for other organ involvement, and treatment responsiveness. Early recognition and initiation of therapy is often crucial for preventing complications due to involvement of pharyngeal and respiratory muscles as well as muscles of the proximal arms and legs.

PATHOPHYSIOLOGY AND RISK FACTORS

DM is a microangiopathy affecting skin and muscle; activation and deposition of complement causes lysis of endomysial capillaries and muscle ischemia. In PM, clonally expanded CD8-positive cytotoxic T cells invade muscle fibers that express major histocompatibility complex class 1 (MHC1) antigens, which leads to fiber necrosis via the perforin pathway.

DM has a bimodal distribution, with one peak at 5 to 15 years and another between 45 and 65 years of age. PM, however, usually occurs between 50 and 60 years of age, and rarely has an onset <15 years of age. The overall female-to-male incidence ratio is 2 to 3 : 1, with equal incidence in juvenile onset DM (JDM). Patient with DM have higher rates of malignancy than those with PM, especially above age 65 years. The highest probability for detection of malignancy was before 2 years and after 3 years of the diagnosis of DM, as well as PM. Malignancies generally associated with the diseases are breast, lung, pancreas, stomach, colon, ovary, and Hodgkin lymphoma.

PRESENTATION

Patients present with symmetric proximal muscle weakness that progresses over weeks to months. Patients report weakness in shoulder and pelvic girdles, and difficulty with everyday tasks such as lifting objects, combing their hair, or rising from a chair (Fig. 108.1). Neck flexor/extensor and trunk muscles are often involved. Less frequently, but more worrisome, is pharyngeal and respiratory muscle involvement, which can lead to voice changes and dysphonia, dysphagia, dyspnea, aspiration, and poor cough leading to risk of pneumonia. Facial and extraocular muscles are almost never affected, and weakness here should prompt consideration of an alternate diagnosis. Pain is not usually a feature of DM/PM but can be a feature of a separate entity called necrotizing myositis. The tendon reflexes are preserved but may be absent in severely weakened or atrophied muscles.

DM is characterized by similar muscle symptoms as well as a variety of skin manifestations. The most pathognomonic are **Gottron papules** and **heliotrope rash** (see Fig. 108.1). Gottron papules are elevated violaceous, pink, or dusky red papules located over the dorsum of the metacarpophalangeal joints or interphalangeal joints. They can also present as macular rash without papules, called Gottron sign. Heliotrope rash is the periorbital red or violaceous erythema of one or both eyelids, often with edema. Other less specific signs are the V sign, shawl sign, Holster sign, pruritic scalp involvement, and nailfold capillary abnormalities. **Amyopathic DM** is a variant in which skin manifestations predominate without clinical or laboratory evidence of myositis.

Another clinical finding is the mechanic's hands, encompassing cracks, fissures, and hyperpigmentation of the hands. This can be seen in either DM or PM and may signify the presence of the **antisynthetase syndrome**. The antisynthetase syndrome is defined by the presence of one or more positive antisynthetase antibodies with two major criteria, or one major and two minor criteria. Major criteria include (1) interstitial lung disease (ILD) and (2) either PM or DM. Minor criteria are (1) inflammatory

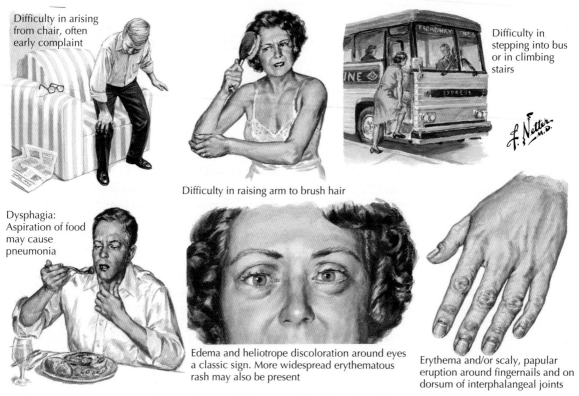

Difficulty in arising from chair, often early complaint

Difficulty in stepping into bus or in climbing stairs

Difficulty in raising arm to brush hair

Dysphagia: Aspiration of food may cause pneumonia

Edema and heliotrope discoloration around eyes a classic sign. More widespread erythematous rash may also be present

Erythema and/or scaly, papular eruption around fingernails and on dorsum of interphalangeal joints

FIG. 108.1 **Symptoms of Inflammatory Myopathies.**

symmetric arthritis, (2) Raynaud phenomenon, and (3) mechanic's hands.

Respiratory involvement in DM and PM can be due to muscle weakness, as outlined earlier, or from parenchymal involvement seen in ILD, especially in the setting of antisynthetase syndrome. The most common type of ILD is nonspecific interstitial pneumonia (NSIP), and in most cases, the changes are present at the time of diagnosis of myositis; they rarely develop after immunosuppressive treatment has started. Cardiac manifestations in PM/DM are most frequently subclinical conduction abnormalities and arrhythmias. The gastrointestinal system can be affected with a variety of symptoms, most commonly weakness of the upper third of the esophagus with trouble swallowing and a risk of aspiration. Patients may have a nasal or weak voice due to pharyngeal weakness, as well as tongue weakness and dysphagia.

EVALUATION AND DIAGNOSIS

The most prominent laboratory finding is elevated muscle enzymes, especially **creatine phosphokinase** (CPK), which is the best marker of muscle damage.

It is typically elevated as much as 50-fold in PM and DM. Other muscle enzymes that are elevated include transaminases (alanine aminotransferase [ALT], aspartate transaminase [AST]), lactate dehydrogenase (LDH), and aldolase.

Autoantibodies are present in 55% to 80% of the cases of PM and DM, and antinuclear antibodies (ANA) are the most common. Myositis-specific antibodies can divide diseases into homogeneous subgroups with distinct clinical features and genotypes, which can facilitate diagnosis and prognostication. Recent studies have shown that the presence of certain antibodies carry a greater risk of malignancy. The specific antibodies and their associated clinical features are described in Table 108.1.

Electromyography shows prominent muscle membrane irritability with increased insertional activity, trains of positive sharp waves, and fibrillations (Fig. 108.2). Polyphasic motor unit action potentials (MUAPs) of short duration and low amplitude, with early recruitment patterns, are also a finding.

MRI can be used to identify affected muscles and areas of focal inflammation, which may be amenable to biopsy (Fig. 108.3).

TABLE 108.1
Myositis Autoantibodies

Autoantibodies	Phenotype	Important Considerations
Antisynthetases (antiaminoacyl tRNA synthetases)—anti Jo1, PL7, PL12, KS, EJ, OJ, Ha, Zo	Myositis, ILD, Raynaud phenomenon, nonerosive symmetric polyarthritis, mechanic's hands	ILD
Anti-Mi2 (nuclear helicase protein)	Classic DM with characteristic skin manifestations	Milder disease, good prognosis
Anti-MDA5 (melanoma differentiation gene 5)	Amyopathic DM, rapidly progressive ILD, severe vasculopathy, mucocutaneous ulcerations, tender palmar papules	Severe disease, poor prognosis
Anti-p155/140 or anti-TIF1γ (transcription intermediary factor-1γ)	Severe cutaneous involvement with cutaneous edema and vasculopathy in children	Risk of malignancy
Anti-NXP2 (nuclear matrix protein 2)	Significant muscle involvement, younger age of onset, calcinosis	Risk of malignancy, persistent disease, muscle contractures, atrophy, worse functional status
Anti-SAE (small ubiquitin-like modifier activating enzyme)	Initially amyopathic DM then progress to muscle weakness with systemic features, including GI involvement with dysphagia	ILD, dysphagia
Anti-SRP (signal recognition particle)	Acute-onset severe necrotizing myopathy, dysphagia	Severe disease, often refractory; cardiac involvement; dysphagia
Anti-HMGCR (3-hydroxy-3-methyl-glutaryl-coenzyme A reductase)	Statin exposure + but not necessary, necrotizing myopathy with high risk in HLA-DR11 carriers	
Anti-PM Scl (polymyositis scleroderma)	Younger age of onset, milder cutaneous SSc features with skin and inflammatory arthritis, Raynaud phenomenon	Overlap, ILD, good response to therapy

DM, Dermatomyositis; *GI,* gastrointestinal; *HLA-DR11,* human leukocyte antigen serotype DR11; *ILD,* interstitial lung disease; *SSc,* systemic sclerosis; *tRNA,* transfer ribonucleic acid.
Reused with permission from Casciola-Rosen L, Mammen AL: Myositis autoantibodies, *Curr Opin Rheumatol* 24:602–608, 2012.

Muscle biopsy is the most specific test. In DM, biopsy shows inflammation with predominantly B cells in blood vessels, the septa between muscle fascicles, and fibroadipose tissue around muscle, as well as vasculitis and perifascicular atrophy (see Fig. 108.2). In PM, muscle biopsy shows endomysial mononuclear cells with fiber size variability, cellular invasion of nonnecrotic muscle fibers expressing MHC1 antigens, and scattered necrotic and regenerating fibers.

The most commonly used criteria for diagnosing DM/PM are the **Bohan and Peter diagnostic criteria** (Box 108.1), which were developed in 1975 and do not consider newer modalities of diagnosis, such as imaging. The International Myositis Assessment and Clinical Studies Group (IMACS) has developed new classification criteria with 16 variables, which are currently under review by the American College of Rheumatology/ European League Against Rheumatism (ACR/EULAR) criteria subcommittee.

Once the diagnosis of DM/PM is confirmed, extramuscular organ system involvement must be assessed. Patients with respiratory involvement, especially those with the antisynthetase syndrome, should undergo high-resolution CT scan of the lungs and pulmonary function testing with spirometry and diffusion capacity to evaluate for ILD. Electrocardiogram (ECG) and echocardiography are recommended to assess cardiac involvement. Swallowing evaluation should be performed if there is suspicion of pharyngeal involvement to determine the critical bulbar muscle involvement.

Age-appropriate malignancy screening should be offered to patients with newly diagnosed DM/PM and

Electromyography

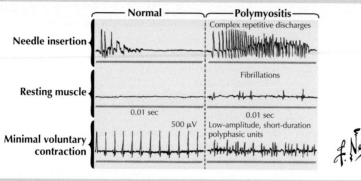

Muscle Biopsy

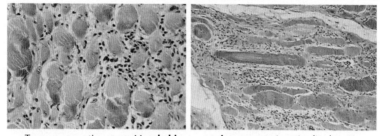

Transverse section ← **Muscle biopsy specimens** → Longitudinal section

Inflammatory reaction: muscle fiber necrosis and regeneration

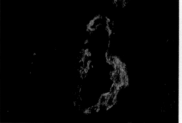

Anti-IgG immuno-fluorescence of frozen muscle section with positive staining within blood vessel wall, indicating immunologic basis of dermatomyositis

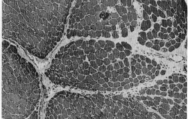

Perifascicular muscle atrophy in child with dermatomyositis

FIG. 108.2 **Investigative Findings of Inflammatory Myopathies: Electromyography and Muscle Biopsy.**

should be continued to be evaluated for the possibility of an underlying malignancy during treatment, the diagnosis of which may involve further imaging. Malignancy screening is especially important in patients with DM, an older age of onset, and with certain autoantibodies (outlined later).

TREATMENT

Effective management of patients with inflammatory myopathies requires a comprehensive multidisciplinary approach, targeting the nonpharmacological aspects of long-term patient outcomes with adequate patient education and rehabilitation considerations.

The primary treatment for DM and PM is immunosuppression, with about a 75% response rate. Systemic corticosteroids are first-line therapy despite there being no controlled trials. Severe cases may require pulse steroid therapy with intravenous methylprednisolone for 3 to 5 days; otherwise, patients are initiated on prednisone with tapering occurring over several weeks guided by serial CPK measurements.

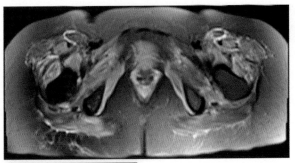

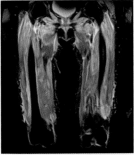

Axial *(top)* and coronal *(bottom)* MR images of femur. Diffuse muscle edema in both anterior and posterior compartments of the thigh, representing inflammation consistent with myositis.

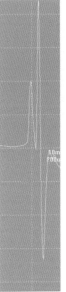

Normal motor unit potential on needle examination

Myopathic motor unit potential changes characterized by polyphasia and reduced amplitude and duration

FIG. 108.3 Investigative Findings of Inflammatory Myopathies: Imaging and Motor Unit Potential Testing.

INDIVIDUAL CRITERIA
1. Symmetric proximal muscle weakness
2. Muscle biopsy evidence of myositis
3. Increase in serum skeletal muscle enzymes
4. Characteristic electromyographic pattern
5. Typical rash of dermatomyositis

DIAGNOSTIC CRITERIA
Polymyositis
Definite: all of 1–4
Probable: any 3 of 1–4
Possible: any 2 of 1–4

Dermatomyositis
Definite: 5 plus any 3 of 1–4
Probable: 5 plus any 2 of 1–4
Possible: 5 plus any 1 of 1–4

Reused with permission from Bohan A, Peter JB: Polymyositis and dermatomyositis (part 1), *N Engl J Med* 292:344–347, 1975; Bohan A, Peter JB: Polymyositis and dermatomyositis (part 2), *N Engl J Med* 292:403–407, 1975.

Steroid-sparing agents can be used as maintenance therapy, as long-term steroid therapy can have unwanted side effects. Methotrexate is used first, with response seen within 2 to 3 months. Azathioprine and mycophenolate mofetil are other options. In cases of refractory DM, especially with skin manifestations and esophageal and respiratory muscle involvement, intravenous immunoglobulin (IVIG) is effective. More evidence exists for its use in DM, but it has shown some efficacy with PM. Randomized, placebo-controlled trials failed to demonstrate a significant effect of either plasmapheresis or leukapheresis over placebo. Nonmuscular manifestations of disease, including arthritis, fatigue, and skin involvement, may benefit from antimalarial therapy, including chloroquine and hydroxychloroquine.

Resistant DM/PM can be treated with cyclophosphamide or rituximab. Cyclosporine and tacrolimus appear to have some role, but data are limited to retrospective case series and anecdotal reports. The limited evidence available suggests that tacrolimus offers some advantage over cyclosporine in efficacy.

CHAPTER 109

Polymyalgia Rheumatica and Temporal Arteritis

SUNENA TEWANI

INTRODUCTION

Polymyalgia rheumatica (PMR) and **temporal arteritis** (also called giant cell arteritis [GCA]) are both rheumatic inflammatory disorders that occur in older age. PMR is an inflammatory disorder that typically affects the shoulders, hip girdles, and neck. Temporal arteritis is a large-vessel and medium-vessel vasculitis involving the major branches of the aorta, the vertebral, subclavian, and extracranial branches of the carotids, and (most commonly) the temporal arteries.

PMR and temporal arteritis are diseases of the elderly. They rarely occur under the age of 50, and the peak age of incidence occurs between ages 70 and 79. Both of these disorders can present individually or may overlap; about 50% to 90% of patients with temporal arteritis show signs of PMR, and about 33% of patients with PMR will show signs of temporal arteritis either on presentation or on biopsy.

PMR and temporal arteritis are two to three times more common in women than men, with the lifetime risk of developing temporal arteritis to be ~1% in women. The annual incidence of temporal arteritis is ~18 in 100,000 people over the age of 50, while the annual incidence of PMR tends to be more variable, ranging anywhere from 12 to 68 in 100,000 people. Both disorders are more common in patients of Northern European descent.

PATHOPHYSIOLOGY

The exact pathogenesis of PMR and temporal arteritis remains unknown, but environmental and genetic factors play a role. Certain viral illnesses, including varicella zoster virus and parvovirus, may play a role, given the cyclical and seasonal pattern as well as clustering of cases of temporal arteritis. Though some studies have purported to show evidence of viral sequences in temporal artery biopsy specimens, a causal relationship has not been proven.

Genetic studies show an increased prevalence of these diseases in both Northern European patients and among siblings. PMR and temporal arteritis have both been found to have a genetic association with the **human leukocyte antigen DR (HLA-DR) gene.** There is a sequence polymorphism in the hypervariable region *HLA-DRB1* gene that is more common in both diseases and that differs from predisposing polymorphisms seen in rheumatoid arthritis.

Both clinical syndromes also show similar inflammatory responses at the cellular level. In temporal arteritis, T-cell activation, perhaps triggered by a specific antigen, results in the release of various cytokines, including interferon-γ (IFN-γ). These cytokines subsequently activate macrophages that migrate to the inner layers of the vessels and result in the inflammatory response and organization of T cells and macrophages into granulomata. In PMR, there is a similar inflammatory response with the release of cytokines and macrophages, but inflammation is limited to the articular and periarticular tissues and does not involve the vasculature. IFN-γ seems to play a key role in the development of vasculitis, as it is found in the arterial walls of inflamed temporal arteries.

PRESENTATION, EVALUATION, AND DIAGNOSIS

Patients with PMR typically present with stiffness in the shoulders, hips, and neck (Fig. 109.1). The stiffness occurs in the mornings, after periods of inactivity, and lasts at least 30 minutes. The stiffness limits patients' abilities to perform activities of daily living, including rising from bed, combing their hair, or dressing themselves. Symptoms slowly improve throughout the day but can recrudesce if patients become sedentary. Typically, there are no physical findings, but some patients will have limitation in active abduction of the shoulders. Polymyalgia is a misnomer in that patients have normal strength and normal musculature; the pathology is in the articular and periarticular structures.

Patients with temporal arteritis may complain of head aches, jaw claudication, or scalp tenderness. Headaches

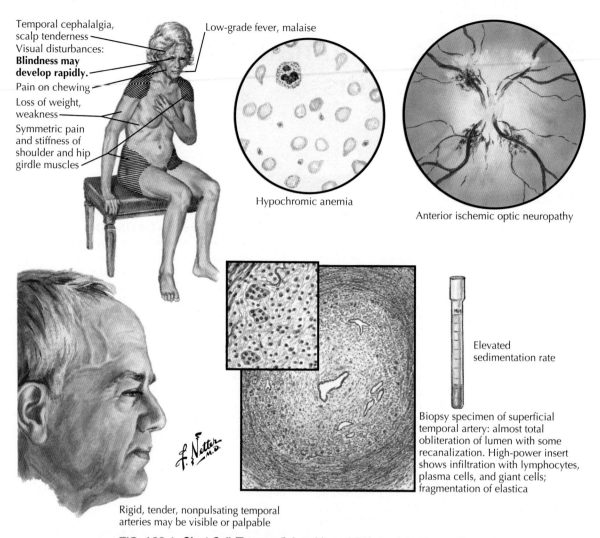

Temporal cephalalgia, scalp tenderness

Visual disturbances: **Blindness may develop rapidly.**

Pain on chewing

Loss of weight, weakness

Symmetric pain and stiffness of shoulder and hip girdle muscles

Low-grade fever, malaise

Hypochromic anemia

Anterior ischemic optic neuropathy

Elevated sedimentation rate

Biopsy specimen of superficial temporal artery: almost total obliteration of lumen with some recanalization. High-power insert shows infiltration with lymphocytes, plasma cells, and giant cells; fragmentation of elastica

Rigid, tender, nonpulsating temporal arteries may be visible or palpable

FIG. 109.1 **Giant Cell (Temporal) Arteritis and Polymyalgia Rheumatica.**

are seen in about two-thirds of patients and can vary in both quality and severity. Patients will sometimes have a tender and visibly swollen temporal artery. About 50% of patients with temporal arteritis will have symptoms of jaw claudication and pain with chewing or talking. Complete, irreversible monocular vision loss is the dreaded complication of temporal arteritis and typically presents without warning. However, rare patients will have transient episodes of altered vision, and these must be treated as an emergency.

Constitutional symptoms, including fatigue, fevers, malaise, and weight loss, are commonly seen in both illnesses. Although there are characteristic symptoms for both PMR and temporal arteritis, other diseases can

mimic these conditions; thus it is important to keep a broad differential diagnosis. Other forms of inflammatory arthritis may present similarly to PMR, while Takayasu arteritis and other small-vessel to medium-vessel vasculitides may sometimes present similarly to temporal arteritis (see Chapter 110 for details). Malignancy and infections should also be considered in the differential.

The workup for patients with PMR or temporal arteritis should include a thorough physical examination, with particular attention to the musculoskeletal, neurological, and vascular examination. If any vascular abnormalities, such as bruits, are found, further evaluation for temporal arteritis should be done. Basic lab workup should include basic chemistries and complete blood count, as well

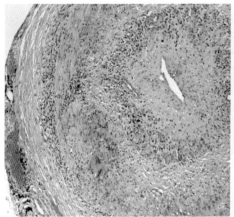

Giant cell arteritis in a temporal artery biopsy stained with H&E. Note the mononuclear cells and giant cells in the infiltrate

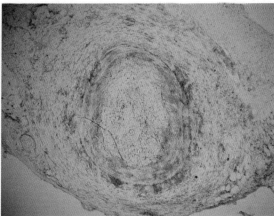

Special stains were used to demonstrate IFN-γ *(brown coloring)*. Other cytokines such as IL17, IL1, IL6, TGF-β, and PDGF are also present but not demonstrated in this example

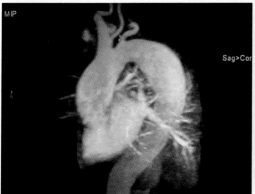

MR angiogram of the aorta and its primary branches in a patient with giant cell arteritis and an aortic root aneurysm

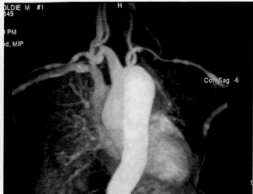

MR image demonstrating bilateral subclavian artery stenosis in a patient with giant cell arteritis

FIG. 109.2 **Imaging of Polymyalgia Rheumatica and Giant Cell Arteritis.** *H&E,* Hematoxylin and eosin; *IFN-γ,* interferon-γ; *IL,* interleukin; *PDGF,* platelet-derived growth factor; *TGF-β;* transforming growth factor-β.

as creatine kinase (CK), thyroid-stimulating hormone (TSH), and serum protein electrophoresis (SPEP) to rule out other causes that may mimic conditions like PMR. Rheumatoid factor and anticyclic citrullinated peptide (anti-CCP) will be negative in PMR patients and point more toward rheumatoid arthritis.

There are no labs that are specific to the diagnosis of PMR or temporal arteritis, but patients almost always have elevated inflammatory markers: **erythrocyte sedimentation rate (ESR)** >40 and/or elevated **C-reactive protein (CRP)**. Patients may also have anemia, leukocytosis, and mildly elevated liver function tests. While elevated inflammatory markers are not specific to either condition, they are sufficiently sensitive that when normal, most often these diseases can be excluded. PMR is usually diagnosed clinically with a characteristic history, the absence of weakness and joint swelling, and elevated inflammatory markers. For temporal arteritis, if the suspicion is high, the gold standard for diagnosis is a temporal artery biopsy. Imaging studies, including Doppler ultrasound, MRI/MR angiography (MRA), and positron-emission tomography (PET)–CT, may be useful in showing signs of vascular inflammation but are not required in diagnosing these conditions (Fig. 109.2).

TREATMENT

The goal of treatment for both PMR and temporal arteritis is to reduce the inflammatory response. Glucocorticoids are the main treatment option. For PMR, treatment with low-dose prednisone (10–20 mg daily) will help control symptoms within a few days and will immediately help improve patient functioning. Patients with temporal arteritis, on the other hand, usually require higher doses of prednisone, sometimes even intravenous (IV) steroids, to control symptoms. Given the risk for blindness, treatment should be started immediately if the concern for temporal arteritis is high and should not be delayed until biopsy results return. High-dose steroids are usually continued for at least 2 to 4 weeks prior to tapering, assuming symptoms are controlled and inflammatory markers normalize. The length and course of treatment depends on clinical symptoms and improvement of inflammatory markers, but often 1 to 2 years of treatment are required.

Steroid-sparing treatments, including methotrexate, cyclophosphamide, and the interleukin-6 (IL6) receptor antibody tocilizumab, have been studied for the treatment of temporal arteritis. Tocilizumab shows promise as a treatment for patients who cannot tolerate high doses of steroids. Low-dose aspirin is also of benefit in reducing ischemic-related complications.

CHAPTER 110

Vasculitides

ELENA K. JOERNS

INTRODUCTION

Vasculitides are potentially life-threatening inflammatory diseases of the vasculature, including arteries, veins, and capillaries. As these vessels reside in every organ, vasculitis can cause a variety of symptoms ranging from limited cutaneous symptoms to severe organ dysfunction and failure. Vasculitides are classified according to the size of the vessel involved, clinical patterns of organ involvement, and characteristic laboratory findings. Treatment usually consists of immunosuppressive medications along with supportive care.

PATHOPHYSIOLOGY

Vasculitis is an invasion of blood vessels by inflammatory cells, leading to luminal narrowing and obstruction, tissue ischemia, and infarction. Vessels of different sizes may be involved, resulting in distinct and characteristic disease manifestations. The mechanisms involved in the pathogenesis of vasculitides include cell-mediated, immune complex–mediated, and antibody-mediated invasion and destruction of involved tissues.

Large-vessel vasculitides include **Takayasu arteritis** and giant cell arteritis (GCA) (see Chapter 109 for further details). **Medium-vessel vasculitides** include **polyarteritis nodosa (PAN)** and **Kawasaki disease.** **Small-vessel vasculitides** comprise several heterogeneous entities, including **Goodpasture disease, antineutrophil cytoplasmic antibody (ANCA)**–associated, and immune complex–mediated vasculitides. **Behçet disease** may involve vessels of any size.

Large-Vessel Vasculitides

Takayasu arteritis and GCA are granulomatous, large-vessel vasculitides that involve the aorta and its major branches. The pathogenesis is as yet unknown, but one hypothesis is that perforin-secreting cytotoxic T lymphocytes that target the media and adventitia of the affected blood vessels may be involved.

Medium-Vessel Vasculitides

Kawasaki disease is a medium-vessel vasculitis affecting children and with predilection for coronary arteries. One of the proposed etiologies for Kawasaki disease is an infectious trigger leading to a cascade of inflammatory cytokines. This inflammatory milieu damages the coronary vessel intima, and dysregulated fibrosis of the inflamed area leads to stenosis and **coronary artery aneurysms** (Fig. 110.1).

PAN is a necrotizing, medium-vessel vasculitis occurring in adults that tends to spare the lungs. Hepatitis B infection is a frequent trigger for the onset of the disease, and immune complexes are believed to play a role in pathogenesis.

Small-Vessel Vasculitides

Goodpasture disease is a small-vessel vasculitis, which results from a pathological antibody directed against basement membranes principally found in the lungs and kidneys and frequently associated with human leukocyte antigen serotype DR15 (HLA-DR15). Immune complexes attach to vascular walls, activate complement, and recruit neutrophils, leading to inflammation and tissue damage. Other small-vessel vasculitides associated with antibodies and immune complexes include **cryoglobulinemic vasculitis, immunoglobulin A (IgA) vasculitis** (or Henoch-Schönlein purpura), and **hypersensitivity** (or urticarial) **vasculitis.**

Cryoglobulinemic vasculitis involves immune complexes with cryoglobulins, or antibodies that precipitate in vitro while at temperatures below body temperature (37°C). There are three classes of cryoglobulins:
- Type I exists in the setting of hematological malignancy.
- Type II is associated with viral infections, such as hepatitis C.
- Type III is more common in autoimmune diseases such as systemic lupus erythematosus (SLE) or rheumatoid arthritis.

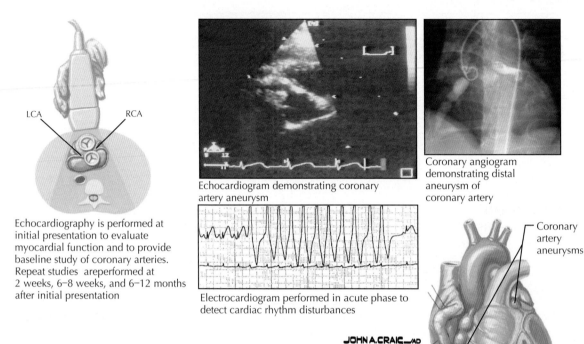

Echocardiogram demonstrating coronary artery aneurysm

Coronary angiogram demonstrating distal aneurysm of coronary artery

Echocardiography is performed at initial presentation to evaluate myocardial function and to provide baseline study of coronary arteries. Repeat studies areperformed at 2 weeks, 6–8 weeks, and 6–12 months after initial presentation

Electrocardiogram performed in acute phase to detect cardiac rhythm disturbances

Coronary artery aneurysms

JOHN A.CRAIG—AD

Coronary angiography is useful in detecting distal aneurysms of coronary arteries not easily detected by echocardiography

FIG. 110.1 **Evaluation in Kawasaki Disease.** *LCA,* Left coronary artery; *RCA,* right coronary artery.

Immune complexes in IgA vasculitis are composed primarily of IgA and usually present after an upper respiratory illness. Hypersensitivity vasculitis features immune complex deposition in response to a known or unknown antigen; eosinophils may be involved early in the disease course.

Pauciimmune small-vessel vasculitides are also known as ANCA-associated vasculitides due to frequent identification of ANCA in the serum of affected patients. Multiple studies have suggested that ANCA play a central role in pathogenesis, but exact details are unclear. Key diseases in this group are **granulomatosis with polyangiitis (GPA, formerly Wegener granulomatosis), microscopic polyangiitis (MPA), and eosinophilic GPA (EGPA, formerly Churg-Strauss syndrome).** The pathological hallmark of GPA is inflammation of small-to-medium vessels with formation of necrotizing granulomas (Fig. 110.2). EGPA also features granulomatous inflammation of blood vessels but demonstrates characteristic hypereosinophilia, suggesting an atopic trigger. MPA is a small-vessel vasculitis that lacks granulomas.

Variable-Vessel Vasculitis

Behçet disease is a necrotizing vasculitis that may involve blood vessels of any size. It is believed to be an autoinflammatory disease triggered by infection in genetically predisposed individuals. In addition to vasculitis, Behçet disease typically causes venous and arterial thromboses, presumably due to vascular inflammation. The exact pathogenesis of Behçet disease is unknown, but there is evidence that immune complex deposition, mediated by Th1 and Th17 lymphocytes and their cytokines, drives vessel damage (Fig. 110.3).

PRESENTATION, EVALUATION, AND DIAGNOSIS

Vasculitides have a range of clinical presentations depending on the organ affected. All vasculitides tend to present with constitutional symptoms such as fevers, fatigue, and weight loss, which are indicative of ongoing inflammatory process. In general, large-vessel vasculitides present with diminished pulses, bruits, asymmetric hypertension, and

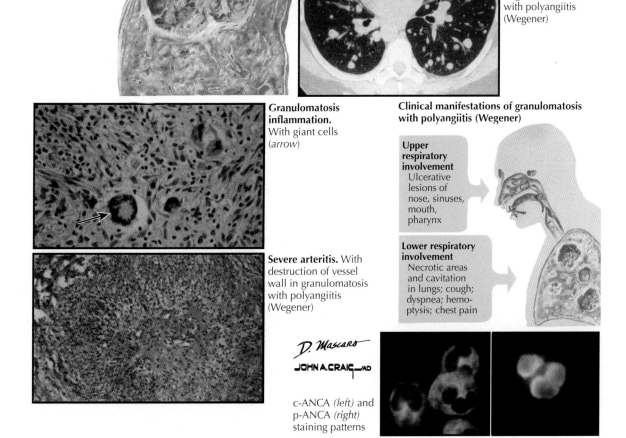

Granulomatosis with polyangiitis (Wegener). Cavity in upper lobe of right lung lined with necrotic material

High-resolution computed tomography pattern of multiple, bilateral pulmonary nodules in granulomatosis with polyangiitis (Wegener)

Granulomatosis inflammation. With giant cells (*arrow*)

Clinical manifestations of granulomatosis with polyangiitis (Wegener)

Upper respiratory involvement Ulcerative lesions of nose, sinuses, mouth, pharynx

Lower respiratory involvement Necrotic areas and cavitation in lungs; cough; dyspnea; hemoptysis; chest pain

Severe arteritis. With destruction of vessel wall in granulomatosis with polyangiitis (Wegener)

D. Mascaro

JOHN A. CRAIG—AD

c-ANCA *(left)* and p-ANCA *(right)* staining patterns

FIG. 110.2 **Clinical and Histological Features of Granulomatosis With Polyangiitis.** *c-ANCA,* Cytoplasmic antineutrophil cytoplasmic antibody; *p-ANCA,* perinuclear antineutrophil cytoplasmic antibody.

limb claudication. Medium-vessel vasculitides tend to manifest with skin ulcers, digital gangrene, hypertension, and mononeuritis multiplex. Small-vessel vasculitides often involve the lung and cause both glomerulonephritis and a purpuric rash.

When evaluating a patient for vasculitis, important things to consider are patient age, demographics, concomitant infection (such as hepatitis B or C), and the organs affected. Given the protean symptoms, multiple other pathological processes are often on the differential diagnosis with vasculitis, including microangiopathic

processes (e.g., disseminated intravascular coagulation), infections (including endocarditis), and malignancies (including lymphoma).

For details on clinical characteristics of the various vasculitides, see Table 110.1.

Symptoms

Skin manifestations are rare in large-vessel vasculitides and may overlap in medium-vessel and small-vessel vasculitides. Skin involvement in medium-vessel vasculitides is frequent and usually presents as **livedo reticularis**

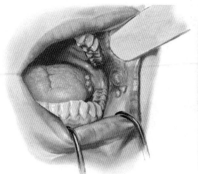

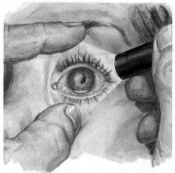

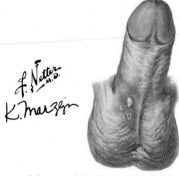

Aphthous ulcers can be found on the lips, tongue, and inside of the cheek. Aphthous ulcers may occur singly or in clusters but occur in virtually all patients with Behçet disease.

Behçet disease may cause anterior uveitis (inflammation in the front of the eye). Anterior uveitis results in pain, blurry vision, light sensitivity, tearing, or redness of the eye.

Painful genital lesions may form on the scrotum, similar to oral lesions, but deeper. Lesions appear as red, ulcerated sores. The genital sores are usually painful and may leave scars.

FIG. 110.3 **Clinical Features of Behçet Disease.**

(lacelike purplish discoloration), cutaneous painful nodules, ulcers, and digital gangrene. Skin findings in small-vessel vasculitides include **palpable purpura** (dark, nonblanching painful rash, more pronounced in dependent areas), necrotizing granulomatous (punched-out) lesions, or urticaria. Musculoskeletal complaints include myalgias, arthralgias, or arthritis in one or more joints. Frank myositis may occur in cases of medium-vessel vasculitis.

Gastrointestinal complaints manifest as abdominal pain, mucosal ulcerations, or mesenteric ischemia. While glomerulonephritis is a typical renal manifestation in small-vessel vasculitides, renovascular hypertension may occur in large-vessel and medium-vessel vasculitides. Other renal manifestations include proteinuria, hematuria, and interstitial nephritis. Neuropathy is a common complaint and can present as mononeuritis multiplex or polyneuropathies of both sensory and motor nerves; peripheral neuropathy is more common than central nervous system (CNS) involvement. Ocular involvement ranges from conjunctivitis and **uveitis** to retinal artery occlusion.

Diagnostic Workup

No single laboratory test can confirm the presence or absence of vasculitis, so diagnosis instead depends on a constellation of symptoms, laboratory findings, and biopsy to differentiate the cause. Erythrocyte sedimentation rate (ESR) and C-reactive protein (CRP) are elevated. Blood counts will frequently show a leukocytosis, anemia of chronic disease, and/or thrombocytosis, but

pancytopenia should prompt concern for underlying SLE. Chemistries can demonstrate renal dysfunction, and liver function tests can show hepatitis from viral infection or autoimmune involvement. Urinalysis can evaluate hematuria, proteinuria, and the presence of casts suggestive of glomerular involvement. Other tests to order include antinuclear antibody (ANA), rheumatoid factor (RF), hepatitis B/C, HIV, Epstein-Barr virus (EBV), herpes simplex virus (HSV) and parvovirus B19 serologies, and cryoglobulin levels.

ANCAs are necessary for the workup of suspected small-vessel vasculitis. ANCAs are separated into **antimyeloperoxidase (MPO,** formerly called p-ANCA) and **antiserine protease 3 (PR3,** formerly called c-ANCA) **antibodies.** Complement levels (C3 and C4) can be low in hypersensitivity vasculitis and cryoglobulinemic vasculitis.

Chest radiography can evaluate for pulmonary involvement such as **diffuse alveolar hemorrhage (DAH).** MRI of the brain should be obtained if one suspects CNS involvement, and MR angiography of the chest/abdomen/pelvis if one suspects involvement of the aorta or of the abdominal vasculature. A biopsy of an affected organ (especially skin, given the ease of biopsy) is tremendously important, as the immunosuppressive regimens are toxic.

TREATMENT

Treatment of systemic forms of vasculitis requires prompt and aggressive immunosuppressive therapy with

TABLE 110.1
Clinical Characteristics of the Various Vasculitides

Disease	Vessel Size/Type Biopsy Findings	Clinical Characteristics	Induction Treatment
Takayasu arteritis	• Large, including aorta and its branches • DX: Granulomatous arteritis with skip lesions	• Women <45 years, often Asian descent • Preceding constitutional symptoms for years • Hypertension • Limb claudication with normal activity • Asymmetric pulses and bruits • Angiography shows stenosis of aorta and its branches	• Corticosteroids
Kawasaki disease	• Medium, with predilection for coronary arteries • BX: Usually not performed; perivascular lymphocytic infiltrate	• Children with fevers unresponsive to antibiotics • Strawberry tongue, rash on trunk, conjunctivitis, cervical lymphadenopathy, desquamative rash on palms/soles • Coronary artery aneurysms • Myopericarditis	• High-dose aspirin • IVIG • Corticosteroids
Polyarteritis nodosa	• Medium, tends to spare the lungs • BX: Focal and segmental fibrinoid necrosis of vessel wall	• Hepatitis B as trigger • Palpable purpura and livedo reticularis • Mononeuritis multiplex • Mesenteric ischemia • Renovascular hypertension, no glomerulonephritis • Testicular tenderness	• Treat hepatitis B in case of HBV-associated PAN • High-dose corticosteroids • Cyclophosphamide, rituximab
Behçet disease	• Variable • BX: Neutrophilic vasculitis	• Mediterranean or Asian descent • Aphthous oral and genital ulcers • Uveitis • Erythema nodosum-like skin lesions • Pulmonary artery aneurysms • Positive pathergy test	• Corticosteroids • Colchicine • Azathioprine • Mycophenolate mofetil • Cyclosporine • Tacrolimus • Infliximab • Rituximab
ANCA-ASSOCIATED VASCULITIS			
GPA (granulomatosis with polyangiitis)	• Small • BX: Necrotizing granulomas, crescents on kidney biopsy	• Upper airway involvement with saddle nose deformity • Sensorineural hearing loss, mononeuritis multiplex • DAH less common than in MPA • Rapidly progressive glomerulonephritis → ESRD • (+) PR3 antibodies	• Corticosteroids • Cyclophosphamide • Rituximab

Continued

TABLE 110.1
Clinical Characteristics of the Various Vasculitides—cont'd

Disease	Vessel Size/Type Biopsy Findings	Clinical Characteristics	Induction Treatment
MPA (microscopic polyangiitis)	• Small • BX: Focal segmental necrotizing vasculitis, crescents on kidney biopsy	• DAH common • Rapidly progressive crescentic glomerulonephritis • (+) MPO antibodies	• Corticosteroids • Cyclophosphamide • Rituximab
EGPA (eosinophilic granulomatosis with polyangiitis)	• Small • BX: Leukocytoclastic vasculitis, eosinophilia; granulomas can be present	• Atopic symptoms, including asthma, atopic dermatitis, or allergic rhinitis • Peripheral eosinophilia • Renal involvement is uncommon	• Corticosteroids • Cyclophosphamide
ANTIBODY-MEDIATED VASCULITIS			
Goodpasture disease	• Small • BX: Linear staining of the IgG and complement deposits along the basement membrane on glomerular immunofluorescence	• Pulmonary-renal syndrome with diffuse alveolar hemorrhage • Rapidly progressive glomerulonephritis	• Plasmapheresis • Corticosteroids • Cyclophosphamide • Rituximab
IMMUNE COMPLEX–MEDIATED VASCULITIS			
IgA vasculitis	• Small • BX: leukocytoclastic vasculitis with IgA and C3 deposits on immunofluorescence	• Children with preceding upper respiratory illness • Purpuric rash primarily on lower extremities and in dependent areas • Abdominal pain from migrating ischemia • Glomerulonephritis • Arthritis	• Frequently self-limited • Corticosteroids for renal involvement. • NSAIDs for arthritis
Hypersensitivity (urticarial) vasculitis	• Small • BX: leukocytoclastic vasculitis in background of dermal edema	• Urticarial-like wheals >24 hours • Angioedema • Complement low-normal	• Antihistamines • NSAIDs • Corticosteroids • Dapsone
Cryoglobulinemic vasculitis	• Small • BX: leukocytoclastic vasculitis, intraluminal cryoglobulin deposits	• Associated with HCV infection and lymphoproliferative disorders • Elevated cryoglobulins in serum • Palpable purpura • Painful sensory polyneuropathy • Glomerulonephritis • Polyarthralgias	• Treat the underlying disease/infection • Corticosteroids • Plasmapheresis • Cyclophosphamide • Rituximab

ANCA, Antineutrophil cytoplasmic antibody; *BX,* biopsy; *DAH,* diffuse alveolar hemorrhage; *ESRD,* end-stage renal disease; *HBV,* hepatitis B virus; *HCV,* hepatitis C virus; *IgA,* immunoglobulin A; *IgG,* immunoglobulin G; *IVIG,* intravenous immunoglobulin; *NSAIDs,* nonsteroidal antiinflammatory drugs; *PAN,* polyarteritis nodosa.

high-dose corticosteroids, as well as additional agents such as rituximab, cyclophosphamide, mycophenolate mofetil, azathioprine, or other immunosuppressive medications. In addition, plasmapheresis for removal of existing autoantibodies is used in antiglomerular basement membrane (anti-GBM) disease and cryoglobulinemic vasculitis. Plasmapheresis was utilized in ANCA-associated vasculitis management with life-threatening complications such as alveolar hemorrhage, but recent data suggest absence of benefit from plasma exchange in ANCA-associated vasculitides.

In cases of vasculitides associated with infection, such as hepatitis B or C, treatment of infection will often result in resolution of vasculitis. Kawasaki disease is treated with high doses of **aspirin** in addition to **intravenous immunoglobulin (IVIG).** Refractory cases may receive high-dose corticosteroids.

CHAPTER 111

Sepsis

DANIEL J. TURNER

INTRODUCTION

Sepsis is a complex clinical syndrome in which a dysregulated host response to infection leads to life-threatening organ dysfunction. The paradigm for understanding sepsis has shifted in recent years in an attempt to distinguish this pathological and maladaptive process from the host's appropriate response to infection.

Sepsis develops after the host detects a microbial pathogen and produces an **inflammatory response** that becomes harmful as it intensifies. The incidence of sepsis and the extent to which it manifests depends on host comorbidities, infectious exposures, and immune system integrity. Sepsis that leads to persistent hypotension despite fluid resuscitation is termed **septic shock,** a distinct clinical entity associated with substantially increased mortality.

With more than 1 million new cases in the United States each year, sepsis is an increasingly recognized public health problem. This is partly attributable to a population that lives longer with chronic diseases and has more exposure to immunosuppressive drugs, indwelling catheters, and medical devices. Because patients with sepsis present across the spectrum of health care settings, all providers should be familiar with its evaluation, diagnosis, and management.

PATHOPHYSIOLOGY

The innate immune system triggers many of the physiological changes encountered in sepsis. Macrophages, granulocytes, and other innate immune cells have surface receptors (e.g., Toll-like receptor 4) that detect molecular microbial markers (e.g., endotoxin on gram-negative bacteria). These interactions activate signal transduction cascades that produce cytokines, recruit immune cells, and activate the endothelium to mount a local inflammatory response. This response includes improved leukocyte adhesion, vasodilation, increased capillary permeability,

and microvascular thrombosis to prevent hematogenous microbial spread (Fig. 111.1).

As inflammation intensifies to control local infection, it may spread systemically and become harmful to the host. Endothelial dysfunction leads to widespread loss of barrier function, precipitating diffuse interstitial edema and lowering systemic vascular resistance resulting in relative hypovolemia and **hypotension**. These circulatory changes produce a compensatory increase in adrenergic tone and heart rate in an attempt to maintain cardiac output. Inflammation-mediated epithelial dysfunction exacerbates this edematous state and promotes organ damage. For example, protein-rich edema leaking from alveolar capillaries fills the interstitial space and eventually the pulmonary airspace. This reduces lung compliance, impairs gas exchange, and induces ventilation-perfusion mismatch that can progress to **acute respiratory distress syndrome (ARDS)** (see Chapter 91 for details). Uncontrolled microvascular thrombosis can lead to consumptive coagulopathy and **disseminated intravascular coagulation. Acute kidney injury** is common, due to microvascular and tubular dysfunction and can progress to renal failure.

Substantial metabolic changes occur as affected patients become critically ill. Heightened adrenergic tone impairs tissue extraction of oxygen and increases anaerobic metabolism, which, along with hypoperfusion, contributes to elevated **lactate**. Patients may become adrenally insufficient and have refractory hypotension. High levels of circulating catecholamine and cytokines produce a catabolic state that, combined with immobility seen in prolonged hospital stays, leads to loss of muscle mass.

Despite the clear role of overactive inflammation in the pathogenesis of sepsis, increasing evidence indicates a more complex underlying interplay between proinflammatory and antiinflammatory responses. The immune system contains capacity to control inflammatory response and prevent injury at distant sites, and these

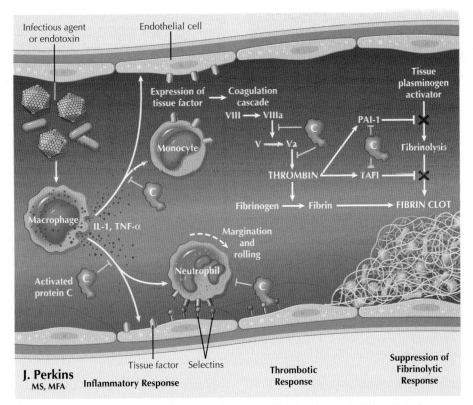

FIG. 111.1 **Dysregulated Immune Response in Sepsis.** *IL-1*, Interleukin-1; *PAI-1*, plasminogen activator inhibitor-1; *TNF-α*, tumor necrosis factor-α.

mechanisms are active within hours of sepsis onset. The mechanism by which this balance becomes dysregulated is a focus of ongoing investigation. Current data indicate that in early sepsis the balance favors inflammation, whereas later in the natural history of disease, antiinflammatory mediators predominate and patients become immunosuppressed. This can lead to a self-perpetuating process with disastrous consequences.

PRESENTATION, EVALUATION, AND DIAGNOSIS

Sepsis can occur in individuals with or without underlying medical comorbidities. Those patients with suboptimal immune function have an increased incidence of sepsis with severe sequelae. This applies especially to patients at the extremes of age and those with comorbidities such as cirrhosis, diabetes, HIV/AIDS, cancer, and autoimmune disease that may disrupt the body's immune response. Alcohol use is a well-documented risk factor for sepsis-related morbidity and mortality.

Patients present with symptoms of specific infection and superimposed signs of systemic illness such as fever or hypothermia, tachycardia, tachypnea, hypotension, and altered mental status without focal deficits. Notably, the presentation is variable and those patients with underlying immune compromise may have subtler presentations. Patients with systemic signs and no obvious source should be evaluated for infection with blood cultures, chest imaging, urinalysis and cultures, and a careful history/physical exam to guide further imaging. Importantly, these signs of systemic illness may be present in noninfectious, yet still life-threatening conditions, including pancreatitis, mesenteric ischemia, vasculitis, malignancy, and thromboembolism.

Laboratory testing commonly reveals leukocytosis or, less commonly, leukopenia. White blood cell differential typically reveals neutrophil predominance or the presence of peripheral bands (a so-called **left shift**). An initial respiratory alkalosis due to hyperventilation gives way to an anion gap metabolic acidosis as lactic acid accumulates. Hyperglycemia is common in diabetic

BOX 111.1
Systemic Inflammatory Response Syndrome (SIRS)

Requires two or more of the following criteria:
- Temperature >38°C or <36°C
- HR >90
- RR >20 or $PaCO_2$ <32 mm Hg
- WBC >12,000, <4000, or >10% bands

HR, Heart rate; *PaCO₂*, partial pressure of oxygen; *RR*, respiratory rate; *SIRS*, systemic inflammatory response syndrome; *WBC*, white blood cell count.
Modified from Bone RC, Balk RA, Cerra FB, et al: American College of Chest Physicians/Society of Critical Care Medicine Consensus Conference: definitions for sepsis and organ failure and guidelines for the use of innovative therapies in sepsis, *Crit Care Med* 20(6):864–874, 1992.

TABLE 111.1
SOFA and qSOFA Scoring Tools

Score	qSOFA	SOFA
Clinical Use	Identify sepsis in non-ICU settings	Recognize organ dysfunction, predict morbidity and mortality in ICU
Positive Test	Two or more criteria	Change of two or more from baseline
Criteria	• AMS • RR ≥22 • Systolic BP ≤100	• PaO_2/FiO_2 • Platelet count • GCS • Bilirubin • Hypotension/pressors • Creatinine/UOP

AMS, Altered mental status; *BP*, blood pressure; *FiO₂*, fraction of inspired oxygen; *GCS*, Glasgow Coma Scale; *ICU*, intensive care unit; *PaO₂*, partial pressure of oxygen; *qSOFA*, Quick Sequential Organ Failure Assessment; *RR*, respiratory rate; *SOFA*, Sequential Organ Failure Assessment score; *UOP*, urine output.
Data from Singer M, Deutschman CS, Seymour CW, et al: The Third International Consensus Definitions for Sepsis and Septic Shock (Sepsis-3), *JAMA* 315(8):801–810, 2016.

patients, while others (especially the elderly) may be hypoglycemic. Other abnormal lab values correlate with the degree of sepsis-related organ dysfunction, such as reduced $PaO_2{:}FiO_2$ ratio on arterial blood gas or elevations in serum creatinine and bilirubin. Transaminases may be elevated in the setting of profound hypotension due to ischemic liver injury.

The diagnosis of sepsis technically requires microbiological confirmation of infection with objective evidence of related organ dysfunction. Because of its high morbidity and mortality in untreated patients, empiric sepsis management is usually initiated while microbiological data are pending. Historically, criteria for the **systemic inflammatory response syndrome (SIRS)** with a suspected infectious source was sufficient to presumptively diagnose sepsis (Box 111.1). While these criteria are still practically helpful, recent guidelines have shifted away from identifying the presence or absence of sepsis toward quickly identifying patients at greatest risk for morbidity and mortality due to potential sepsis. The **quick Sequential Organ Failure Assessment (qSOFA) score** is helpful in the non–intensive care unit (ICU) setting, while the full **SOFA score** helps identify organ dysfunction and predict prognosis in the ICU (Table 111.1).

TREATMENT

Sepsis management has been marked by significant advances in recent decades. In 2001, the landmark study by Rivers et al. on **early goal-directed therapy (EGDT)** played a critical role in propagating a vision for standardized treatment algorithm. Questions arose as to which component of EGDT was most responsible

for improved mortality, and the increased interest in sepsis spurred the development of the Surviving Sepsis Campaign in 2002. That campaign's subsequent guidelines and emphasis on bundles of care has led to significant improvement in outcomes, and subsequent trials (including PROCESS [2014], ARISE [2014], and PROMISE [2015]) have supported the principles of rapid identification, fluid resuscitation, and early antibiotics (Table 111.2).

Broad-spectrum intravenous antibiotics should be administered immediately after cultures are drawn (preferably within 1 hour of identifying sepsis), as delaying antibiotics has a well-documented association with increased mortality. Antibiotics should be chosen based on the patient's symptoms, local resistance patterns, and host-specific risk factors such as level of immunosuppression or unique infectious exposures. Infectious source control is critical, and appropriate attention should be given to the need for abscess drainage or device removal.

Resuscitation with isotonic crystalloid solution should be initiated immediately. The recommended initial quantity is 30 mL/kg (to be given in the first 3 hours) but total requirement varies per patient, and additional volume should be given based on hemodynamic reassessment. Resuscitation can be titrated to surrogate markers for adequate end-organ perfusion, including lactate clearance, urine output (UOP) of 0.5 mL/kg/hr,

TABLE 111.2
Surviving Sepsis Campaign Bundles 2016

To be completed within 3 hours	1. Measure lactate level 2. Obtain blood cultures prior to antibiotics 3. Administer broad-spectrum antibiotics 4. Administer 30 mL/kg crystalloid for hypotension or lactate ≥4 mmol/L

To be completed within 6 hours	5. Apply vasopressors (for refractory hypotension) to maintain MAP ≥65 mm Hg
	6. In the event of persistent hypotension or initial lactate ≥4 mmol/L, reassess volume status and tissue perfusion with one of the following:
	  a. Serial focused exam findings
	  b. CVP
	  c. Central venous oxygen saturation
	  d. Bedside IVC ultrasound
	  e. Passive leg raise or fluid challenge
	7. Remeasure lactate if initial lactate was elevated

CVP, Central venous pressure; *IVC,* inferior vena cava; *MAP,* mean arterial pressure.
Data from Rhodes A, Evans LE, Alhazzani W, et al: Surviving Sepsis Campaign: International Guidelines for Management of Sepsis and Septic Shock: 2016, *Crit Care Med* 45(3):486–552, 2017.

central venous oxygen saturation ($ScVO_2$), and central venous pressure (CVP) of 8 to 12 mm Hg. However, dynamic measures, including ultrasound of the inferior vena cava (IVC) and passive leg raise to simulate a fluid bolus, are increasingly accepted. The goal mean arterial pressure (MAP) for patients with sepsis is >65 mm Hg, and patients with a suboptimal MAP despite fluid resuscitation may require the addition of vasopressors, with norepinephrine as a first-line agent. Multiple studies have shown that increasing oxygen delivery with red blood cell transfusions and routine use of inotropes, part of the original EGDT algorithm, did not improve outcomes.

Some patients will require organ-specific support, such as low tidal volume mechanical ventilation for respiratory failure and ARDS or continuous renal replacement therapy for renal failure. Intravenous corticosteroids are recommended for persistent hypotension despite vasopressors, but studies have shown only hastened recovery from hypotension and no mortality benefit. Insulin should be used as needed to maintain blood glucose <180, and while the optimal nutrition strategy remains unclear, current consensus is to administer enteral feeding as early as tolerated.

Prognosis in sepsis is highly variable, and mortality rates correlate with age and the burden of preexisting illness. Thirty-day mortality ranges from 10% to 35%, but increases to 40% to 60% in septic shock. Further developments in the care of septic patients, including a better understanding of the underlying pathophysiology, novel therapeutics based on this understanding, and optimization of care delivery models, will be crucial to improving outcomes.

CHAPTER 112

Cellulitis

MATTHEW R. MCCULLOCH

INTRODUCTION

Cellulitis and superficial skin abscesses are among the most common infectious processes encountered in clinical medicine. Cellulitis is defined as bacterial infection of the soft tissue of the deep dermis and superficial fascia, with the epidermis generally spared.

PATHOPHYSIOLOGY

Skin and skin structure infections generally begin with a disruption of the cutaneous barrier that allows for the introduction of bacteria into normally sterile tissue. The disruption may be the result of an acute event such as an insect bite, intravenous (IV) line insertion, or trauma; it may also be the result of a more chronic process undermining skin integrity such as venous stasis ulcers (Fig. 112.1). Importantly, the disruption may be of insufficient magnitude to be noticeable to the patient or the physician.

Once pathogens enter the skin or subcutaneous tissue, they may proliferate while avoiding the integumentary immune system. The vast majority of cellulitis cases yield negative cultures of both the blood and affected site. This may be due to the relatively small infectious burden triggering the inflammatory response or to the effective control of bacteria through host defenses. In contrast to skin abscesses, cellulitis generally does not produce purulent discharge, so superficial skin cultures are largely uninterpretable.

The most common causative pathogens are *Streptococcus pyogenes* (group A streptococcus) and *S. aureus*. In immunocompromised hosts, including those with diabetes, pathogens such as *Pseudomonas aeruginosa* become more likely, though streptococcal and staphylococcal species remain predominant. *Pasteurella multocida* and *Capnocytophaga canimorsus* are common causes of cellulitis associated with animal bites, while *Aeromonas hydrophila* and *Vibrio vulnificus* can cause cellulitis associated with trauma sustained in fresh or brackish water.

RISK FACTORS

Recent studies have clarified that immunocompromised patients and diabetics are not at increased risk of acute cellulitis, even though the causative pathogens may differ as described earlier. Edema, particularly lymphedema, is the most common risk factor, as it allows bacterial proliferation in static fluid. Additional risk factors include age, obesity, homelessness (due to poor foot care and hygiene), and chronic causes of barrier disruption, such as ulcers or trauma.

PRESENTATION AND DIAGNOSIS

The diagnosis of cellulitis is primarily established based on history and physical examination. Cellulitis causes skin edema, erythema, warmth, and tenderness (Fig. 112.2). Pitting edema and bullae may sometimes occur. Providers should look for signs of purulence (pustules, abscess, or drainage), which increases the likelihood of *S. aureus* infection. In contrast, lymphangitis, or lymphatic inflammation proximal to the affected area, is more likely to be noted in cases of streptococcal infection. In cases of cellulitis of the lower extremity, a careful examination should be performed to assess for superficial causes of bacterial introduction, such as interdigital infections or skin breakdown, as these must be treated to reduce the risk of recurrence.

It is essential to distinguish cellulitis from a group of similar conditions, together known as **pseudocellulitis.** This group includes common disorders, such as stasis dermatitis, hematoma, and deep venous thrombosis, as well as the less common calciphylaxis and erythema migrans. Stasis dermatitis is usually bilateral, unlike cellulitis. Hematomas are often found in patients with a history of extremity trauma, especially those on anticoagulants, and can be confirmed by ultrasound. Deep venous thrombosis should be considered in immobile patients with unilateral pain and swelling; this can be confirmed by ultrasound. Calciphylaxis is often much

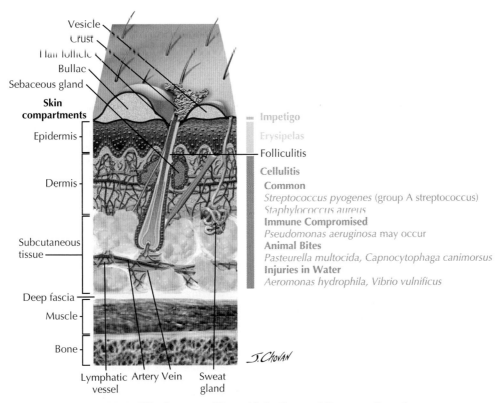

Vesicle
Crust
Hair follicle
Bullae
Sebaceous gland
Skin compartments
Epidermis
Dermis
Subcutaneous tissue
Deep fascia
Muscle
Bone

Impetigo
Erysipelas
Folliculitis
Cellulitis
Common
Streptococcus pyogenes (group A streptococcus)
Staphylococcus aureus
Immune Compromised
Pseudomonas aeruginosa may occur
Animal Bites
Pasteurella multocida, Capnocytophaga canimorsus
Injuries in Water
Aeromonas hydrophila, Vibrio vulnificus

Lymphatic vessel Artery Vein Sweat gland

J.Chovan

FIG. 112.1 **Skin Anatomy, Sites of Infection, and Common Organisms.**

more painful than cellulitis and presents as retiform purpura, as opposed to diffuse erythema; it should be considered in patients with end-stage renal disease or those taking warfarin. Erythema migrans usually causes skin erythema in a targetoid distribution, though it may present only with homogenous swelling; in either case, it should have more clearly defined borders than cellulitis.

Cellulitis should also be distinguished from other types of soft tissue infections, such as **impetigo, erysipelas,** and **ecthyma.** Impetigo, an infection of the outer keratin of the skin, is the most superficial and results in crusty lesions. Erysipelas is a slightly deeper infection involving the epidermis; however, it is still relatively superficial, and lesion borders are often quite visually sharp. In contrast, the borders of cellulitis are often vague because the epidermis itself is not directly infected. Ecthyma refers to a deep form of impetigo that descends to the dermis with a scaly, ulcerated cap.

Blood or tissue cultures, as well as swabs and biopsies, are not recommended for the routine evaluation of cellulitis. If purulence is noted, however, wound culture and

susceptibility testing should be performed to assess for methicillin-resistant *S. aureus* (MRSA) infection. Blood cultures should also be obtained in patients with immune compromise, animal bites, pain out of proportion to physical examination, crepitus, edema beyond the erythematous area, or severe disease (hypotension or rapid progression) as these may be predictive of systemic infection.

TREATMENT

The treatment of cellulitis is intended to relieve symptoms, prevent progression to necrotizing infection, and reduce the risk of complications such as disseminated infection (bacteremia, endocarditis, osteomyelitis), glomerulonephritis, toxic shock syndrome, and lymphedema.

In most cases, antibiotics are prescribed for 5 to 10 days, with longer courses reserved for immunocompromised patients or severe disease. If clinical improvement does not occur within 24 to 48 hours, treatment should be extended and possibly escalated, and alternative

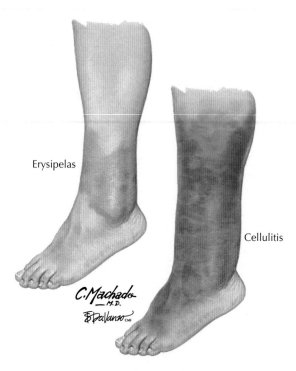

Erysipelas

Cellulitis

FIG. 112.2 **Appearance of Skin Infections.**

diagnoses should be considered. Patients meeting two or more systemic inflammatory response syndrome (SIRS) criteria (fever or hypothermia, tachycardia, tachypnea, leukocytosis, or leukopenia) or with an elevated qSOFA score may have sepsis and should be admitted and treated with IV antibiotics (see Chapter 111 for details).

Patients with nonpurulent cellulitis and no evidence of sepsis can receive outpatient oral therapy with penicillin, cephalexin, or amoxicillin-clavulanate. Those allergic to penicillin should receive clindamycin. Patients with nonpurulent cellulitis complicated by sepsis physiology requiring hospitalization and IV therapy should receive cefazolin, ceftriaxone, or penicillin G.

Patients with penetrating trauma, known staphylococcal infection, IV drug use, or purulent infection require staphylococcal coverage in addition to streptococcal coverage. The choice of therapy depends on the severity of the infection as well as the local epidemiology of community-associated MRSA. Patients with purulent cellulitis but no evidence of sepsis or known MRSA infection should receive oral cephalexin, dicloxacillin, or amoxicillin-clavulanate. If MRSA is suspected, preferred agents include trimethoprim-sulfamethoxazole or doxycycline. Clindamycin is also a reasonable alternative. Patients requiring IV therapy but without evidence of MRSA should receive oxacillin, nafcillin, or cefazolin; those with evidence of MRSA should receive vancomycin or daptomycin.

Patients with pain out of proportion to physical examination, crepitus, edema beyond the erythematous area, or severe disease require imaging and a surgical evaluation for possible necrotizing infection. The preferred antibiotic is vancomycin, with the addition of piperacillin-tazobactam for nonpurulent cases. Protein synthesis inhibitors (i.e., clindamycin) are often included as adjuvant therapy to reduce toxin formation.

CHAPTER 113

Meningitis

LAUREN PISCHEL

INTRODUCTION

Meningitis refers to inflammation of the meningeal lining of the brain and typically occurs when bacteria or viruses gain access to the immune-privileged compartment of the subarachnoid space. Less often, meningitis results from infection with parasites, spirochetes, or fungi, or from noninfectious causes such as autoimmune diseases, neoplasms, and medications. Meningitis is distinct from but can occur alongside encephalitis (inflammation of the brain parenchyma itself).

Based on initial analysis of cerebrospinal fluid (CSF), meningitis is generally classified as **acute bacterial** or **aseptic** (most often viral). The incidence of acute bacterial meningitis in 2006 to 2007 was 1.38 cases per 100,000 individuals in the United States, a decrease from the rate of 2.0 per 100,000 from 1998 to 1999. Such improvements are most likely attributable to increasing vaccination against major pathogens.

PATHOPHYSIOLOGY

The pathogens responsible for acute bacterial meningitis depend on the patient's age (Fig. 113.1), but the most frequent are *Streptococcus pneumoniae* and *Neisseria meningitidis*. These bacteria often colonize the nasopharynx and, in the setting of nasal trauma, can be transported in the bloodstream to the intraventricular choroid plexus and gain access to the subarachnoid space. Far less often, meningitis occurs by direct inoculation of bacteria during neurosurgery or from hematological dissemination of other primary infections.

Both *S. pneumoniae* and *N. meningitidis* possess a polysaccharide capsule that helps prevent phagocytosis. Once in the subarachnoid space, the bacteria easily proliferate because low levels of complement and immunoglobulins allow the bacteria to evade opsonization. The consequent release of cytokines and chemokines produces an inflammatory response that disrupts the integrity of the blood-brain barrier, permitting fluid and proteins to enter the subarachnoid space. The resulting purulent exudate occludes the subarachnoid granules, leading to hydrocephalus, cerebral edema, and increased intracranial pressure. Without prompt treatment, cerebral herniation and death may occur.

The major risk factors for *S. pneumoniae* meningitis are chronic nasal colonization, minor infection (e.g., chronic rhinosinusitis or otitis media), and immune compromise (e.g., alcoholism, complement deficiency). *N. meningitidis* typically affects individuals <30 years of age living in close quarters, such as military barracks or college dorms.

Group B streptococcus primarily affects infants and adults >50 years of age. *Haemophilus influenzae* meningitis was once relatively common in children but has become rare owing to increased vaccination rates. Among adults, risk factors for *H. influenzae* meningitis include immune compromise, chronic obstructive pulmonary disease, and alcoholism. *Listeria monocytogenes* mostly infects those at the extremes of ages, individuals with altered immune function, and pregnant women. As soft cheeses and deli meats are a major source of exposure, women are generally advised to avoid these products throughout pregnancy.

Aseptic meningitis is most often caused by viral infection, and common pathogens include herpes simplex virus (HSV), enteroviruses, arboviruses, and echoviruses. Infection is more frequent in the warmer months, correlating with increased transmission of enteroviruses and arboviruses. Subacute or chronic symptoms may suggest infection with atypical pathogens (spirochetes, mycobacteria) or noninfectious processes (malignancy, autoimmune disease, medication effects).

PRESENTATION, EVALUATION, AND DIAGNOSIS

Meningitis presents acutely (over hours) or subacutely (over days). Nearly all patients with acute bacterial meningitis will experience at least two of the following symptoms: fever, headache, neck stiffness, and altered mental status. Additional symptoms may include

485

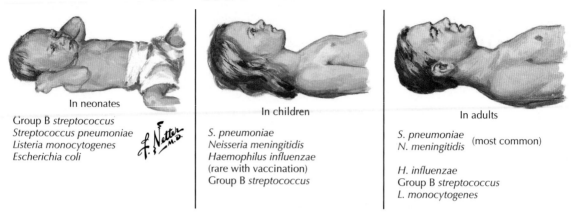

In neonates

Group B *streptococcus*
Streptococcus pneumoniae
Listeria monocytogenes
Escherichia coli

In children

S. pneumoniae
Neisseria meningitidis
Haemophilus influenzae
(rare with vaccination)
Group B *streptococcus*

In adults

S. pneumoniae
N. meningitidis (most common)

H. influenzae
Group B *streptococcus*
L. monocytogenes

FIG. 113.1 **Acute Bacterial Meningitis: Major Pathogens.**

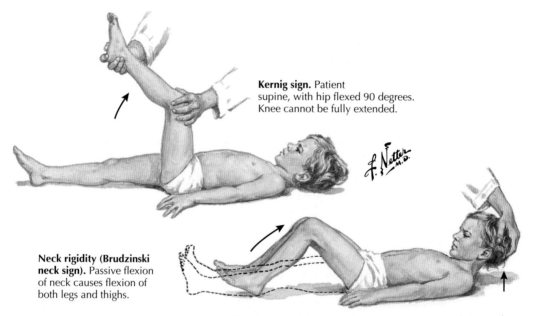

Kernig sign. Patient supine, with hip flexed 90 degrees. Knee cannot be fully extended.

Neck rigidity (Brudzinski neck sign). Passive flexion of neck causes flexion of both legs and thighs.

FIG. 113.2 **Physical Exam Maneuvers.**

photosensitivity, nausea, vomiting, focal neurological deficits, and (in rare cases) seizures.

Patients with aseptic meningitis usually have a milder presentation consisting of a frontal headache, nausea, vomiting, malaise, and myalgias. Nuchal rigidity is also less common. Elderly patients and those with immune compromise may also have subtle presentations, owing to milder degrees of meningeal inflammation.

The classic physical examination maneuvers to evaluate for meningitis are the **Kernig and Brudzinski signs**

(Fig. 113.2). The Kernig sign is noted when a supine patient with a flexed hip is reluctant to extend the knee, since doing so would increase meningeal tension. The Brudzinksi sign is noted when a supine patient flexes his or her hips or knees in response to flexion of the neck, so as to reduce meningeal tension. Although neither test is particularly sensitive, their specificity is high.

Certain pathogens also produce characteristic physical exam findings. Early in the course of *N. meningitis* infection, for example, a classic petechial rash may be noted

TABLE 113.1
Cerebrospinal Fluid Analysis

	Acute Bacterial Meningitis	Aseptic Meningitis
Opening pressure	High (>180 mm H_2O)	Normal or minimally elevated
White blood cell count	10–10,000 cells/μL with a neutrophilic predominance	10–300 cells/μL with a lymphocytic predominance
Glucose concentration	Low (<45 mg/dL)	Normal or slightly elevated (50–100 mg/dL)
Protein concentration	Elevated (100–1000 mg/dL)	Slightly elevated (50–100 mg/dL)

on the trunk and extremities. These lesions may coalesce into larger purpuric and ecchymotic lesions.

Diagnosis

Acute bacterial meningitis is a medical emergency. If the diagnosis is suspected, a **lumbar puncture (LP)** should be performed as soon as possible (see Chapter 51 for details). Those at risk of having increased intracranial pressure, however, should undergo head CT prior to LP; such patients include those with known central nervous system (CNS) malignancy, immune compromise, papilledema on exam, seizures, altered mental status, focal neurological deficits, or recent head trauma.

Patients who do not require a CT scan should receive antibiotics as soon as the LP is completed. If a CT scan is required, antibiotics should not be delayed until after the LP. As long as the duration between the initiation of antibiotics and the LP is <4 hours, the results should not be significantly altered. Two sets of blood cultures, however, should always be obtained before antibiotics are administered; in acute bacterial meningitis, peripheral blood cultures are positive in as many as 50% to 90% of cases.

The individual performing the LP should use a manometer to note the opening pressure. CSF should be submitted to the laboratory for cell count, total protein concentration, glucose concentration, Gram stain, and culture. Many laboratories now offer multiplex polymerase chain reaction (PCR) panels to rapidly assess for common bacterial, viral, and fungal pathogens. The initial CSF analyses can usually distinguish between acute bacterial and aseptic meningitis (Table 113.1); however, HSV meningitis may have a profile suggestive of acute bacterial meningitis. In cases of aseptic meningitis, useful additional analyses may include multiplex PCR panels, acid-fast bacilli (AFB) stain and culture, cryptococcal antigen and culture, Lyme antibody testing, and venereal disease research laboratory (VDRL) testing.

In aseptic meningitis, the LP results are variable and depend on the etiology. In general, the opening pressure is normal or minimally elevated, the white blood cell (WBC) count is 10 to 300 cells/μL with a lymphocytic predominance, glucose is normal to slightly elevated, and total protein is slightly elevated.

TREATMENT

The rapid initiation of empiric antibiotics is essential to reduce the morbidity and mortality of acute bacterial meningitis. Antibiotics should be selected based on likely organisms, taking into account risk factors for antimicrobial-resistant pathogens (based on local epidemiology and health care exposure) and unusual organisms (based on immune status and unique community exposures).

A common regimen in nonimmunocompromised adults is ceftriaxone or ceftazidime (depending on local resistance patterns) and vancomycin. Acyclovir is often initiated alongside antibacterials and can be discontinued if HSV PCR testing of the CSF is negative. If the patient is immunosuppressed or at the extremes of age, the regimen should also include ampicillin to cover *Listeria*. Patients with known or suspected pneumococcal meningitis should receive dexamethasone ~20 minutes prior to antibiotic initiation to limit inflammation and cerebral edema in response to bacterial death and breakdown.

In cases of confirmed infection with *N. meningitidis*, close contacts should receive primary prophylaxis with rifampin. Meanwhile, the patient should be placed on droplet isolation while hospitalized to prevent infection of providers and other patients.

Even with appropriate treatment, the overall mortality associated with meningitis remains high. The mortality rate for *S. pneumoniae* is ~20%, with about one in three survivors experiencing long-term neurological sequelae such as deafness, seizures, or intellectual disability.

CHAPTER 114

Pneumonia

PRANAY SINHA

INTRODUCTION

Infectious pneumonia refers to pulmonary inflammation that occurs when microbes enter the lungs through inhalation or aspiration and overwhelm the local immune system. Termed the "captain of the men of death" by Sir William Osler, pneumonia remains the leading infectious cause of death worldwide.

The three distinct pneumonia syndromes are **community-acquired pneumonia** (CAP), **hospital-acquired pneumonia** (HAP), and **ventilator-associated pneumonia** (VAP) (Fig. 114.1). CAP refers to pneumonia contracted by patients dwelling in the community. HAP is defined as pneumonia that is contracted by a patient at least 48 hours after hospital admission. VAP is defined as pneumonia contracted after 48 hours of mechanical ventilation.

PATHOPHYSIOLOGY

The branching anatomy of the respiratory tract normally prevents most inhaled pathogens from reaching the alveoli. The epithelium of the respiratory tract is ciliated and produces a thin layer of mucus. Inhaled particles are bound by mucus and moved toward the pharynx through the coordinated movement of the cilia, a system known as the **mucociliary escalator.** Pathogens that manage to evade these structural barriers and reach the alveoli are recognized and phagocytosed by alveolar macrophages. When alveolar macrophages are overwhelmed by a large inoculum of pathogens, they release cytokines and initiate an inflammatory cascade. Leukocytes invade the lung tissue, filling infected alveoli with purulent exudates that impair effective gas exchange.

CAP is most commonly caused by bacteria or viruses. As the sensitivity of sputum culture is highly variable, and a significant proportion (~25%–40%) of cases result from viral infections, the causative agent is not identified in the majority of cases. Overall, however, *Streptococcus pneumoniae* and *Haemophilus influenzae* are the most common causes and are considered typical pathogens. The atypical organisms that can cause CAP include *Mycoplasma pneumoniae, Legionella pneumophila,* and *Chlamydophila pneumoniae;* these organisms are traditionally intracellular and lack a cell wall, rendering β-lactam antibiotics ineffective. *Staphylococcus aureus,* including methicillin-resistant *S. aureus* (MRSA), can also cause infection, often accompanying or following a viral respiratory illness. Anaerobes, *Pseudomonas aeruginosa,* and *Moraxella catarrhalis* are less common pathogens. Only 2% to 3% of cases result from mycobacterial, fungal, or rickettsial organisms.

HAP is most commonly caused by gram-negative bacilli (*Escherichia coli, Enterobacter* spp., *Klebsiella* spp., *Serratia marcescens, Acinetobacter baumannii, Pseudomonas aeruginosa, Stenotrophomonas maltophilia, Burkholderia cepacia*) and gram-positive cocci (*S. aureus, Streptococcus* spp.). Anaerobic infections, generally resulting from aspiration of large volumes of oral secretions or gastric contents, are also more common among hospitalized patients. The causes of VAP are similar to those of HAP, although the higher oxygen levels in intubated lungs make anaerobic infections less common.

In the past, the term healthcare-associated pneumonia (HCAP) was used to describe pneumonias occurring in community-dwelling patients with significant exposures to the health care environment, which was thought to confer increased risk of infection with multidrug-resistant organisms (MDROs). Several studies, however, have challenged this underlying assumption, and thus HCAP has been excluded from Infectious Diseases Society of America/American Thoracic Society (IDSA/ATS) guidelines.

RISK FACTORS

The major risk factors for pneumonia can be classified as follows:
- Increased aspiration risk: seizure, delirium, dementia, stroke, neuromuscular disorder, endotracheal intubation, alcoholism
- Decreased clearance of inhaled pathogens: mechanical ventilation, chronic obstructive pulmonary disease

Community-acquired pneumonia (CAP)	Hospital-acquired pneumonia (HAP)	Ventilator-associated pneumonia (VAP)
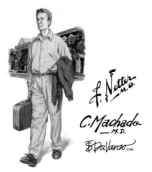	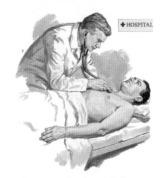	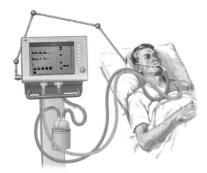
Predominant organisms are *Streptococcus pneumoniae* and *Haemophilus influenzae*	Contracted at least 48 hours after hospital admission	Contracted at least 48 hours after initiation of mechanical ventilation

Increased frequency of gram-negative bacilli (*Escherichia coli*, *Klebsiella*) and gram-positive cocci (*Staphylococcus*, *Streptococcus*)

FIG. 114.1 Pneumonia Syndromes.

(COPD), and asthma (impaired mucociliary clearance due to mucous hypersecretion and airway inflammation); smoking (destruction of cilia); obstruction of bronchial tree (tumors, lymph nodes, or foreign bodies); ciliary dysfunction (i.e., Kartagener syndrome); cystic fibrosis (inspissated mucous trapping microbes); neuromuscular weakness (weakened cough)

- Immune compromise: congenital immunological deficiency, iatrogenic immunosuppression (e.g., transplant and chemotherapy), HIV infection, malignancy (particularly hematological malignancies), alcoholism (impaired macrophages, decreased chemokine production, and leukopenia), cirrhosis

PRESENTATION, EVALUATION, AND DIAGNOSIS

The usual symptoms include fever, chills, dyspnea, and cough productive of purulent sputum. Extension of inflammation to the adjacent pleura can produce sharp, pleuritic pain. About 15% of patients with pneumonia experience hemoptysis. The presentation can vary, however, based on the pathogen, host factors, and stage of presentation.

A detailed history of recent exposures (including sick contacts, travel, animal exposures, and unique hobbies/behaviors) may help identify the causative pathogen (Table 114.1). On physical exam, nearly all patients have fever/hypothermia, tachycardia, tachypnea, and/or hypoxemia. Many patients have labored breathing and use accessory muscles. Asymmetric chest excursion is a rare but specific finding. Abnormal lung sounds are often present and include bronchial breath sounds, egophony, and crackles. Dullness and flatness on chest percussion are associated with consolidation and effusion, respectively. Tactile fremitus and whispered pectoriloquy are well-known signs of consolidation, but are rare and have poor interrater reliability. Older and immunosuppressed patients often have atypical examinations.

Chest radiography (CXR) is required to confirm the diagnosis and may reveal consolidation in either a lobar (Fig. 114.2) or more diffuse pattern (see Chapter 39 for details). Chest CT can reveal additional details, such as structural airway defects, effusions, obstructing masses, abscesses, and enlarged lymph nodes; however, CT should generally be reserved for patients with immune compromise, atypical clinical presentations, recurrent infection, or failure to improve with appropriate treatment.

On laboratory evaluation, leukocytosis is common, though leukopenia may also occur and is generally a sign of more severe illness. Sputum Gram stain and culture should be collected when possible (Fig. 114.3), though a significant number of patients are unable to produce an adequate sample, defined as having >25 leukocytes and <10 epithelial cells per low-power field. Excess epithelial cells indicate contamination with oral flora. Blood cultures are only positive in 5% to 14% of patients and rarely change therapies or outcomes. Thus the IDSA does not recommend routine blood cultures for all patients with CAP. They are recommended, however, for patients with CAP requiring intensive care unit (ICU)

TABLE 114.1
Selected Examples of Associations Between Exposures and Pathogens

Exposure	Organism
COMORBIDITIES	
Cystic fibrosis, bronchiectasis	*Pseudomonas aeruginosa, Burkholderia cepacia, Staphylococcus aureus, Mycobacterium avium* complex
Alcoholism	Oral anaerobes, *Klebsiella pneumoniae, M. tuberculosis, Acinetobacter* spp.
COPD	*Haemophilus influenza, P. aeruginosa, Legionella* spp., *Moraxella catarrhalis, Chlamydophila pneumoniae*
Dementia	Oral anaerobes and gram-negative enteric bacteria
HIV	*M. tuberculosis, Pneumocystis jirovecii, Nocardia asteroides*
TRAVEL	
South America	Tuberculosis, hantavirus
Southwestern United States	*Coccidioides* spp.
Ohio, St. Lawrence, or Mississippi river valleys	*Histoplasma* spp., *Blastomyces* spp.
Southeast Asia	*B. pseudomallei, M. tuberculosis*
Sub-Saharan Africa	*M. tuberculosis*
Arabian Peninsula	Middle East respiratory syndrome coronavirus
ANIMAL	
Sheep, goats, cattle	*Coxiella burnetii*
Palm civet	Severe acute respiratory syndrome (SARS)
Rats	Hantavirus, *Yersinia pestis*
Rabbits and hares	*Francisella tularensis*
Sheep, goats, camels, horses, pigs	*Bacillus anthracis*
Horses	*B. mallei*, Hendra virus
Pigs	Influenza virus, Nipah virus
HOBBIES	
Cave exploration	*Histoplasma capsulatum*
Hiking	*Y. pestis, F. tularensis*
Birdkeeping	*Chlamydia psittaci*
Global health volunteering	*M. tuberculosis*
Desert rock collectors	*Coccidioides* spp.
Hunters	*Blastomyces dermatitidis*

COPD, Chronic obstructive pulmonary disease.

care and for patients with HAP or VAP. For critically ill patients, urinary antigen testing for *L. pneumophila* (serotype 1) and *S. pneumoniae* is recommended.

The **pneumonia severity index (PSI)** and **CURB-65** score can be used to triage patients and determine their overall risk. The PSI score is calculated based on patient demographics, comorbidities, severity of vital sign abnormalities, laboratory values, and radiographic findings; several online calculators are available. In the CURB-65 score, the patient receives 1 point each for confusion, uremia (blood urea nitrogen [BUN] >19), respiratory rate >30, blood pressure <90/60 mm Hg, and age >65 years; patients with a score of 1 can receive outpatient care, those with a score of ≥2 should receive

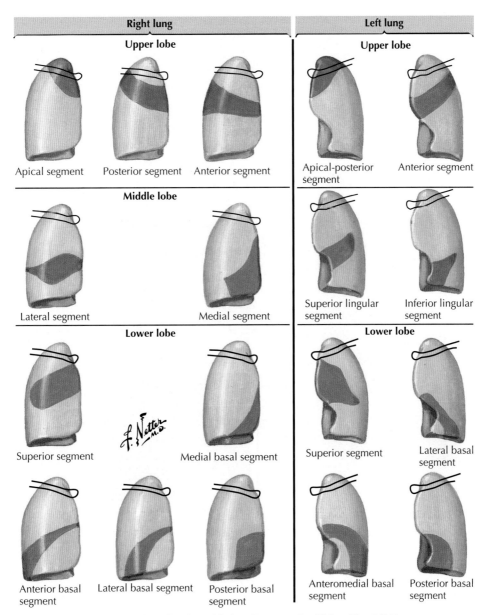

	Right lung			Left lung	

FIG. 114.2 Localization of Lobar Pneumonias Using Chest X-Ray.

inpatient care, and those with a score of ≥3 generally require ICU care.

TREATMENT

The choice of empiric antibiotics is based on the likely pathogens, the patient's previous microbiological history (from both infection and colonization), and regional resistance patterns. Treatment should be narrowed as soon as cultures reveal a causative pathogen and its antibiotic susceptibilities.

Community-Acquired Pneumonia

Outpatients with a low suspicion for resistant organisms can receive a macrolide (azithromycin, clarithromycin, or erythromycin). Risk factors for resistance include age

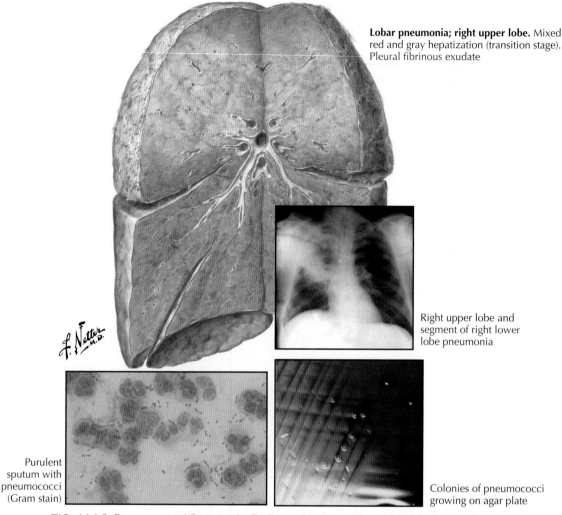

Lobar pneumonia; right upper lobe. Mixed red and gray hepatization (transition stage). Pleural fibrinous exudate

Right upper lobe and segment of right lower lobe pneumonia

Purulent sputum with pneumococci (Gram stain)

Colonies of pneumococci growing on agar plate

FIG. 114.3 **Pneumococcal Pneumonia: Radiographic Appearance, Gram Stain, and Culture.**

>65 years, receipt of β-lactam therapy in past 90 days, immune compromise, multiple medical comorbidities, or exposure to institutional care (e.g., child in day care). Patients with such risk factors should receive respiratory quinolones (moxifloxacin or levofloxacin). Inpatients can be treated with either fluoroquinolone monotherapy or a combination of antistreptococcal cephalosporin/β-lactam (e.g., ceftriaxone, cefotaxime, or amoxicillin-clavulanate) plus a macrolide or doxycycline for coverage of atypical organisms. For all patients, 5 to 7 days of therapy is generally adequate.

Patients with suspected or proven influenza coinfection should receive oseltamivir. Those with a history of MRSA colonization or infection may be treated with vancomycin or linezolid; daptomycin is generally inappropriate as it is inactivated by pulmonary surfactant.

Finally, recent studies have shown that systemic steroids may decrease the duration of symptoms and hospital length of stay for patients with severe CAP (PSI >III or CURB-65 >2). The ideal integration of such therapy into standard care has yet to be established.

Hospital-Acquired Pneumonia and Ventilator-Associated Pneumonia

An appropriate empiric regimen for HAP generally includes coverage for both MRSA and *P. aeruginosa*. As noted, vancomycin or linezolid can be used to cover MRSA. Piperacillin-tazobactam, advanced generation cephalosporins (ceftazidime, cefepime), carbepenems (meropenem, imipenem), and fluoroquinolones (levofloxacin, ciprofloxacin) are appropriate for gram-negative coverage. Aminoglycosides (amikacin, tobramycin, gentamicin) can be used for additional pseudomonal coverage (i.e., double coverage), especially in patients with risk factors for MDROs, though they should not be used alone for respiratory infections. After antimicrobial susceptibility patterns are obtained, antibiotics can be narrowed to a single agent, and double coverage is no longer necessary.

Serum procalcitonin is a biomarker that can be used to monitor the effect of treatment and potentially decrease its duration. Procalcitonin is a peptide produced in response to interleukin-1β (IL-1β), tumor necrosis factor-α (TNF-α), and lipopolysaccharide from gram-negative bacteria; it is inhibited by interferon-γ (IFN-γ), produced during viral infections. Serum levels peak 6 hours after infection onset and fall with resolution. Renal disease, trauma, surgery, rhabdomyolysis, various immunotherapies, cocaine, amphetamines, cardiogenic shock, and various malignancies can result in false positives. Viral pneumonia should be suspected if procalcitonin levels are <0.25 µg/L at presentation. For bacterial pneumonias, procalcitonin levels should be measured at least every other day. Antibiotics can be stopped once procalcitonin levels either fall below 0.25 µg/L or decrease by ≥80% from their peak value. The use of procalcitonin as a biomarker continues to evolve, and more studies are necessary.

Despite appropriate antibiotics, patients with pneumonia often continue to have fevers, tachycardia, and hypoxemia until the third or fourth day of therapy and may also have other vital sign abnormalities. These findings should not generally prompt broadening of antibiotics, but patients with more severe vital sign abnormalities and clinical decompensation, especially hypotension requiring vasopressor support, should be considered for broader empiric antibiotic coverage. Supplemental oxygen, chest physiotherapy, mucolytic agents, and bronchodilators may be used to improve oxygenation, clear secretions, and improve symptoms.

CHAPTER 115

Tuberculosis

SASHA A. FAHME

INTRODUCTION

Infection with *Mycobacterium tuberculosis* (MTB), also known as **tuberculosis (TB)**, is a leading cause of mortality worldwide, resulting in ~1.4 million deaths in 2015. According to the latest World Health Organization (WHO) report, 10.4 million new cases of **active TB** occurred in 2015, with the largest burden of disease occurring in six countries: India, Indonesia, China, Nigeria, Pakistan, and South Africa. In contrast, the annual incidence of active TB in the United States is only 0.03%, with most infections occurring in immigrants and socioeconomically disadvantaged populations. Recent advances in the detection and treatment of TB have blunted its global impact, with 49 million deaths prevented between the years 2000 and 2015.

TB infection is classified as latent or active. **Latent TB** infection refers to the presence of viable bacteria in the absence of clinical disease secondary to suppression by the body's native immune defenses. Active disease occurs when, for uncertain reasons, the bacillus is able to overcome host defenses and produce symptoms once more.

An estimated 2 to 3 billion people worldwide have latent TB, and ~5% to 15% of these cases are expected to progress to active infection. The reactivation of latent TB is not entirely understood though it is thought to be secondary to both host-specific factors (e.g., age, immune suppression, recurrent exposure) and pathogen-specific characteristics (including MTB strain and initial bacterial load).

PATHOPHYSIOLOGY

Although infection can occur in virtually any organ system, pulmonary disease is the most common. Active pulmonary TB can be subclassified into symptomatic **primary disease** (<10% of cases) and **secondary,** or cavitary, **disease** (>90% of cases). In both cases, infection begins with inhalation of aerosolized bacteria-containing droplets, followed by prompt phagocytosis of the bacilli by alveolar macrophages. The bacteria then replicate within macrophages and subsequently disseminate, through lymphatic drainage and/or the bloodstream, to potentially seed distant organs, though rarely leading to extrapulmonary infection (Fig. 115.1).

Caseating granulomas (or **tuberculomas**) form in the lungs, most commonly in the middle and lower lobes, and may be small enough to evade radiographic detection. Once these tuberculomas undergo fibrosis and calcification, they are termed **Ghon** focuses and become visible on chest radiographs. A Ghon focus in the presence of hilar lymphadenopathy is termed a Ghon complex (Fig. 115.2).

This process, which generally occurs in childhood, represents the natural history of primary TB. Approximately 90% of cases are entirely asymptomatic and identified in adulthood, commonly by small calcified lesions on chest imaging suggestive of prior granulomatous exposure. Less than 10% of patients will develop symptomatic primary TB, typically of the lower lobes, following initial exposure; this risk is generally limited to those at extremes of age or with significant immune suppression.

In immune-competent hosts, the risk of TB reactivation (i.e., the development of secondary TB) is ~5% during the first 18 months following exposure, then 5% for the remainder of their lifetime. The exact pathophysiology of reactivation is unknown, although it may reflect deficiencies in cell-mediated immunity. Unlike in primary infection, reactivated pulmonary disease has a predilection for the upper lobes where the partial pressure of oxygen is greater.

RISK FACTORS

HIV infection is the most significant risk factor for active TB infection. Patients with latent TB who become coinfected with HIV have a reactivation risk of ~10% per year. Medications that inhibit cell-mediated immunity also increase the reactivation risk; common agents include tumor necrosis factor-α inhibitors (e.g., infliximab and

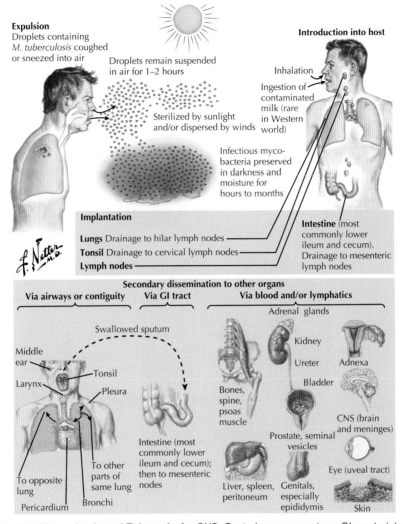

Expulsion
Droplets containing *M. tuberculosis* coughed or sneezed into air

Droplets remain suspended in air for 1–2 hours

Sterilized by sunlight and/or dispersed by winds

Introduction into host

Inhalation

Ingestion of contaminated milk (rare in Western world)

Infectious myco-bacteria preserved in darkness and moisture for hours to months

Implantation

Lungs Drainage to hilar lymph nodes

Tonsil Drainage to cervical lymph nodes

Lymph nodes

Intestine (most commonly lower ileum and cecum). Drainage to mesenteric lymph nodes

Secondary dissemination to other organs

Via airways or contiguity | **Via GI tract** | **Via blood and/or lymphatics**

Swallowed sputum

Middle ear
Larynx
Tonsil
Pleura

To opposite lung
Pericardium
Bronchi
To other parts of same lung

Intestine (most commonly lower ileum and cecum); then to mesenteric nodes

Adrenal glands
Kidney
Ureter
Adnexa
Bladder
Bones, spine, psoas muscle
Prostate, seminal vesicles
CNS (brain and meninges)
Eye (uveal tract)
Liver, spleen, peritoneum
Genitals, especially epididymis
Skin

FIG. 115.1 **Dissemination of Tuberculosis.** *CNS,* Central nervous system; *GI,* gastrointestinal.

adalimumab, both of which carry the highest risk of reactivation, as well as etanercept) and glucocorticoids; patients should be screened for latent TB prior to initiating such agents. Silicosis is another important risk factor, possibly due to inhibition of pulmonary macrophages by silica particles, particularly among coal mine workers in endemic areas. Additional risk factors include solid organ and hematopoietic stem cell transplantation, end-stage renal disease, recent immigration from an endemic country, significant health care exposures, household exposure to an infected source, and living in crowded quarters, such as a prison or homeless shelter.

CLINICAL PRESENTATION, EVALUATION, AND DIAGNOSIS

Latent Tuberculosis

Adults with latent TB are, by definition, asymptomatic. The diagnosis depends on routine evaluation with one of two screening tests: the Mantoux tuberculin skin test (TST) or an **interferon-γ release assay (IGRA)**. The skin test assesses the immune response to a **purified protein derivative (PPD)** of the bacillus, which induces a T-cell–mediated hypersensitivity reaction, while the IGRA measures the serum concentration of interferon-γ after in vitro exposure to antigen. Thus both tests assess the host's

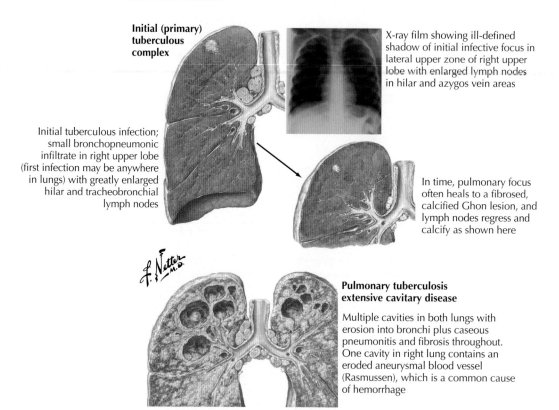

Initial (primary) tuberculous complex

X-ray film showing ill-defined shadow of initial infective focus in lateral upper zone of right upper lobe with enlarged lymph nodes in hilar and azygos vein areas

Initial tuberculous infection; small bronchopneumonic infiltrate in right upper lobe (first infection may be anywhere in lungs) with greatly enlarged hilar and tracheobronchial lymph nodes

In time, pulmonary focus often heals to a fibrosed, calcified Ghon lesion, and lymph nodes regress and calcify as shown here

Pulmonary tuberculosis extensive cavitary disease

Multiple cavities in both lungs with erosion into bronchi plus caseous pneumonitis and fibrosis throughout. One cavity in right lung contains an eroded aneurysmal blood vessel (Rasmussen), which is a common cause of hemorrhage

FIG. 115.2 **Pulmonary Tuberculosis.**

immune response to the bacillus and are challenging to interpret in immunocompromised patients and, in the case of the skin test, those who have received the **bacillus Calmette-Guerin (BCG) vaccine.** This is because, unlike the PPD, the IGRA antigens are specific to MTB and are not associated with the strains contained in the BCG vaccine (Fig. 115.3).

Any patient with a positive screening test should have a chest radiograph to evaluate for evidence of latent disease; most of these return normal. There are several radiographic characteristics that help risk stratify patients with respect to likelihood of reactivation. For instance, individuals with nodular or fibrotic lesions are at greater risk of reactivation, whereas those with focal, entirely calcified granulomas are not. Of note, chest radiographs should never be used as a primary diagnostic tool in patients with symptomatic disease, as x-rays carry only an estimated 73% to 79% sensitivity and 60% to 63% specificity for active TB.

Active Tuberculosis

Active pulmonary TB is a chronic illness characterized by cough, hemoptysis, drenching night sweats, weight loss, and fevers. The clinical presentation may be subtle in patients with poorly controlled HIV; those with CD4 counts <75 cells/mm^3 may present only with nonspecific constitutional symptoms.

Extrapulmonary TB refers to disease outside of the lungs and can involve a number of organ systems, with the most common being thoracolumbar osteomyelitis (Pott disease), cervical lymphadenitis (scrofula), renal disease, and subacute meningitis.

Miliary TB refers to the multiorgan disease that occurs following hematogenous dissemination of MTB and is characterized by small tuberculomas throughout affected systems. (The name miliary reflects the resemblance of the tuberculomas to millet seeds.) In addition to constitutional and pulmonary symptoms, the presentation often features hepatic involvement manifested by right upper quadrant tenderness, nausea, vomiting, jaundice, and (rarely) fulminant hepatic failure, splenomegaly, and adrenal insufficiency. Optic nerve involvement, characterized by choroiditis, neuroretinitis, retinal vasculitis, and/or panuveitis, may also be present. Visualization of choroidal tubercles on funduscopic examination is diagnostic of acute miliary TB.

0.1-mL tuberculin (5 TU) injected just under skin surface of forearm. Pale elevation results. Needle bevel directed upward to prevent too deep penetration.

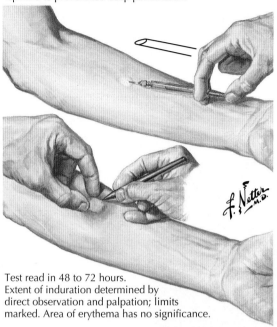

Test read in 48 to 72 hours.
Extent of induration determined by
direct observation and palpation; limits
marked. Area of erythema has no significance.

FIG. 115.3 **Tuberculin Skin Testing.**

Only patients with untreated pulmonary or laryngeal TB are infectious. Additionally, infectiousness rapidly declines after the initiation of appropriate treatment. Any patient with suspected pulmonary TB should be placed under airborne isolation precautions during the diagnostic evaluation. Isolation precautions may be lifted once a patient is deemed noninfectious, which occurs when the following three criteria are met: at least 2 weeks of appropriate treatment, clinical improvement (the most sensitive marker is weight gain), and consecutively obtained negative sputum smears.

Active TB is diagnosed using one of three laboratory methods: **smear microscopy, sputum culture,** and **rapid nucleic acid amplification (NAA) testing.** The combination of positive sputum culture and microscopy is the gold standard for the diagnosis of pulmonary TB. The Centers for Disease Control and Prevention (CDC) recommends that three sputum samples be collected at intervals between 8 and 24 hours for culture and smear. The analysis of a second respiratory specimen has been estimated to improve sensitivity by 30%; however, studies have found only a minimal benefit to testing a third sputum sample, thereby questioning the diagnostic utility of testing three specimens (Fig. 115.4).

As compared to **acid-fast bacilli (AFB) smear and culture,** NAA testing has comparatively greater positive predictive value among populations in which nontuberculous *Mycobacteria* are common. When it was first introduced, NAA testing was shown to have particular clinical utility in patients with AFB smear-negative and culture-positive sputum, confirming infection in ~50% to 80% of such cases. Currently, however, the CDC recommends molecular testing on at least one sputum sample from any patient undergoing testing for TB in whom a diagnosis has not yet been confirmed and for whom the diagnosis would have treatment or public health implications.

Bronchoscopy is generally not indicated in the diagnosis of active TB unless respiratory specimens are otherwise unable to be obtained or are repeatedly negative despite high clinical suspicion of TB.

The screening tests administered in latent TB have no utility in this setting, as these can be falsely negative in the context of active infection.

Once the diagnosis has been established, it is important to assess susceptibility to the first-line agents: rifampicin (RIF), isoniazid (INH), ethambutol (EMB), and pyrazinamide (PZA). **Drug-susceptible TB** is fully susceptible to all four of these agents. **Multidrug-resistant (MDR) TB** is resistant to at least INH and RIF. **Extensively drug-resistant (XDR) TB** is a subgroup of MDR TB that is also resistant to any fluoroquinolone and at least one injectable second-line agent. Drug resistance can be acquired or primary. Acquired resistance refers to infection by strains that are initially susceptible but undergo spontaneous mutations in the setting of inappropriate treatment regimens (e.g., by failing to use all four first-line agents or by treating for a shorter duration than that which is recommended). In contrast, primary resistance refers to infection with an already resistant strain.

The CDC recommends resistance testing to second-line agents only in specific, high-risk subpopulations, including those who have had prior TB, known exposure to MDR TB (including living in endemic regions), resistance to first-line agents, or persistence of positive cultures despite 3 months of therapy.

TREATMENT
Latent Disease

The preferred therapy is either INH monotherapy for 6 to 9 months or a combination of INH and rifampin or rifapentine for 3 to 4 months. Patients with HIV coinfection require longer treatment courses. Patients should also receive pyridoxine (vitamin B_6) to prevent INH-associated peripheral neuropathy.

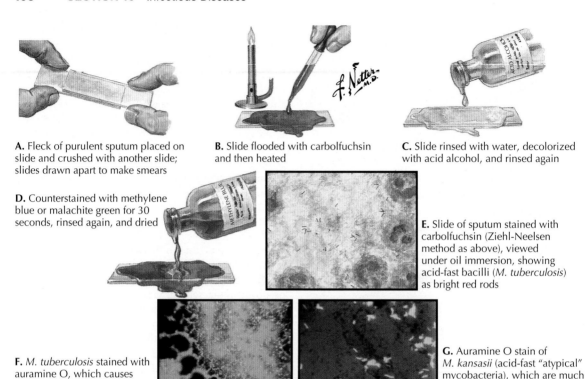

A. Fleck of purulent sputum placed on slide and crushed with another slide; slides drawn apart to make smears

B. Slide flooded with carbolfuchsin and then heated

C. Slide rinsed with water, decolorized with acid alcohol, and rinsed again

D. Counterstained with methylene blue or malachite green for 30 seconds, rinsed again, and dried

E. Slide of sputum stained with carbolfuchsin (Ziehl-Neelsen method as above), viewed under oil immersion, showing acid-fast bacilli (*M. tuberculosis*) as bright red rods

F. *M. tuberculosis* stained with auramine O, which causes acid-fast bacilli to fluoresce (×200)

G. Auramine O stain of *M. kansasii* (acid-fast "atypical" mycobacteria), which are much larger than *M. tuberculosis* (×200)

FIG. 115.4 **Sputum Examination in Tuberculosis.**

Active Disease

Drug-susceptible active TB is generally treated with the four first-line agents for 2 months in an intensive phase, then with INH and rifampin for at least 4 additional months during the continuation phase. In patients with HIV coinfection, there is a benefit from early initiation of antiretroviral (ARV) therapy (i.e., within 2–8 weeks of initiating anti-TB treatment). An important exception is patients with TB meningitis, who experience higher rates of adverse events with ARVs. In addition, there is a risk of **immune reconstitution inflammation syndrome (IRIS)** upon initiating ARVs that is typically manifested as worsening lymphadenopathy and pulmonary symptoms. Furthermore, common drug-drug interactions between ARVs and the rifamycins may alter serum drug concentrations of the antimycobacterial agents and thereby increase the risk of MTB becoming drug resistant.

The treatment of MDR TB depends on local resistance patterns and the results of individual susceptibility testing. A typical regimen includes four drugs to which the isolate is susceptible, along with pyrazinamide for

an induction phase of 6 to 8 months, followed by a prolonged continuation phase for a total duration of therapy of at least 20 months. Shorter courses are currently being evaluated. Pyrazinamide is empirically included in the treatment regimen as MTB susceptibility testing has classically been challenging to perform. However, newer polymerase chain reaction–deoxyribonucleic acid (PCR-DNA) sequencing assays evaluating specific mutations are being developed such that pyrazinamide resistance testing will likely be incorporated into future standard practice.

Second-line agents frequently used in this setting include fluoroquinolones, injectable agents (amikacin, capreomycin, kanamycin, and streptomycin), and newer oral agents such as bedaquiline and delamanid.

Overall clinical improvement is a critical marker of successful TB treatment; however, culture conversion is the gold standard, and the CDC recommends serial sputum analyses at monthly intervals during treatment until two consecutive specimens demonstrate negative cultures.

CHAPTER 116

Infective Endocarditis

JUSTIN G. AARON

INTRODUCTION

Infective endocarditis (IE) refers to an infection of the endothelial surface of the heart. Most cases result from bacterial infection and involve the valves. IE is associated with significant morbidity and mortality, with both cardiac and extracardiac manifestations.

The annual incidence of IE in developed countries is 3 to 15 cases per 100,000 persons. Although the disease was classically described in injection drug users, its epidemiology has changed significantly over time. Healthcare-associated endocarditis has risen in incidence, partly due to the increasing use of **cardiovascular implantable electronic devices (CIED)** in the aging population, and is now responsible for over one-third of IE cases in the United States.

Infections were previously classified as acute or subacute based on the duration of symptoms preceding diagnosis, but they are now preferentially classified by location, organism, and whether a native valve or prosthesis is involved. The mortality can range from <10% for right-sided, native valve endocarditis (NVE) associated with *Streptococcus* to >40% for left-sided, prosthetic valve endocarditis (PVE) associated with *Staphylococcus aureus*.

PATHOPHYSIOLOGY

Normal heart valves are resistant to bacterial colonization; however, the native endothelial surface can become damaged because of degeneration, instrumentation, or contact with solid particles introduced during injection drug use. Platelet and fibrin deposits form on the damaged endothelium and facilitate bacterial adhesion (Fig. 116.1). **Prosthetic valves** are also susceptible to bacterial adhesion and biofilm formation, particularly in the first few months after surgery when endothelialization has not yet occurred. Bacterial proliferation promotes further deposition of platelets and fibrin, ultimately forming a valvular mass or **vegetation.**

As a vegetation forms, it may disrupt normal valve function and cause valvular insufficiency. In addition, infection can extend to the perivalvular area and form an abscess, which can disrupt the electrical conduction system and induce heart block; aortic valve infections are most likely to result in this complication. Large, mobile, left-sided vegetations, particularly those on the mitral valve, are prone to embolization. Emboli to the systemic circulation (including to the brain and kidneys) are most common from left-sided vegetations; emboli to the pulmonic circulation are most common from right-sided vegetations.

Over 80% of cases of IE are caused by *Staphylococcus* or *Streptococcus* species. In the past, NVE resulted primarily from oral flora introduced during gingival manipulation, such as the viridans group streptococci. In injection drug users, the main pathogen was *S. aureus* originating from a skin source. With the rise in healthcare-associated cases, however, a greater number of infections are now from *S. aureus*, coagulase-negative staphylococci, and enterococci. Early PVE (within the 2 months after surgery) is commonly due to staphylococcal species introduced during the operation or from hematogenous spread. After the early postoperative period, the organisms responsible for PVE are similar to those seen with NVE.

In ~10% of IE cases, no causative organism is identified. Culture-negative endocarditis usually occurs when antibiotics are administered prior to drawing the appropriate number of blood cultures. Less frequently, culture-negative endocarditis reflects infection with a fastidious organism that is difficult to grow in culture; however, modern microbiological techniques are better able to isolate organisms that were previously implicated in these cases, including fungi (most commonly *Candida* species) and the gram-negative **HACEK** group: *Haemophilus* (now *Aggregatibacter*) *aphrophilus, Actinobacillus* (now *Aggregatibacter*) *actinomycetemcomitans, Cardiobacterium hominis, Eikenella corrodens,* and *Kingella kingae.* With unusual epidemiological exposures, other organisms such as *Bartonella, Brucella, Coxiella,* and *Tropheryma whipplei* can be considered as causes of culture-negative endocarditis.

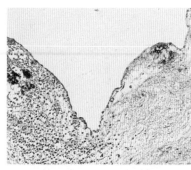

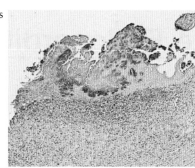

Deposit of platelets and organisms (stained dark), edema, and leukocytic infiltration in very early bacterial endocarditis of aortic valve

Development of vegetations containing clumps of bacteria on tricuspid valve

Early vegetations of bacterial endocarditis on bicuspid aortic valve

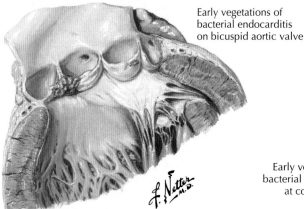

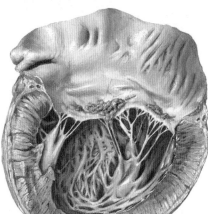

Early vegetations of bacterial endocarditis at contact line of mitral valve

FIG. 116.1 **Pathology of Endocarditis.**

RISK FACTORS

The greatest risk factors for IE are prosthetic heart valves, CIEDs, unrepaired congenital cyanotic heart disease (reflecting a predisposition to endothelial damage), and a prior history of IE. Other risk factors include rheumatic heart disease, age-related degenerative valve disease, injection drug use, end-stage renal disease (from frequent intravascular access and immune compromise), diabetes mellitus (from immune compromise), HIV infection, and poor dentition. Half of IE cases occur in individuals with no known history of valvular disease.

PRESENTATION, EVALUATION, AND DIAGNOSIS

Fever is the most common symptom of IE. Other common symptoms include malaise, myalgias, night sweats, headache, and dyspnea. A new or worsened murmur may be noted on physical exam. Less common findings can include peripheral stigmata of endocarditis from emboli, such as splinter hemorrhages and **Janeway lesions** (nontender erythematous lesions on the palms or soles), as well as immunological phenomena, such as **Osler nodes** (tender raised lesions on the hands or feet) and **Roth spots** (retinal hemorrhages) (Fig. 116.2).

Patients can also present with sepsis, heart failure, and/or manifestations of systemic embolization, including stroke, meningitis, renal failure, septic pulmonary emboli, septic arthritis, acute peripheral arterial occlusions, and myocardial infarction from coronary artery embolization. Cerebral complications are the most severe and most common extracardiac manifestations of endocarditis, occurring in approximately one in five cases.

The stratified diagnosis of IE is often established using the modified **Duke criteria** (Box 116.1), which include clinical, microbiological, and echocardiographic data and have a sensitivity and specificity >80%.

Because symptoms of IE are often nonspecific, clinicians must maintain a high index of suspicion.

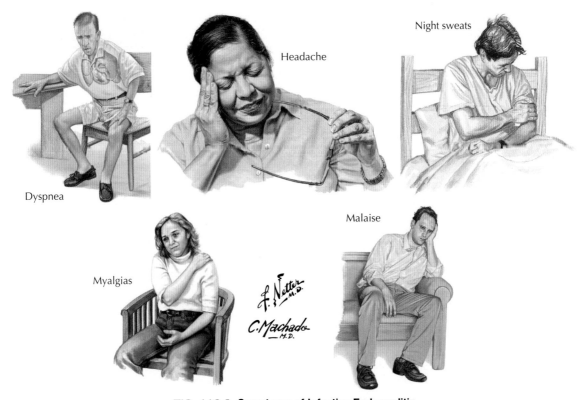

FIG. 116.2 **Symptoms of Infective Endocarditis.**

Any patient with potential endocarditis should have at least three sets of blood cultures drawn from different venipuncture sites (the first and last at least 1 hour apart) before receiving antibiotics. Serological testing may help identify rare causes of culture-negative endocarditis, such as *Bartonella*, *Brucella*, and *Coxiella burnetii*, in individuals with unique epidemiological exposures.

Transthoracic echocardiography (TTE) is often the first imaging study performed for visualization of vegetations (Fig. 116.3), although transesophageal echocardiography (TEE) is more sensitive. Patients with a negative TTE with known significant risk factors for IE, including prosthetic valves or prior IE, as well as those with high clinical suspicion of IE, should undergo TEE. Individuals with a positive TTE with high-risk features, including large mobile vegetations, valvular insufficiency, or potential perivalvular extension, should still receive a TEE for additional imaging to assess the need for valve surgery. If clinical suspicion remains high despite a negative TEE, the test should be repeated in 3 to 5 days.

TREATMENT

Patients with IE require a prolonged course of bactericidal intravenous antibiotics, given the high burden of organisms and difficulty accessing bacteria deep within a vegetation. The choice and duration of antibiotics depends on the organism, antibiotic susceptibilities, and whether a native or prosthetic valve is involved. NVE is typically treated for 4 to 6 weeks and PVE for 6 weeks. Gentamicin is often combined with a β-lactam antibiotic for synergy in the treatment of PVE but is infrequently recommended in NVE (with the exception of enterococcal infections). Professional societies provide regularly updated guidelines.

In some cases, surgical valve replacement may be required. Indications for valve surgery include acute heart failure secondary to valve insufficiency or a fistula into a cardiac chamber, heart block secondary to infection, penetrating lesions, uncontrolled source of infection (fungal infection, highly resistant organism, paravalvular abscess, prosthetic material, recurrent embolization,

BOX 116.1
Modified Duke Criteria for Infective Endocarditis

Definite diagnosis of IE: 2 major, 1 major and 3 minor, or 5 minor criteria fulfilled

Possible diagnosis of IE: 1 major and 1 minor or 3 minor criteria fulfilled

MAJOR CRITERIA
- Positive Blood Cultures
  - Typical organism associated with IE in 2 separate blood cultures (*Staphylococcus aureus*, viridans group streptococci, *Streptococcus gallolyticus*, HACEK group, Enterococci) *or*
  - Persistently positive blood cultures with a consistent organism from 2 separate cultures drawn at least 12 hours apart *or* at least 3 or a majority of ≥4 blood cultures *or*
  - Single positive blood culture for *Coxiella burnetii* or phase I IgG antibody titer >1:800
- Evidence of Endocardial Involvement
  - Positive echocardiogram with vegetation or abscess or dehisced prosthetic valve *or*

- New valvular regurgitation (new or worsened murmur on exam is insufficient)

MINOR CRITERIA
- Predisposition: Intravenous drug use or predisposing heart condition (including a prosthetic valve or significant valvular regurgitation)
- Fever (T ≥38°C)
- Vascular phenomena: Major arterial emboli, septic pulmonary infarcts, mycotic aneurysm, intracranial hemorrhage, conjunctival hemorrhage, Janeway lesions
- Immunologic phenomena: Glomerulonephritis, Osler nodes, Roth spots, rheumatoid factor
- Microbiologic evidence: Positive blood culture that does not meet major clinical criterion *or* serologic evidence of active infection with an organism consistent with IE

IE, Infective endocarditis; *IgG,* immunoglobulin G; *T,* temperature.
Reused with permission from Li JS, Sexton DJ, Mick N, et al: Proposed modifications to the Duke criteria for the diagnosis of infective endocarditis, *Clin Infect Dis* 30:633–638, 2000.

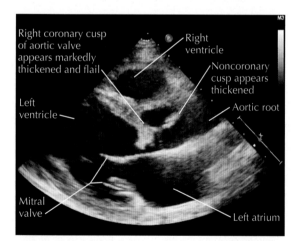

FIG. 116.3 Echocardiogram Findings in Severe Infective Endocarditis of Aortic Valve.

persistently positive cultures), or high risk of embolic events (greatest in vegetations >10 mm). The optimal timing for valve replacement remains unclear. In CIED-related endocarditis, the device should be removed, when possible, for source control.

Antibiotic prophylaxis to reduce the risk of IE associated with invasive dental procedures is currently recommended for certain high-risk individuals with prosthetic heart valves, a history of IE, or unrepaired cyanotic congenital heart disease. A single dose of 2 g oral amoxicillin 30 to 60 minutes prior to the procedure is the first-line prophylactic regimen.

CHAPTER 117

Gastroenteritis

ELIEZER SHINNAR

INTRODUCTION

Gastroenteritis, or inflammation of the mucous membranes of the gastrointestinal tract, is one of the leading causes of global mortality and is ubiquitously found in all types of communities. It can present with varying degrees of diarrhea, nausea, and vomiting. The World Health Organization defines acute gastroenteritis as having a rapid onset and duration of <14 days, distinguishing it from chronic diarrheal illnesses.

In developed nations, gastroenteritis rarely causes death, but its high prevalence takes a heavy toll on the health care system. Most people experience multiple episodes of gastroenteritis of varying severities throughout their lifetimes. Although the majority of presentations can be treated with simple rehydration, health care providers must be able to recognize and appropriately triage cases that require more intensive treatment and support.

PATHOPHYSIOLOGY

Gastroenteritis encompasses a large spectrum of processes caused by a diverse array of pathogens. The major symptom of gastroenteritis is diarrhea, which can be defined by increased stool mass (>200 g/day), increased stool frequency (>3 times/day), decreased stool consistency, and increased tenesmus (see Chapter 13 for details).

Diarrhea is often classified pathophysiologically as secretory, osmotic, functional, or inflammatory. In infectious gastroenteritis, several of these mechanisms may contribute to the clinical manifestations of disease. Enteric pathogens may directly affect epithelial ion transporters and intestinal barrier function through elaboration of toxins. They may also alter the flow of ions and water indirectly through the generation of inflammation, the modulation of neuropeptides, and the loss of the absorptive surface (i.e., shortening or effacement of intestinal villi).

For example, some gastrointestinal pathogens, such as *Vibrio cholerae,* elaborate enterotoxins that increase the secretion of water from the small intestine, usually by promoting efflux through the chloride channel (Fig. 117.1). Other pathogens, such as *Shigella,* cause a more inflammatory diarrhea from the elaboration of cytotoxins that cause cell death and mucosal damage. The resulting diarrhea may be visibly bloody or, on microscopy, contain a large number of leukocytes. Still other pathogens, such as the parasite *Giardia,* impair absorption by shortening intestinal villi and reducing the brush border absorptive surface.

While most infectious causes of diarrhea remain localized to the gut, certain organisms can penetrate into the reticuloendothelial system and cause systemic disease. *Salmonella typhi* (responsible for typhoid fever) and *Yersinia* (responsible for enteric fever) invade the intestinal mucosa and reproduce in the lymphatic or reticuloendothelial resulting in fevers, mesenteric adenitis, and weight loss. Pathogens that remain localized to the intestine may still have profound effects on overall health due to their effects on fluid homeostasis and nutritional status. Secondary bacteremias from translocation of gut flora can also cause significant morbidity and mortality.

RISK FACTORS

The main risk factors for gastroenteritis include international travel, institutionalized care (day care, long-term care facilities), recent antibiotic use, hospitalization, HIV infection, and blood group antigen. Some pathogens have been linked to specific environmental exposures (Table 117.1).

PRESENTATION, EVALUATION, AND DIAGNOSIS

The sequence and timing of gastrointestinal symptoms varies greatly on the infecting organism and the underlying host. Symptoms often begin with abdominal cramping and bloating, followed by diarrhea and possibly nausea and vomiting. Most patients with gastroenteritis experience minor symptoms and do not seek a treatment. Some pathogens, however, can cause more serious

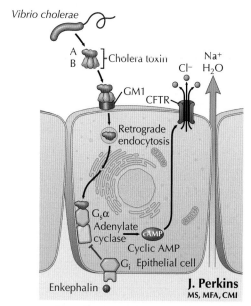

FIG. 117.1 Mechanism of Secretory Diarrhea in Cholera.

TABLE 117.1
Exposures and Associated Pathogens

Uncooked poultry	*Salmonella*, *Campylobacter*, and *Shigella*
Seafood	*Vibrio cholera*, *V. parahaemolyticus*, *V. vulnificus*, *Salmonella*, *Shigella*, hepatitis A, tapeworm, anisakiasis
Unpasteurized cheese	*Listeria monocytogenes*
Contaminated mayonnaise	*Staphylococcus* and *Clostridium*
Reheated fried rice (previously left at room temperature)	*Bacillus cereus*
Improperly canned food	*C. botulinum*
Unpurified fresh water	*Giardia* and *Cryptosporidium*

presentations, resulting in fever, dehydration, and severe abdominal pain. Immunocompromised patients, infants, and the elderly are also more prone to severe disease.

A thorough history and examination is necessary to rule out systemic illness. The nature of the symptoms should be recorded, including the number, approximate volume, and consistency of stools. The clinical history should also focus on recent food intake and pertinent exposures, including travel, hobbies, health care exposures, sick contacts, medication changes, antibiotic use, and food intolerances.

The physical exam must assess the degree of dehydration, which can be done by checking for orthostasis and examining the oral mucosa and axillae. The abdominal exam should assess for hepatic tenderness and peritonitis (rebound, guarding).

Most patients will not require further diagnostic workup, as their history and physical will be sufficient for the diagnosis of mild, noninflammatory gastroenteritis. For those patients with severe volume depletion, significant rectal bleeding, severe abdominal pain, weight loss, prolonged symptoms, or high-risk host factors (extremes of age, immunosuppression, pregnancy), additional testing and/or hospital admission may be warranted.

Specific tests that can be considered include serum chemistries, liver function tests, a complete blood count, and pancreatic enzymes. The stool itself can be examined macroscopically and microscopically to assess for inflammation (fecal leukocytes), bleeding, and specific pathogens (particularly ova and parasites). While stool culture was traditionally used, some centers now utilize enzyme immunoassays and multiplex polymerase chain reaction (PCR) panels to identify various bacterial, viral, and parasitic pathogens.

TREATMENT

The mortality associated with gastroenteritis results from the sequelae of dehydration. In alert patients without severe dehydration, replacement of lost volume with **oral rehydration solution** is generally sufficient. Severely dehydrated patients should receive intravenous fluids. Patients with significant malnourishment may require additional vitamin supplementation (i.e., zinc and vitamin A).

Diarrhea can be reduced using antimotility agents, the most common being bismuth subsalicylate. Loperamide, an opiate, has also been shown to be safe for many forms of acute diarrhea, especially when combined with antibiotics. For inflammatory and toxin-mediated processes, such agents are often not recommended as decreased motility allows toxins to remain in the colon longer, potentially causing further damage.

There is growing evidence that a variety of probiotics, specifically lactobacilli, are safe in diarrheal illnesses and can shorten the average length of symptoms. These are often avoided in immunosuppressed patient populations, however, as they have the potential to cause iatrogenic disease.

The role of antibiotics in diarrheal illness is variable. While antibacterials may shorten the duration of travelers' diarrhea, they can also contribute to antimicrobial resistance, alter gut flora, and cause medication-specific adverse events. In general, antibiotics are indicated to treat severe diarrhea (more than four episodes per day), especially in the presence of inflammatory symptoms (fever or pus, blood, or mucus in the stool). Patients with immune compromise and those at the extremes of age are also treated with antibiotics.

Empirically, azithromycin or fluoroquinolones are the first-line antibiotics of choice, followed by trimethoprim-sulfamethoxazole. Many pathogens (especially viral etiologies) will not respond to antibiotic therapies. It should be noted that antibiotic treatment of Shiga toxin–producing *Escherichia coli* strains (including serotype O157:H7) is contraindicated, as it can increase the risk of toxin release and hemolytic-uremic syndrome.

CHAPTER 118

Cholangitis

SAMAN NEMATOLLAHI

INTRODUCTION

Acute cholangitis describes the clinical syndrome of biliary inflammation resulting from bacterial infection and obstruction of bile ducts. In Western countries, biliary obstruction most often results from **choledocholithiasis** (presence of a stone in the common bile duct).

The incidence of symptomatic acute cholangitis is low, ranging from 0.3% to 1.6% among patients with asymptomatic gallstones. Mortality rates, previously as high as 50% in the 1970s, have decreased to 10% with wider and prompter access to endoscopic therapies to relieve obstruction and facilitate the clearance of infection.

PATHOPHYSIOLOGY

Bile is normally sterile, but bacteria can infect the biliary system by ascending from the duodenum through the ampulla. Hematogenous dissemination from the portal vein is also possible but less common. Apart from normal barrier mechanisms protecting the biliary tree (e.g., the sphincter of Oddi), the continuous flushing action of bile flow and antibacterial properties of bile salts usually prevent ascending bacterial contamination. Secretory biliary immunoglobulin A (IgA) and biliary mucus also act as antiadherence factors limiting the ability of bacteria to colonize the biliary system. In the setting of biliary obstruction and high intraductal pressures, these defense mechanisms may fail, resulting in overt infection.

The usual causes of biliary obstruction include choledocholithiasis, biliary strictures, sclerosing cholangitis, obstructing duodenal diverticula, pancreatitis (causing pancreatic edema and obstruction of the biliary tract), and bile duct injuries following direct instrumentation (Fig. 118.1). In addition to such anatomical processes, weakened host defenses and specific bacterial virulence factors may also contribute to the pathogenesis of acute cholangitis.

The most common pathogens causing acute cholangitis are from gram-negative bacilli (including *Escherichia coli*, *Klebsiella* spp., and *Enterobacter* spp.) as well as *Enterococcus* spp. Less common pathogens are anaerobic organisms, such as *Clostridium* spp. and *Bacteroides fragilis*. Infection with *Pseudomonas aeruginosa* generally occurs in the setting of improperly disinfected endoscopic equipment. Parasitic cholangitis is rare in the United States but can result from infection with *Ascaris lumbricoides*, *Clonorchis sinensis*, *Fasciola hepatica*, *Opisthorchis felineus*, and *Opisthorchis viverrini*.

RISK FACTORS

In the general population, the main risk factors for cholangitis are gallstones, active smoking, diabetes mellitus (due to increased risk of gallstone formation and systemic infections), and advanced age (>70 years). Endoscopic biliary procedures can result in ascending cholangitis, particularly when they fail to achieve drainage of an obstructed biliary system.

PRESENTATION, EVALUATION, AND DIAGNOSIS

In 1877, Dr. Jean-Martin Charcot first described cholangitis as "hepatic fever," characterized by fever, right upper quadrant pain, and jaundice—a presentation later termed **Charcot triad** (Fig. 118.2). In 1959, Drs. B.M. Reynolds and Everett Dargan expanded the definition to include altered mental status and hypotension **(Reynold pentad)**. Despite these historic descriptions, only a subset of patients fulfill all componements of Charcot triad. Fever is the most common manifestation of acute cholangitis (90%) followed by abdominal pain (70%) and jaundice (60%). Hypotension occurs in 30% of patients, and mental status changes (often mediated by hypotension) occur in 10% to 20%. Elderly and immune-compromised patients may present with nonfocal findings of sepsis.

Other conditions that can present with similar symptoms include acute cholecystitis, liver abscesses, pancreatitis, hepatitis, diverticulitis, appendicitis, infected choledochal cysts (congenital dilation of a bile duct), recurrent pyogenic cholangitis (cholangitis from

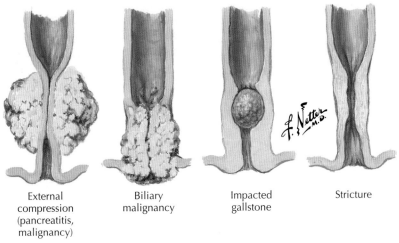

External
compression
(pancreatitis,
malignancy)

Biliary
malignancy

Impacted
gallstone

Stricture

FIG. 118.1 **Common Mechanisms of Biliary Obstruction.**

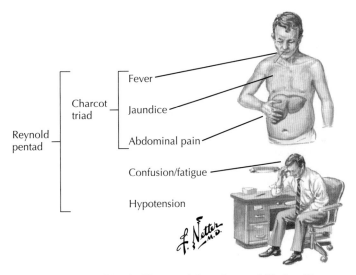

FIG. 118.2 **Classic Signs and Symptoms of Cholangitis.**

intrahepatic pigment stones), **Mirizzi syndrome** (impacted stone in cystic duct or gallbladder neck causing extrinsic compression of the common bile or hepatic ducts), and right lower lobe pneumonias.

Given the low sensitivity of Charcot triad and the importance of prompt identification and treatment of cholangitis, the Tokyo Guidelines (TG), first published in 2007 and revised in 2018 (TG18), provide criteria for both suspected and definite diagnosis. A related grading system can help determine the severity of cholangitis and guide treatment (Boxes 118.1 and 118.2).

Biliary imaging is often used in the diagnosis of acute cholangitis. Abdominal ultrasound is the preferred initial screening test since it is widely available, noninvasive, and has high diagnostic accuracy for evaluating bile duct dilation. **Magnetic resonance cholangiopancreatography (MRCP)** is highly sensitive but time consuming, expensive, and not widely available. Endoscopic ultrasound (EUS) and **endoscopic retrograde cholangiopancreatography (ERCP)** are also very sensitive for bile duct stones but require instrumentation.

TREATMENT

The treatment of cholangitis includes both systemic antibiotics and biliary drainage.

BOX 118.1
TG18/TG13 Diagnostic Criteria for Acute Cholangitis

A. Systemic inflammation
  A-1. Fever and/or shaking chills
  A-2. Laboratory data: evidence of inflammatory response
B. Cholestasis
  B-1. Jaundice
  B-2. Laboratory data: abnormal liver function tests
C. Imaging
  C-1. Biliary dilatation
  C-2. Evidence of the etiology on imaging (stricture, stone, stent)

Suspected diagnosis: One item in A + one item in either B or C

Definite diagnosis: One item in A, one item in B, and one item in C

Note:

A-2: Abnormal white blood cell counts, increase of serum C-reactive protein levels, and other changes indicating inflammation

B-2: Increased serum ALP, r-GTP (GGT), AST, and ALT levels

ALP, Alkaline phosphatase; *ALT,* alanine aminotransferase; *AST,* aspartate aminotransferase; *r-GTP (GGT),* r-glutamyltransferase. Reused with permission from Kiriyama S, Kozaka K, Takada T, et al: Tokyo Guidelines 2018: diagnostic criteria and severity grading of acute cholangitis (with videos), *J Hepatobiliary Pancreat Sci* 25(1):17–30, 2018.

BOX 118.2
TG18/TG13 Severity Assessment Criteria for Acute Cholangitis

GRADE III (SEVERE) ACUTE CHOLANGITIS
- Grade III acute cholangitis is defined as acute cholangitis that is associated with the onset of dysfunction in at least one of any of the following organs/systems:
  1. Cardiovascular dysfunction: Hypotension requiring dopamine ≥5 µg/kg per min, or any dose of norepinephrine
  2. Neurological dysfunction: Disturbance of consciousness
  3. Respiratory dysfunction: PaO_2/FiO_2 ratio <300
  4. Renal dysfunction: Oliguria, serum creatinine >2.0 mg/dL
  5. Hepatic dysfunction: PT-INR >1.5
  6. Hematological dysfunction: Platelet count <100,000/mm^3

GRADE II (MODERATE) ACUTE CHOLANGITIS
- Grade II acute cholangitis is associated with any two of the following conditions:
  1. Abnormal WBC count (>12,000/mm^3, <4,000/mm^3)
  2. High fever (≥39°C)
  3. Age (≥75 years old)
  4. Hyperbilirubinemia (total bilirubin ≥5 mg/dL)
  5. Hypoalbuminemia (<STD × 0.7)

GRADE I (MILD) ACUTE CHOLANGITIS
- Grade I acute cholangitis does not meet the criteria of Grade III (severe) or Grade II (moderate) acute cholangitis at initial diagnosis.

FiO₂, Fraction of inspired oxygen; *PaO₂,* partial pressure of oxygen; *PT-INR,* prothrombin time–international normalized ratio; *STD,* lower limit of normal value; *WBC,* white blood cell. Reused with permission from Kiriyama S, Kozaka K, Takada T, et al: Tokyo Guidelines 2018: diagnostic criteria and severity grading of acute cholangitis (with videos), *J Hepatobiliary Pancreat Sci* 25(1):17–30, 2018.

Antibiotics

Antibiotics should be started promptly with the specific agents selected based on risk factors, local susceptibility patterns, prior culture data, and disease severity.

The TG18 and Infectious Diseases Society of America (IDSA) 2010 guidelines on the diagnosis and management of complicated intraabdominal infection in adults and children recommend empiric antibiotic regimens for both community-associated and healthcare-associated infections. For comminuty-associated infections, combination β-lactam/β-lactam inhibitors or cephalosporins are often used. These may be used alone or combined with an aminoglycoside if local antibiotic susceptibility patterns suggest an increased burden of gram-negative resistance. For more severe cases, or for immunosuppressed individuals, vancomycin may be added to cover *Enterococcus* spp. If patients fail to improve with initial treatment, carbapenems should be used. Fluoroquinolones may be considered but used with caution given rising gram-negative bacilli resistance and potential serious adverse effects. Anaerobic coverage, such as metronidazole, is not indicated unless a biliary-enteric anastomosis is present.

For healthcare-associated cholangitis, both TG18 and IDSA recommend selecting antibiotics that cover polymicrobial infections and resistant organisms, such as *P. aeruginosa,* methicillin-resistant *Staphylococcus aureus* (MRSA), and/or vancomycin-resistant *Enterococcus* (VRE). Local antimicrobial resistance patterns, the patient's past

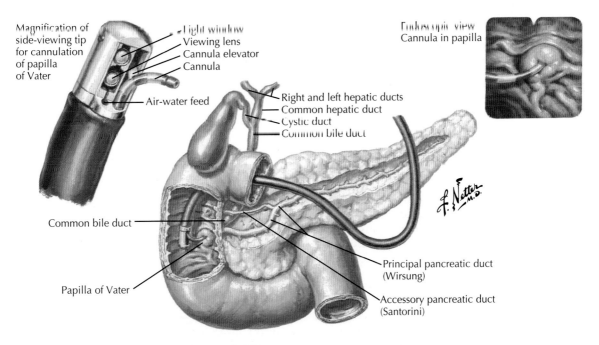

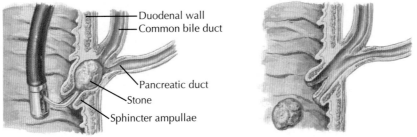

Sphincterotomy for Release of Stone Trapped in Ampulla

Stone retained in ampulla of Vater after cholecystectomy. Cutting wire introduced into ampulla via endoscope

Sphincterotomy performed. Stone released into duodenum

FIG. 118.3 **Endoscopic Cholangiopancreatography and Stone Extraction.**

culture data, and the patient's known colonization status (MRSA, VRE, multidrug-resistant gram-negative rods) can be used to determine the antibiotic regimen. If a specific organism is identified, the antibiotic regimen should be narrowed as appropriate and may eventually be transitioned to an oral agent with good bioavailability.

IDSA guidelines recommend 4 to 7 days of therapy after source control is established. In cases complicated by bacteremia, antibiotics should be continued for a minimum of 1 to 2 weeks, particularly if the organism involved is prone to cause endocarditis.

Biliary Drainage

Biliary drainage and relief of obstruction are also required to achieve source control. Early biliary drainage (within 12 hours) is recommended for grade 2 (moderate) infections while urgent drainage (within 6 hours) is recommended for grade 3 (severe) infections.

The standard methods for biliary drainage include ERCP (Fig. 118.3), EUS-guided drainage, percutaneous transhepatic cholangiography (PTC), and open surgical drainage. PTC involves transhepatic insertion of a needle into a bile duct using contrast material to opacify the bile ducts. ERCP is preferred over PTC and surgery as it is less invasive and safer. After resolution of acute cholangitis (with antibiotics and biliary drainage as described), definitive therapy with laparoscopic cholecystectomy may be indicated to eliminate the risk of recurrent disease.

CHAPTER 119

Clostridioides (Formerly *Clostridium*) *difficile* Colitis

JUSTIN G. AARON

INTRODUCTION

Clostridioides (formerly *Clostridium*) *difficile* is an anaerobic, spore-forming, gram-positive bacillus named for being historically difficult to grow on routine culture media. *C. difficile* causes a toxin-mediated **colitis** that typically develops after the normal gastrointestinal (GI) flora has been altered by antibiotics.

Infections with *C. difficile* have been increasing worldwide, and it is currently the most frequent nosocomial pathogen in the United States, with over 453,000 cases and 29,000 attributed deaths in 2011. In severe infections, all-cause mortality can be in excess of 15%. Although most cases are healthcare-associated events, about one in four occur in the community.

PATHOPHYSIOLOGY

C. difficile spores spread from person to person through the fecal-oral route and then colonize the large intestine of susceptible individuals. These spores are resistant to heat, acidity, and most antibiotics. Spores are found throughout the environment of health care facilities, which may facilitate nosocomial spread independent of person-to-person transmission. They are also found in low levels in the food supply, possibly contributing to transmission in the community setting.

The diversity of normal GI flora is protective against both colonization with ingested *C. difficile* spores and the development of infection among those already colonized. Exposure to antibiotics, however, eliminates many normal commensal organisms, facilitating *C. difficile* colonization, proliferation, and toxin elaboration.

Clinical infection is mediated by toxin production since the organism itself is noninvasive and rarely causes extraintestinal infection. Pathogenic strains of *C. difficile* produce two major toxins, TcdA (toxin A, an enterotoxin) and TcdB (toxin B, a cytotoxin), with the latter being more potent. The toxins bind to receptors on colonocytes (the epithelial cells of the colon) and inactivate members of the Rho GTPase family, leading to colonocyte death, loss of the normal intestinal barrier,

and development of a neutrophilic colitis. An increase in *C. difficile* infection (CDI) severity was noted in the early 2000s, attributed to increased prevalence of the BI/NAP1/027 strain that is more efficient at spore formation and has markedly higher toxin production. While *C. difficile* strains lacking toxin production can colonize the GI tract, they are unlikely to cause clinical infection.

Individuals with immune systems able to mount a sufficient antitoxin response will remain asymptomatically colonized, but those with an inadequate response will develop clinical infection. Many human infants are colonized with *C. difficile* but are asymptomatic, as they lack toxin receptors. Recurrent infections are common and result from either new exposure or spore reactivation in patients with impaired immune function or a persistently abnormal colonic microbiota. The risk of disease recurrence is 20% after an initial episode and as high as 60% after multiple prior recurrences.

RISK FACTORS

The most important risk factor for overt CDI is antibiotic exposure. Although the initial cases of CDI were described after exposure to clindamycin, any antibiotic that can disrupt the normal colonic microbiota can precipitate infection. Penicillins, cephalosporins, clindamycin, and fluoroquinolones are the most commonly implicated drug classes in current use.

Another major risk factor is exposure to another person known to be colonized or infected with *C. difficile*. In hospitals and health care facilities, 20% to 50% of patients are asymptomatic carriers capable of spreading infection.

Other risk factors include older age, immunosuppression (including chemotherapy and organ transplantation), inflammatory bowel disease, prior GI surgery, and chronic kidney disease. Even though spores are acid resistant, proton-pump inhibitor use also appears to be a risk factor for *C. difficile*, as gastric acid can kill the organism in its vegetative state and neutralize toxin. Risk

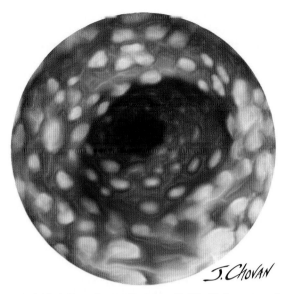

FIG. 119.1 **Pseudomembranous Colitis (Colonoscopy).**

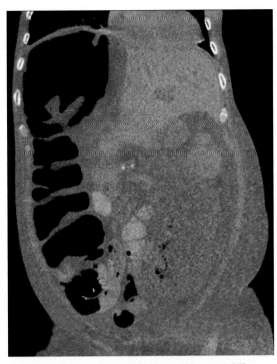

FIG. 119.2 **Toxic Megacolon (Coronal CT).**

factors for severe infection include prolonged antibiotic exposure, older age, and immunosuppression.

PRESENTATION, EVALUATION, AND DIAGNOSIS

Symptoms typically develop 5 to 10 days after antibiotic exposure but can occur up to 10 weeks later. Infections are classified by severity, with important implications for prognosis and treatment. Mild and moderate cases are characterized by diarrhea with abdominal discomfort/tenderness, leukocytosis, and, in some cases, fevers. Severe infections are characterized by heavy, possibly bloody diarrhea, along with significant abdominal pain, fevers, marked leukocytosis, acute kidney injury (typically from dehydration), and hypoalbuminemia (sometimes due to a protein-losing enteropathy). In severe cases, endoscopic examination may reveal **pseudomembranes** (raised yellowish plaques with severe inflammation of the inner bowel lining) characteristic of *C. difficile* colitis (Fig. 119.1). The exact definition of severe infection is controversial, but current guidelines have suggested a white blood cell count >15,000 cells/mm³ or an elevation in serum creatinine >1.5 times baseline as supportive data. The complications of severe infection can include shock, ileus, and **toxic megacolon** (marked distention of the large bowel with risk of perforation) (Fig. 119.2).

Infection is typically diagnosed using enzyme immunoassay (EIA) to directly detect toxin in the stool, or deoxyribonucleic acid (DNA)–based tests to detect toxin-producing genes in stool. Polymerase chain reaction (PCR) has a higher sensitivity than EIA but may also identify colonization or clinically insignificant infections that do not require treatment. Testing is only recommended for individuals with diarrhea, and it should not be repeated after completion of therapy as a test of cure because recently treated individuals may continue to test positive. Anaerobic stool culture is not recommended for routine clinical diagnosis given the long incubation time, high labor requirements, and poor yield.

TREATMENT

Asymptomatic individuals with a positive stool *C. difficile* assay are likely colonized and should not receive treatment. Patients with symptoms and a positive stool test require antibiotics. Oral vancomycin is generally the recommended first-line therapy for CDI. Oral vancomycin is not absorbed and remains in the gut lumen at the site of infection, while intravenous vancomycin does not reach therapeutic levels within the intestine and is not useful for the treatment of *C. difficile*. Fidaxomicin, a poorly absorbed macrolide, is also a recommended treatment option, but its use is limited in some settings by its high cost. Metronidazole is an alternative antibiotic when vancomycin or fidaxomicin are unavailable, generally recommended orally, but intravenous administration can achieve therapeutic fecal levels for patients unable to tolerate medication by mouth.

Patients with an initial or first recurrence of nonsevere infection should receive a course of oral vancomycin or fidaxomicin, or consideration of a prolonged vancomycin taper. Of note, antimicrobial resistance to either drug is thought to be uncommon but is not routinely assessed, as culture-based diagnostics are rarely used. Patients with severe infection should receive oral vancomycin or fidaxomicin as the initial therapy, as metronidazole has been associated with worse outcomes in severe infections. For cases complicated by ileus, high-dose oral vancomycin may be combined with intravenous metronidazole. Rectally administered vancomycin may also be useful in cases of complete ileus. Severe fulminant cases of *C. difficile* colitis, including toxic megacolon, may require surgical resection of the affected colon.

Individuals with more than one recurrent infection remain at high risk for additional recurrences. For such cases, oral vancomycin remains a treatment option, often administered as a prolonged taper over several weeks with pulsed dosing (every 2–3 days for the last 3 weeks) to eliminate any remaining spores in the colon. Fidaxomicin is also effective for recurrent infections.

In addition to providing therapeutic antibiotics, it is also essential to terminate all other antibiotics as soon as possible, so as to promote restoration of the normal colonic microbiota. If other antibiotics are still needed, therapy for *C. difficile* is often extended for at least 1 week beyond the stop date of other agents. Full recovery of the colonic microbiota can take >12 weeks after termination of other antibiotics, contributing to the high recurrence rate.

Fecal microbiota transplant (FMT) from a screened stool donor can help restore a balanced enteric flora and has emerged as an effective treatment for individuals with recurrent infection, with success rates >90%. The utility of FMT in acute infection remains unclear.

Initiatives for the prevention of CDI include antimicrobial stewardship and preventing nosocomial spread by appropriate hand hygiene and isolation practices. Alcohol-based hand sanitizers do not eradicate *C. difficile* spores, so health care workers should wash with soap and water when caring for infected patients, as the mechanical act of scrubbing is more effective for spore removal. Patients with suspected or confirmed infection should be placed on contact precautions (gloves and gown) and isolated or, when necessary, cohorted with other infected patients. Environmental decontamination is also emerging as a possible prevention strategy, given the ability of spores to persist on fomites in the hospital setting. The benefit of probiotics to help maintain or restore the colonic microbiota remains unclear.

CHAPTER 120

Urinary Tract Infection

JONATHAN R. KOMISAR

INTRODUCTION

Urinary tract infections (UTIs) are subdivided into infections of the bladder **(cystitis)** and of the kidneys **(pyelonephritis).** The diagnosis of UTI requires the presence of bacteriuria combined with symptoms and physiological signs consistent with infection; the presence of bacteriuria without infectious signs or symptoms is known as **asymptomatic bacteriuria** and generally does not require treatment.

UTI can be further categorized as complicated or uncomplicated. **Complicated UTI** is defined as a UTI in a patient with characteristics that increase the risk of treatment failure, including diabetes mellitus, pregnancy, renal failure, urinary tract obstruction, indwelling urinary device (e.g., urethral catheter, ureteral stent, nephrostomy tube), renal transplantation, immunosuppression, functional or anatomical abnormality of the genitourinary (GU) tract, hospital-acquired infection, prolonged duration of symptoms prior to the initiation of appropriate treatment, and failure to respond to appropriate treatment within 48 to 72 hours.

PATHOPHYSIOLOGY

UTIs most commonly occur when bacteria are introduced into and ascend the GU tract. Less often, the GU tract becomes infected from hematogenous dissemination in the setting of bacteremia. The ascension of bacteria through the urethra into the bladder results in cystitis, while further ascension through the ureters into the renal parenchyma results in pyelonephritis. The most common uropathogens include *Escherichia coli, Proteus mirabilis, Klebsiella pneumoniae,* and Enterobacteriaceae. In complicated UTIs, additional uropathogens include *Serratia* spp., enterococci, staphylococci, *Pseudomonas* spp., and fungi (e.g., *Candida* spp.).

RISK FACTORS

Females are at greater risk of UTI than males, owing both to the proximity of the urethra to the anus and to the shorter length of the urethra. Such anatomy allows for vaginal and periurethral colonization with enteric bacteria, especially following sexual intercourse. In women, spermicide use has also been shown to increase UTI risk since the active ingredients are toxic to normal vaginal flora and increase the risk of colonization with pathogenic species.

In contrast, the risk is lower among males because of longer urethral length, antimicrobial properties of prostatic fluid, and decreased periurethral colonization (owing to a drier environment). The risk for males increases with age, however, as the increased prevalence of benign prostatic hyperplasia (BPH) causes bladder outlet obstruction and urinary stasis. Uncircumcised males are also at higher risk because of periurethral colonization with enteric flora.

Processes associated with **urinary stasis** further increase the risk of UTI. Urinary stasis may occur secondary to anatomical obstruction or detrusor muscle dysfunction and impaired bladder contraction. Common causes of obstruction include BPH, fecal impaction, pregnancy, and malignancy, while common causes of detrusor dysfunction include neurological disorders (demyelinating processes, spinal cord trauma, or stroke), diabetes mellitus (owing to autonomic neuropathy), and aging (muscle atrophy and reduced bladder sensitivity) (Fig. 120.1).

Indwelling catheters and renal stones can serve as niduses for bacterial colonization. Anatomical abnormalities that promote retrograde passage of urine, such as vesicoureteral reflux, also increase the risk of infection.

PRESENTATION, EVALUATION, AND DIAGNOSIS

The clinical history is invaluable for guiding the diagnosis, localization, and management of UTI. Patients with cystitis typically report dysuria, increased urinary frequency, increased urinary urgency, and/or suprapubic pain. They may also describe changes in the color, smell, or turbidity of their urine. In contrast, patients with

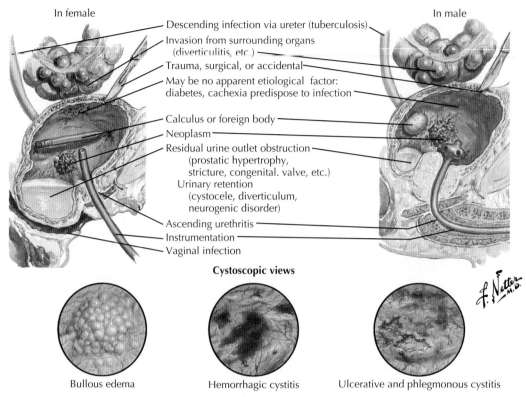

In female

In male

Descending infection via ureter (tuberculosis)

Invasion from surrounding organs (diverticulitis, etc.)

Trauma, surgical, or accidental

May be no apparent etiological factor: diabetes, cachexia predispose to infection

Calculus or foreign body

Neoplasm

Residual urine outlet obstruction (prostatic hypertrophy, stricture, congenital. valve, etc.)

Urinary retention (cystocele, diverticulum, neurogenic disorder)

Ascending urethritis

Instrumentation

Vaginal infection

Cystoscopic views

Bullous edema

Hemorrhagic cystitis

Ulcerative and phlegmonous cystitis

FIG. 120.1 **Risk Factors for Cystitis.**

pyelonephritis often report constitutional symptoms (e.g., fever, chills, nausea, vomiting) combined with flank pain, sometimes without symptoms of cystitis. If UTI is the likely diagnosis, it is important to assess for prior GU procedures, recent instrumentation, and comorbid medical conditions that could predispose to infection with specific uropathogens.

Several conditions can have similar presentations and should be differentiated from UTIs. Men should be evaluated for prostatitis if they report symptoms of cystitis combined with constitutional symptoms, acute changes in bladder voiding (retention, hesitancy, and dribbling), pain at the tip of the penis, perineal pain, or pelvic pain. Meanwhile, a sexual history can help clarify the risk of such infections as urethritis, vaginitis, cervicitis, and/or pelvic inflammatory disease.

It is also important to note that elderly patients with UTI may present with nonspecific complaints, poorly localizing symptoms (e.g., lethargy, confusion), and chronic issues with dysuria (e.g., GU syndrome of menopause), urinary retention, and urinary hesitancy (i.e., BPH).

The physical examination should begin with an assessment of vital signs. The presence of fever, hypotension, tachypnea, and/or tachycardia should prompt immediate evaluation for complicated UTI and possible **sepsis.** A thorough abdominal examination should be performed, with special attention to suprapubic tenderness and assessment of the bladder, which may be palpable in the setting of urinary retention. Gentle percussion of both flanks should be performed to assess for costovertebral angle tenderness, which would suggest pyelonephritis (Fig. 120.2). Pelvic examination should be considered in women with symptoms suggestive of vaginitis or cervicitis. Likewise, digital rectal examination should be considered in men with symptoms suggestive of prostatitis.

In young, healthy, nonpregnant females with symptoms consistent with uncomplicated cystitis, empiric treatment is appropriate without any laboratory testing. Urine culture should be collected if symptoms do not resolve or if there is concern for resistance.

In contrast, all other patients should have urinalysis and urine culture to document infection and identify the

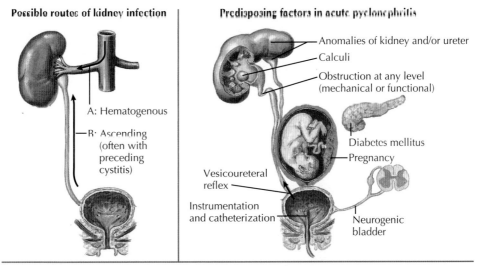

Possible routes of kidney infection

A: Hematogenous

B: Ascending (often with preceding cystitis)

Predisposing factors in acute pyelonephritis

Anomalies of kidney and/or ureter

Calculi

Obstruction at any level (mechanical or functional)

Diabetes mellitus

Pregnancy

Vesicoureteral reflex

Instrumentation and catheterization

Neurogenic bladder

Common clinical and laboratory features of acute pyelonephritis

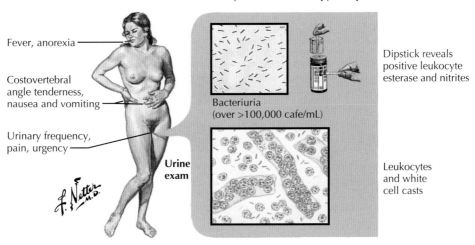

Fever, anorexia

Costovertebral angle tenderness, nausea and vomiting

Urinary frequency, pain, urgency

Urine exam

Bacteriuria (over >100,000 cafe/mL)

Dipstick reveals positive leukocyte esterase and nitrites

Leukocytes and white cell casts

FIG. 120.2 **Pyelonephritis: Risk Factors and Major Findings.**

responsible pathogen and its antibiotic sensitivities. A positive urinalysis may show elevated **leukocyte esterase,** which is produced by white blood cells (WBCs) in the urine **(pyuria),** and elevated nitrites, which are converted from nitrates by Enterobacteriaceae. Microscopic analysis can further quantify the number of WBCs in the urine; >5 WBCs qualifies as pyuria. Urine cultures are considered positive if the colony count exceeds 10^4 cfu/mL. Imaging of the urinary tract using ultrasound or CT is appropriate in patients with persistent symptoms despite appropriate antimicrobial treatment after 48 to 72 hours and in patients who present with severe illness (Fig. 120.3).

TREATMENT

The selection of antimicrobial agents depends on the severity and type of UTI, local resistance patterns, and prior culture data from the patient, when available.

For uncomplicated cystitis in women, appropriate antimicrobials include nitrofurantoin, fosfomycin, trimethoprim-sulfamethoxazole, and pivmecillinam, with the time course depending on the specific agent selected. If these are not available or tolerated, second-line options include β-lactams (amoxicillin-clavulanate, cefdinir, cefaclor, cefpodoxime) and fluoroquinolones (ciprofloxacin, levofloxacin). For uncomplicated cystitis in

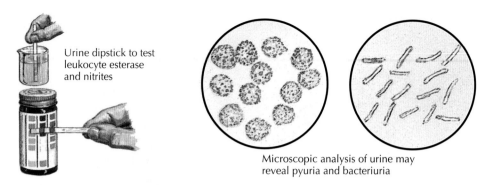

Urine dipstick to test leukocyte esterase and nitrites

Microscopic analysis of urine may reveal pyuria and bacteriuria

Urine culture quantifies degree of infection and characterizes pathogen

Dip slides

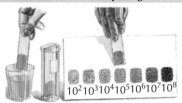

$10^2 10^3 10^4 10^5 10^6 10^7 10^8$

The slide is dipped in urine, allowed to dry, and then incubated in a plastic bottle. One side of the slide contains a general soy agar, which grows both gram-positive and gram-negative bacteria, while the other side contains eosin methylene blue (EMB) agar or MacConkey agar, which grows gram-negative bacteria. After several days, the growth is compared with a visual reference.

Direct plating

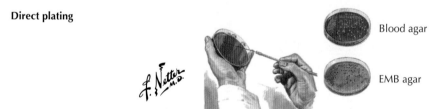

Blood agar

EMB agar

Agar plates are inoculated with urine. A calibrated loop is used to deliver a precise quantity of urine to each plate. Blood agar grows gram-positive and gram-negative bacteria, while EMB agar grows gram-negative bacteria. By counting the number of colonies that grow, the number of colonies that would form per milliliter of urine can be estimated. For example, if 100 colonies appear after 0.001 mL of urine is transferred to the plate, the reported colony count is 100,000 cfu/mL. The colonies can subsequently be sub cultured for identification and determination of antibiotic susceptibilities.

FIG. 120.3 **Evaluation of Lower Urinary Tract Infection.**

men, appropriate antimicrobials include trimethoprim-sulfamethoxazole and fluoroquinolones.

For cases of acute uncomplicated pyelonephritis, empiric therapy should be prescribed until culture data are available. The choice of empiric therapy depends on the severity of illness. In stable patients with mild-to-moderate disease, outpatient treatment with fluoroquinolones is appropriate. In cases of moderate-to-severe illness, inpatient treatment with an intravenous fluoroquinolone, an extended-spectrum cephalosporin, an extended-spectrum penicillin, carbapenem, or an aminoglycoside is recommended.

For cases of acute complicated cystitis, empiric therapy with oral fluoroquinolone is appropriate. If the patient cannot tolerate oral therapy (e.g., due to recurrent nausea and vomiting), parenteral treatment options include levofloxacin, ceftriaxone, gentamicin, tobramycin, or a carbapenem, especially if an extended-spectrum β-lactamase (ESBL)–producing organism is suspected. Rapid clinical deterioration despite appropriate antimicrobial therapy with a β-lactam in a patient with a history of nosocomial-acquired infections or pathogens with known high rates of ESBL-producing activity (*E. coli, K. pneumoniae*) should prompt broadening of antimicrobial treatment to a carbapenem.

All cases of acute complicated pyelonephritis should be initially managed in the inpatient setting using broad-spectrum parenteral antimicrobials. Appropriate agents include aztreonam, ciprofloxacin, levofloxacin, and ceftriaxone for mild to moderate pyelonephritis, and carbapenems (meropenem, imipenem, ertapenem, doripenem), cefepime, and piperacillin-tazobactam for severe pyelonephritis. The duration of treatment varies depending on the underlying risk factors.

Of note, patients with asymptomatic bacteriuria do not generally require antimicrobials unless they are pregnant or are undergoing urological procedures with a high risk of mucosal bleeding. In particular, the treatment of asymptomatic bacteriuria in individuals with indwelling catheters or spinal cord injury should be avoided unless there are physiological signs consistent with infection.

CHAPTER 121

Urethritis

JUSTIN C. LARACY

INTRODUCTION

The term **urethritis** describes any process resulting in inflammation of the male or female urethra. Most cases are infectious and associated with sexually transmitted pathogens. Lack of barrier contraception and recent new sexual partners are important risk factors for infection.

The most common causes of infectious urethritis are *Neisseria gonorrhoeae* and *Chlamydia trachomatis.* Thus urethritis is traditionally classified as gonococcal urethritis (GU) or nongonococcal urethritis (NGU). Besides *C. trachomatis*, additional causes of NGU include other bacteria *(Mycoplasma genitalium)*, protozoa *(Trichomonas vaginalis)*, and viruses (herpes simplex virus, adenovirus). Coinfection with two or more pathogens can occur, with important implications for management. In approximately half of NGU cases, no specific pathogen is identified.

PRESENTATION, EVALUATION, AND DIAGNOSIS

Dysuria (painful urination) is the most common symptom of urethritis. Other symptoms include itching, burning, and discharge at the urethral meatus. Urethral discharge may or may not be present, and its appearance can vary from thin and watery to thick and purulent (Fig. 121.1). The clinical presentations of GU and NGU overlap and cannot be reliably distinguished based on signs or symptoms; nonetheless, thick purulent urethral discharge is more suggestive of GU, whereas dysuria alone without urethral discharge is more suggestive of NGU. Up to 10% of patients with GU, and >40% of patients with NGU, may be asymptomatic.

It is important to consider alternative causes of dysuria, especially in men with no sexual risk factors. The differential diagnosis should include noninfectious causes of urethritis (e.g., chemical or physical irritation) and infections (e.g., cystitis, epididymitis, prostatitis).

The diagnosis of urethritis is confirmed by Gram strain of a urethral swab and urine studies (see Fig. 121.1). The urethral swab can establish the presence of white blood cells (WBCs) and may reveal a causative organism. The US Centers for Disease Control and Prevention (CDC) recommends a threshold of ≥2 WBCs per oil immersion field to diagnose urethritis; higher WBC counts are more suggestive of GU, specifically. The presence of gram-negative intracellular diplococci is diagnostic of GU, whereas the absence of visible organisms instead suggests NGU.

Given the discomfort associated with urethral swabs, urine specimens are often used in the diagnosis of urethritis. These should be tested with a dipstick, microscopic evaluation, and nucleic acid amplification testing (NAAT), if available. A dipstick positive for leukocyte esterase, as well as the presence of ≥10 WBCs per high-power field on microscopy, suggests the presence of an inflammatory process.

NAAT testing is available for *N. gonorrhoeae* and *C. trachomatis* at most laboratories and is highly sensitive and specific. If gram-negative intracellular diplococci are found on Gram stain, NAAT testing for *N. gonorrhoeae* is superfluous; however, NAAT testing for *C. trachomatis* should still be performed since these two infections often coexist. If no organisms are seen on Gram stain, or if Gram staining is unavailable, NAAT testing for both *N. gonorrhoeae* and *C. trachomatis* is appropriate. By identifying the exact organism(s) responsible for symptoms, NAAT testing facilitates the treatment of both the patient and his or her recent sexual partners. It is also essential because *N. gonorrhoeae* and *C. trachomatis* are reportable diseases in the United States and should be documented with the appropriate local authorities, which can facilitate partner identification and notification. Of note, because urethritis is generally a **sexually transmitted infection** (STI), patients with a confirmed diagnosis should be offered testing for other STIs, such as syphilis and HIV.

Finally, urethritis can occur in conjunction with infection at other anatomical sites (Fig. 121.2), such as the lower urogenital tract, rectum, and pharynx. Thus patients with urethritis should be evaluated for infection at these sites.

Clinical findings

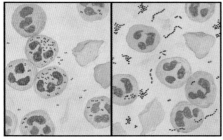

Mild urethritis

Severe urethritis
(usually gonococcal)

Urethritis and skenitis

Microscopic findings

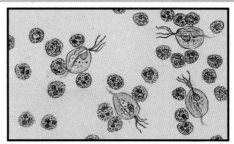

Gonorrheal infection   Non specific infection

Trichomonas vaginalis as seen in fresh specimen
from urethral discharge

FIG. 121.1 **Gonococcal Urethritis: Clinical and Microscopic Findings.**

TREATMENT

The antimicrobial regimen for urethritis is often empirical and depends on the clinical evidence for GU and/or NGU. Any man with high clinical suspicion for urethritis (dysuria, purulent discharge, known exposure) and supporting microscopic evidence should be treated. When urethritis is diagnosed but no intracellular diplococci are detected, presumptive treatment of NGU can be initiated while awaiting NAAT results. If there is a high suspicion for GU (i.e., known exposure, high-risk behavior) despite negative microscopy findings, empiric GU treatment should also be given.

The treatment for GU must address antibiotic resistance among *N. gonorrhoeae* strains and typically consists of a single intramuscular dose of ceftriaxone and a single oral dose of azithromycin, which has the added benefit of treating potential *C. trachomatis* coinfection if present. Of note, combination therapy for GU is still required even when coinfection with *C. trachomatis* has been ruled out.

The treatment for NGU specifically targets *C. trachomatis*. The preferred regimens are either a single oral

dose of azithromycin or a 7-day course of doxycycline. Azithromycin is preferred when possible because it can be given as a single, observed dose and it is more effective against other possible causes of NGU, such as *M. genitalium*.

Potential causes of recurrent or persistent symptoms despite treatment include reinfection, poor adherence, antimicrobial resistance, and niche organisms that were not covered with the original regimen. A patient with persistent symptoms should be reevaluated and retested as described earlier. Any patient who was reexposed or not adherent can be treated a second time. If the patient was adherent and there is minimal concern for reexposure, then antimicrobial resistance, alternative organisms, and alternative diagnoses should be considered. In that setting, the cause for treatment failure should be considered on a case-by-case basis. For example, in areas with high levels of *N. gonorrhoeae* resistance, the treatment regimen should be modified to include a higher dose of ceftriaxone and/or azithromycin. If the patient continues to have symptoms despite retreatment with higher doses, an aminoglycoside or fluoroquinolone can be substituted

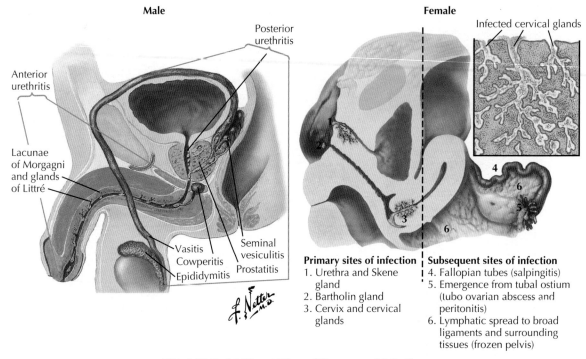

Male

Posterior
urethritis

Anterior
urethritis

Lacunae
of Morgagni
and glands
of Littré

Vasitis
Cowperitis
Epididymitis

Seminal
vesiculitis
Prostatitis

Female

Infected cervical glands

Primary sites of infection
1. Urethra and Skene
   gland
2. Bartholin gland
3. Cervix and cervical
   glands

Subsequent sites of infection
4. Fallopian tubes (salpingitis)
5. Emergence from tubal ostium
   (tubo ovarian abscess and
   peritonitis)
6. Lymphatic spread to broad
   ligaments and surrounding
   tissues (frozen pelvis)

FIG. 121.2 Additional Sites of Gonococcal Infection.

for ceftriaxone. In addition, metronidazole can be used to cover *T. vaginalis.*

To prevent transmission to sexual partners, men should be advised to refrain from sexual activity for at least 7 days from the initiation of antimicrobial therapy and for as long as symptoms persist. A test of cure (performed 1–3 weeks following treatment) is not needed in cases treated with first-line therapy; however, all patients should undergo repeat NAAT testing 3 to 6 months after treatment regardless of clinical condition to detect reinfection, which is common in the 6 months after initial *N. gonorrhoeae* or *C. trachomatis* infection.

CHAPTER 122

Osteomyelitis

CATHERINE DEVOE

INTRODUCTION

Osteomyelitis (OM) is an infection of bone that leads to an inflammatory response and, ultimately, to bone destruction. Given that bone, compared to other possible sites of infection, is relatively inaccessible from both a tissue sampling and an antibiotic delivery perspective, OM poses a significant diagnostic and therapeutic challenge. Further complicating management of these infections, randomized controlled trials in this area are few, and most recommendations are based on expert opinion and common practice.

Multiple classification schemes for OM have been proposed. Two of the most common are the Lew-Waldvogel classification, which breaks down OM by duration of illness and mechanism of spread, and the Cierny-Mader classification, which takes into account the affected portion of bone, the physiological status of the host, and local factors that may affect healing. Practically speaking, it is useful to categorize OM as acute (developing over a few days or weeks) or chronic (developing over more than a few weeks), as this has an effect on both treatment and prognosis. It is also important to consider the site of infection, the development of local complications such as adjacent abscesses or joint space infections, and whether a prosthesis or foreign material is involved, as these, too, will have treatment implications.

PATHOPHYSIOLOGY

OM occurs via one of three primary mechanisms: hematogenous spread, contiguous spread, or secondary infection of damaged tissue, generally in areas of vascular or neurological compromise. In hematogenous spread, bacteria travel through the blood from the primary site of infection and seed the bone. In children, this mechanism most commonly results in OM of the metaphyses of long bones, particularly the tibia and the femur; in adults, it most frequently causes OM of the vertebral column (Fig. 122.1). In contiguous spread, bacteria are inoculated at a site of bony injury or surgical intervention. This mode

of infection may result in sternal OM after cardiovascular surgery, OM of the long bones following fracture or trauma, or periarticular OM following prosthetic joint insertion. Finally, chronic vascular and/or neurological compromise can lead to soft tissue breakdown, infection and necrosis, and finally to OM. This pathway is classic for the development of OM complicating diabetic foot infections or pressure ulcers (Fig. 122.2).

Regardless of the mechanism of infection, the invasion of bacteria into bone in acute OM leads to a suppurative inflammatory process, in which both inflammatory factors and leukocytes contribute directly to tissue necrosis and breakdown of bone matrix. Inflammation can also cause compression and obliteration of local vasculature, leading to ischemia and further necrosis. When the vascular supply to small regions of bone is destroyed, discrete areas of avascular necrosis, known as **sequestra,** can result. These may harbor bacteria that are inaccessible to systemically delivered antibiotics. The formation of sequestra is one of the developments that separate acute from chronic OM, and it partially explains why antibiotic treatment alone, which may be sufficient in acute OM, is generally not effective in chronic cases.

Hematogenously acquired OM is usually monomicrobial, while OM acquired via contiguous spread or secondary infection may be either monomicrobial or polymicrobial. The most common causative pathogens in OM vary somewhat by site and mechanism of infection. Despite this variation, *Staphylococcus aureus* (both methicillin susceptible and resistant) is the most frequent etiology overall. Coagulase-negative staphylococcal species are also common, especially in prosthetic joint infections. Streptococcal species and gram negative organisms, including *Pseudomonas,* are responsible for a significant number of cases, while anaerobes and fungi are less common. *Mycobacterium tuberculosis* should be considered as a possible cause of OM in patients from endemic areas and is particularly known for causing spondylitis and OM of the spine (**Pott disease**). *Salmonella* is notorious for causing OM in patients with sickle cell disease.

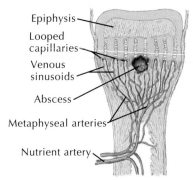

Epiphysis

Looped capillaries

Venous sinusoids

Abscess

Metaphyseal arteries

Nutrient artery

Terminal branches of metaphyseal arteries form loops at growth plate and enter irregular afferent venous sinusoids. Blood flow slowed and turbulent, predisposing to bacterial seeding. In addition, lining cells have little or no phagocytic activity. Area is catch basin for bacteria, and abscess may form.

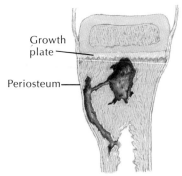

Growth plate

Periosteum

Abscess, limited by growth plate, spreads transversely along Volkmann canals and elevates periosteum; extends subperiosteally and may invade shaft. In infants under 1 year of age, some metaphyseal arterial branches pass through growth plate, and infection may invade epiphysis and joint.

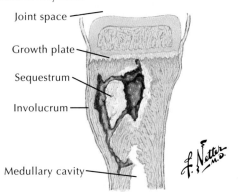

Joint space

Growth plate

Sequestrum

Involucrum

Medullary cavity

As abscess spreads, segment of devitalized bone (sequestrum) remains within it. Elevated periosteum may also lay down bone to form encasing shell (involucrum). Occasionally, abscess walled off by fibrosis and bone sclerosis to form Brodie abscess.

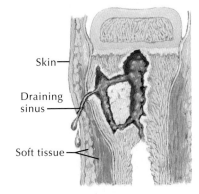

Skin

Draining sinus

Soft tissue

Infectious process may erode periosteum and form sinus through soft tissues and skin to drain externally. Process influenced by virulence of organism, resistance of host, administration of antibiotics, and fibrotic and sclerotic responses.

FIG. 122.1 **Pathogenesis of Hematogenous Osteomyelitis.**

PRESENTATION, EVALUATION, AND DIAGNOSIS

The most common presentation of OM involves pain at the site of infection. Systemic signs of infection, most commonly low-grade fever, may also be present but are frequently absent in subacute or chronic OM. Leukocytosis may or may not be present. Elevations in **erythrocyte sedimentation rate (ESR)** and **C-reactive protein (CRP)** have a high sensitivity for the presence of OM and can therefore serve as a useful screening tool; if these inflammatory markers are normal, OM is less likely. On examination of suspected OM associated with foot or pressure ulcers, the **probe-to-bone test,** in which a blunt metal instrument is inserted and a hard gritty

surface is felt for, has been found to be 87% sensitive and 83% specific.

Regarding imaging, MRI has the greatest sensitivity for the detection of OM and is considered the gold standard. It has the ability to detect bone marrow edema early in infection and can also evaluate the extent of cortical destruction (Fig. 122.3). CT is less sensitive than MRI but is also an acceptable modality for the evaluation of bony destruction (including sequestra) and surrounding soft tissue abnormalities. Patients with metal hardware who may be unable to undergo MRI or have an unacceptable amount of artifact on CT can undergo nuclear scan. Radiographic plain films may be suggestive of OM in patients with at least 2 weeks of clinical symptoms

Secondary to contiguous focus of infection

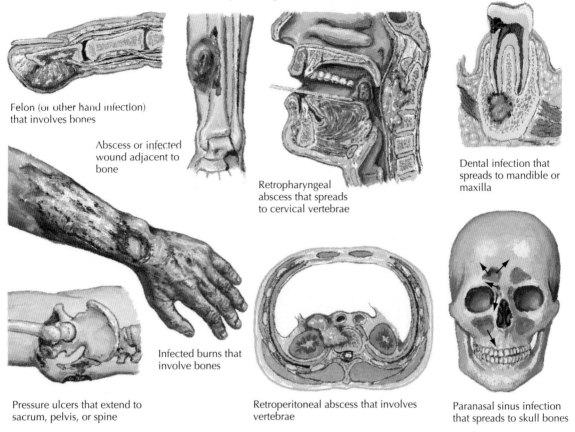

Felon (or other hand infection) that involves bones

Abscess or infected wound adjacent to bone

Retropharyngeal abscess that spreads to cervical vertebrae

Dental infection that spreads to mandible or maxilla

Infected burns that involve bones

Pressure ulcers that extend to sacrum, pelvis, or spine

Retroperitoneal abscess that involves vertebrae

Paranasal sinus infection that spreads to skull bones

Contributory or predisposing factors

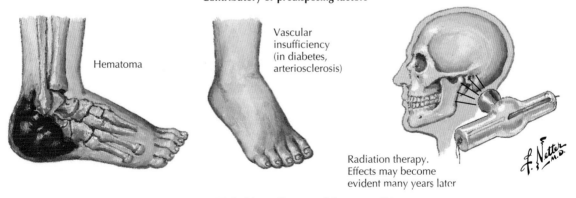

Hematoma

Vascular insufficiency (in diabetes, arteriosclerosis)

Radiation therapy. Effects may become evident many years later

FIG. 122.2 **Direct Causes of Osteomyelitis.**

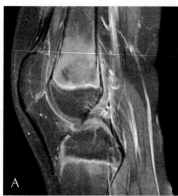

(A) Lateral T2-weighted MRI of distal femur with early acute osteomyelitis. 10-year-old female with progressive pain in left knee region and difficulty walking. Plain radiographs normal. MRI showed signal changes of distal femur metaphyseal region consistent with osteomyelitis.

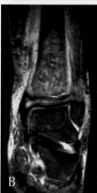

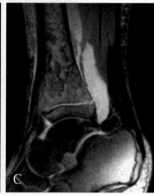

Anteroposterior (B) and lateral (C) of T2-weighted MRI of the distal tibia with late acute osteomyelitis. Note the inflammatory changes in the distal tibia metaphysis, the signal changes beneath the elevated periosteum, and the large posterior abscess from pus breaking through the periosteum.

FIG. 122.3 MRI Findings in Early and Late Acute Osteomyelitis.

and are a reasonable first test in that setting; however, plain films are insufficient for exclusion of OM due to their low sensitivity (variably reported at 22%–75%), and patients with negative plain films should therefore proceed to a more definitive test.

For all cases of OM, an attempt should be made to identify the causative pathogen, both to confirm the diagnosis and to allow tailoring of the antibiotic regimen. If blood cultures are positive—as they are in about half of acute cases—this is often sufficient, especially if imaging is characteristic and the organism is a frequent cause of OM. If blood cultures are negative and clinical suspicion for OM remains high, the patient should proceed to bone biopsy, which can be either CT guided or open. If there is a contiguous abscess (e.g., a paravertebral abscess complicating a vertebral OM) or synovial fluid infection, sampling of these can also provide a causative pathogen. Superficial wound swabs and cultures are not useful; in fact, they can be misleading and should be avoided. Pretreatment with antibiotics significantly reduces the yield of both blood cultures and bone biopsy; antibiotics should therefore be withheld in clinically stable, nonseptic patients until

an organism has been identified or a bone sample has been obtained.

TREATMENT

OM is generally treated with a prolonged course of antibiotics along with debridement or removal of infected bone, if feasible. For cases of acute OM without soft tissue complications or involvement of foreign material, antibiotics alone are appropriate initial treatment. The recommended length of treatment is at least 4 weeks, but more often 6 to 8 weeks. Traditionally, antibiotics are administered intravenously (IV) for at least the first 2 weeks, and in the past, many clinicians preferred to give the entire course IV. However, this practice is now changing, largely based on a 2019 randomized controlled trial that found that switching to oral therapy within the first 7 days of treatment was noninferior to completing an entire course IV. The agent chosen is guided by the susceptibilities of the responsible pathogen, but frequently is a β-lactam followed by a fluoroquinolone (owing to superior absorption and bioavailability) if and when the switch is made to oral therapy. For infections due to methicillin-resistant *S. aureus* (MRSA), treatment with IV vancomycin or daptomycin, with or without adjunctive rifampin, is often required.

Some cases of acute OM require surgical intervention in addition to antibiotics. This is the general rule when devices or prostheses are involved. Usually, the infected device should be removed and can either be immediately replaced or (more commonly) replaced following a weeks-long course of antibiotics. In cases of secondary infections of diabetic foot ulcers or pressure ulcers, debridement should generally be attempted; if debridement plus antibiotics fails, then amputation may be necessary. Soft tissue complications of OM, such as abscesses, often require surgical intervention as well.

In cases of chronic OM, the management should be primarily surgical: Removal of as much infected bone as possible is required for eradication. If complete removal of infected bone is achieved (e.g., via amputation of an infected limb), surgery can be followed by a much shorter course of antibiotics. In cases where comorbidities, overall functional status, or patient preference preclude surgical management, chronic suppressive antibiotics can be given, but this should be done with the understanding that it is not curative.

CHAPTER 123

HIV/AIDS: Infection and Treatment

COLIN M. SMITH

INTRODUCTION

HIV is a bloodborne, cytopathic retrovirus that targets a subset of human helper T cells (CD4+ T lymphocytes). If untreated, HIV infection causes profound immune dysfunction that eventually results in the opportunistic infections and malignancies characteristic of **AIDS.**

Since the initial reports of "gay-related immune deficiency" in the early 1980s, HIV has infected >75 million people worldwide, and ~35 million have died from HIV-related complications. In 2015, the estimated prevalence of HIV infection among adults age 15 to 49 years was 0.8%, ranging from 0.1% in the Western Pacific to 4.4% in sub-Saharan Africa. In the United States, >50,000 new infections occur each year, with the greatest number occurring in men who have sex with men.

Two types of HIV have been characterized, known as HIV1 and HIV2; however, HIV1 is more virulent and transmissible, and has been responsible for nearly all cases of HIV infection in the United States. Thus HIV1 is the focus of this chapter.

PATHOPHYSIOLOGY

HIV infects specific body fluids (blood, semen, preseminal fluid, rectal fluids, vaginal fluids, and breast milk) and is transmitted either by exposure to mucosal tissue or direct inoculation into the bloodstream.

HIV has tropism for several immune cells, including CD4+ T lymphocytes, monocytes, macrophages, and dendritic cells. In most cases, new infection results from virus tropic to macrophages (Fig. 123.1). The HIV envelope glycoprotein gp120 binds to the macrophage CD4 receptor and CCR5 chemokine coreceptor, inducing a conformational change in the HIV transmembrane protein gp41 that facilitates fusion and subsequent entry into the host cell. Some individuals lack CCR5 receptors and have near-complete protection from HIV acquisition.

Once inside the host cell, single-stranded HIV ribonucleic acid (RNA) undergoes reverse transcription to deoxyribonucleic acid (DNA) and then integration into the host genome. The host cell then transcribes the virus DNA to produce RNA, which is translated into HIV proteins. The RNA and proteins assemble to form immature virions. These virions are released from the host cell and undergo further maturation, including the cleavage of a polyprotein into mature proteins by a viral protease.

The infection then spreads to lymph nodes, where it further replicates and disseminates into blood and lymphoid tissue. Gut-associated lymphatic tissue (GALT) becomes depleted, even as peripheral T-cell counts are initially preserved. The loss of GALT causes relative immune deficiency and has also been hypothesized to alter intestinal mucosal function, increasing the translocation of gut flora and thereby generating the chronic immune activation typical of HIV infection.

The initial mucosal infection and viremia are followed by a chronic, clinically latent phase of infection, characterized by continued viral replication in lymph nodes and other lymphoid tissues. Over time, the progressive depletion of CD4+ cells and rise in HIV viral load create a state of immune deficiency/dysregulation associated with opportunistic (AIDS-defining infections and malignancies) and nonopportunistic complications (cardiovascular disease, solid tumors, nephropathy, etc.).

AIDS is diagnosed when the patient experiences specific **opportunistic infections** (see Box 123.1 and Chapter 124 for further details) or when the CD4 count falls to <200 cells/μL.

RISK FACTORS

HIV transmission occurs primarily through sexual contact but can also occur from direct inoculation of blood (i.e., intravenous [IV] drug use or blood transfusion) and from vertical transmission (i.e., childbirth and breastfeeding). There is a small risk of healthcare-associated exposure. There is no evidence of HIV transmission from casual contact. Those at greatest risk of infection are men who have sex with men, commercial sex workers, transgender individuals, IV drug users, infants of HIV-positive mothers, and incarcerated individuals.

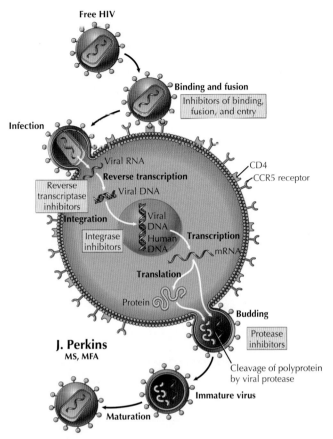

FIG. 123.1 HIV Lifecycle and Mechanisms of Antiretroviral Medications. *DNA,* Deoxyribonucleic acid; *mRNA,* messenger RNA; *RNA,* ribonucleic acid.

PRESENTATION, EVALUATION, AND DIAGNOSIS

Acute HIV infection commonly causes a mononucleosis-like syndrome (termed **acute retroviral syndrome**) about 3 to 6 weeks after viral acquisition. Initial symptoms typically include fever, lymphadenopathy, pharyngitis, rash, and myalgias. Physical exam findings are similarly nonspecific, though painful mucocutaneous ulcerations and hepatosplenomegaly are sometimes noted. Symptoms usually persist for at least 1 week but may be present for much longer. Superimposed opportunistic processes can rarely occur during acute infection, complicating the clinical presentation.

As patients with acute HIV infection may not yet have antibodies to the virus, the diagnostic tests of choice are a fourth-generation combined immunoassay for HIV antibody/p24 antigen and an HIV1 RNA quantitative real-time polymerase chain reaction (PCR). If these initial tests are negative but a high-risk exposure occurred, then the tests should be repeated after 1 to 2 weeks.

A positive test should generally prompt genotypic resistance testing, although empiric **antiretroviral therapy (ART)** can be initiated while awaiting the results. Additional laboratory studies for all newly diagnosed patients should include a quantitative viral load, a **CD4 count**, a complete blood count, a comprehensive metabolic panel, a fasting lipid profile, and a urinalysis. Patients should also be screened for other sexually transmitted infections and latent tuberculosis. These laboratory tests should be closely followed during the first 3 months of ART to ensure its safety and efficacy, then periodically reassessed once the viral load becomes undetectable and the CD4 count normalizes.

BOX 123.1
AIDS-Defining Opportunistic Complications

- Bacterial infections, multiple or recurrent[a]
- Candidiasis of bronchi, trachea, or lungs
- Candidiasis of esophagus[b]
- Cervical cancer, invasive[c]
- Coccidioidomycosis, disseminated or extrapulmonary
- Cryptococcosis, extrapulmonary
- Cryptosporidiosis, chronic intestinal (>1-month duration)
- Cytomegalovirus disease (other than liver, spleen, or nodes), onset at age >1 month
- Cytomegalovirus retinitis (with loss of vision)[b]
- Encephalopathy, HIV related
- Herpes simplex: chronic ulcers (>1-month duration) or bronchitis, pneumonitis, or esophagitis (onset at age >1 month)
- Histoplasmosis, disseminated or extrapulmonary
- Isosporiasis, chronic intestinal (>1-month duration)
- Kaposi sarcoma[b]

- Lymphoid interstitial pneumonia or pulmonary lymphoid hyperplasia complex[a,b]
- Lymphoma, Burkitt (or equivalent term)
- Lymphoma, immunoblastic (or equivalent term)
- Lymphoma, primary, of brain
- *Mycobacterium avium* complex or *M. kansasii*, disseminated or extrapulmonary[b]
- *Mycobacterium tuberculosis* of any site, pulmonary,[b,c] disseminated,[b] or extrapulmonary[b]
- *Mycobacterium*, other species or unidentified species, disseminated[b] or extrapulmonary[b]
- *Pneumocystis jirovecii* pneumonia[b]
- Pneumonia, recurrent[b,c]
- Progressive multifocal leukoencephalopathy
- *Salmonella* septicemia, recurrent
- Toxoplasmosis of brain, onset at age >1 month[b]
- Wasting syndrome attributed to HIV

[a]Only among children aged <13 years. (Centers for Disease Control and Prevention: 1994 revised classification system for human immunodeficiency virus infection in children less than 13 years of age, *MMWR* 43[RR-12], 1994.)
[b]Condition that might be diagnosed presumptively.
[c]Only among adults and adolescents aged ≥13 years. (Centers for Disease Control and Prevention: 1993 revised classification system for HIV infection and expanded surveillance case definition for AIDS among adolescents and adults, *MMWR* 41[RR-17], 1992.)
Reused from Schneider E, Whitmore S, Glynn KM, et al: Revised surveillance case definitions for HIV infection among adults, adolescents, and children aged <18 months and for HIV infection and AIDS among children aged 18 months to <13 years—United States, 2008, *MMWR Recomm Rep* 57(RR-10):1–12, 2008.

TREATMENT

The US Department of Health and Human Services (DHHS) recommends initiating indefinite ART in all HIV-infected individuals regardless of CD4 count, both to reduce the morbidity associated with HIV infection and to decrease the risk of transmission to others. The DHHS guidelines also highlight the importance of educating patients about ART and reviewing strategies to optimize adherence. Since effective ART requires sustained effort from patients, it is essential for them to be involved in the decision to begin therapy.

The goal of HIV treatment is to maintain viral suppression while minimizing the risk of resistance. Most regimens use three drugs from two different classes (Table 123.1), including a backbone of two nucleoside reverse transcriptase inhibitors (often tenofovir/emtricitabine or abacavir/lamivudine) combined with a protease inhibitor (darunavir) or integrase inhibitor (dolutegravir, elvitegravir, or raltegravir). Agents such as ritonavir and cobicistat, both potent inhibitors of CYP3A4, are commonly added to boost the blood concentrations of certain antiretrovirals. The response should be monitored by checking the viral load. Persistently detectable virus 3 to 4 months after ART initiation generally indicates treatment failure, and resistance testing should occur before changing the regimen.

Individuals with known exposure to HIV should immediately begin a three-drug postexposure prophylaxis regimen for a period of 4 weeks while undergoing serial testing (at the time of exposure and again at 6 weeks, 12 weeks, and 6 months, though these intervals may vary depending on the specific assay used).

SCREENING AND PREVENTION

The US Preventive Services Task Force recommends that all persons between the ages of 15 and 65 receive HIV testing at least once, with high-risk groups tested more often. The Centers for Disease Control and Prevention recommends screening with the fourth-generation

TABLE 123.1
Antiretroviral Medications

Class	Brand Name	Generic Name(s)
Nucleoside reverse transcriptase inhibitors (NRTIs)	Emtriva	emtricitabine (FTC)
	Epivir	lamivudine (3TC)
	Retrovir	zidovudine (ZDV) (also known as azidothymidine [AZT])
	Videx	didanosine (ddI)
	Viread	tenofovir disoproxil fumarate (TDF)
	Zerit	stavudine (d4T)
	Ziagen	abacavir sulfate (ABC)
Combination NRTIs	Combivir	lamivudine, zidovudine
	Epzicom	abacavir, lamivudine
	Trizivir	abacavir, lamivudine, zidovudine
	Truvada	tenofovir disoproxil fumarate, emtricitabine
Nonnucleoside reverse transcriptase inhibitors (NNRTIs)	Edurant	rilpivirine (RPV)
	Intelence	etravirine (ETR)
	Rescriptor	delavirdine (DLV)
	Sustiva	efavirenz (EFV)
	Viramune	nevirapine (NVP)
Protease inhibitors	Aptivus	tipranavir (TPV)
	Crixivan	indinavir (IDV)
	Invirase	saquinavir mesylate (SQV)
	Kaletra	lopinavir and ritonavir (LPV/RTV)
	Lexiva	fosamprenavir calcium (FOS-APV)
	Norvir	ritonavir (RTV)
	Prezista	darunavir (DRV)
	Reyataz	atazanavir sulfate (ATV)
	Viracept	nelfinavir mesylate (NFV)
Fusion inhibitors	Fuzeon	enfuvirtide (T20)
Entry inhibitors	Selzentry	maraviroc (MVC)
Integrase inhibitors	Isentress	raltegravir (RAL)
	Tivicay	dolutegravir (DTG)
	Vitekta	elvitegravir (EVG)
Multiclass combination therapy	Atripla	efavirenz, emtricitabine, tenofovir disoproxil fumarate
	Complera	emtricitabine, rilpivirine, tenofovir disoproxil fumarate
	Evotaz	atazanavir sulfate, cobicistat
	Prezcobix	cobicistat, darunavir
	Stribild	elvitegravir, cobicistat, emtricitabine, tenofovir disoproxil fumarate

Data from U.S. Food & Drug Administration: *Antiretroviral drugs used in the treatment of HIV infection.* https://www.fda.gov/patients/hiv-treatment/antiretroviral-drugs-used-treatment-hiv-infection.

antigen/antibody test. A positive result should be followed by an HIV1/HIV2 antibody differentiation assay. If the antibody test is positive, the diagnosis is confirmed. If it is negative, a nucleic acid amplification test (NAAT) should be performed to assess for acute (i.e., antibody-negative) infection.

Preexposure prophylaxis (PrEP) with daily tenofovir-emtricitabine is recommended in individuals from high-risk groups, such as men who have sex with men, injection drug users, and partners of HIV-infected persons. Mounting evidence suggests preexposure prophylaxis is generally safe and effective among adherent patients.

CHAPTER 124

HIV/AIDS: Common Opportunistic Infections

ERIC J. BURNETT

INTRODUCTION

Opportunistic infections (OIs) occur in patients with severe immune compromise, whether from congenital immunodeficiencies, malnutrition, malignancy, chemotherapy, immunosuppressive medications (i.e., for prevention of organ transplant rejection), or **HIV/AIDS.**

OIs most frequently occur in the context of HIV/AIDS and were commonplace prior to the introduction of effective **antiretroviral therapy (ART)** and standardized OI prophylaxis. In the modern era, however, they occur primarily among those who are unable to receive adequate care. In HIV infection, the risk of acquiring OIs depends primarily on the degree of immune suppression (often reflected by the CD4 count).

COCCIDIOIDOMYCOSIS

Coccidioidomycosis is a fungal infection endemic to the Southwestern United States that can affect both immunocompetent and immunocompromised individuals, with the greatest risk occurring in HIV-positive patients with CD4 counts <250 cells/μL.

Although coccidioidomycosis may have a wide range of clinical manifestations, it typically presents as a pulmonary infection causing shortness of breath, fevers, chills, and cough. Patients with advanced AIDS may have disseminated disease and present with fevers, weight loss, meningitis, and rash. Serological testing may be useful but is often unreliable in patients with HIV; blood or sputum cultures are usually required for definitive diagnosis.

Disseminated coccidioidomycosis is treated with amphotericin B until clinical improvement occurs, then with an azole antifungal (fluconazole or itraconazole) for a total of 1 year of treatment. Less severe forms of coccidioidomycosis, such as pneumonia, can be treated with fluconazole in combination with ART.

Patients with CD4 counts <250 cells/μL who live in endemic regions and have positive serum antibodies should receive daily fluconazole prophylaxis. If serological testing is negative, it should be repeated on an annual basis.

PNEUMOCYSTIS PNEUMONIA

The risk of *Pneumocystis jirovecii* **pneumonia** (still abbreviated PCP to remain in line with the former diagnosis of *Pneumocystis carinii* pneumonia) (Fig. 124.1) increases as CD4 cell counts fall to <200 cells/μL. Patients often present with acute or subacute shortness of breath, typically followed by fever and a nonproductive cough. As the disease progresses, however, severe hypoxemia and respiratory failure can occur.

The laboratory findings of PCP infection are nonspecific but may include an elevated lactate dehydrogenase level. Chest x-ray may demonstrate diffuse bilateral interstitial infiltrates, but they may also be normal early in the disease course. CT imaging is more sensitive and may be performed when there is a high clinical suspicion, but the chest x-ray is normal; the typical finding is diffuse ground-glass opacities.

The gold standard for diagnosis is bronchoalveolar lavage, which has nearly 100% sensitivity and specificity. Given the significant hypoxemia associated with PCP infection, it is not always available or well tolerated. The serum $(1,3)$ β-D-glucan assay has been investigated as a potential alternative to invasive testing, with sensitivity and specificity reported as 95% and 84%. It should be noted, however, that other fungal infections (notably candidiasis and aspergillosis) can also cause this assay to become positive.

The preferred treatment for PCP is a 3-week course of trimethoprim-sulfamethoxazole. Patients with allergies to sulfa medications may instead be treated with either intravenous pentamidine or a combination of oral primaquine and clindamycin for 3 weeks. Patients with significant hypoxemia (defined as PaO_2 <70 mm Hg on room air or alveolar-arterial (A-a) gradient >35 mm Hg) should also receive a course of prednisone to reduce pulmonary inflammation resulting from dying *Pneumocystis* organisms.

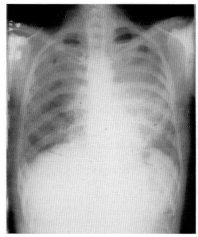

Diffuse bilateral pulmonary infiltrates

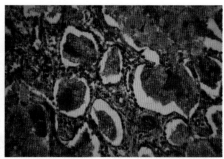

Interstitial lymphocyte and plasma cell
infiltration with foamy exudate in alveoli

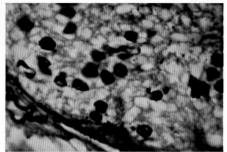

Methenamine AgNO$_3$ stain showing
Pneumocystis organisms in lung *(black spots)*

FIG. 124.1 **Pneumocystis Pneumonia.**

Given their high risk of PCP, patients with HIV infection and CD4 counts <200 cells/μL should be treated with prophylactic trimethoprim-sulfamethoxazole. In cases of sulfa allergies, atovaquone or dapsone is an appropriate alternative.

HISTOPLASMOSIS

The risk of **histoplasmosis** increases when the CD4 count is <150 cells/μL and the patient lives in an endemic area, such as the Ohio/Mississippi river valleys, southern Mexico, Central/South America, and China.

Histoplasmosis can present as a mild pulmonary infection, resulting in fever and cough, or as a more disseminated infection, resulting in fever, weight loss, nausea, vomiting, and dyspnea. Physical exam may reveal hepatosplenomegaly, lymphadenopathy, and cutaneous lesions. Laboratory evaluation may show pancytopenia as a manifestation of bone marrow infiltration.

The *Histoplasma capsulatum* antigen assay is the most sensitive and specific test for histoplasmosis and can be performed with urine, serum, and cerebrospinal fluid (CSF). Among patients with advanced AIDS, urine assays are the most sensitive. Although culture is the gold standard for diagnosis, results may be delayed for several weeks, and thus treatment should begin empirically.

Amphotericin B is the preferred initial therapy for patients with severe immune compromise and disseminated disease. Following an initial induction period (often 14 days), patients can be transitioned to an azole antifungal (usually itraconazole) for a total of 1 year of therapy. Antigen levels should be checked every 3 months while on treatment to assess response, and then every 6 to 12 months after therapy is completed.

Patients in hyperendemic areas with CD4 counts <150 cell/μL are often treated with itraconazole for prophylaxis.

TOXOPLASMOSIS

The risk of **toxoplasmosis** (Fig. 124.2) increases once the CD4 cell count is <100 cells/μL. Although toxoplasmosis typically causes encephalitis with masslike lesions, extracerebral manifestations (including pneumonitis and chorioretinitis) can also occur. The encephalitis usually presents with fever, headache, and mental status changes, sometimes with focal neurological deficits or seizures. A presumptive diagnosis can usually be established if the patient has not received adequate prophylaxis, has

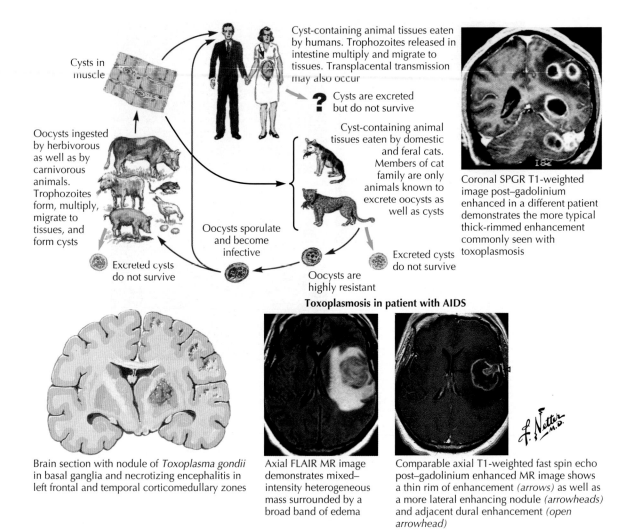

Coronal SPGR T1-weighted image post–gadolinium enhanced in a different patient demonstrates the more typical thick-rimmed enhancement commonly seen with toxoplasmosis

Toxoplasmosis in patient with AIDS

Brain section with nodule of *Toxoplasma gondii* in basal ganglia and necrotizing encephalitis in left frontal and temporal corticomedullary zones

Axial FLAIR MR image demonstrates mixed–intensity heterogeneous mass surrounded by a broad band of edema

Comparable axial T1-weighted fast spin echo post–gadolinium enhanced MR image shows a thin rim of enhancement *(arrows)* as well as a more lateral enhancing nodule *(arrowheads)* and adjacent dural enhancement *(open arrowhead)*

FIG. 124.2 Toxoplasmosis. *SPGR,* Spoiled gradient.

a consistent clinical syndrome, has positive *Toxoplasma gondii* immunoglobulin G (IgG) antibodies, and has brain imaging that demonstrates multiple, ring-enhancing lesions. A definitive diagnosis of toxoplasmosis requires brain biopsy, although this is generally only pursued when the patient has not responded to the appropriate antibiotic therapy.

The preferred treatment for toxoplasmosis is pyrimethamine and sulfadiazine for 6 weeks. The course should be prolonged further if there is incomplete resolution based on surveillance radiographic imaging performed 2 to 3 weeks after treatment begins. Clindamycin can be substituted for sulfadiazine if the patient is allergic to sulfa medications.

HIV-infected patients with CD4 counts <100 cells/uL should receive toxoplasmosis prophylaxis. Options include trimethoprim-sulfamethoxazole, dapsone plus pyrimethamine, or atovaquone plus pyrimethamine.

CRYPTOSPORIDIOSIS

Cryptosporidium parvum is a waterborne parasite that causes gastroenteritis in immunocompromised and immunocompetent hosts. Intestinal cryptosporidiosis presents with severe watery diarrhea, abdominal cramping, nausea, and vomiting. While the symptoms are self-limited in immunocompetent hosts, they can last for weeks in HIV-positive patients. The diagnosis is established based on stool culture or the use of a stool multiplex polymerase chain reaction (PCR) panel. The treatment is mostly supportive, consisting primarily of reconstituting the immune system with antiretroviral therapies. The disease can be much more severe in patients with CD4 counts <50 cells/μL, to whom nitazoxanide, paromomycin, or azithromycin can also be administered.

CRYPTOCOCCOSIS

Cryptococcus neoformans is a yeast that can cause meningitis, pneumonia, and disseminated disease in HIV-infected patients with severe immune deficiencies (generally CD4 count <100 cells/μL). Cryptococcal meningitis may have a similar clinical presentation to toxoplasmic encephalitis, causing fever, altered mental status, and focal neurological deficits. The diagnosis should be considered if brain imaging fails to reveal space-occupying lesions. A lumbar puncture should be performed to assess for CSF pleocytosis (which may be absent in severe immunosuppression), direct visualization of yeast (using the **India ink** capsule stain), and assessment of the CSF cryptococcal antigen, which has slightly better sensitivity than the serum assay.

For cryptococcal meningitis, the treatment of choice is amphotericin B and flucytosine for 2 weeks, followed by high-dose fluconazole for 8 weeks, then lower-dose fluconazole for a total of 1 year of therapy. For isolated pulmonary disease, fluconazole monotherapy may be appropriate.

CYTOMEGALOVIRUS

Cytomegalovirus (CMV) infections generally occur in patients with CD4 counts <50 cells/μL. The manifestations can range from a nonspecific viral syndrome to organ-invasive disease, including encephalitis, chorioretinitis, pneumonitis, esophagitis, colitis, and hepatitis. The infection can be confirmed using a quantitative serum PCR assay.

Traditionally, the most common manifestation of invasive AIDS associated CMV disease was chorioretinitis, manifested by decreased visual acuity, floaters, and visual field loss. Ophthalmological examination typically demonstrates perivascular hemorrhage and exudates. The treatment depends on disease severity and may include oral valganciclovir or intravenous ganciclovir, foscarnet, or cidofovir.

Esophagitis usually presents with odynophagia, whereas colitis presents with bloody diarrhea. Both diagnoses are confirmed with biopsy, which reveals CMV inclusion bodies. The treatment is ganciclovir or foscarnet.

Pneumonitis presents with dyspnea, nonproductive cough, and fever. Chest x-ray may reveal diffuse interstitial infiltrates. The preferred treatment is ganciclovir. Adjuvant CMV-specific Ig therapy may also be used in organ-invasive and/or refractory CMV disease.

Routine prophylaxis against CMV is generally not given to HIV-infected patients, as valganciclovir and ganciclovir may cause bone marrow suppression; however, CMV prophylaxis is routinely utilized in solid organ transplant recipients.

MYCOBACTERIUM AVIUM COMPLEX

Mycobacterium avium **complex** (MAC) infection generally occurs in patients with CD4 counts <50 cells/μL and causes nonspecific symptoms, including fevers, chills, night sweats, diarrhea, and weight loss. The laboratory abnormalities are also nonspecific and generally include anemia (due to bone marrow infiltration), elevated alkaline phosphatase (due to liver infiltration), and elevated lactate dehydrogenase. MAC is diagnosed through isolation of the organism in culture, typically from blood but sometimes from lymph nodes or bone marrow. The treatment of choice is clarithromycin and ethambutol. Rifabutin may also be added to enhance the efficacy of the standard regimen. Patients with CD4 counts <50 cells/μL are commonly treated with a macrolide antibiotic (i.e., azithromycin or clarithromycin) for prophylaxis.

CHAPTER 125

Gastrointestinal System Anatomy Review

MONICA SAUMOY • YECHESKEL SCHNEIDER

INTRODUCTION

The gastrointestinal (GI) system consists of several connecting organs forming a continuous tube from mouth to anus, spanning multiple cavities, including the neck, thorax, and abdomen. The GI system can be divided into **luminal** and **nonluminal** portions. The **luminal** portion contains the esophagus, stomach, small intestine (duodenum, jejunum, and ileum), large intestine (cecum, ascending colon, transverse colon, descending colon, and sigmoid colon), and rectum. The **nonluminal** portion consists of the liver, gallbladder, and pancreas.

ESOPHAGUS

The esophagus begins in the neck and extends to the diaphragm, connecting the oropharynx to the stomach (Fig. 125.1). In the thorax, the esophagus lies posterior to the trachea and the heart. The most distal centimeter of the esophagus is located in the abdomen. The lower esophageal sphincter consists of circular smooth muscle and is usually closed at rest, preventing the reflux of gastric contents into the esophagus. As a food bolus advances through the esophagus, propagated by peristalsis, the sphincter opens to allow passage into the stomach.

STOMACH

The stomach is a muscular, J-shaped organ that begins at the gastroesophageal (GE) junction and extends to the pylorus, where it empties into the duodenum (the first part of the small intestine) (Fig. 125.2). The stomach is mobile and dilates to accommodate ingested material. The primary function of the stomach is to initiate digestion by transforming food into a semiliquid mass known as chyme. The stomach does so by acidifying and mechanically breaking down its contents.

The stomach has two curvatures: a lesser curvature, which lies superiorly, and a greater curvature, which lies inferiorly. The stomach is divided into multiple portions, including the cardia (at the GE junction), fundus (blind sac adjacent to the cardia), body (the largest portion of the stomach), antrum (the area between the body and the pylorus), and pylorus (where the stomach and duodenum meet).

The stomach receives blood from the celiac artery, which supplies the left and right gastric arteries to the lesser curvature, the short gastric arteries to the fundus, and the left and right gastroomental (gastroepiploic) arteries to the greater curvature.

SMALL INTESTINE
Duodenum

The duodenum is the first portion of the small intestine. This 12-inch-long, C-shaped portion can be divided into four parts: a superior segment, a descending segment, an inferior or horizontal segment, and an ascending segment (Fig. 125.3). The superior segment is intraperitoneal, while the others are retroperitoneal. The major duodenal papilla (of Vater), formed by the common bile and pancreatic ducts, is in the descending segment. The minor duodenal papilla, if present, contains the accessory pancreatic duct.

The luminal surface of the duodenum is covered by villi, fingerlike projections of mucosa that assist with digestion and absorption by greatly increasing the overall

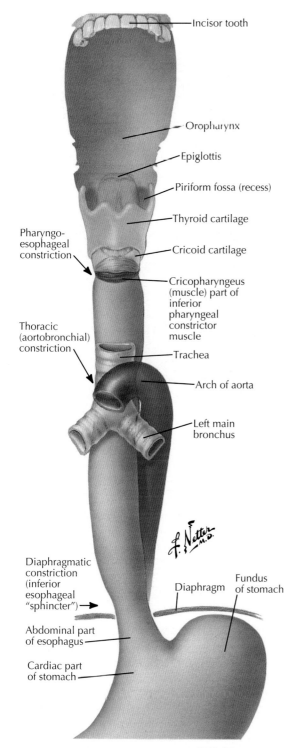

Incisor tooth

Oropharynx

Epiglottis

Piriform fossa (recess)

Thyroid cartilage

Pharyngo-
esophageal
constriction

Cricoid cartilage

Cricopharyngeus
(muscle) part of
inferior
pharyngeal
constrictor
muscle

Thoracic
(aortobronchial)
constriction

Trachea

Arch of aorta

Left main
bronchus

Diaphragmatic
constriction
(inferior
esophageal
"sphincter")

Fundus
of stomach

Diaphragm

Abdominal part
of esophagus

Cardiac part
of stomach

FIG. 125.1 Anatomical Relations of the Esophagus.

surface area. Brunner glands are submucosal mucous glands that are present in high concentrations.

The superior segment of the duodenum receives blood from the supraduodenal artery, a branch of the gastroduodenal artery. The remainder of the duodenum receives blood along the pancreatic surface from the pancreaticoduodenal arteries.

The ligament of Treitz, located at the duodenojejunal flexure, divides the upper and lower GI tracts, with important implications for GI bleeding (see Chapter 11).

Jejunum and Ileum

The jejunum and ileum are the second and third portions of the small intestine. The ileum ends at the ileocecal valve, where it meets the cecum, the first portion of the large intestine.

The jejunum is mostly in the central upper abdomen, whereas the ileum is mostly in the lower abdomen and partially in the pelvis. The jejunum is also wider and has a thicker wall than the ileum. The jejunum is more vascular than the ileum, which gives it a redder gross appearance. The jejunum has more rapid peristalsis than the ileum. Finally, the jejunum has lymphatic capillaries in the mucosa, known as lacteals, whereas the ileum has more lymph nodes in the submucosal layer, known as Peyer patches.

The jejunum and ileum receive blood from the intestinal branches of the superior mesenteric artery, which courses through the mesentery to reach the intestine. Within the mesentery, the arteries form loops and arcades that terminate as end arteries to supply the intestine. Occlusion of these end arteries can result in intestinal ischemia and infarct.

LARGE INTESTINE/COLON

The main function of the colon is the absorption of water and salt. The colon consists of multiple segments, including the cecum, ascending (right) colon, transverse colon, descending (left) colon, and sigmoid colon (Fig. 125.4). As the colon progresses from the ascending colon to the sigmoid colon, its diameter narrows.

The colon wall contains longitudinal and circular layers of smooth muscle. The relatively shorter length of the longitudinal smooth muscle in relation to the actual length of the colon results in sacculations, known as haustra. The colon also has sacs of fat on its peritoneal surfaces, known as omental (epiploic) appendices.

The cecum, the first portion of the large intestine, is a blind pouch in the right lower quadrant of the abdomen immediately distal to the ileocecal valve. It

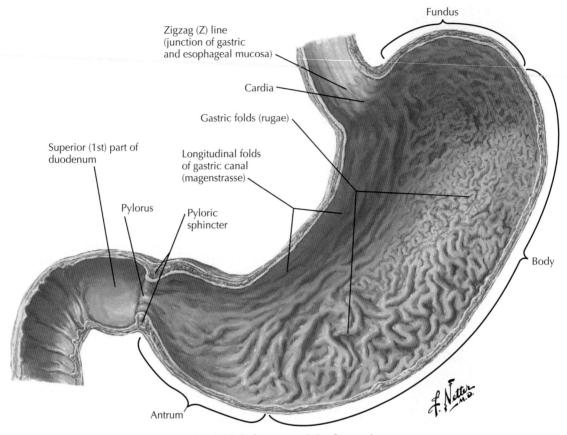

FIG. 125.2 **Anatomy of the Stomach.**

does not contribute to the major functions of the colon. The cecum gives rise to the appendix, a vestigial organ rich in lymphoid tissue. The appendix receives blood from a branch of the ileocolic artery, known as the appendicular artery.

The ascending colon begins adjacent to the ileocecal valve and extends along the right side of the abdomen to the right colic (hepatic) flexure, where it meets the transverse colon. The transverse colon extends to the left colic (splenic) flexure, where it meets the descending colon. The descending colon courses along the left side of the abdomen to the sigmoid colon, which continues toward the midline and joins the rectum in the pelvis. The ascending colon and most of the descending colon are retroperitoneal, while the transverse and sigmoid colon are intraperitoneal.

The colon receives blood from branches of the superior mesenteric artery (to the cecum, appendix, ascending colon, and proximal portion of the transverse colon)

and inferior mesenteric artery (to the distal portion of the transverse colon, descending colon, and sigmoid colon). The venous drainage is through the superior mesenteric and inferior mesenteric veins. The superior mesenteric and splenic veins join to form the portal vein. The inferior mesenteric vein can join the splenic, superior mesenteric, or portal vein.

RECTUM/ANAL CANAL/ANUS

The final portion of the GI tract is the rectum, anal canal, and anus (Fig. 125.5). The anorectal line is at the level where the puborectalis muscle meets the rectum, though this may be difficult to identify. The lumen of the rectum contains three valves, typically with two on the left and one on the right in an alternating fashion. The rectum receives blood from the superior rectal artery, which arises from the inferior mesenteric artery.

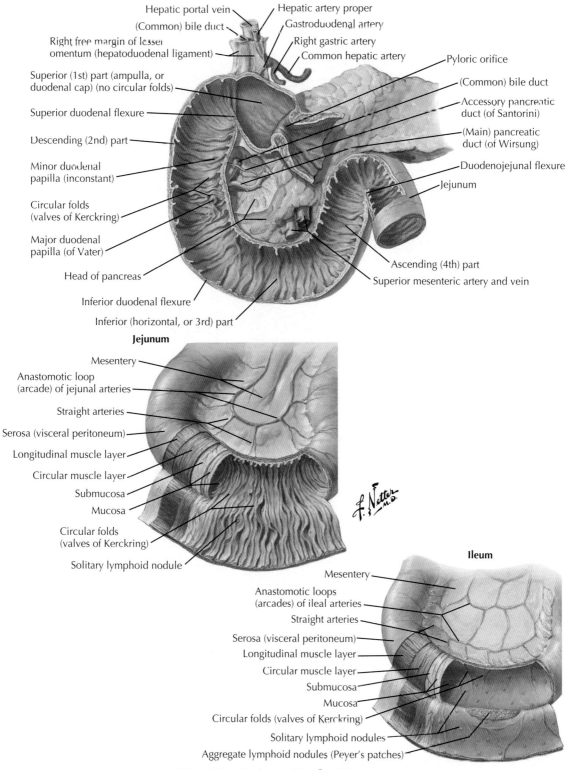

Hepatic portal vein
(Common) bile duct
Right free margin of lesser omentum (hepatoduodenal ligament)
Superior (1st) part (ampulla, or duodenal cap) (no circular folds)
Superior duodenal flexure
Descending (2nd) part
Minor duodenal papilla (inconstant)
Circular folds (valves of Kerckring)
Major duodenal papilla (of Vater)
Head of pancreas
Inferior duodenal flexure
Inferior (horizontal, or 3rd) part

Hepatic artery proper
Gastroduodenal artery
Right gastric artery
Common hepatic artery
Pyloric orifice
(Common) bile duct
Accessory pancreatic duct (of Santorini)
(Main) pancreatic duct (of Wirsung)
Duodenojejunal flexure
Jejunum
Ascending (4th) part
Superior mesenteric artery and vein

Jejunum

Mesentery
Anastomotic loop (arcade) of jejunal arteries
Straight arteries
Serosa (visceral peritoneum)
Longitudinal muscle layer
Circular muscle layer
Submucosa
Mucosa
Circular folds (valves of Kerckring)
Solitary lymphoid nodule

Ileum

Mesentery
Anastomotic loops (arcades) of ileal arteries
Straight arteries
Serosa (visceral peritoneum)
Longitudinal muscle layer
Circular muscle layer
Submucosa
Mucosa
Circular folds (valves of Kerckring)
Solitary lymphoid nodules
Aggregate lymphoid nodules (Peyer's patches)

FIG. 125.3 **Anatomy of the Small Intestine.**

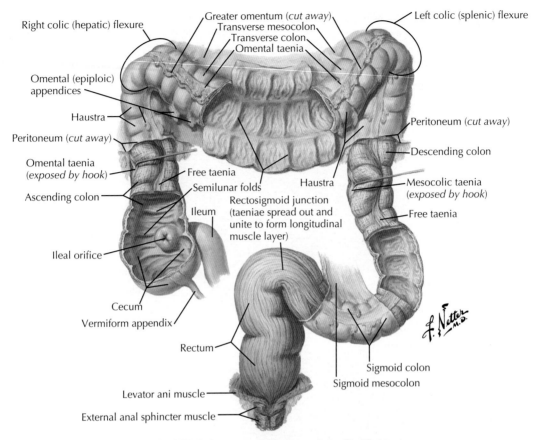

Right colic (hepatic) flexure

Greater omentum (*cut away*)
Transverse mesocolon
Transverse colon
Omental taenia

Left colic (splenic) flexure

Omental (epiploic) appendices

Haustra

Peritoneum (*cut away*)

Omental taenia (*exposed by hook*)

Ascending colon

Free taenia

Semilunar folds

Ileum

Ileal orifice

Cecum

Vermiform appendix

Rectum

Levator ani muscle

External anal sphincter muscle

Rectosigmoid junction (taeniae spread out and unite to form longitudinal muscle layer)

Haustra

Peritoneum (*cut away*)

Descending colon

Mesocolic taenia (*exposed by hook*)

Free taenia

Sigmoid colon

Sigmoid mesocolon

FIG. 125.4 Anatomy of the Large Intestine/Colon.

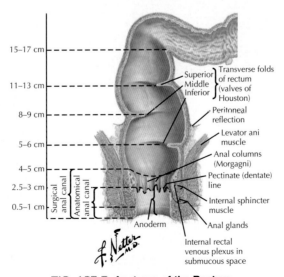

15–17 cm

11–13 cm

8–9 cm

5–6 cm

4–5 cm

2.5–3 cm

0.5–1 cm

Surgical anal canal

Anatomical anal canal

Superior
Middle
Inferior

Transverse folds of rectum (valves of Houston)

Peritoneal reflection

Levator ani muscle

Anal columns (Morgagni)

Pectinate (dentate) line

Internal sphincter muscle

Anoderm

Anal glands

Internal rectal venous plexus in submucous space

FIG. 125.5 Anatomy of the Rectum.

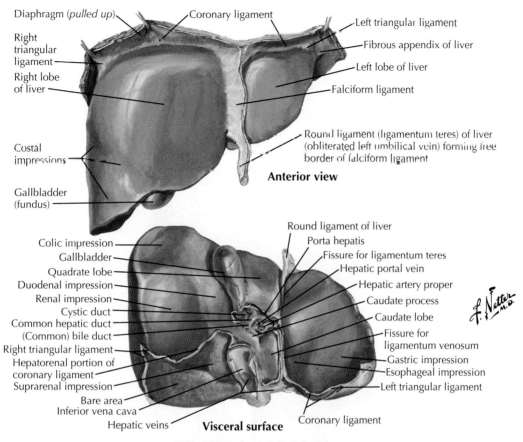

FIG. 125.6 Anatomy of the Liver.

The anal canal is continuous with the rectum and terminates at the anus. The anal canal is divided into upper and lower portions; separating them is the pectinate line, the site of the anal valves. The internal anal sphincter consists of smooth muscle, whereas the external anal sphincter consists of skeletal muscle. The upper portion of the anal canal receives blood from the superior rectal artery, while the lower portion receives blood from the inferior rectal artery.

LIVER AND GALLBLADDER

The liver is in the right upper quadrant of the abdomen, just beneath the diaphragm, and is the largest gland in the body (Fig. 125.6). The liver can be divided into four anatomical lobes: right, left, caudate, and quadrate. The left and right lobes are separated by the falciform

ligament. The caudate and quadrate lobes are on the inferior surface. The liver has a dual blood supply, with 75% of the blood volume coming from the portal vein and 25% from the hepatic artery. Each makes a similar contribution, however, to the overall oxygenation of the liver. The bile ducts are perfused predominantly by the arterial system, rather than branches of the portal vein. The three hepatic veins drain blood to the inferior vena cava.

The gallbladder lies posterior to the liver and is responsible for storing and concentrating bile. The gallbladder has three distinct parts: the fundus, body, and neck. The fundus is a blind pouch that connects with the body. The S-shaped neck connects with the cystic duct. The left and right hepatic ducts join to form the common hepatic duct, which joins the cystic duct to form the common bile duct (CBD). Bile is conjugated

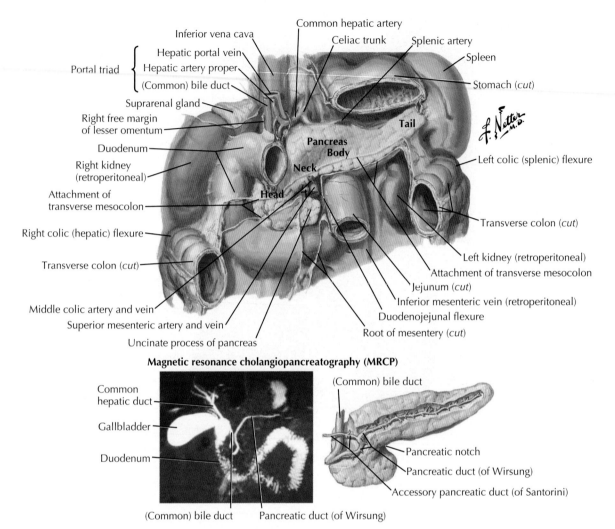

Common hepatic artery
Celiac trunk
Splenic artery
Inferior vena cava
Hepatic portal vein
Hepatic artery proper
(Common) bile duct
Portal triad
Spleen
Stomach (*cut*)
Suprarenal gland
Right free margin
of lesser omentum
Tail
Pancreas
Body
Duodenum
Right kidney
(retroperitoneal)
Neck
Left colic (splenic) flexure
Attachment of
transverse mesocolon
Head
Right colic (hepatic) flexure
Transverse colon (*cut*)
Transverse colon (*cut*)
Left kidney (retroperitoneal)
Attachment of transverse mesocolon
Jejunum (*cut*)
Inferior mesenteric vein (retroperitoneal)
Middle colic artery and vein
Duodenojejunal flexure
Superior mesenteric artery and vein
Root of mesentery (*cut*)
Uncinate process of pancreas

Magnetic resonance cholangiopancreatography (MRCP)

(Common) bile duct
Common
hepatic duct
Gallbladder
Duodenum
Pancreatic notch
Pancreatic duct (of Wirsung)
Accessory pancreatic duct (of Santorini)
(Common) bile duct
Pancreatic duct (of Wirsung)

FIG. 125.7 **Anatomy of the Pancreas.**

in the liver parenchyma and conveyed though canaliculi and ductules until it reaches the hepatic ducts, then it enters the gallbladder through the cystic duct. When the gallbladder is stimulated to contract, it expels bile into the CBD, which conveys it through the ampulla of Vater into the duodenum. The cystic artery is a branch of the right hepatic artery and supplies blood to the gallbladder.

PANCREAS

The pancreas is a retroperitoneal gland, lobulated in appearance, with four distinct parts: the head, neck, body, and tail (Fig. 125.7). The head lies adjacent to the duodenum, where the pancreatic duct (which traverses the length of the pancreas) meets the CBD and drains into the duodenum. The head is joined to the body via the neck. The tail of the pancreas lies in the splenic hilum.

CHAPTER 126

Gastrointestinal System Physiology Review

MONICA SAUMOY • YECHESKEL SCHNEIDER

MOTILITY

The **luminal gastrointestinal (GI) tract** contains muscular walls responsible for propelling food from the mouth to the anus, while also mechanically breaking it down and mixing it with digestive enzymes. Most of the GI tract contains longitudinal and circular smooth muscle; exceptions are the upper third of the esophagus and the external anal sphincter, which contain striated muscle.

Several neuroendocrine hormones and neurotransmitters regulate GI motility. Acetylcholine causes contraction of smooth muscle and relaxation of sphincters, whereas norepinephrine has the opposite effect. Vasoactive-intestinal peptide (VIP) promotes relaxation of the lower esophageal sphincter, stomach, and gallbladder, while substance P promotes contraction of longitudinal muscles and sphincters.

The **contraction** of circular muscle decreases the diameter of the lumen, while the contraction of longitudinal muscle shortens the GI tract. Two main types of contractions are observed: **phasic contractions,** which are brief and followed by a period of relaxation, and **tonic contractions,** which are more sustained. Phasic contractions occur in the esophagus, part of the stomach, and small intestine, while tonic contractions occur in sphincters and valves (e.g., the gastroesophageal junction, ileocecal valve, and internal anal sphincter).

When a person swallows, the upper esophageal sphincter briefly opens and allows the food bolus to enter. A series of successive contractions, known as **peristalsis,** guides the bolus toward the lower esophageal sphincter, which relaxes and allows the bolus to enter the fundus. The fundus dilates to accept the food in a process known as receptive relaxation. The stomach then contracts to mechanically break down the food and mix it with gastric acid, producing chyme.

Ultimately, the stomach empties chyme into the duodenum for further digestion. Notably, as gastric contractions approach the pylorus, much of the chyme is retropulsed back into the stomach for further grinding, since particles larger than 1 mm^3 are unable to traverse the pyloric sphincter. The stomach requires ~3 hours to clear its contents. The rate of gastric emptying is accelerated by increased gastric volume, liquid versus solid foods, and protein over fat content (via **cholecystokinin [CCK]** release); it is slowed by duodenal distention, acidity, and osmolarity (via sympathetic nerve reflexes and secretin).

In the fed state, small bowel motility consists of contractions of longitudinal muscle, which generate peristaltic waves that propel chyme forward, and contractions of circular muscle that mix it with digestive enzymes. In the fasting state, waves of electrical activity known as migrating motor complexes serve as a so-called housekeeper, to sweep luminal contents from the stomach to the colon every 90 to 120 minutes.

Once the intestinal contents pass through the ileocecal valve and reach the large intestine, or colon, they become known as feces. The ileocecal valve contracts after ileal contents enter the cecum, preventing reflux. Like the small intestine, the large intestine has contractions to facilitate mixing of its contents and the absorption of water and nutrients; however, the colon does not have muscular contractions to promote the forward movement of feces. Instead, feces move through the colon because of mass effect, which increases as the colon becomes more distended.

As the rectum fills with feces, its walls contract and the internal anal sphincter relaxes. Once the rectum fills to about 25% capacity, a person experiences the urge to defecate. The external sphincter consists of striated muscle and is under voluntary control.

DIGESTION AND ABSORPTION OF FOOD

The **digestion** of food begins in the mouth, where salivary lipase and amylase initiate the metabolism of fats and carbohydrates. In the stomach (Fig. 126.1), parietal cells secrete **intrinsic factor,** which is essential

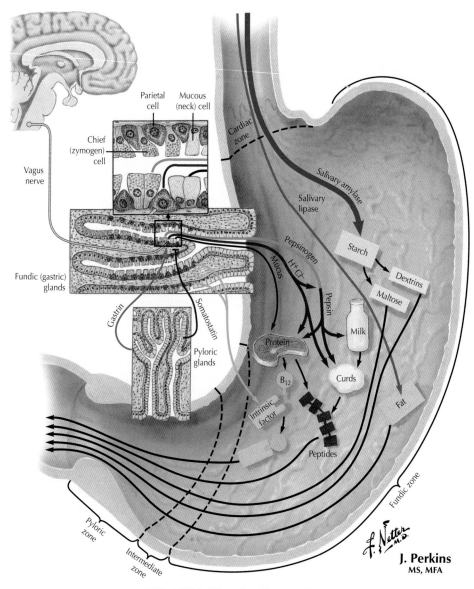

FIG. 126.1 **Digestion (Stomach).**

for vitamin B$_{12}$ absorption, and **hydrochloric acid (HCl),** which accelerates the breakdown of food. HCl secretion is promoted by gastrin, histamine, and acetylcholine. **Gastrin** is produced by G cells of the stomach in response to gastric distention, vagal stimulation, and the presence of amino acids. When the gastric pH reaches a target level, somatostatin is released from gastric D cells and inhibits further HCl secretion. The chief cells of the stomach secrete pepsinogen to facilitate protein digestion.

The chyme produced in the stomach enters the duodenum for further digestion and absorption. In the duodenum (Fig. 126.2), the presence of chyme triggers the release of **secretin** and CCK. Secretin is produced in the duodenum in response to acid and fatty acids, and it promotes bicarbonate secretion from the pancreas and biliary system and a decrease in gastric HCl production. CCK is produced in the duodenum and jejunum in response to fatty acids or amino acids. CCK promotes

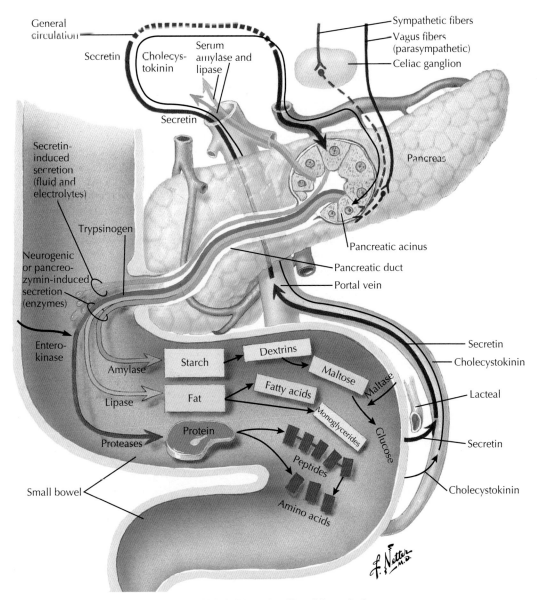

FIG. 126.2 Digestion (Small Intestine).

an increase in pancreatic enzyme and bicarbonate secretion, contraction of the gallbladder, relaxation of the sphincter of Oddi, and inhibition of gastric emptying, which allows duodenal contents more time to mix with digestive enzymes.

The pancreatic enzymes released in response to CCK include lipase (lipid digestion), amylase (carbohydrate digestion), and proteases (protein digestion). The proteases include trypsin, chymotrypsin, elastase, and

carboxypeptidase. The end products of protein digestion are amino acids, dipeptides, and tripeptides, which are absorbed on sodium–amino acid cotransporters, as well as on hydrogen ion dipeptide and tripeptide cotransporters.

The small intestinal mucosal surface area is structured into rugae with villi and microvilli that vastly increase surface area and maximize the absorption of nutrients, vitamins, and minerals. The mucosa also contains many different brush border enzymes (such as lactase, sucrose, maltase) that help further digest carbohydrates into end products that include glucose, galactose, and fructose. These sugars are then absorbed on cotransporters with sodium (glucose and galactose) or absorbed by diffusion (fructose).

Lipid digestion is aided by the pancreas (via lipase, as mentioned earlier) and by the gallbladder, which secretes bile salts, bilirubin, and cholesterol. In the small intestine, lipids are digested and emulsified by pancreatic enzymes and bile salts. The end products of this process include fatty acids, monoglycerides, and cholesterol. Bile salts emulsify fats to form micelles (small lipid droplets), which have a hydrophilic exterior and hydrophobic core, allowing them to be soluble in chyme and carried to the brush border. The end products of lipid metabolism then diffuse directly into intestinal cells, where they undergo reesterification to triglycerides and phospholipids. Chylomicrons then form and are transferred to lymph. Bile salts are reabsorbed in the ileum via sodium–bile salt cotransporters and recycled back to the liver, a process known as **enterohepatic circulation**.

WATER ABSORPTION

The GI tract is responsible for the absorption of almost 8 to 9 L of fluid per day, consisting of 1 to 2 L from oral ingestion and 6 to 8 L from GI secretions. Most of this water (~6–8 L) is absorbed in the small bowel. Afterward, the colon absorbs 90% of the remaining fluid, amounting to another 1 to 2 L of water, resulting in 150 to 200 mL of feces. The intestinal absorption of water is a passive process and depends on the movement of solutes, primarily sodium. Coupled transport of water and sodium depends on specialized mechanisms that pump sodium into the paracellular spaces, establishing high osmotic pressure in that region. Water then follows this osmotic gradient across the intestinal mucosa through transcellular and paracellular pathways.

CHAPTER 127

Achalasia

MONICA SAUMOY • YECHESKEL SCHNEIDER

INTRODUCTION

Achalasia is a primary motility disorder of the esophagus characterized by impaired relaxation of the **lower esophageal sphincter (LES)** and a loss of peristalsis in the distal esophagus. The annual incidence is ~1.6 cases per 100,000, while the prevalence is 1 in 10,000. Most cases occur in adults between the ages of 25 and 60 years. Older patients are more likely to have **pseudoachalasia** (secondary achalasia), which occurs secondary to a specific cause, such as malignancy or Chagas disease.

PATHOPHYSIOLOGY

Achalasia occurs when degeneration of the ganglion cells in the esophageal myenteric plexus causes failure of LES relaxation and loss of peristalsis. The upper esophageal sphincter (UES) may also exhibit increased tone.

In primary achalasia the underlying cause of the neuron degeneration is unknown. There is some evidence that an underlying autoimmune disorder is responsible for the destruction of enteric neurons, though the precise cause and mechanism remain unknown.

As stated, the major causes of pseudoachalasia are Chagas disease and malignancy. In Chagas disease, *Trypanosoma cruzi* infection causes degeneration and depopulation of autonomic neurons. With certain malignancies, such as gastric cancer, tumor cells can directly invade the esophageal neural plexus or cause a paraneoplastic syndrome that interferes with esophageal motility.

PRESENTATION

The onset of symptoms is typically gradual and progresses for years prior to diagnosis. Most patients first complain of heartburn that is unresponsive to proton-pump inhibitors. As the disease severity increases, patients develop dysphagia to both solids and liquids. Impaired LES relaxation leads to accumulation and regurgitation of undigested food, which can be complicated by aspiration. Patients will also complain of difficulty belching, secondary to impaired UES relaxation.

Because of these issues, patients often change their eating habits, switching to soft or primarily liquid foods to facilitate passage through the LES. Patients may also adopt maneuvers to aid esophageal emptying, such as extending the neck and shoulders or drinking large amounts of water. Because of changes in diet, patients can develop associated weight loss. Of note, however, rapid weight loss should raise concern for pseudoachalasia due to an underlying malignancy.

When a patient presents with dysphagia and/or regurgitation, appropriate initial tests include a barium esophagram and upper endoscopy. A barium esophagram provides real-time images of esophageal motility and emptying. The characteristic sign of achalasia is the "bird's beak esophagus," which is dilated proximally and tapers at the LES (Fig. 127.1). As the disease progresses, the dilation can worsen and assume a sigmoid, tortuous shape. An upper endoscopy should be performed to rule out malignancy at the gastroesophageal (GE) junction. Patients without any signs of mechanical obstruction should undergo esophageal manometry to confirm impaired LES relaxation and distal esophageal aperistalsis, and to rule out other motility disorders (e.g., diffuse esophageal spasm).

Achalasia is categorized into three types based on the manometric findings, as defined by the Chicago Classification system. All types of achalasia are associated with an elevated mean integrated relaxation pressure (IRP) of >15 mm Hg. Type I achalasia (classic) is defined as minimal contractility in the esophageal body, a.k.a. 100% failed peristalsis. Type II achalasia is defined as intermittent periods of panesophageal pressurization, a.k.a. panesophageal pressurization in 20% or more of swallows. And type III achalasia (spastic) is associated with premature or spastic distal esophageal contractions in 20% or more of swallows. Finally, the Eckardt symptom score (a self-reported clinical assessment tool) has been used to assess achalasia severity, as well as follow symptom resolution after treatment.

TREATMENT

The treatment of achalasia focuses on decreasing LES pressure to facilitate passage of food into the stomach.

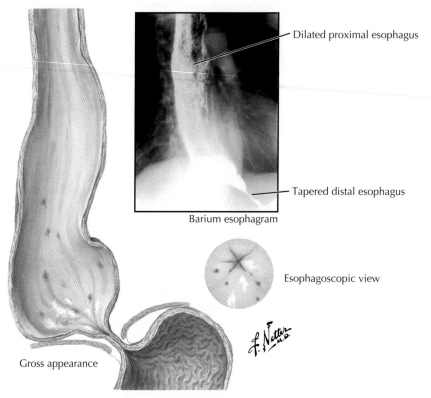

Dilated proximal esophagus

Tapered distal esophagus

Barium esophagram

Esophagoscopic view

Gross appearance

FIG. 127.1 **Achalasia.**

The three classes of therapy are pharmacological, endoscopic, and surgical.

Pharmacological Therapy
Calcium channel blockers (e.g., nifedipine) and long-acting nitrates (e.g., isosorbide dinitrate) can improve smooth muscle relaxation and reduce LES pressure; however, symptom improvement is often incomplete, and side effects are common.

Endoscopic Therapy
Pneumatic dilation can mechanically dilate the LES and disrupt the circular muscle fibers. One-third of patients, however, will experience symptom relapse, especially those with thicker LES musculature at the time of the procedure. The most serious complication from pneumatic dilation is esophageal perforation, which requires endoscopic or possibly surgical repair.

A newer technique is a peroral endoscopic myotomy (POEM), in which endoscopic dissection of the esophageal submucosa is performed to expose the muscular layer. A myotomy is performed, then the esophageal

mucosal defect is closed. Although most patients experience relief of achalasia-related symptoms, GE reflux is a common complication.

Patients who are poor candidates for these procedures may instead undergo endoscopic injection of botulinum toxin into the LES to cause short-term paralysis. About half of patients, however, will experience recurring symptoms requiring retreatment. Moreover, the use of botulinum toxin can complicate subsequent attempts at myotomy, as the layers of the esophageal wall become fibrotic.

Surgical Therapy
A surgical (Heller) myotomy is a laparoscopic procedure in which the muscle fibers of the LES are divided from a transabdominal approach. To prevent postoperative GE reflux, surgeons often perform a simultaneous fundoplication, in which the upper portion of the stomach is wrapped around the lower end of the esophagus. Patients with end-stage, refractory achalasia may be candidates for esophagectomy, though it is associated with significant morbidity and mortality and is therefore a last-resort treatment.

CHAPTER 128

Gastroesophageal Reflux Disease (GERD) and Barrett Esophagus

ALEKSEY NOVIKOV • YUNSEOK NAMN

INTRODUCTION

Gastroesophageal reflux disease (GERD) is a chronic disorder in which gastroduodenal contents flow retrograde into the esophagus and produce symptoms. The short-term effects include pain and discomfort, while long-term complications include esophagitis, esophageal scarring/stricture formation, ulceration, and **Barrett esophagus (BE)**. BE, a premalignant condition, occurs in 10% to 15% of patients and is diagnosed based on the presence of at least 1 cm of metaplastic columnar epithelium replacing the stratified squamous epithelium that normally lines the esophagus. BE can progress from **intestinal metaplasia (IM)** to low-grade dysplasia (LGD) to high-grade dysplasia (HGD) and eventually to an invasive adenocarcinoma. The incidence of GERD/BE-related adenocarcinomas has been increasing, underscoring the need for regular follow-up and treatment of symptomatic individuals (see Chapter 158 for details).

PATHOPHYSIOLOGY

GERD results from a combination of factors, including the structural and functional integrity of the **lower esophageal sphincter (LES),** gastric acidity, esophageal mucosal defenses, and sensory mechanisms.

GERD occurs when intragastric pressure exceeds LES pressure (Fig. 128.1). The esophagus enters the abdominal cavity through a hiatus in the diaphragm, forming a sling that creates an angle at the gastroesophageal (GE) junction. This LES is composed of at least two muscles: a circular clasp muscle that forms a partial ring and a gastric sling that completes the ring. Patients with GERD have been shown to have decreased distal esophageal pressures, poor contractility of the gastric clasp/gastric sling muscle complex, generalized increased distensibility of the LES, ineffective esophageal motility, and excessive relaxation in response to nicotinic stimulation. The consequent reflux of acidic stomach contents (including pepsin, bile salts, and pancreatic enzymes) into the distal esophagus causes erosion, pain, and inflammation.

In some individuals, chronic reflux results in transformation of the stratified squamous epithelium into metaplastic columnar epithelium, the phenomenon known as BE (Fig. 128.2). Three types of columnar epithelium are seen in BE: gastric fundus type, cardia type, and intestinal type (goblet cells). With time, metaplasia can progress to cancer. The intestinal-type transformation has the highest risk of malignant progression into esophageal adenocarcinoma at a rate of about 0.3% to 0.5% per year.

RISK FACTORS

Risk factors for GERD include Caucasian race, male gender, central obesity, increased body mass index (BMI), age >50 years, tobacco use, and the presence of a hiatal hernia. Smoking can cause GERD, presumably through nicotine-mediated relaxation of the smooth muscle complex. Patients with systemic sclerosis frequently have GERD and BE due to decreased pressures at the LES and decreased esophageal motility. Obesity may cause GERD through extrinsic gastric compression, leading to an increase in intragastric pressures and subsequent relaxation of the LES. Patients with hiatal hernias often have GERD secondary to disruption of the normal anatomical structure of the LES. The risk of BE increases with prolonged duration of GERD, lack of effective therapy, and family history of BE.

PRESENTATION, EVALUATION, AND DIAGNOSIS

GERD often presents as heartburn and regurgitation that increase after meals and in a supine position. Patients may also present with atypical symptoms, however, such as nausea, bloating, chronic cough, asthma, laryngitis, and globus pharyngeus. The extraesophageal manifestations of GERD are generally attributable to laryngopharyngeal reflux (LPR). The differential diagnosis includes

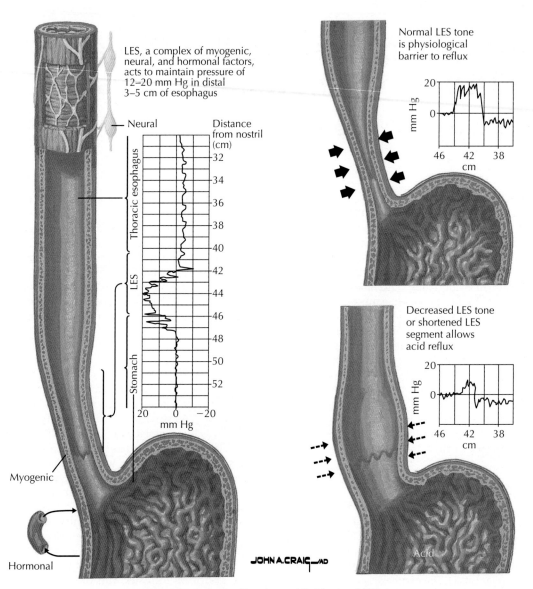

LES, a complex of myogenic, neural, and hormonal factors, acts to maintain pressure of 12–20 mm Hg in distal 3–5 cm of esophagus

Normal LES tone is physiological barrier to reflux

Decreased LES tone or shortened LES segment allows acid reflux

FIG. 128.1 **Lower Esophageal Sphincter (LES).**

peptic ulcer disease, achalasia, gastritis, dyspepsia, and gastroparesis.

A careful history and a physical exam are often sufficient for the presumptive diagnosis of GERD. A positive response to a trial of a **proton-pump inhibitor (PPI)** further supports the diagnosis. Patients who do not respond to therapy or who have red flags such as odynophagia, dysphagia, hematemesis, weight loss, and iron-deficiency anemia should undergo esophagogastroduodenoscopy (EGD) to evaluate the esophageal

and gastric mucosa. Of note, the EGD may be normal despite heartburn and reflux symptoms, in which case esophageal pH monitoring and/or manometry may be helpful to establish the diagnosis.

The diagnosis of BE can be established when EGD reveals extension of salmon-colored mucosa into the tubular esophagus ≥1 cm above the GE junction (Z line), and biopsies show intestinal metaplasia. The presence and a degree of dysplasia are determined based on the presence of goblet cells and disruption of cellular

Gastroesophageal junction

Esophageal epithelium

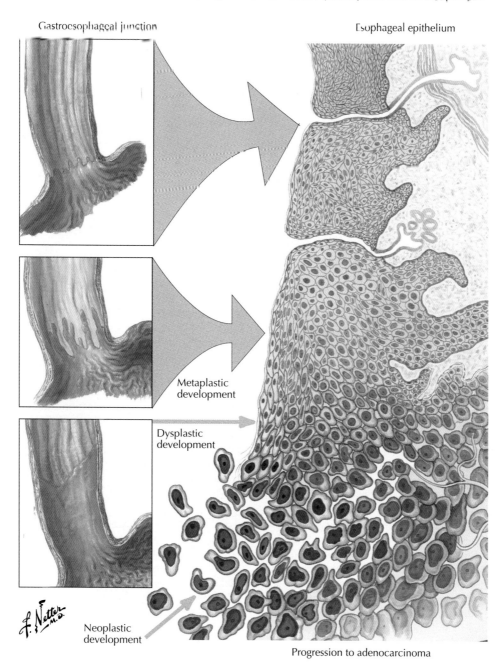

Metaplastic
development

Dysplastic
development

Neoplastic
development

Progression to adenocarcinoma

FIG. 128.2 **Barrett Esophagus.**

architecture. Screening for BE is challenging because up to 50% of patients with BE do not have any symptoms, and active reflux symptoms do not predict the presence of BE. Thus the current recommendation is to offer one-time, EGD-based screening to men with a history of GERD for >5 years regardless of symptoms and two or more risk factors, which include age >50 years, Caucasian race, chronic and/or frequent GERD, central obesity, current or past history of smoking, and a confirmed family history of BE or esophageal cancer in a first-degree relative.

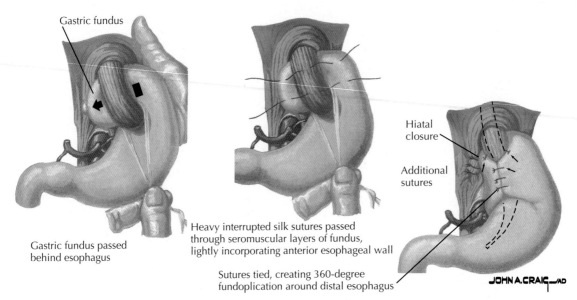

Gastric fundus

Gastric fundus passed behind esophagus

Heavy interrupted silk sutures passed through seromuscular layers of fundus, lightly incorporating anterior esophageal wall

Sutures tied, creating 360-degree fundoplication around distal esophagus

Hiatal closure

Additional sutures

JOHN A.CRAIG—AD

FIG. 128.3 **Nissen Fundoplication.**

TREATMENT

The initial therapy should focus on weight loss, elevation of the head of the bed, and avoidance of meals 3 hours before bedtime. Patients may also start empiric therapy with an 8-week course of a daily PPI. If symptoms persist, PPI frequency can be increased to twice daily, or second-line agents can be added, such as antacids or nocturnal histamine receptor antagonists (H2RA). This method can help manage nighttime acid breakthrough symptoms, which affect up to 73% of patients with GERD despite twice-daily PPI.

If an EGD is performed and shows severe erosive disease, the test should be repeated after 8 weeks to evaluate for BE that may have been obscured by inflammation. Patients who improve with PPI therapy should be maintained on the lowest effective dose, as PPI therapy has been rarely associated with *Clostridioides* (formerly *Clostridium*) *difficile* infection, pneumonia, dementia, renal insufficiency, hypocalcemia, hypomagnesemia, and hip fractures.

Patients who are unwilling to remain on lifelong medical therapy, are intolerant of medical therapy, have medically refractory symptoms, or have a large hiatal hernia are candidates for surgery. In the **Nissen fundoplication** (Fig. 128.3), the distal esophagus is surgically plicated to prevent reflux. Gas-bloat syndrome, resulting from excessive tightness of the plicated esophagus, is the most frequent complication and occurs in 20% of patients. Other potential complications include dysphagia, infection, and hemorrhage. Alternatives to Nissen fundoplication include novel, minimally invasive endoscopic and surgical procedures for LES augmentation, such as transoral incisionless fundoplication (TIF) and magnetic bead sphincter augmentation.

The management of BE depends on the presence or degree of dysplasia. If the initial biopsy is negative for dysplasia, a repeat endoscopic exam should be performed 1 year later, then again at intervals of 3 to 5 years. Low-grade dysplasia warrants either yearly endoscopic surveillance or endoscopic therapy, and the presence of high-grade dysplasia necessitates endoscopic therapy. Available endoscopic therapies include endoscopic mucosal resection, submucosal dissection, tissue ablation, radiofrequency ablation, and cryotherapy. These therapies aim to resect or ablate the dysplastic mucosa and permit reepithelialization, which reduces the probability of malignant transformation. Surgical therapies are reserved for those with an incomplete endoscopic mucosal resection, adenocarcinoma that extends into submucosa, and lymphovascular invasion and poor cellular differentiation.

CHAPTER 129

Peptic Ulcer Disease and *Helicobacter pylori*

GAURAV GHOSH • SHAWN L. SHAH

INTRODUCTION

Peptic ulcer disease (PUD), defined as the presence of ulcerations in the gastric and duodenal mucosa, is associated with significant morbidity and mortality worldwide. Nearly 2% of the global population has peptic ulcers, with >500,000 new cases reported each year in the United States alone.

The understanding of PUD shifted dramatically in the early 1980s after the discovery that *Helicobacter pylori,* a gram-negative bacterium, was responsible for a large number of cases. *H. pylori* infects the gastrointestinal (GI) epithelium and is one of the most pervasive bacterial pathogens worldwide, with the highest burden in developing countries. Infection generally occurs early in life. Because *H. pylori* can survive the acidic environment of the stomach, it is estimated that over half of the world's population has been infected, with a prevalence of 30% to 40% in the United States. Of note, however, only 5% to 10% of those infected with *H. pylori* will develop ulcers.

PATHOPHYSIOLOGY AND RISK FACTORS

A peptic ulcer contains necrotic debris overlying layers of fibrinoid necrosis, granulation tissue, and fibrous tissue that can extend into the muscular layers of the stomach or duodenum (Fig. 129.1). If the ulcer extends into the serosa, there is a high risk of frank perforation into the peritoneal space. If the ulcer erodes into an overlying artery, life-threatening GI hemorrhage can occur.

Many environmental and host risk factors contribute to ulcer development by increasing acid secretion and weakening the normal mucosal barrier. The most important environmental exposures are *H. pylori* infection and NSAID use.

H. pylori (Fig. 129.2) colonizes the gastric epithelium and can promote a robust immune-mediated response, leading to severe inflammation. In addition, the urease activity of *H. pylori* can produce ammonia, which prevents glands in the stomach from sensing the true gastric pH,

leading to inappropriate gastrin release. The resulting hypergastrinemia promotes hyperplasia of acid-secreting parietal cells and increased acid secretion. In the duodenum, the low pH promotes gastric metaplasia, which further promotes colonization of *H. pylori* due to its predisposition for gastric epithelial cells.

Infection with *H. pylori* is also associated with an increased risk of gastric malignancy. The role of *H. pylori* carcinogenesis is incompletely understood, but bacterial properties, host response, and environmental factors are thought to play a role. Eventually, through the path of chronic active and atrophic gastritis, patients can develop adenocarcinoma. In addition, chronic stimulation of T and B cells can lead to gastric mucosa-associated lymphoid tissue (MALT) lymphomas.

Meanwhile, NSAIDs damage the gastric mucosa primarily by inhibiting mucosal cyclooxygenase (COX), thereby impairing production of the prostaglandins central to mucosal defense. Because mucosa-protecting prostaglandins are produced primarily by COX-1, selective inhibitors of COX-2 (e.g., celecoxib) can help lower (but not eliminate) the risk of mucosal injury.

Smoking, excessive alcohol consumption, and emotional stress increase the risk of ulcer formation, but are usually not sufficient in the absence of *H. pylori* infection or NSAID use. Less common causes of peptic ulcers include **Zollinger-Ellison syndrome,** in which gastrin-secreting tumors in the pancreas or duodenum cause excess gastric acidification resulting in extensive ulcerations at high risk of bleeding, and critical illness (e.g., traumatic brain injury, severe burns, hemorrhage, sepsis), which can cause stress ulcers.

PRESENTATION, EVALUATION, AND DIAGNOSIS

Many patients with PUD, particularly those with chronic or NSAID-induced ulcers, do not experience pain, and GI bleeding or perforation may be the first presenting manifestation. In others, the predominant symptom of

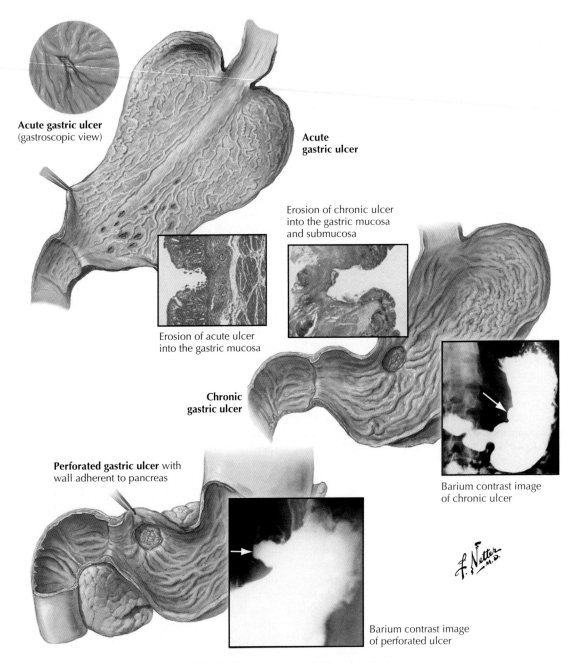

Acute gastric ulcer
(gastroscopic view)

Acute
gastric ulcer

Erosion of chronic ulcer
into the gastric mucosa
and submucosa

Erosion of acute ulcer
into the gastric mucosa

Chronic
gastric ulcer

Barium contrast image
of chronic ulcer

Perforated gastric ulcer with
wall adherent to pancreas

Barium contrast image
of perforated ulcer

FIG. 129.1 **Peptic Ulcer: Gross and Microscopic Appearance.**

uncomplicated PUD is a dull, hungerlike epigastric pain, often associated with nausea and bloating. In patients with gastric ulcers, food intake typically exacerbates epigastric pain secondary to increased acid production. In patients with duodenal ulcers, food intake tends to relieve the pain secondary to increased alkaline secretions from the pancreas.

Testing for *H. pylori* is beneficial only in select populations, including patients with known ulcers, gastric cancer, or gastric MALT lymphoma. More recent guidelines also

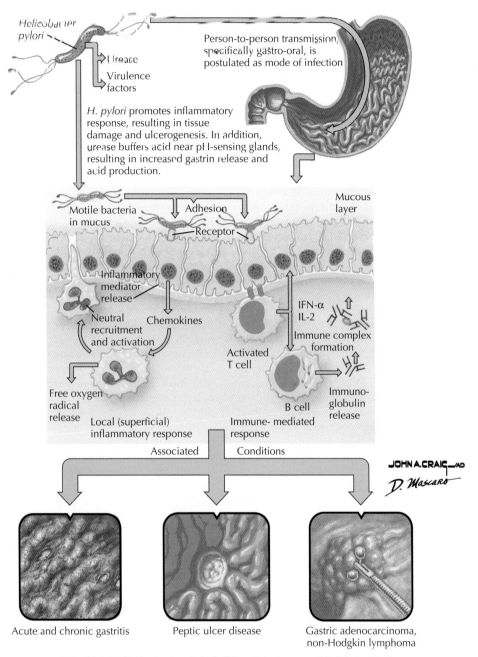

Helicobacter pylori

Urease

Virulence factors

Person-to-person transmission, specifically gastro-oral, is postulated as mode of infection

H. pylori promotes inflammatory response, resulting in tissue damage and ulcerogenesis. In addition, urease buffers acid near pH-sensing glands, resulting in increased gastrin release and acid production.

Motile bacteria in mucus

Adhesion

Mucous layer

Receptor

Inflammatory mediator release

Chemokines

IFN-α
IL-2

Immune complex formation

Neutral recruitment and activation

Activated T cell

Free oxygen radical release

Local (superficial) inflammatory response

B cell

Immune- mediated response

Immuno-globulin release

Associated   Conditions

JOHN A.CRAIG—AD

D. Mascaro

Acute and chronic gastritis

Peptic ulcer disease

Gastric adenocarcinoma, non-Hodgkin lymphoma

FIG. 129.2 **Helicobacter pylori.** *IFN-α,* Interferon-α; *IL2,* interleukin-2.

recommend testing for *H. pylori* before the initiation of low-dose aspirin and in patients with chronic NSAID use, iron-deficiency anemia, and idiopathic thrombocytopenic purpura.

Initial testing usually consists of either ^{13}C-**urea breath testing** or stool antigen testing. Although serum tests for immunoglobulin G (IgG) antibodies to *H. pylori* are frequently ordered, a positive result cannot differentiate between prior and current infection.

In the ^{13}C-urea breath test, the patient drinks urea containing radiolabeled carbon. The urease in *H. pylori* produces radiolabeled carbon dioxide, which is measured in the breath. The test is logistically cumbersome but has high specificity (95%–100%) and sensitivity (88%–95%). It is important to note that proton-pump inhibitors (PPIs), H2 receptor antagonists (H2RA), antibiotics, and bismuth can all increase the probability of false-negative results from both breath and stool antigen tests, and should be discontinued at least 2 to 4 weeks before testing.

Endoscopic evaluation is recommended for patients who report epigastric pain and are >60 years, have prolonged NSAID use, or have alarm symptoms such as new-onset dyspepsia, weight loss, intractable nausea, or GI bleeding. A mucosal break >5 mm with overlying fibrin confirms the diagnosis of PUD. *H. pylori* infection can be assessed by obtaining biopsies of the gastric antrum and body, then using either a rapid urease-based method or immunofluorescence. Direct histological examination or biopsy-based urease testing is especially preferred over noninvasive tests for patients on acid-suppressing medications.

TREATMENT

PPIs, which reduce acid secretion by selectively blocking hydrogen-potassium ATPases in parietal cells, are the most effective agents both for preventing and treating PUD. More than 90% of peptic ulcers resolve with 8 weeks of PPI therapy. Patients must also modify underlying risk factors (e.g., discontinuing NSAIDs).

Other agents include H2RAs, which are weaker antisecretory agents; misoprostol, a prostaglandin analogue that increases mucosal resistance by reducing acid secretion and stimulating mucous and bicarbonate production; bismuth salts, which form complexes with epithelial cells to create a physical barrier; and sucralfate, which binds to glycoproteins and increases mucous secretion to protect ulcerated areas. These agents can be used as adjuncts to PPIs or for those patients who cannot accept the potential side effects from PPIs.

H. pylori infection should be treated not only to improve symptoms, but also to reduce the risk of gastric malignancy. The treatment regimens generally include a PPI or H2RA, antibiotics, and occasionally bismuth. A recent expert consensus for the treatment of *H. pylori* infection in adults recommended a first-line regimen of either 14 days of nonbismuth quadruple therapy (PPI, amoxicillin, metronidazole, clarithromycin) or traditional bismuth quadruple therapy (PPI, bismuth, metronidazole, tetracycline). The guidelines recommend that PPI triple therapy (PPI, clarithromycin, either amoxicillin or metronidazole) be reserved for areas with low clarithromycin resistance. Rescue regimens for patients with three failed treatment attempts include rifabutin or levofloxacin (e.g., PPI, amoxicillin, either levofloxacin or rifabutin).

Because of increasing antibiotic resistance, many patients will have persistent *H. pylori* infection despite treatment and remain at risk for complications. As a result, posttreatment testing for *H. pylori* is recommended, despite little evidence to date that it is cost effective. Posttreatment testing can be particularly helpful in patients with a documented *H. pylori*–associated ulcer, ongoing dyspepsia, gastric MALT lymphoma, or gastric cancer. A urea breath test or stool antigen test should be performed at least 4 weeks after completing treatment.

CHAPTER 130

Biliary Disease

ALEKSEY NOVIKOV • YUNSEOK NAMN

INTRODUCTION

The biliary system is a complex network of small intrahepatic and larger extrahepatic ducts that convey bile produced by the liver or stored in the gallbladder to the small intestine, where it is excreted or aids in the digestion of cholesterol and fat. **Cholestasis** refers to any process that obstructs biliary flow. Over 95% of cases are attributable to gallstones or biliary sludge, which are present in 10% to 20% of people in developed countries. Most gallstones are asymptomatic and found incidentally on abdominal ultrasound; however, the risk of developing symptoms is substantial, averaging 2% to 2.6% per year. Symptoms occur when gallstones obstruct the cystic duct or common bile duct, resulting in ductal spasms that cause painful **biliary colic.** Sustained obstruction can result in complications such as **acute cholecystitis** or cholangitis, depending on stone location.

Less commonly, cholestasis can result from obstruction of bile flow, either extrinsic or intrinsic to the bile duct. These include tumors of the bile duct (cholangiocarcinoma), pancreas, and gallbladder; congenital malformations; primary adenomas and polyps; metastases from other primary tumors; and chronic autoimmune inflammatory conditions leading to strictures **(primary biliary cholangitis [PBC]** and **primary sclerosing cholangitis [PSC]).**

PATHOPHYSIOLOGY

Approximately 80% of gallstones are known as cholesterol stones (Fig. 130.1), composed of long, thin cholesterol monohydrate crystals mixed with a small amount of phospholipids and bile acids. Increased cholesterol secretion and/or gallbladder hypomotility create an environment that predisposes cholesterol monohydrate crystals to conglomerate and form macroscopic stones, a process known as nucleation.

Much less common are pigmented stones (see Fig 130.1), which can be further described as black or brown. Black-pigmented (bilirubin) stones consist of bilirubin conjugate polymers and result from chronic hemolysis, cirrhosis, cholesterol malabsorption in the terminal ileum, and inherited conditions such as Gilbert syndrome. Brown-pigmented (or "mixed") stones consist of calcium bilirubinate and are usually associated with biliary infections.

PBC is a chronic progressive autoimmune disorder in which intralobular bile ducts are gradually destroyed, leading to signs and symptoms of cholestasis. Retained bile acids eventually result in cirrhosis and liver failure (Fig. 130.2). PBC is more common in women and carries an increased risk for hepatocellular carcinoma, hypothyroidism, metabolic bone disease, and anemia. PSC is an idiopathic cholestatic disease characterized by chronic inflammation and fibrosis of the medium and large bile ducts, but rarely also the small bile ducts. It is particularly associated with inflammatory bowel disease and, like PBC, can eventually result in liver failure.

RISK FACTORS

The incidence of gallstones is twice as great among younger women compared to men, though the difference does not persist beyond age 50. First-degree relatives of patients with gallstone disease are 4.5 times more likely to also have gallstones. Other major risk factors include ethnicity (Native American, Mexican American, and Northern European), advanced age, obesity, rapid weight loss, pregnancy, and the use of contraceptive hormones, total parenteral nutrition (TPN), ceftriaxone, and octreotide.

PRESENTATION, EVALUATION, AND DIAGNOSIS

Biliary colic is episodic, severe pain in the epigastrium and right upper quadrant (RUQ) that occurs when biliary contractions cause a gallstone to become transiently impacted in the cystic duct (Fig. 130.3). Once the gallbladder relaxes, the stone disengages or passes, and the obstruction is relieved. Symptoms are often precipitated by large and fatty meals, which promote the release of cholecystokinin, a hormone that facilitates digestion by increasing hepatic bile production and contracting the

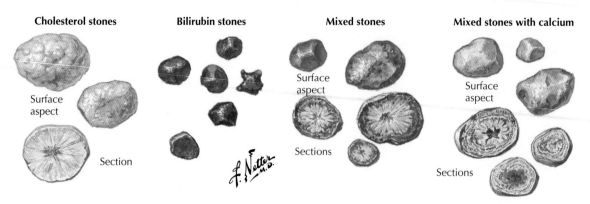

FIG. 130.1 **Gallstone Subtypes.**

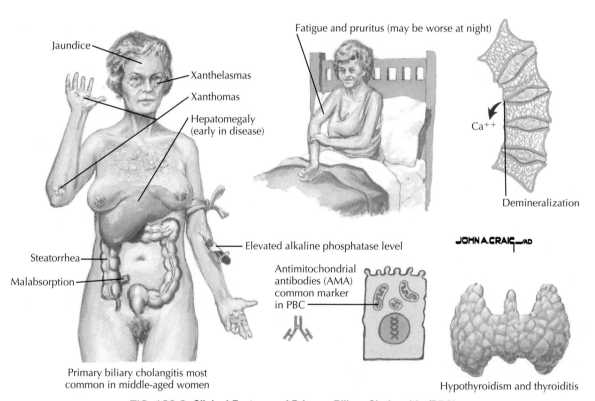

FIG. 130.2 **Clinical Features of Primary Biliary Cholangitis** *(PBC).*

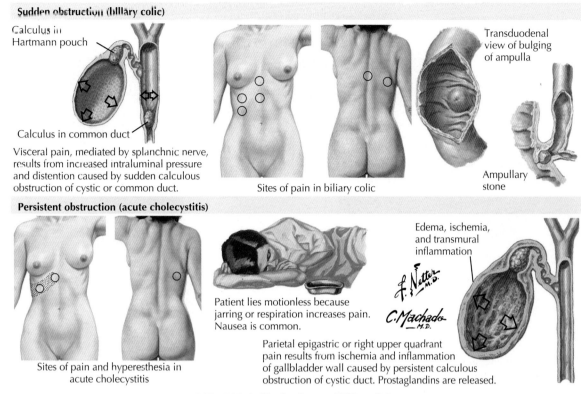

Sudden obstruction (biliary colic)

Calculus in Hartmann pouch

Calculus in common duct

Visceral pain, mediated by splanchnic nerve, results from increased intraluminal pressure and distention caused by sudden calculous obstruction of cystic or common duct.

Sites of pain in biliary colic

Transduodenal view of bulging of ampulla

Ampullary stone

Persistent obstruction (acute cholecystitis)

Sites of pain and hyperesthesia in acute cholecystitis

Patient lies motionless because jarring or respiration increases pain. Nausea is common.

Parietal epigastric or right upper quadrant pain results from ischemia and inflammation of gallbladder wall caused by persistent calculous obstruction of cystic duct. Prostaglandins are released.

Edema, ischemia, and transmural inflammation

FIG. 130.3 **Mechanisms of Biliary Pain.**

gallbladder. Patients are symptom free and have normal laboratory studies between episodes.

Acute cholecystitis occurs in the setting of sustained cystic duct obstruction and should be suspected if RUQ pain lasts >6 hours and is associated with fever (Fig. 130.4). A diagnostic evaluation should begin with a thorough history, focusing on risk factors, and a physical exam to locate and better characterize the pain. The principal diagnostic test is the RUQ ultrasound (see Fig. 130.4); supportive findings include pericholecystic fluid, gallbladder wall thickening >3 mm, and a positive Murphy sign (see Chapter 44 for details). Laboratory evaluation usually reveals leukocytosis and may also feature elevated serum aminotransferases and alkaline phosphatase levels, secondary to gallbladder edema causing partial obstruction of the common bile duct.

Choledocholithiasis, or a stone in the common bile duct (CBD), causes dull RUQ pain similar to that experienced with biliary colic and cholecystitis; however, early laboratory abnormalities include elevated transaminases, and later findings include elevated alkaline phosphatase and direct hyperbilirubinemia >1.5 times the upper limit

of normal. Acute pancreatitis may also be present (see Chapter 131 for further details). The differential diagnosis should also include CBD obstruction from a cyst, sludge, obstructed stent (in patients with prior endoscopic biliary procedures), or mass. In the emergent setting, an RUQ ultrasound is the initial imaging modality because of its rapid availability; however, if it is nondiagnostic or negative, a magnetic resonance cholangiopancreatography (MRCP) should be performed, as it is more sensitive for the detection of CBD obstruction. If there is a high suspicion for an obstructive tumor, contrast-enhanced CT or MRI of the abdomen and pelvis should be performed, with any suspicious findings assessed using endoscopic ultrasound (EUS) and fine-needle aspiration (FNA).

Ascending cholangitis, or superinfection of an obstructed biliary system, should be considered in patients with fever, hemodynamic instability, or confusion in addition to the pain syndrome described earlier (see Chapter 118 for further details). Urgent diagnostic tests should be performed to locate the cause of biliary obstruction and plan for possible intervention, such as endoscopic retrograde cholangiopancreatography (ERCP).

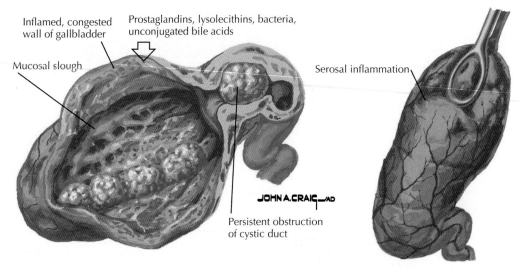

Inflamed, congested wall of gallbladder

Prostaglandins, lysolecithins, bacteria, unconjugated bile acids

Mucosal slough

Serosal inflammation

JOHN A.CRAIG—AD

Persistent obstruction of cystic duct

FIG. 130.4 Acute Calculous Cholecystitis.

Patients with PBC and PSC can have elevated bilirubin, and especially alkaline phosphatase, and present with jaundice, pruritus, and fatigue. Workup for PBC includes imaging to rule out extrahepatic biliary obstruction and analysis for **antimitochondrial antibodies,** which are present in 90% to 95% of affected patients. Patients with suspected PSC should undergo cholangiography, often with MRCP or ERCP, which visualizes multifocal strictures and dilatations of both intrahepatic and extrahepatic bile ducts. Note that gallstones may be present in PSC. Liver biopsy can help support the diagnosis of either PBC or PSC but may not be necessary.

TREATMENT

Patients with biliary colic should be referred to a surgeon for elective cholecystectomy, as most will continue to have pain episodes and are at risk for complications.

Patients with acute cholecystitis should be hospitalized and referred for early **cholecystectomy.** Although a 2013 Cochrane review found no difference in mortality with early (within 7 days from onset of symptoms) compared to delayed (6 weeks from onset of symptoms) laparoscopic cholecystectomy, patients in the early cholecystectomy group had shorter operative times and a shorter hospital stay. Patients who are poor surgical candidates can receive a percutaneous cholecystostomy drain to relieve biliary stasis and achieve source control.

Newer endoscopic techniques allow for internal drainage of the gallbladder using endoscopic ultrasound-guided placement of self-expanding, fully covered metal stents that directly connect the dilated gallbladder to the adjacent stomach or duodenum. The advantages of this technique include its high rate of success, reduced pain, and a reduced length of stay in the hospital; however, prospective trials are needed to fully evaluate its benefit over percutaneous drainage.

Patients with possible acute ascending cholangitis should be resuscitated and stabilized with intravenous (IV) fluids and antibiotics, then undergo ERCP to relieve any obstruction emergently. Patients with confirmed choledocholithiasis should undergo ERCP to relieve the obstruction (Fig. 130.5). In patients with concomitant pancreatitis in the absence of cholangitis, the timing and even role of ERCP is debated.

Patients with PBC should receive ursodeoxycholic acid (UDCA), a nontoxic bile acid that improves liver function tests and reduces disease progression; patients refractory to UDCA can receive obeticholic acid. In PSC, immunosuppressive and antiinflammatory medications have yielded few benefits. UDCA can improve liver function tests but has yet to show reduction in disease progression. Extrahepatic strictures may be treated with stenting via ERCP. Patients with advanced PBC or PSC should undergo evaluation for liver transplantation.

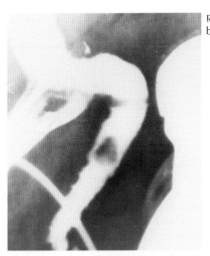

T-tube cholangiogram shows retained stone in common duct

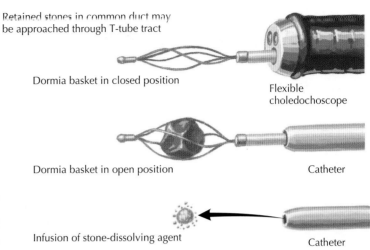

Retained stones in common duct may be approached through T-tube tract

Dormia basket in closed position

Flexible choledochoscope

Dormia basket in open position

Catheter

Infusion of stone-dissolving agent

Catheter

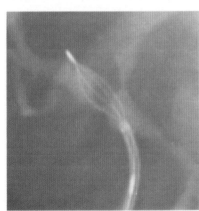

Radiograph shows stone in Dormia basket (retrograde approach)

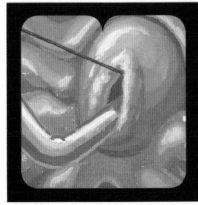

If trapping techniques fail, stone may be removed by sphincterotomy at ampulla

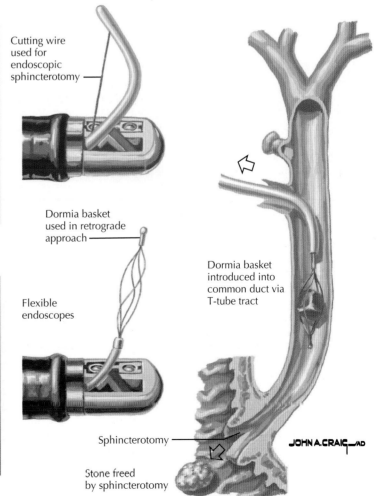

Cutting wire used for endoscopic sphincterotomy

Dormia basket used in retrograde approach

Flexible endoscopes

Dormia basket introduced into common duct via T-tube tract

Sphincterotomy

Stone freed by sphincterotomy

JOHN A. CRAIG—AD

FIG. 130.5 **Management of Choledocholithiasis.**

CHAPTER 131

Acute Pancreatitis

MONICA SAUMOY • YECHESKEL SCHNEIDER

INTRODUCTION

Acute pancreatitis is an inflammatory process of the pancreas that typically causes severe abdominal pain. It is the third most common inpatient gastrointestinal diagnosis in the United States, with a mortality rate ranging from 3% to 17%. The two most common causes of **acute pancreatitis** are **gallstones** and **excess alcohol consumption,** which are together responsible for 70% to 80% of cases of acute pancreatitis in the United States.

PATHOPHYSIOLOGY

The pancreas produces zymogens, or proenzymes, that are activated in the duodenum to facilitate the digestion of carbohydrates, proteins, and lipids. The premature activation of these enzymes, particularly trypsinogen, leads to pancreatic autodigestion and acinar cell injury, prompting a release of cytokines that recruit neutrophils and macrophages. The ensuing inflammation produces the symptoms of acute pancreatitis. If severe enough, inflammation can cause hemorrhage and necrosis, which may be complicated by infection (Fig. 131.1).

Gallstone pancreatitis is the most common cause of pancreatitis. Though the exact mechanism is unclear, an obstructing stone at the ampulla of Vater increases pancreatic ductal pressures and causes bile to reflux into the pancreatic duct, likely activating digestive enzymes and the inflammatory cascade.

The exact mechanism of alcohol-related pancreatitis is also unclear, as only a small proportion of alcohol abusers will develop this complication. One proposed mechanism is that the pancreas metabolizes alcohol via the nonoxidative pathway (as compared to the oxidative pathway within the liver). The nonoxidative breakdown of alcohol leads to the formation of fatty acid ethanol esters, which accumulate and may cause pancreatitis. Another proposed mechanism is that alcohol alters cell permeability, destabilizes intracellular membranes, and increases lysosomal fragility, making the pancreas more susceptible to injury.

RISK FACTORS

Gallstone pancreatitis can result from both large gallstones and microlithiasis (sludge), though the risk is greater with smaller stones. The incidence of gallstone pancreatitis is higher in women, secondary to their greater burden of gallstones, but the risk of developing acute pancreatitis from gallstones is higher in men. Overall, pancreatitis occurs in only 3% to 7% of those with gallstones. Meanwhile, alcohol-induced pancreatitis typically occurs after many years of alcohol abuse.

Other etiologies of and risk factors for pancreatitis include pancreatic duct obstruction (e.g., pancreatic or ampullary tumor), structural abnormalities (e.g., pancreatic divisum, choledochocele), hypertriglyceridemia (serum triglycerides usually >1000 mg/dL), medication use (particularly α-methyldopa, dapsone, enalapril, furosemide, isoniazid, mesalamine, metronidazole, simvastatin, sulfamethoxazole, tetracycline, and valproic acid), certain infections (ascariasis, clonorchiasis, coxsackievirus, cytomegalovirus, tuberculosis), toxin exposures (organophosphates, scorpion venom), endoscopic retrograde cholangiopancreatography (ERCP), and direct physical trauma. Several genetic mutations are also associated with pancreatitis, including mutations in *PRSS1* (hereditary pancreatitis), mutations in *CFTR* (cystic fibrosis), and mutations in *SPINK7* (blocks the feedback inhibitor of trypsin, predisposing to pancreatitis).

PRESENTATION

Patients typically present with acute-onset epigastric abdominal pain that radiates to the back and may be partially improved by bending forward. Nausea and vomiting are common. In severe cases of hemorrhagic pancreatitis, patients may have periumbilical ecchymosis (Cullen sign) or flank ecchymoses (Grey Turner sign).

The major laboratory finding is elevation of serum **amylase** and/or **lipase** concentrations of more than three times the upper limit of normal. Lipase elevations are more sensitive for pancreatitis than amylase elevations. The degree of elevation does not correlate with disease severity, and trending levels are not useful for assessing

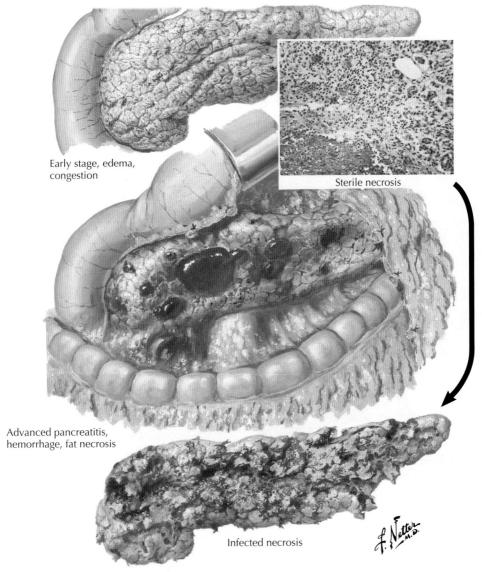

Early stage, edema, congestion

Sterile necrosis

Advanced pancreatitis, hemorrhage, fat necrosis

Infected necrosis

FIG. 131.1 **Gross Appearance of Organ Damage From Pancreatitis.** Pancreatitis can range from edema and congestion of the pancreas, to fat necrosis/hemorrhage and infected necrosis.

disease resolution. Gallstone pancreatitis is often associated with marked initial elevation of aminotransferases, followed by elevated conjugated bilirubin and alkaline phosphatase levels.

Pancreatitis results in characteristic findings of inflammation on CT or MRI, such as diffuse parenchymal enlargement with indistinct margins and surrounding retroperitoneal fat stranding (Fig. 131.2). Imaging is not required for the diagnosis of acute pancreatitis, though it can be useful to evaluate for local complications of severe pancreatitis, such as pancreatic fluid collections or walled-off necrosis, in patients with severe illness or who fail to improve with supportive care.

Risk stratification is important for triage and determining the need for intensive care admission. Multiple scoring systems have been developed (e.g., Ranson criteria,

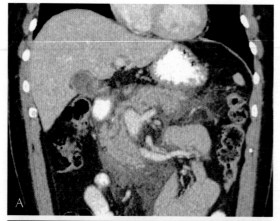

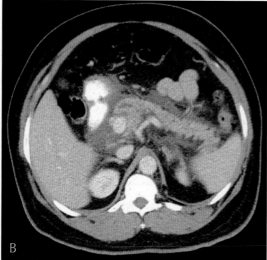

FIG. 131.2 **Radiographic Image of Pancreatitis With Edema of the Pancreas as Well as Around the Organ.**

Balthazar, Atlanta, BISAP). The revised Atlanta criteria of 2012 categorizes pancreatitis as mild, moderately severe, and severe. Mild pancreatitis is not associated with organ failure or other complications such as peripancreatic fluid collections or pancreatic/peripancreatic necrosis. Moderately severe acute pancreatitis can be associated with transient organ failure, such as acute kidney injury, that resolves within 48 hours, or local complications.

Severe acute pancreatitis is associated with persistent organ failure.

TREATMENT

The initial treatment of pancreatitis focuses on aggressive hydration (to prevent hypoperfusion), pain control (frequently with parenteral opioids), and bowel rest (to prevent pancreatic stimulation).

Pancreatitis is associated with third spacing of fluids and effective arterial volume depletion, so it is essential to establish and maintain adequate hydration to reduce morbidity and mortality. **Lactated Ringer** crystalloid solution is preferred over normal saline for fluid resuscitation, as it appears to cause less systemic inflammation. Patients should receive fluids with a goal urine output of 0.5 to 1 mL/kg/h and a decrease in hematocrit or blood urea nitrogen (BUN) by 5 mg/dL in the first 24 hours (secondary to hemodilution).

Patients with moderately severe or severe pancreatitis must be monitored for acute respiratory distress syndrome (ARDS) resulting from systemic inflammation. Other potential complications include hypocalcemia and hypomagnesemia, which occurs because pancreatic enzymes cause saponification of mesenteric fat, with chelation of these cations.

Fever is common, though febrile patients should not receive empiric antibiotics unless they have positive blood cultures, radiographic evidence of infected necrosis, or clinical evidence of another infection (e.g., cholangitis, pneumonia).

Once a patient has been initially resuscitated, identification and management of the underlying cause of pancreatitis are necessary to prevent further attacks. Many patients require ERCP, either to manage pancreatic duct obstruction from stones/tumor or to manage other structural disruptions of the pancreatic duct. For other patients, removing the offending agent (such as alcohol or a medication) will prevent additional episodes of pancreatitis.

As the patient clinically improves, a liquid diet can slowly be reintroduced and then transitioned to a low fat and then regular diet. If a patient has moderately severe or severe pancreatitis and oral feeding cannot be resumed within a few days, then enteral nutrition through a feeding tube should be considered.

CHAPTER 132

Irritable Bowel Syndrome

ZACHARY SHERMAN • JOSÉPHINE A. COOL • VIKAS GUPTA

INTRODUCTION

Irritable bowel syndrome (IBS) is a disorder of the gastrointestinal (GI) tract that often presents in early adulthood and is characterized by abdominal pain, **bloating,** diarrhea, and/or constipation. It is a global problem, affecting up to 15% of the population, with varying geographic prevalence. Patterns suggest that developed countries have a higher incidence of IBS; however, access to care, reporting, and social stigmata likely underestimate the burden of disease in undeveloped countries. The prevalence is so great that even though only a small minority of patients with IBS seek medical attention, it nonetheless accounts for 25% to 50% of all gastroenterology referrals.

PATHOPHYSIOLOGY

The pathophysiological mechanisms underlying IBS have not been fully elucidated, but contributing factors appear to include visceral hypersensitivity, abnormalities in GI motility, immune dysfunction, alterations in fecal microbiota, small bowel overgrowth, food sensitivity, familial predisposition, and psychosocial factors.

IBS is classified as **constipation predominant, diarrhea predominant,** or **mixed.** In constipation-predominant IBS, patients have irregular luminal contractions and slow colonic transit. In diarrhea-predominant IBS, patients have accelerated transit time and abnormally strong colonic contractions. In both, bowel wall pain receptors are hypersensitive.

Underlying psychosocial stressors can alter intestinal motor function and contribute to worsened symptoms. For example, stress-related elevations in corticotropin-releasing hormone levels are associated with increased bowel permeability, which results in increased colonic motility and abdominal pain.

Recent research has also highlighted the role of an exaggerated inflammatory response in IBS. Studies have found that some patients have increased numbers of lymphocytes and mast cells in the small intestine and colon, as well as higher plasma levels of proinflammatory cytokines. Through uncertain mechanisms, these immune cells can release proteins that stimulate the enteric nervous system and thereby cause abnormal colonic motility and spasms.

RISK FACTORS

Risk factors for IBS include age <50 years, female sex, psychiatric disease, and prior abdominal surgery. Studies have shown familial aggregation and higher rates of disease among monozygotic twins compared to dizygotic twins; however, specific genetic or environmental risk factors have not yet been identified.

PRESENTATION, EVALUATION, AND DIAGNOSIS

There is no one sign, symptom, or test that is pathognomonic for IBS. Rather, it is important to consider the severity, duration, and overall constellation of symptoms, and to rule out other diseases with similar presentations, such as celiac sprue (Fig. 132.1) (see Chapter 133), inflammatory bowel disease (IBD) (see Chapter 134), microscopic colitis, pancreatic insufficiency, bile malabsorption, lactose intolerance, small bowel overgrowth, and chronic *Clostridioides* (formerly *Clostridium*) *difficile* infection (see Chapter 119).

The abdominal pain of IBS tends to be crampy and episodic, frequently triggered by food ingestion or emotional stress. Alteration of bowel habits, whether constipation or diarrhea, is also common. Patients with diarrhea have frequent, small-to-midsize bowel movements, often in the morning or after meals, that are preceded by crampy abdominal pain and urgency that improve with defecation. Patients with constipation have hard, pelletlike stools.

Other common symptoms include bloating and gas production, dyspepsia, reflux, and early satiety. It is important to inquire about alarm symptoms (e.g., weight loss, rectal bleeding, laboratory abnormalities such as elevated inflammatory markers, a family history of colon cancer or IBD) that could suggest an alternative diagnosis.

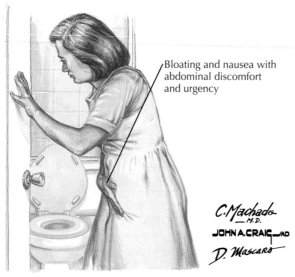

Bloating and nausea with abdominal discomfort and urgency

C. Machado
— M.D.

JOHN A. CRAIG —AD

D. Mascaro

Irritable bowel syndrome is a syndrome of intermittent abdominal pain, diarrhea, and constipation related to hypermotility of the gut. Clinical variants include:

1) Spastic colitis characterized by chronic abdominal pain and constipation
2) Intermittent diarrhea that is usually painless
3) Combination of both with alternating diarrhea and constipation

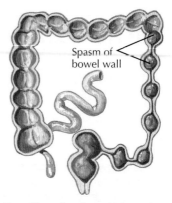

Spasm of bowel wall

Altered bowel wall sensitivity and motility result in IBS symptom complex

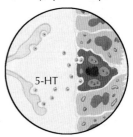

5-HT

Potential causes include abnormalities in serotonin (5HT) transmission, immune dysfunction, microbiota disturbances

Rome IV Criteria for Diagnosis	Symptoms suggestive of diagnoses beyond functional bowel disease

Recurrent abdominal pain for at least 1 day per week in the last 3 months associated with two or more of the following features:
  1) Improvement with defecation
  2) Change in stool frequency
  3) Change in stool consistency
	1) Anemia
	2) Fever
	3) Persistent diarrhea
	4) Rectal bleeding
	5) Severe constipation
	6) Weight loss
	7) Nocturnal GI symptoms
	8) Family history of GI cancer, inflammatory bowel disease, or celiac disease
	9) New onset of symptoms after age 50

FIG. 132.1   **Irritable Bowel Syndrome *(IBS).*** *GI,* Gastrointestinal.

Because there is no single diagnostic test, IBS is a clinical diagnosis that is established according to the Rome IV criteria. According to these criteria, patients have IBS if they experience abdominal pain for at least 1 day per week for 3 months along with at least two of the following: improvement with defecation, change in stool frequency, or change in stool consistency. Symptoms also must have started at least 6 months ago. Based on symptoms, the disease is further classified as constipation predominant (IBS-C), diarrhea predominant (IBS-D), or mixed.

Experts often state that IBS is not a diagnosis of exclusion; however, because its symptoms overlap with those of many other GI conditions, patients should follow age-appropriate colorectal cancer screening. A laboratory evaluation, including a complete metabolic profile, complete blood count, serum inflammatory markers (erythrocyte sedimentation rate or C-reactive protein), fecal calprotectin (an indicator of stool inflammation), and immunoglobulin A (IgA) antitissue transglutaminase antibodies, can help rule out other disorders.

Patients with IBS-D should undergo colonoscopy with random biopsies from each segment of the colon to evaluate for microscopic colitis. Patients with IBS-C and suspicion for a structural lesion (e.g., change in stool caliber) should also undergo colonoscopy.

TREATMENT

Patients with **mild to moderate disease** that does not interfere with overall quality of life should attempt dietary and lifestyle modifications to improve symptoms. A food diary can help identify certain foods most likely to trigger symptoms. Empiric dietary changes may also be helpful. A low-**FODMAP** diet is low in fermentable oligosaccharides, disaccharides, and monosaccharides as well as polyols. A more traditional IBS diet includes a regular meal pattern, avoidance of large meals, and low intake of fat, insoluble fibers, caffeine, and gas-producing foods (e.g., beans, cabbage, and onions). Studies have shown that both diets are equally effective in reducing symptom severity after 4 weeks. Patients with persistent symptoms can also lower their intake of lactose, gluten, and fiber. Finally, 20 to 60 minutes of vigorous physical activity 3 to 5 days per week can also improve symptoms.

For patients with **moderate to severe symptoms,** pharmacological therapy is used in addition to lifestyle interventions.

Patients with IBS-C may be treated with polyethylene glycol (PEG), lubiprostone, or guanylate cyclase agonists. PEG, a nonabsorbable osmotic laxative, is the least expensive and best tolerated. Lubiprostone is a locally acting chloride channel activator that increases intestinal fluid secretion. Guanylate cyclase agonists, such as linaclotide, stimulate intestinal fluid secretion and transit; however, their long-term effects are not yet known, and they are thus reserved for patients who have failed PEG. All of these agents can improve constipation, but lubiprostone and linaclotide are more effective for treating bloating and abdominal pain.

Patients with IBS-D can be treated with antidiarrheal agents, bile acid sequestrants, and serotonin-3 receptor antagonists. Loperamide is the only antidiarrheal agent evaluated in randomized trials of patients with IBS-D and was found to decrease stool frequency and consistency, though it did not improve bloating or abdominal discomfort. Eluxadoline, another antidiarrheal, combines a μ-opioid receptor agonist with a δ-opioid receptor antagonist; it had a greater effect than placebo on abdominal pain and stool consistency but can cause pancreatitis in patients with biliary disorders or alcohol use.

Patients who fail antidiarrheal agents may use bile acid sequestrants to increase colonic transit time, though side effects of bloating, flatulence, abdominal discomfort, and constipation are often limiting. A serotonin-3 receptor antagonist, alosetron, is approved for the treatment of severe IBS-D in women who have failed other agents; further studies have found a benefit in men as well. This medication decreases colonic motility and secretion by acting on GI visceral afferents. Its use is restricted, however, due to the risk of ischemic colitis. Finally, ondansetron has been shown to improve stool consistency, frequency, and urgency, though it does not relieve abdominal pain.

Patients with abdominal pain and bloating may experience relief with antispasmodics, such as dicyclomine, hyoscyamine, and peppermint oil. Antidepressants, such as tricyclic antidepressants, can also improve abdominal pain because of anticholinergic properties that slow intestinal transit time. Selective serotonin reuptake inhibitors (SSRIs) and serotonin-norepinephrine reuptake inhibitors (SNRIs) are sometimes given to patients with underlying depression, but there is no evidence they are helpful in patients without depression. Finally, a 2-week course of rifaximin was shown to decrease bloating and diarrhea with a decreasing but durable response over 10 weeks.

CHAPTER 133

Celiac Disease

SHIRLEY COHEN-MEKELBURG • STEPHANIE L. GOLD

INTRODUCTION

Celiac disease is a chronic, systemic autoimmune disorder triggered by the ingestion of dietary gluten, a protein found in wheat, barley, and rye. The global prevalence has been rising and is now ~1%, though even this figure is likely an underestimate because many individuals are undiagnosed.

The greatest burden of celiac disease is in the industrialized world, where wheat is heavily processed and constitutes a large portion of the diet. The highest prevalence is in Sweden and Finland. Although celiac disease was once considered a disease that caused diarrhea primarily in young, white children, it is now known to affect individuals of any age, gender, or ethnicity.

PATHOPHYSIOLOGY

Gluten, the environmental trigger of celiac disease, is a protein contained in many grains, including wheat, barley, and rye. Gluten contains a glycoprotein known as gliadin, which stimulates enterocytes to release a protein known as zonulin, which loosens tight junctions and permits gluten fragments to enter the lamina propria. Gluten then stimulates the release of interleukin-15, which attracts intraepithelial lymphocytes.

Tissue transglutaminase (TTG) crosslinks and deamidates gliadin, facilitating its binding to the human leukocyte antigen (HLA)–DQ receptor on antigen-presenting cells (APCs). The HLA-DQ receptor presents foreign antigens to T cells and is also central to the process of self-recognition and tolerance. Nearly all patients with celiac disease have the HLA-DQ2 or HLA-DQ8 haplotype. These haplotypes are also found in the normal population, however, and are therefore not sufficient to cause the disease.

Helper T cells recognize APC-bound gliadin and initiate a robust immune response, which damages enterocytes and stimulates production of anti-TTG antibodies. The resulting histological findings may vary from an isolated increase in intraepithelial lymphocytes to complete villous atrophy with associated epithelial apoptosis and crypt hyperplasia.

Small bowel inflammation and loss of villi limit the absorptive capacity of the small intestine, leading to malabsorption and nutrient deficiencies. Furthermore, untreated or refractory celiac disease significantly increases the risk of both non-Hodgkin lymphoma and small bowel adenocarcinoma through a mechanism that is largely unknown.

PRESENTATION, EVALUATION, AND DIAGNOSIS

The clinical presentation of celiac disease is variable and often nonspecific. Young children often present with diarrhea and failure to thrive. Older children are less likely to present with diarrhea, instead coming to medical attention because of short stature, difficulty gaining weight, anemia, or abdominal pain.

Adults can present with a wide range of manifestations (Fig. 133.1), including bloating, diarrhea, flatulence, borborygmi (hyperactive bowel sounds), foul smelling and greasy stools, weight loss, anemia, neuropathy, vitamin deficiencies, alopecia, osteopenic bone disease, and amenorrhea. The gastrointestinal symptoms of celiac disease reflect malabsorption in the diseased small bowel. The loss of nutrients—especially iron, folate, and vitamins such as B_{12}, A, D, E, and K—results in many of the other complications. Other rare manifestations include headache, ataxia, depression, dysthymia, anxiety, epilepsy, arthritis, and mild elevations in serum aminotransferase levels.

The dermatological manifestations of celiac disease include dermatitis herpetiformis, glossitis, cheilosis, and stomatitis. Dermatitis herpetiformis is a vesicular rash typically distributed over the extensor areas of the shins, elbows, knees, and buttocks. Cheilosis refers to inflammation of the corners of the mouth, which can cause red, fissured, or painful lesions. Glossitis is characterized by tongue inflammation, while stomatitis

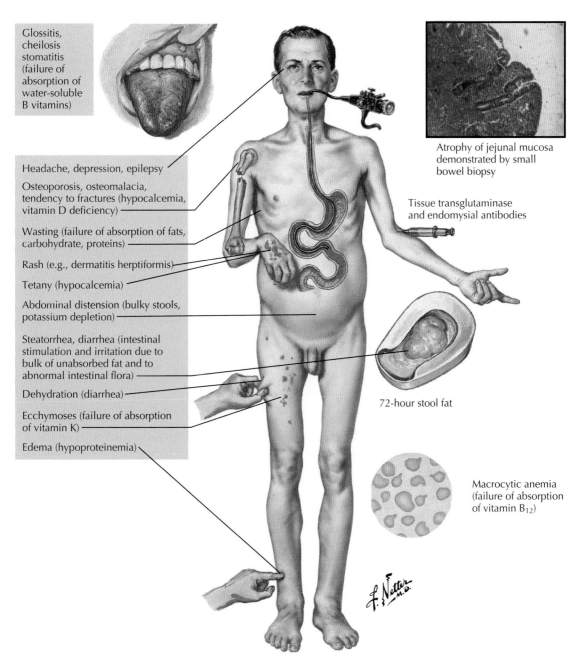

Glossitis, cheilosis stomatitis (failure of absorption of water-soluble B vitamins)

Atrophy of jejunal mucosa demonstrated by small bowel biopsy

Headache, depression, epilepsy

Osteoporosis, osteomalacia, tendency to fractures (hypocalcemia, vitamin D deficiency)

Wasting (failure of absorption of fats, carbohydrate, proteins)

Rash (e.g., dermatitis herptiformis)

Tetany (hypocalcemia)

Abdominal distension (bulky stools, potassium depletion)

Steatorrhea, diarrhea (intestinal stimulation and irritation due to bulk of unabsorbed fat and to abnormal intestinal flora)

Dehydration (diarrhea)

Ecchymoses (failure of absorption of vitamin K)

Edema (hypoproteinemia)

Tissue transglutaminase and endomysial antibodies

72-hour stool fat

Macrocytic anemia (failure of absorption of vitamin B_{12})

FIG. 133.1 **Celiac Disease.**

refers to inflammation and ulceration of the mucous membranes in the oropharynx.

Evaluation and Diagnosis

The current guidelines recommend testing for celiac disease in patients with symptoms suggestive of malabsorption, including chronic diarrhea, unexplained weight loss, or steatorrhea. Patients with affected first-degree family members should also be tested, even if asymptomatic. Finally, patients with dyspepsia who fail first-line therapy and require upper endoscopy should have mucosal biopsies of the duodenum to rule out celiac disease.

Testing for serum immunoglobulin A (IgA) anti-TTG antibodies is the preferred screening method in patients >2 years of age, with a sensitivity of 94% and specificity of 97%. In individuals with IgA deficiency, serum IgG anti-TTG antibodies and serum IgG antibodies targeting deamidated gliadin peptides can be measured instead. In patients with borderline positive IgA or IgG anti-TTG antibodies and an uncertain diagnosis, **IgA antiendomysial antibodies** can be checked, since elevated levels are very specific to celiac disease.

Once gluten is removed from the diet, the sensitivity of serological testing drops significantly. Therefore all serological testing should be done while on a gluten-rich diet. If serological tests are positive, duodenal biopsies are performed to confirm the diagnosis. The histological findings consistent with celiac disease include partial to total villous atrophy, increased number of intraepithelial lymphocytes, and crypt hyperplasia. In inconclusive cases, double immunofluorescence can identify subepithelial anti-TTG antibodies in the lamina propria.

Testing for HLA-DQ2 and HLA-DQ8 is not recommended as part of the initial workup, since the healthy population also expresses these haplotypes; however, in specific populations (such as those with equivocal histological findings or a diet already free of gluten) HLA testing can be helpful to rule out celiac disease, given its high negative predictive value.

Wheat Allergies and Gluten Sensitivities

It is not always straightforward to differentiate celiac disease from gluten sensitivity or wheat allergy; however, because only celiac disease carries a long-term risk of malignancy, the distinction is crucial. The presence of the autoantibodies described earlier and histological findings of villous blunting are unique to celiac disease. In patients without these findings, the timing of symptoms can help distinguish between allergy and sensitivity. Patients with wheat allergies often experience symptoms within minutes to hours of wheat ingestion, while those with gluten sensitivities develop symptoms after hours to days. Wheat allergies can also be confirmed with skin testing.

TREATMENT

The only currently approved treatment for celiac disease is a strict **gluten-free diet.** Patients generally report symptom improvement within 4 weeks, and mucosal healing and elimination of antibodies is generally seen within 6 to 24 months. Adherence to a gluten-free diet, however, is expensive, challenging, and can be socially isolating.

To date, two investigational drugs (larazotide and ALV003) have been evaluated for the treatment of celiac disease. These drugs increase the strength of the tight junctions between enterocytes, potentially decreasing the movement of gluten into the lamina propria.

When patients experience persistent symptoms despite a reportedly gluten-free diet, the usual cause is noncompliance or inadvertent exposure to gluten. In other cases, symptoms may be secondary to concomitant irritable bowel syndrome, lactose intolerance, small bowel bacterial overgrowth, pancreatic insufficiency, or microscopic colitis (see Chapter 13 for details). About 0.1% to 1% of patients, however, have true refractory celiac disease despite perfect adherence to a gluten-free diet for at least 1 year. The treatment of refractory celiac disease involves corticosteroids and, in some cases, steroid-sparing agents such as thiopurines or cyclosporine.

CHAPTER 134

Inflammatory Bowel Disease

SHIRLEY COHEN-MEKELBURG • STEPHANIE L. GOLD

INTRODUCTION

Inflammatory bowel disease (IBD) encompasses both **ulcerative colitis** (UC) and **Crohn disease** (CD). UC is defined by mucosal inflammation in a continuous distribution that is limited to the colon (Fig. 134.1). Depending on the extent, UC is described as proctitis, proctosigmoiditis, left-sided colitis, extensive colitis, or pancolitis. CD, in contrast, is defined by transmural inflammation in a patchy distribution that can occur in any part of the gastrointestinal (GI) tract. CD is further characterized by disease behavior as nonpenetrating/nonstricturing, stricturing, or fistulizing, and furthermore as having or not having perianal involvement. One in 20 patients with IBD have an overlap presentation, known as indeterminate colitis. The North American prevalence of UC is 249 per 100,000, while that of CD is 319 per 100,000.

PATHOPHYSIOLOGY

The pathogenesis of IBD is complex and thought to result from an inappropriate cellular immune response to luminal bacteria. Multiple genetic mutations have been associated with increased risk; for example, a mutation in *NOD2*, which encodes a protein that acts as an intracellular sensor of bacterial components, is responsible for an estimated one-third of CD cases. An imbalance between T-helper and regulatory cells, along with excessive and persistent CD4 T-helper cell type 1 activity, also contribute to disease development. Lastly, commensal bacteria in the intestinal lumen are thought to prime the immune system and cause exaggerated inflammatory responses directed at other resident dysbiotic luminal bacteria.

RISK FACTORS

The peak incidence of both UC and CD is in the second and third decades of life, with a smaller peak from age 50 to 70 years. IBD primarily affects Caucasians, with the next highest incidence among African Americans, and the lowest incidence among Asians and Hispanics. IBD is more common in industrialized nations.

PRESENTATION

The overlapping and often variable presentations of UC and CD can lead to delays and challenges in diagnosis. Both feature **chronic diarrhea,** abdominal pain, hematochezia, fever, and weight loss. UC typically presents more acutely, with bloody diarrhea. CD can be more indolent and usually presents with abdominal pain as the predominant symptom, sometimes with nonbloody diarrhea. The presence of nocturnal diarrhea is consistent with bowel inflammation since in noninflammatory conditions (e.g., irritable bowel syndrome), diarrhea abates during periods of fasting.

Patients with CD can also present with nausea and vomiting, a draining perianal **fistula,** or rectal pain secondary to a perianal abscess. Extraintestinal manifestations (Fig. 134.2) include primary sclerosing cholangitis, uveitis, episcleritis, oral aphthous ulcers, pyoderma gangrenosum, erythema nodosum, and arthritis. These are more common in CD than UC, with the exceptions of primary sclerosing cholangitis and pyoderma gangrenosum, which are more common in UC. UC and CD can both cause anemia (from decreased iron absorption and chronic blood loss), while in CD, fat malabsorption can lead to nephrolithiasis (from increased oxalate absorption), cholelithiasis (from bile salt malabsorption), or metabolic bone disease (from decreased vitamin D absorption). Lastly, long-standing UC or Crohn colitis can lead to colorectal dysplasia and adenocarcinoma.

Physical examination may reveal cachexia, pallor, abdominal tenderness, or an abdominal mass. In the case of CD, rectal examination may reveal a perianal skin tag, abscess, fissure, or fistula. Serum inflammatory markers, such as erythrocyte sedimentation rate (ESR) or C-reactive protein (CRP), may be elevated; a more specific marker of intestinal inflammation is **fecal calprotectin,** which has recently become commercially available. Stool

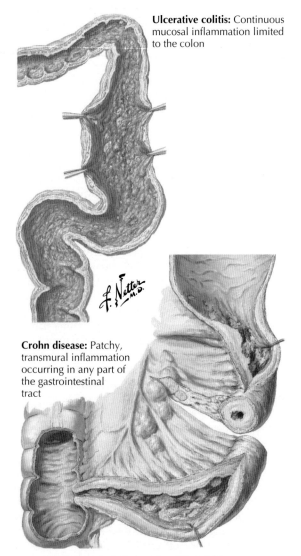

Ulcerative colitis: Continuous mucosal inflammation limited to the colon

Crohn disease: Patchy, transmural inflammation occurring in any part of the gastrointestinal tract

FIG. 134.1 **Inflammatory Bowel Disease.**

should be sent for *Clostridioides* (formerly *Clostridium*) *difficile* toxin testing, ova and parasites screening, and culture to rule out infection.

The diagnosis of IBD relies on findings from the history and physical exam as well as radiographic, endoscopic, and histological examinations of the GI tract. A CT scan (Fig. 134.3) may help define the extent of active inflammation and evaluate for **strictures,** fistulas, and abscesses. If the diagnosis of IBD seems plausible, the patient should undergo colonoscopy with tissue sampling. An upper endoscopy should be performed if there is a concern for upper GI involvement. UC features continuous inflammation starting at the rectum and

extending proximally throughout (but not beyond) the colon. CD is associated with rectal sparing, skip lesions (patchy inflammation separated by normal mucosa), and cobblestoning (nodular appearing mucosa from submucosal edema and crossing linear ulcerations).

In both UC and CD, biopsies will reveal chronic inflammation, with cryptitis, crypt distortion, and crypt abscesses, though in CD alone inflammation may be transmural. The presence of **noncaseating granulomas** is pathognomonic for CD.

Serological markers have low sensitivity and specificity, but they can be helpful when the diagnosis is indeterminate and distinguishing UC from CD would change management (e.g., consideration of a curative total proctocolectomy for UC). Anti-*Saccharomyces cerevisiae* antibody (ASCA) is associated with CD, while antiperinuclear-antineutrophil cytoplasmic antibody (p-ANCA) is associated with UC.

TREATMENT

The treatment for IBD is divided into induction and maintenance strategies, with the choice of agent dependent on the extent and severity of disease. IBD can be classified as mild, moderate, or severe using various indices. The Mayo score for UC classifies disease severity based on stool frequency, rectal bleeding, global assessment, and endoscopic findings. The Harvey-Bradshaw Index for CD considers general well-being, abdominal pain, stool frequency, presence of a palpable mass, and complications (fistulas, extraintestinal manifestations).

In mild-moderate UC, oral aminosalicylates (also known as 5-aminosalicylic acid [5ASA] agents), such as sulfasalazine or mesalamine, have historically been used for both induction and maintenance of remission. Newer 5ASA agents (e.g., Apriso, Lialda, and Asacol) are formulated to release their active drug in certain parts of the GI tract, sometimes through a pH-dependent mechanism. In mild-moderate CD, 5ASAs are ineffective.

For mild-moderate UC and CD, oral budesonide (a corticosteroid formulation with controlled release in the distal ileum and right colon) is more effective than 5ASAs for induction. Antibiotics, such as metronidazole and ciprofloxacin, can also reduce inflammation but there is less evidence to support their use, and long-term tolerance is difficult.

For moderate-to-severe UC and CD, conventional corticosteroids can effectively control inflammation, but their long-term adverse effects limit their use to the induction phase. **Immunomodulators,** including the thiopurines (6-mercaptopurine and azathioprine) and parenteral methotrexate, can be used for maintenance

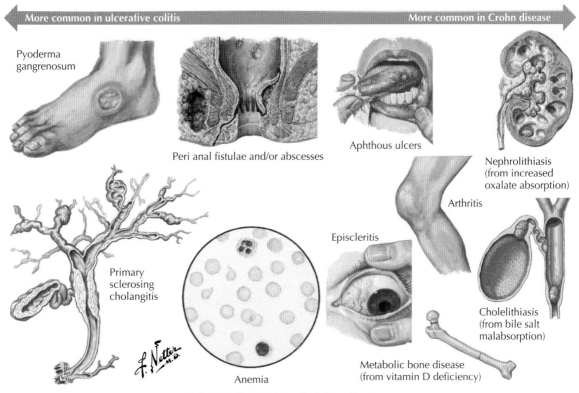

FIG. 134.2 **Extraintestinal Complications.**

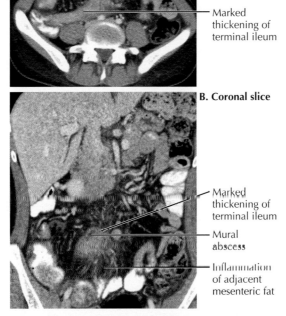

FIG. 134.3 **Radiographic Findings: Crohn Disease.**

of remission and are often preferred for moderate disease.

Thiopurine methyltransferase (TPMT) is an enzyme involved in thiopurine metabolism; as some patients have complete or partial deficiency, activity levels should be checked to guide dosage. In addition, allopurinol can be carefully used to shift thiopurine metabolism from toxic metabolites to therapeutic metabolites in patients with a relative excess of the former.

Cyclosporine can be used as rescue induction therapy in patients with UC who do not respond to corticosteroids; however, patients should be carefully selected, given the potential adverse effects and need for close monitoring of drug levels. For moderate-to-severe UC and CD, the preferred treatment is **biological agents,** which include antitumor necrosis factor (anti-TNF) antibodies and antiintegrins. The anti-TNF antibodies include infliximab (a chimeric monoclonal antibody), adalimumab and golimumab (humanized monoclonal antibodies), and certolizumab (a pegylated monoclonal antibody). These can be combined with immunomodulators for even greater efficacy. Side effects include infusion reactions, infection (including reactivation), and lymphoma. Patients should be tested for tuberculosis and hepatitis B virus infection before initiating treatment.

The antiintegrins, a newer class of biologics, include natalizumab and vedolizumab. Natalizumab, a nonselective α4 antiintegrin, is no longer used owing to the risk of **progressive multifocal leukoencephalopathy** associated with John Cunningham (JC) virus reactivation. Vedolizumab, a safer, gut-selective α4β7 antiintegrin, has shown promise as both first-line and salvage therapy, though with greater efficacy in UC than in CD. Ustekinumab, a fully humanized monoclonal antiinterleukin-12/23 (anti–IL-12/23) antibody, was approved for use in CD in 2016 and for UC in 2019. In 2018, tofacitinib, an oral Janus-kinase inhibitor, was approved for the treatment of UC.

Many patients with IBD require surgery. In UC, surgery can be curative. In CD, postsurgical recurrences can occur; however, small randomized controlled trials have shown efficacy of infliximab and adalimumab in preventing CD recurrence after surgical resection.

CHAPTER 135

Acute Liver Failure

DAVID B. SNELL • RUSSELL ROSENBLATT

INTRODUCTION

Acute liver failure (ALF) is a rare but highly lethal condition in which patients without preexisting liver disease experience a rapid deterioration of liver function. There are ~2000 cases of ALF each year in the United States, and survival in the absence of liver transplant can be as low as 15%, depending on the cause.

ALF is defined as any elevation in aminotransferases (aspartate aminotransferase [AST]/ alanine aminotransferase [ALT]), an international normalized ratio (INR) ≥1.5, and any degree of encephalopathy in a patient without preexisting liver disease occurring within the span of <26 weeks. ALF can be further categorized based on the time from jaundice to encephalopathy as fulminant—consisting of hyperacute (<1 week) and acute (1–3 weeks)—or subfulminant/subacute (3–26 weeks).

All health care providers should have a high index of suspicion for the diagnosis of ALF, since the condition can progress rapidly to coma and death. Patients with ALF should be transferred to an intensive care unit (ICU) and referred to a liver transplant center.

PATHOPHYSIOLOGY AND RISK FACTORS

The most common cause of ALF in the United States is drug-induced liver injury (60%), with **acetaminophen** (APAP) overdose (>4 g) accounting for nearly half of all cases. Normally, 90% of APAP is metabolized in the liver to sulfate and glucuronide conjugates, which are excreted in the urine, while the remainder is metabolized by the cytochrome P450 (CYP2E1, CYP1A2, CYP3A4) pathway into a toxic intermediate, NAPQI. In normal circumstances, NAPQI is conjugated with hepatic glutathione and safely excreted in urine. With toxic APAP overdoses, however, the sulfation and glucuronidation pathways become saturated and NAPQI accumulates. Once glutathione stores are depleted, NAPQI causes hepatic injury. Factors that predispose patients to APAP toxicity include chronic alcohol ingestion (induces CYP2E1), tobacco use (induces CYP1A2), malnutrition (resulting in decreased glucuronidation and increased NAPQI production), and older age (associated with decreased glutathione stores).

Several other medications can also cause idiosyncratic drug reactions and ALF, including aspirin, NSAIDs, statins, certain antibiotics and antifungal drugs, antiepileptics, and antiretrovirals. Herbal supplements that can cause ALF include comfrey, greater celandine, he shou wu, Herbalife, Hydroxycut, LipoKinetix, kava, and ma huang. Other important causes include acute hepatitis A virus (HAV), acute hepatitis B virus (HBV), and autoimmune hepatitis. Less common causes include toxins such as Amanita mushrooms, other viral infections (acute hepatitis E, herpes simplex virus [HSV], varicella zoster virus [VZV]), Wilson disease, ischemic hepatopathy, Budd-Chiari syndrome (hepatic vein thrombosis), malignant infiltration, venoocclusive disease, illicit drugs (i.e., cocaine, methamphetamine), and acute fatty liver of pregnancy/HELLP syndrome. In ~15% of cases, no clear etiology is identified.

Cerebral edema and **intracranial hypertension** are the most serious complications of ALF and manifest as variable degrees of encephalopathy. The pathogenic mechanisms are not completely understood but thought to include loss of cerebrovascular autoregulation, osmotic imbalances, inflammation, and/or infection.

PRESENTATION, EVALUATION, AND DIAGNOSIS

The initial symptoms of ALF include jaundice, confusion, lethargy, fatigue, anorexia, nausea, vomiting, right upper quadrant abdominal pain, pruritus, and abdominal distention. **Hepatic encephalopathy** (Fig. 135.1) follows a grading system from I to IV (Table 135.1); cerebral edema becomes more common and severe at higher grades of hepatic encephalopathy.

Patients presenting with possible ALF should undergo a thorough evaluation to clarify the underlying etiology, since it is the most important prognostic indicator. It is crucial to identify any recent exposures to medications,

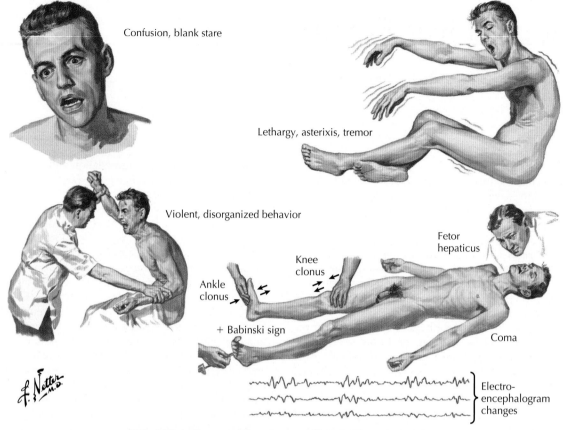

Confusion, blank stare

Lethargy, asterixis, tremor

Violent, disorganized behavior

Fetor hepaticus

Knee clonus

Ankle clonus

+ Babinski sign

Coma

Electro-encephalogram changes

FIG. 135.1 **Signs and Symptoms of Hepatic Encephalopathy.**

TABLE 135.1
West Haven Criteria for Hepatic Encephalopathy

Grade	Definition
I	Mild unawareness, euphoria, anxiety, shortened attention span, impairment of calculation ability
II	Lethargy or apathy, disorientation to time, obvious personality change, inappropriate behavior, asterixis
III	Somnolence to stupor, responsiveness to stimuli, confusion, gross disorientation, bizarre behavior
IV	Comatose

Modified from Vilstrup H, Amodio P, Bajaj J, et al: Hepatic encephalopathy in chronic liver disease: 2014 Practice Guideline by the American Association for the Study of Liver Diseases and the European Association for the Study of the Liver, *Hepatology* 60(2):715–735, 2014.

herbal supplements, or toxins (as described earlier). Patients should also be queried about the timing of symptoms, the presence of personal or family history of liver disease, or other comorbidities (e.g., substance abuse, depression) that could affect transplant candidacy.

The patient's transplant candidacy should be assessed as early as possible, according to institutional protocols.

The physical examination is usually nonspecific. Patients should be assessed for encephalopathy, which manifests as irritability, reversal of sleep-wake cycle, asterixis, and confusion. The typical stigmata of chronic liver disease (i.e., ascites, caput medusae, and spider angiomata) are usually not present given the acuity of liver dysfunction.

The laboratory evaluation should include a complete metabolic panel, coagulation studies, complete blood count, APAP level, drug toxicology screen, viral hepatitis serologies and polymerase chain reaction (PCR), serum pregnancy test when appropriate, and autoimmune markers (antinuclear antibodies, anti–smooth muscle antibodies, immunoglobulin G (IgG) levels, anti–liver-kidney antibodies). An arterial blood gas and ammonia level should be measured; an arterial pH ≤7.3 indicates a poor prognosis, and an ammonia concentration >150 μmol/L indicates increased risk of herniation. Additional testing may include ceruloplasmin and urine copper for those age <40 years or with findings suggestive of Wilson disease, HSV serologies and PCR for those with suspected HSV, hepatitis E antibodies for pregnant women and those who have traveled to endemic areas, and urinalysis (in pregnant women) to assess for proteinuria consistent with preeclampsia/HELLP syndrome.

Abdominal Doppler ultrasonography should be performed to evaluate for Budd-Chiari syndrome, portal hypertension, hepatic congestion, malignant infiltration, and underlying cirrhosis. A head CT without intravenous (IV) contrast can be obtained to exclude alternative causes for altered mental status. An echocardiogram is essential for transplant evaluation.

Certain presentations are classic for specific diseases. For example, vesicular skin lesions can be seen in HSV, while tender hepatomegaly and significant ascites are typical in Budd-Chiari syndrome. Wilson disease features hemolytic anemia, low alkaline phosphatase, and Kayser-Fleischer rings. APAP overdose usually causes marked transaminase elevations (in the thousands), very elevated INR, and renal failure with relatively mild bilirubin elevation.

Rarely, a liver biopsy can be performed to help determine the underlying etiology and predict mortality (i.e., when >50% hepatic necrosis is seen). Biopsy should not be done routinely, however, as the results typically do not change management, the bleeding risk is often significant, and the results do not offer additional prognostic value beyond clinical scoring systems.

TREATMENT

Patients with suspected ALF should be monitored in an ICU and transferred to a liver transplant center as soon as feasible. Although all patients require supportive care, the specific treatment varies according to the suspected etiology.

Patients with suspected APAP overdose should receive activated charcoal within 4 hours of ingestion time, if known, and a prompt infusion of N-acetylcysteine (NAC), an APAP antidote. NAC restores hepatic glutathione by acting as a glutathione substitute. It appears to also be beneficial for drug-induced ALF even when not secondary to APAP if given before the onset of severe encephalopathy.

Patients with viral hepatitis should receive antiviral agents when appropriate: either tenofovir or entecavir for HBV, and acyclovir for HSV or VZV. Patients with autoimmune hepatitis may receive a trial of corticosteroids if there is severe liver injury and the MELD score is under 28. Patients with acute fatty liver of pregnancy or HELLP syndrome should undergo prompt delivery, which sometimes leads to improvement of liver dysfunction. If Budd-Chiari syndrome is identified, the patient must be evaluated for thrombolysis, transjugular intrahepatic portosystemic shunt, and malignancy before potential liver transplantation.

The major causes of death in ALF are infection and cerebral herniation due to edema. Thus blood cultures should be obtained and broad-spectrum antibiotics initiated if there is any evidence of infection. Patients may require serial neurological exams and/or intracranial monitoring devices to monitor for development of cerebral edema and intracranial hypertension. Lactulose generally does not improve the encephalopathy of ALF, as it does in more chronic liver disease, since it does not reduce cerebral edema. Instead, hypertonic saline and mannitol can be administered to reduce the risk of herniation. Hypertonic saline is recommended prophylactically in those at high risk for developing cerebral edema. IV mannitol and/or hyperventilation can provide transient improvement of nonsevere intracranial hypertension.

Spontaneous bleeding is relatively rare, and blood products should only be administered in response to active bleeding or before invasive procedures. Prophylaxis against gastrointestinal bleeding with proton-pump inhibitors or H2 receptor antagonists is strongly recommended.

In many cases, the only definitive therapy is orthotopic liver transplantation (OLT). The King's College criteria is a scoring system to predict prognosis in both APAP and non-APAP–induced ALF. A high score indicates a more urgent need for OLT. The most important parameters include arterial lactate >3 mmol/L, arterial pH <7.3, presence of grade 3/4 encephalopathy, and markedly elevated INR and Cr. Patients with ALF receive priority on the transplant list, as transplantation increases the survival rate to nearly 80% at 1 year.

Experimental alternatives to OLT, such as artificial hepatic assist devices and auxiliary liver transplantation, have not yet demonstrated any benefit. Artificial hepatic assist devices support some of the major functions of the failing liver, just as hemodialysis does for the kidneys. In auxiliary liver transplant, a smaller or partial liver graft is implanted next to the patient's native liver with the hope that it will bridge the native liver to recovery.

CHAPTER 136

Viral Hepatitis

NICOLE T. SHEN

HEPATITIS A

Hepatitis A virus (HAV) is a nonenveloped ribonucleic acid (RNA) picornavirus that causes acute liver disease. HAV is highly endemic in Asia and Africa, where infection typically occurs in childhood, and intermediately endemic in Central and South America and Eastern Europe, where it is more likely to occur in adulthood. The mortality of HAV infection is 0.3% overall, with a higher rate (1.8%) among adults.

Transmission occurs through direct person-to-person contact, with an incubation period of about 28 days (range, 15–50 days). Infected individuals shed the virus in their feces and can contaminate frozen or inadequately cooked foods, drinks, and ice. Patients are most infectious in the 1 to 2 weeks preceding the onset of symptoms, when the viral load is highest and antibodies are lowest. As antibody levels increase and viral clearance occurs, patients become more symptomatic and less infectious. An exception is children and infants, who can remain contagious for up to 6 months.

The clinical presentation depends on age. Most infants and young children remain asymptomatic. In contrast, adults usually become jaundiced. Symptoms can last for up to 2 months. A minority (10%–15%) have a relapsing, remitting course lasting 6 to 9 months. Chronic infection has not been reported. Fulminant hepatitis and liver failure occur very rarely in older adults and in those with other chronic liver diseases.

The diagnosis is established by measuring HAV antibodies (anti-HAV). Both infected and immunized patients are anti-HAV positive, but only those with acute infection have anti-HAV immunoglobulin M (IgM) antibodies. A positive viral load, which may be checked in cases of fulminant hepatitis and liver failure, also indicates active infection. The treatment is supportive, usually consisting of hydration and symptom management. Travelers to endemic countries can receive a vaccination to prevent infection.

HEPATITIS B

Hepatitis B virus (HBV), a deoxyribonucleic acid (DNA) virus, causes both acute and chronic liver disease. Chronic disease, defined as the presence of hepatitis B surface antigen (HBsAg) in the blood for >6 months, affects nearly 250 million people worldwide. Chronic disease can be either active or inactive, as described later. Childhood infection often results in chronic disease, whereas adult infection usually does not (Fig. 136.1). Patients with active chronic disease are at risk of developing cirrhosis and **hepatocellular carcinoma (HCC)** (see Chapter 162 for details).

Though temporal trends suggest a decrease in the overall global burden, the prevalence remains high in sub-Saharan Africa (8.3%) and the Western Pacific region (5.26%). Areas with intermediate endemicity (prevalence 2%–5%) include Eastern Europe, Middle East, India, and parts of South America. Areas with low endemicity (<2%) include North America and Western Europe.

In highly endemic countries, most infections result from perinatal (mother-to-child) and horizontal (exposure to infected blood) transmission during childhood. In less endemic countries, infection usually results from sexual contact or the reuse of objects with contaminated blood (e.g., needles, razors).

The majority of HBV infections do not cause acute symptoms. A minority of patients experience fatigue, malaise, fevers, chills, nausea, vomiting, poor appetite, abdominal pain, dark urine, joint pain, and/or jaundice, typically about 90 days after infection. In rare cases, acute HBV infection results in fulminant hepatitis. The symptoms usually last for a few weeks but may persist for up to 6 months. About half of patients are no longer infectious 7 weeks after the onset of symptoms, owing to low HBV DNA viral levels and the formation of hepatitis B surface antibodies (HBsAb).

Both acute and chronic infections are diagnosed based on serological testing (Fig. 136.2). Acute infections are associated with elevated levels of HBsAg (within 4 weeks of exposure), hepatitis B core IgM antibodies (IgM HBcAb), and hepatitis B early antigen (HBeAg). Chronic infections are associated with elevated HBsAg and IgG HBcAb, with no detectable levels of HBsAb. Finally, immunity is indicated by the presence of HBsAb; patients with cleared infection also have HBcAb, while those with prior vaccination do not.

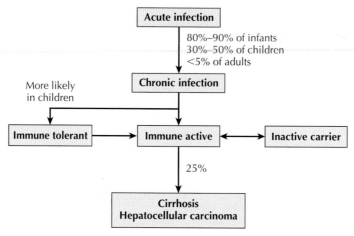

FIG. 136.1 **Hepatitis B Infection: Phases and Progression.**

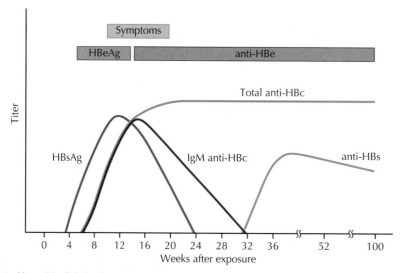

FIG. 136.2 **Hepatitis B Infection: Typical Time Course of Serological Tests.** *HBeAg,* Hepatitis B early antigen; *HBsAg,* hepatitis B surface antigen; *HBc,* hepatitis B core; *IgM,* immunoglobulin M.

Chronically infected patients can be further characterized as **immune tolerant, immune active, or inactive carriers** (Table 136.1)

All patients with chronic HBV and significant fibrosis should receive treatment. Patients with chronic HBV who lack significant fibrosis should be treated if they are immune active, and they should be carefully monitored with consideration of treatment if they are immune tolerant. Inactive carriers without significant fibrosis are not treated. The standard treatment is tenofovir or entecavir, both antiviral agents. Lamivudine and interferon-α2b are no longer in wide use, owing

to increased resistance and poor patient tolerance, respectively.

Patients with chronic HBV in specific demographic groups (Asian males age >40 years, Asian females age >50 years, or African males or females age >20 years) should undergo biannual screening for HCC, which can develop even in the absence of cirrhosis.

Vaccination prevents infection in 95% of exposures and should begin within 24 hours of birth. HBV infection rates have significantly declined in high-income and middle-income countries with effective vaccination policies.

TABLE 136.1
Phases of Chronic Hepatitis B Infection

	HBeAg	HBV Viral Load	Aminotransferases	Biopsy Findings
Immune Tolerant	Positive	>20,000 IU/mL	Normal	Minimal to no inflammation or fibrosis
Immune Active	Positive or negative	>2000 IU/mL	Elevated ALT (>20 IU/L for women or >30 IU/L for men)	Inflammation and/or fibrosis
Inactive Carrier	Negative	<2000 IU/mL	Normal	Minimal to no inflammation or fibrosis

ALT, Alanine aminotransferase; *HBeAg,* hepatitis B early antigen; *HBV,* hepatitis B virus.
Modified from Terrault NA, Bzowej NH, Chang KM, et al: AASLD guidelines for treatment of chronic hepatitis B, *Hepatology* 63(1)261–283, 2016.

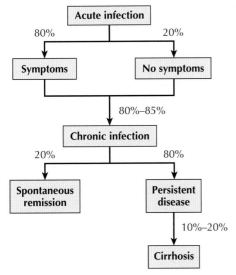

FIG. 136.3 Hepatitis C Infection: Phases and Progression.

HEPATITIS C

Hepatitis C virus (HCV) is a small, single-stranded RNA virus from the Flaviviridae family. HCV is divided into six main genotypes, each with different subtypes. Genotype 1 is the most common genotype in the United States. The highest infection rates are reported in Egypt, where the prevalence is ~10%. In Africa, the Middle East, and Eastern Europe the prevalence is 2% to 10%. In the United States and Western Europe, the prevalence is <2%.

HCV can cause acute or chronic hepatitis, with ~80% to 85% of patients developing chronic hepatitis (Fig. 136.3). About 10% to 20% of chronic HCV cases eventually progress to end-stage liver disease.

The transmission of HCV is primarily from expo-sure to contaminated blood, though HCV can also be transmitted through mucosal injuries (e.g., from sharing toothbrushes). Individuals at increased risk for infection include intravenous (IV) drug users, health care workers, transfusion recipients in areas that do not adequately screen blood products, and men who have sex with men. Tattooing and acupuncture are also associated with increased risk.

After infection, the average incubation period is 6 to 7 weeks. Of newly infected patients, 80% are asymp-tomatic. The remainder experience nonspecific symptoms (e.g., malaise, fevers, nausea, vomiting, abdominal pain) and/or jaundice. In addition to hepatic disease, HCV can also have extrahepatic manifestations, includ-ing renal (membranoproliferative glomerulonephritis, membranous nephropathy), hematological (lymphoma), dermatological (porphyria cutanea tarda), and rheuma-tological (mixed cryoglobulinemia) manifestations.

HCV is diagnosed by antibody testing and HCV RNA quantification. Current guidelines recommend that all individuals born between 1945 and 1965 have a screening antibody test. If the test is positive, HCV RNA polymerase chain reaction (PCR) is performed. A positive HCV antibody test with undetectable HCV RNA implies previously cleared infection, passively acquired antibodies through blood transfusions or vertical transmission, or viral load below the detectable limit. A positive HCV RNA PCR indicates active infection and should prompt genotype testing.

About one in five infected patients achieves sponta-neous clearance. Those with persistently elevated HCV RNA levels for 3 months should receive treatment with the goal of sustained viral response (SVR), defined as an undetectable HCV RNA for at least 12 weeks after therapy.

Previously, HCV treatments included peginterferon-α and ribavirin for 24 weeks. Response rates were dismal (only 45% for genotype 1 and 70%–80% for genotypes 2 and 3), with significant adverse effects and multiple contraindications. The newer **direct-acting antivirals** (DAAs) have fewer side effects and significantly improved SVR rate (>95%) for all genotypes. DAAs include protein inhibitors, protease inhibitors, and polymerase inhibitors, which inhibit the enzymes needed for viral replication. Multiple combinations of DAAs have been approved for every genotype, and most involve a combination of a polymerase inhibitor plus a protein or protease inhibitor. One example is the combination of ledipasvir (HCV protein inhibitor) and sofosbuvir (polymerase inhibitor), which has cure rates of 97% in treatment-naïve genotype 1a patients. The treatment duration is 8 to 12 weeks in noncirrhotic patients and 12 weeks in cirrhotic patients.

HEPATITIS D

Hepatitis D virus (HDV) is a defective RNA virus dependent on HBV coinfection for virion assembly and secretion. Thus all individuals with HDV infection have concurrent HBV infection. HDV is rare in developed countries, where it is mainly associated with IV drug use. Infection rates are highest in the Middle East, Africa, and southern Italy. About 5% of patients with chronic HBV infection have concurrent HDV infection and should be screened appropriately.

The transmission of HDV is similar to that of HBV and can occur simultaneously (coinfection) or in the setting of existing HBV infection (superinfection). The consequences of infection can range from fulminant liver failure to an asymptomatic carrier state. The symptoms of acute infection are similar to those seen with HBV infection. In chronic infection, HDV exacerbates the liver damage caused by HBV and can hasten progression to cirrhosis.

The diagnosis is established in acute infection by measuring HDV antigen (HDVAg), which is most readily detectable within 2 weeks of infection. HDV antibodies (anti-HDV) are detectable in patients presenting later. Patients with coinfection are more likely to clear HDV than those with superinfection. The treatment should focus on controlling HBV replication. There is no effective vaccine against HDV, but vaccination against HBV can prevent HDV transmission.

HEPATITIS E

Hepatitis E virus (HEV) is a single-stranded RNA virus that causes acute hepatitis. HEV infection is most common in low-income areas, with the highest incidence in the Middle East, Asia, Central America, and Africa. HEV is transmitted through fecal contamination of water and food, or blood transfusions in areas with poor screening. The incubation period ranges from 15 to 60 days. HEV infection is usually self-limited but in rare cases can progress to fulminant liver failure. For unclear reasons the mortality is highest in pregnant woman (usually in the third trimester), in whom infection is more likely to progress to fulminant liver failure. The diagnosis is established using PCR-based detection of virus in the stool or serum. IgM anti-HEV antibodies can be checked, but false positives and negatives are common. A vaccine against HEV has been used in China but is not currently available elsewhere.

CHAPTER 137

Nonalcoholic Fatty Liver Disease (NAFLD)

AMIT MEHTA • RUSSELL ROSENBLATT

INTRODUCTION

Nonalcoholic fatty liver disease (NAFLD) represents a spectrum of conditions that ranges from simple steatosis to more advanced liver injury. The diagnosis of NAFLD requires both evidence of abnormal retention of lipids within hepatic cells (i.e. hepatic steatosis), either by imaging or histology, and the exclusion of other secondary causes of hepatic fat accumulation, such as excessive alcohol consumption, steatogenic medications (i.e., amiodarone, methotrexate, corticosteroids, and tamoxifen), or hereditary disorders.

NAFLD can be further subcategorized based on histological features into **nonalcoholic fatty liver (NAFL)** or **nonalcoholic steatohepatitis (NASH)**. NAFL is defined as the presence of hepatic steatosis with no evidence of hepatocellular injury (i.e., ballooning of hepatocytes). NASH is defined as the presence of hepatic steatosis along with hepatocellular injury, which can progress over time to cirrhosis.

NAFLD is currently the most common cause of liver disease in the United States. The prevalence of NAFLD in the general population of industrialized countries ranges from 20% to 51%, with most estimates around 33%. NASH occurs in ~10% of patients with NAFLD, or about 3% to 5% of the population overall.

PATHOPHYSIOLOGY

The mechanisms underlying the development of NAFLD and NASH are not well understood but involve multiple factors.

The traditional understanding of NAFLD was based on a two-hit hypothesis. The initial event, or first hit, was hepatic fat accumulation or steatosis, which occurs due to triglyceride deposition in the liver from either increased import or decreased export of free fatty acids, with insulin resistance playing a key role. This steatosis then increases the susceptibility of the liver to injury mediated by second hits, such as inflammatory cytokines, mitochondrial dysfunction, and oxidative stress, which would cause steatohepatitis and fibrosis (Fig. 137.1).

The two-hit hypothesis, however, has become largely obsolete, as there is increasing recognition of multiple molecular and metabolic insults that likely act in concert on genetically susceptible subjects to induce NAFLD. These additional hits include nutritional factors, gut microbiota and dysbiosis, and mutations in genes such as *PNPLA3* and *TM6SF2*.

Although simple steatosis progresses slowly, with only 3% experiencing cirrhosis within 10 years, NASH progresses more rapidly, with 15% to 20% reaching advanced fibrosis and cirrhosis within 10 years.

DEMOGRAPHICS AND RISK FACTORS

Advanced age, male gender, and Hispanic and South Asian ethnicity are all associated with increased risk of NAFLD. Obesity and type 2 diabetes mellitus are also both well-established risk factors. Multiple studies have found that up to 69% of patients with type 2 diabetes mellitus had evidence of fatty infiltration. Furthermore, ~80% of patients with NAFLD have some evidence of hyperlipidemia, and there is a strong association with the metabolic syndrome. Furthermore, compared to patients with NAFLD in general, patients with NASH are more likely to be older, more obese, and have diabetes and metabolic syndrome.

PRESENTATION, EVALUATION, AND DIAGNOSIS

The presumptive diagnosis of NAFLD is established based on the abnormal radiographic appearance of the liver (Fig. 137.2) in a patient with risk factors, such as diabetes and metabolic syndrome. Because patients lack symptoms, the finding is typically incidental.

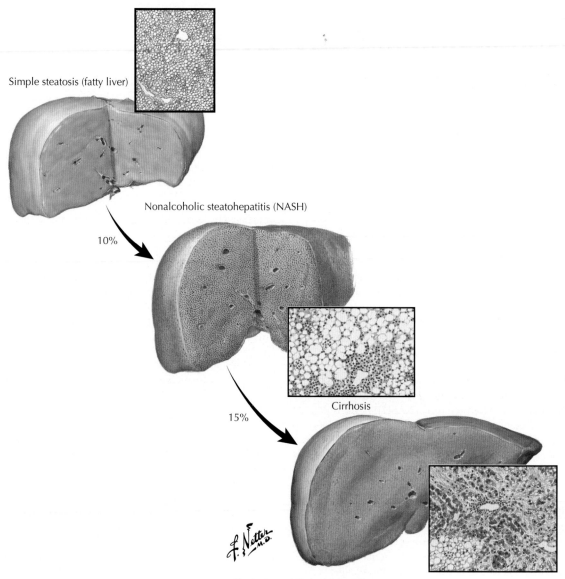

FIG. 137.1 Evolution of Fatty Liver Disease.

As stated, confirmation of the diagnosis requires the exclusion of excessive alcohol consumption (see Chapter 138) and other causes of chronic liver disease, such as medications (i.e., corticosteroids, amiodarone, methotrexate, and tamoxifen), stimulant abuse, hepatitis B virus (HBV) and hepatitis C virus (HCV) infection, hemochromatosis, autoimmune liver disease, and Wilson disease.

The combination of NAFLD and elevated transaminases is more of NASH but not diagnostic. Likewise, transaminases can be normal in NASH, advanced fibrosis, and even cirrhosis. The gold standard test for these conditions remains liver biopsy. Recently, however, there has been an increased use of noninvasive tests to assess for liver fibrosis, including **transient elastography (TE)** and the **NAFLD fibrosis score.** TE is currently the most widely used noninvasive measurement of fibrosis, with sensitivity and specificity both approaching 90%. The NAFLD fibrosis score is calculated using six common variables (age, body mass index [BMI], hyperglycemia, platelet count, albumin, and aspartate aminotransferase

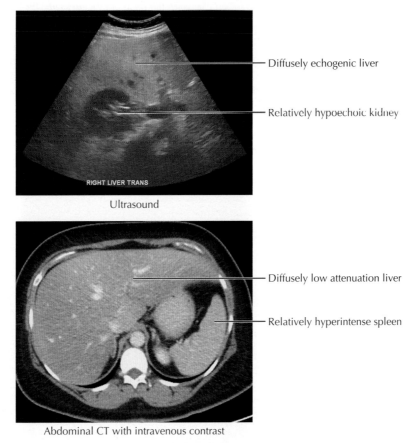

Ultrasound

— Diffusely echogenic liver

— Relatively hypoechoic kidney

RIGHT LIVER TRANS

— Diffusely low attenuation liver

— Relatively hyperintense spleen

Abdominal CT with intravenous contrast

FIG. 137.2 **Radiographic Findings.**

[AST]/alanine aminotransferase [ALT] ratio) and is useful for predicting advanced fibrosis or cirrhosis.

TREATMENT

There are few established treatments for NAFLD. The best-studied therapy is weight loss, with a goal of at least a 10% weight reduction, which has been associated with the resolution of histological findings such as lobular steatosis, necroinflammatory changes, and even fibrosis. Bariatric surgery can be an effective means of achieving weight loss goals. Of note, however, rapid weight loss after bariatric surgery can rapidly worsen hepatic function, secondary to rapid mobilization and metabolism of hepatic fat stores, causing an inflammatory response. The mechanism underlying this effect involves increased metabolic stress and inflammation, as well as excessive fat mobilization resulting in increased free fatty acid levels and fat deposition.

Pharmacological therapy for NAFLD is recommended only for patients with NASH and fibrosis. Currently, there are only two approved pharmacological therapies for NASH: **vitamin E** and **pioglitazone.** The PIVENS study assessed the benefit of these two therapies in a cohort of patients with NASH without diabetes. Both therapies significantly reduced hepatic steatosis and lobular inflammation. Pioglitazone improved insulin resistance, whereas vitamin E did not. Of note, in some but not all studies, vitamin E was also associated with increased all-cause mortality attributed mostly to cardiovascular causes. One major criticism of the PIVENS trial is its limited applicability, as most patients with NASH have diabetes; however, several trials have demonstrated that pioglitazone improves histological findings in patients with both NASH and diabetes and can be used in that setting. Newer medications, such as **obeticholic acid** (a farnesoid X receptor agonist), are under active investigation. As with other causes of liver disease, liver transplantation is an option for patients with complications from cirrhosis, such as hepatocellular carcinoma (see Chapter 162 for details).

Among patients with NAFLD, the most common cause of mortality is cardiovascular disease. Though this is mostly due to the high prevalence of metabolic syndrome and diabetes, recent studies have shown that NAFLD is also an independent risk factor for atherosclerosis. As the stage of hepatic fibrosis progresses, however, patients become more likely to die from complications of cirrhosis, such as hepatocellular carcinoma.

CHAPTER 138

Alcohol-Associated Liver Disease

NICOLE T. SHEN • MADISON DENNIS

INTRODUCTION

Alcohol-associated liver disease (ALD) encompasses a spectrum of histopathological abnormalities that include **steatosis** (fat infiltration), **steatohepatitis** (steatosis along with neutrophil-predominant inflammatory infiltrate resulting in hepatocyte injury), **fibrosis**, and cirrhosis with or without hepatocellular carcinoma. Patients can present clinically with alcohol-associated hepatitis characterized by jaundice and other signs of liver failure, or they can remain asymptomatic until liver fibrosis becomes advanced and the sequelae of cirrhosis emerge.

ALD typically occurs in the setting of high-risk drinking and/or alcohol use disorder. High-risk drinking involves consumption of ≥4 and 5 drinks in a day for women and men, respectively. The prevalence of high-risk drinking and alcohol use disorder has increased over the past decade.

In the Western world, ALD is the most common cause of cirrhosis. In the United States, 14 million people consume pathological quantities of alcohol, and 10% to 20% develop cirrhosis. The majority of patients with ALD are 40 to 50 years of age. Each year 70,000 to 100,000 patients warrant transplant referral, but for various reasons <4000 are listed. In 2013, an estimated 18,000 patients in the United States died of ALD.

PATHOPHYSIOLOGY

The pathogenesis of alcohol-associated steatosis and steatohepatitis remains incompletely understood.

In the liver, both alcohol dehydrogenase (ADH) and cytochrome P450 2E1 (CYP2E1) metabolize ethanol to acetaldehyde, which is in turn converted to acetate. These processes increase levels of nicotinamide adenine dinucleotide hydrogen (NADH), which shifts the reduction oxidation potential, inhibiting the oxidation and metabolism of fatty acids and triglycerides. Alcohol also increases hepatic lipogenesis and decreases lipolysis through inhibition of adenosine monophosphate activated kinase (AMPK) and peroxisome proliferator-activated

receptor-α (PPAR-α). These processes promote increased fat storage in the liver, known as steatosis.

A subset of patients develops steatohepatitis, characterized by a neutrophil-predominant infiltrate that injures hepatocytes and accelerates fibrosis. This condition is thought to occur via proinflammatory cytokines, oxidative stress, and toxic metabolic products of alcohol. The inflammation may arise in part from reactive oxygen species produced by CYP2E1 and antigenic adducts during alcohol metabolism. There is also evidence that chronic alcohol exposure increases translocation of bacteria-derived endotoxin from the intestinal lumen into the portal venous system. Endotoxin stimulates Kupffer cells to produce tumor necrosis factor-α (TNF-α), which, in addition to other proinflammatory cytokines and cells of the innate immune system, initiate and maintain hepatic inflammation.

About 10% to 20% of patients with steatosis (small to large droplet fat) will progress to fibrosis, and then 8% to 20% of those with fibrosis will progress to cirrhosis. The subset of patients with steatohepatitis is at increased risk of fibrosis and may experience marked hepatic inflammation that presents clinically with acute hepatitis.

On liver biopsy (Fig. 138.1), the presence of both small and large fat droplets in hepatocytes indicates steatosis. The additional presence of Mallory-Denk bodies (eosinophilic hepatocyte inclusion bodies), hepatocyte ballooning, and neutrophil infiltration indicates steatohepatitis. Patients with ALD frequently have perivenular and pericellular fibrosis (often described as being in a chicken wire–fence pattern), along with central-central or central-portal fibrous septa. The histological changes are most prominent in the centrilobular region (zone 3), likely because it has the lowest oxygen tension and is therefore most susceptible to oxidative stress.

RISK FACTORS

Both environmental and genetic factors can predispose patients to ALD and increase the risk of experiencing severe alcohol-associated hepatitis (SAH) or progressing

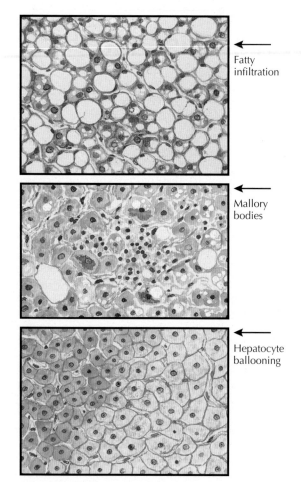

Fatty infiltration

Mallory bodies

Hepatocyte ballooning

FIG. 138.1 Pathological Findings in Alcohol-associated Steatosis and Steatohepatitis.

to cirrhosis. The quantity of alcohol ingested appears to be the greatest risk factor for ALD. The risk is increased further if alcohol is consumed outside of mealtimes. A diet high in saturated fat is thought to be protective, while a diet high in polyunsaturated fats promotes ALD. Vitamin A and E deficiencies may increase the risk of ALD. Patients with other causes of liver disease (viral hepatitis, autoimmune hepatitis, nonalcoholic fatty liver disease, nonalcoholic steatohepatitis) are also at increased risk.

PRESENTATION, EVALUATION, AND DIAGNOSIS

Patients with alcohol-associated hepatitis typically present with jaundice, tender hepatomegaly, ascites, hepatic encephalopathy, and/or constitutional symptoms such as anorexia and fever. Those with underlying cirrhosis may also have stigmata of chronic liver disease, including ascites, palmar erythema, spider nevi, gynecomastia, and asterixis. The most common laboratory findings are moderate elevations of aspartate aminotransferase (AST) and alanine aminotransferase (ALT) (typically <300), and an AST:ALT ratio ≥2. Other findings may include elevated levels of direct bilirubin and γ-glutamyltransferase (GGT), leukocytosis, hypoalbuminemia, thrombocytopenia, and a prolonged prothrombin time (PT). Hepatic ultrasound may reveal steatosis or cirrhosis and ascites, which is helpful for excluding other causes of liver injury, such as biliary obstruction or hepatic or portal vein thrombosis.

The diagnosis of ALD requires a thorough alcohol history that documents the presence of high-risk drinking or alcohol use disorder, but patients may not be forthcoming. The AUDIT questionnaire is widely validated but involves multiple questions; the AUDIT-C is a shortened screening tool with growing data for efficacy. The traditional CAGE questionnaire is no longer thought to be an adequate screening tool, being insensitive to the gamut of unhealthy alcohol use, but may be used as an adjunct for patients who screen positive on another screening tool. Collateral history from family members or friends may be helpful.

The diagnosis of ALD also requires the exclusion of other causes of hepatitis, including infectious (viral), autoimmune, and obstructive hepatitis. When patients have multiple potential reasons for liver injury, a biopsy may help identify the predominant pathology and guide therapy.

TREATMENT

The mainstay of treatment for ALD in general is abstinence counseling and supportive care. Abstinence results in histological normalization in 27% of patients over an 18-month follow-up period, improved overall survival, and a lower risk of cirrhosis. Pharmacological agents that can help reduce alcohol cravings and consumption include baclofen, naltrexone (an opioid antagonist), and acamprosate. Patients require nutritional support to ensure adequate caloric intake and electrolyte repletion; supplementation of thiamine, folate, and vitamin B_6 is common.

Patients with alcohol-associated hepatitis present on a spectrum of clinical severity, and the Maddrey discriminant function (mDF) helps distinguish those with SAH, who may benefit from treatment with corticosteroids (Table 138.1). The usual dose of corticosteroids is prednisolone 40 mg daily. Prednisolone is preferred over prednisone because the latter requires hepatic conversion to prednisolone. Pentoxifylline can be considered when

TABLE 138.1
Risk-Stratification Scoring Systems

	Equation	Interpretation
Maddrey Discriminant Function (calculated upon diagnosis of alcohol-associated hepatitis)	4.6 * (Prothrombin Time [s] – Control Prothrombin Time [s]) + Total Bilirubin (mg/dL)[a]	Score of ≥32 indicates severe alcohol-associated hepatitis, an indication for corticosteroids
Lille Model (calculated after 7 days of corticosteroids for severe alcohol-associated hepatitis)	$e^{-R} / 1 + e^{-R}$ $R = 3.19 - 0.101 *$ (age in years) $+ 0.147 *$ (albumin at day 0 [g/L]) $+ 0.0165 *$ (change in total bilirubin level from day 0 to 7 [μmol/L]) $-$ ($0.206 *$ creatinine [μmol/L]) $- 0.0065 *$ (bilirubin on day 0 [μmol/L]) $- 0.0096 *$ (prothrombin time [s]) (calculator available at www.lillemodel.com)[b]	Score of >0.45 indicates corticosteroid treatment failure and poor prognosis (6-month survival of 25%)

[a]*Maddrey equation:* Maddrey WC, Boitnott JK, et al: Corticosteroid therapy of alcoholic hepatitis, *Gastroenterology* 75(2):193–199, 1978.
[b]*Lille equation:* Louvet A, Naveau S, Abdelnour M, et al: The Lille model: a new tool for therapeutic strategy in patients with severe alcoholic hepatitis treated with steroids, *Hepatology* 45(6):1348–1354, 2007.

steroids are contraindicated; however, studies have found that it is inferior, and one large randomized controlled trial showed no benefit over placebo.

The Lille model score (see Table 138.1) assesses the response to steroid therapy at 7 days and determines the appropriateness of continuing treatment. A score of <0.45 indicates adequate treatment response, and patients are continued on steroids for a total of 28 days, with subsequent tapering over 2 to 3 weeks. A Lille score >0.45 suggests treatment failure and a very poor prognosis, so steroids are stopped.

Failure to improve with steroids predicts a mortality rate >70% at 2 months. In this case, liver transplant should be considered. A recent trial demonstrated that in highly selective patients, liver transplant resulted in a 6-month survival of 77%, significantly greater than the rate of 22% among nontransplanted controls. Alcohol relapse occurred in only 3 of the 26 transplanted patients over 2-year follow-up. Despite this trial, there are ongoing ethical concerns about performing transplantation in patients with active alcohol abuse, with a need for more long-term data.

CHAPTER 139

Cirrhosis and Portal Hypertension

VIKAS GUPTA

INTRODUCTION

Although the liver has a remarkable ability to regenerate, chronic damage from alcohol, viral hepatitis, fatty liver disease, or other causes can result in progressive hepatic fibrosis and distortion of liver architecture. Advanced, irreversible fibrosis is known as cirrhosis, a condition that affects >600,000 Americans.

The complications of cirrhosis result from decreased hepatocellular function and **portal hypertension** (Fig. 139.1). The loss of hepatocytes reduces the synthetic and detoxification capacity of the liver, resulting in decreased production of coagulation factors and impaired clearance of bilirubin. In addition, the accumulation of toxins can lead to **hepatic encephalopathy** and **asterixis** (transient losses of muscle tone often seen when wrists are extended), while impaired sex hormone metabolism can lead to gynecomastia, testicular atrophy, and other findings.

Meanwhile, portal venous hypertension results in complications such as **ascites,** splenomegaly, peripheral edema, and the formation of portosystemic venous shunts known as **varices.** Portal hypertension can also cause dysfunction of other organs (e.g., hepatorenal syndrome, portopulmonary hypertension, hepatopulmonary syndrome, and cirrhotic cardiomyopathy).

PATHOPHYSIOLOGY

Chronic hepatocyte injury, death, and replication lead to liver fibrosis through an exaggeration of the normal wound-healing process. Hepatic stellate cells, which line the space of Disse, become activated upon hepatocyte death and deposit extracellular matrix (ECM) proteins. After months to years of chronic liver injury, this ultimately leads to scar tissue in the space of Disse and the loss of endothelial fenestrations, such that blood in the liver sinusoids can no longer contact surrounding hepatocytes. Regenerating hepatocytes become trapped by this scar tissue, forming the regenerative nodules that histologically characterize cirrhosis.

The loss of hepatocyte mass and entrapment of remaining hepatocytes causes loss of normal synthetic function and detoxification processes. Portal hypertension is believed to result from three separate mechanisms. The first is severe architectural distortion of the liver parenchyma, which increases resistance to blood flow from the portal vein to the central hepatic vein (Fig. 139.2). Another is increased intrahepatic vascular tone, which accounts for 20% to 30% of the increased portal pressure. The third is local release of splanchnic circulation vasodilators, which increase portal blood flow and thereby further worsen portal hypertension.

The complications of portal hypertension start to develop once the pressure gradient across the liver reaches 10 mm Hg. To divert blood flow around the fibrotic liver, preexisting anastomoses between the portal and systemic venous system (portosystemic collaterals or varices) begin to enlarge. Such connections are most prominent in the left gastric–distal esophageal, splenorenal, and umbilical veins. Dilated submucosal esophageal and gastric varices can rupture into the lumen, causing severe gastrointestinal (GI) bleeding.

Ascites is often the first clinically evident complication of cirrhosis and derives not only from portal hypertension, but also from progressive volume overload. The opening of portosystemic collaterals and the increase in circulating systemic vasodilators cause profound peripheral vasodilatation. The consequent activation of vascular baroreceptors stimulates the release of norepinephrine, aldosterone, and antidiuretic hormone, which promote avid sodium and water retention. The rising portal pressures, decreased overall oncotic pressure (from impaired albumin synthesis), and volume overload cause fluid to leak from the surface of the liver and the mesenteric vessels into the peritoneum.

PRESENTATION, EVALUATION, AND DIAGNOSIS

The development of cirrhosis is an insidious process, and thus the presentation can range from nonspecific constitutional complaints to incidentally discovered laboratory abnormalities to hepatic decompensation

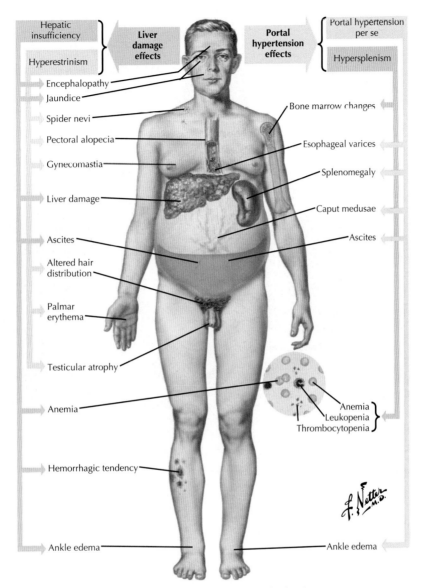

FIG. 139.1 **Complications of Cirrhosis.**

(e.g., GI bleeding, ascites, hepatic encephalopathy or jaundice) requiring hospitalization.

Although the gold standard for diagnosing cirrhosis remains liver biopsy, the combination of history, physical examination, laboratory, and imaging findings are often considered sufficient for a presumptive diagnosis.

The clinical history can reveal risk factors for cirrhosis, including excessive alcoholic intake, intravenous drug use (a major risk factor for hepatitis C infection), obesity and/or uncontrolled diabetes (which can cause fatty liver disease), and family history.

The physical examination can reveal signs of altered sex hormone metabolism, manifesting as palmar erythema, spider nevi/telangiectasias (dilated blood vessels under the skin), gynecomastia, and testicular atrophy. The signs of portal hypertension include dilated abdominal wall veins (caput medusae), ascites, splenomegaly, and peripheral edema. With worsening liver function, jaundice and encephalopathy become common.

Laboratory testing often reveals mildly elevated liver aminotransferases; however, moderate elevation can occur in those with ongoing hepatocellular damage.

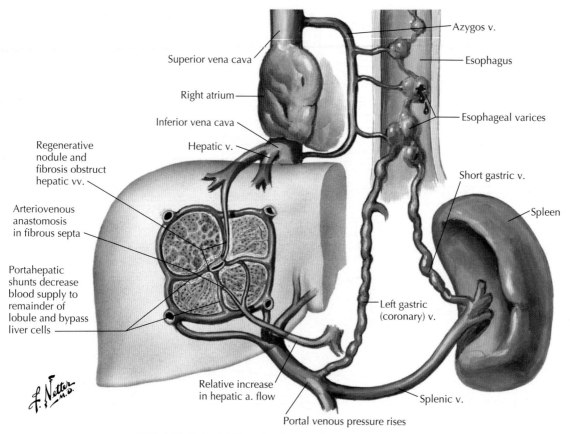

Superior vena cava

Right atrium

Inferior vena cava

Hepatic v.

Regenerative
nodule and
fibrosis obstruct
hepatic vv.

Arteriovenous
anastomosis
in fibrous septa

Portahepatic
shunts decrease
blood supply to
remainder of
lobule and bypass
liver cells

Relative increase
in hepatic a. flow

Portal venous pressure rises

Azygos v.

Esophagus

Esophageal varices

Short gastric v.

Spleen

Left gastric
(coronary) v.

Splenic v.

FIG. 139.2 **Portal Hypertension.** *a.*, Artery; *v.* or *vv.*, vein(s).

Normal aminotransferases do not rule out cirrhosis and are seen with the cessation of underlying hepatocellular damage. Mild elevations in alkaline phosphatase are common, with higher levels seen in patients with underlying cholestatic disease. Tests of liver function (albumin, prothrombin time, clearance of bilirubin) are often abnormal, with the degree dependent on the presence of acute decompensation, amount of fibrosis, and residual hepatocyte mass. Hematological abnormalities are also common. Portal hypertension causes splenomegaly, which leads to sequestration of platelets and thrombocytopenia. Decreased levels of thrombopoietin, which is normally produced by the liver, further contributes to thrombocytopenia. Anemia is multifactorial and results from acute and chronic GI blood losses as well as iron sequestration from chronic inflammation.

A liver ultrasound provides a rapid, noninvasive means of assessing hepatic structure. In cirrhosis, the liver is nodular and highly echogenic (secondary to the

increase in extracellular fibrosis) (Fig. 139.3). Ultrasound and color Doppler imaging help identify complications of portal hypertension, such as ascites, splenomegaly, portal vein flow, and portal vein thrombosis. Additionally, newer technologies can noninvasively stage fibrosis using magnetic resonance or ultrasound elastography to measure liver stiffness.

TREATMENT

The treatment of cirrhosis is focused primarily on managing ascites, varices, and hepatic encephalopathy.

Ascites

The initial treatment for ascites is sodium restriction and diuretics. Spironolactone and furosemide are started at low doses and titrated to keep ascites at a minimum and maintain normokalemia. Although this strategy is effective in most patients, those with diuretic-refractory ascites may require regular large-volume **paracenteses,**

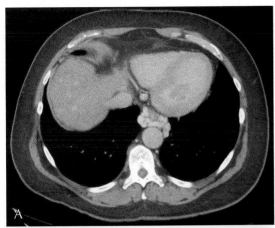

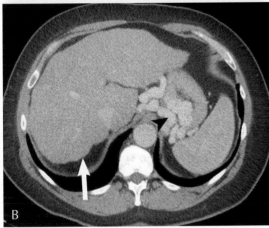

Compared with a normal liver, the cirrhotic liver has an irregular contour *(arrow)*. Additionally, the veins of the portal vasculature are dilated *(arrowhead),* indicating portal hypertension.

FIG. 139.3 **Radiographic Findings in Cirrhosis.**

with albumin replacement given to prevent postparacentesis circulatory dysfunction secondary to volume shifts (see Chapter 53 for details). If paracenteses become too frequent and no contraindications exist, patients can undergo placement of a **transjugular intrahepatic portosystemic shunt (TIPS).** In this procedure, a mesh stent is placed in the liver that connects one of the hepatic veins to an intrahepatic branch of the portal vein, decompressing the portal circulation and reducing the complications of portal hypertension.

Spontaneous bacterial peritonitis (SBP), which results from translocation of gut flora through the intestinal wall into the mesenteric lymph nodes and ascites fluid, is a major cause of mortality. Patients may present with fever, abdominal pain, or altered mental status, or they can be asymptomatic. Thus all patients with decompensated cirrhosis and ascites warrant a diagnostic paracentesis. A positive ascites fluid culture, or a fluid total neutrophil count >250 cells/mm³, confirms the diagnosis. Patients with SBP should receive antibiotics with excellent penetration into the peritoneum, such as cefotaxime or ceftriaxone, for at least 5 days. Because of the risk of renal dysfunction secondary to SBP, patients should also receive albumin (1.5 g/kg of body weight on day 1 and 1 g/kg on day 3).

Patients with prior episodes of SBP should receive ongoing antibiotic prophylaxis, as the 1-year risk of reoccurrence is as high as 70%. Patients with an ascitic fluid protein concentration ≤1.5 g/dL along with renal dysfunction (creatinine ≥1.2 mg/dL, blood urea nitrogen ≥25 mg/dL, or serum sodium ≤130 mEq/L) or liver dysfunction (bilirubin ≥3 mg/dL) should also receive prophylaxis. Prophylaxis regimens consist typically of a fluoroquinolone or trimethoprim-sulfamethoxazole.

Varices

Any patient with cirrhosis should undergo a screening upper endoscopy to evaluate for the presence of varices, which should be defined as small or medium/large, with the former being collapsible upon esophageal insufflation. Small varices in a compensated cirrhotic without any high-risk features of bleeding, such as red spots, can be managed expectantly with screening repeated at 2-year intervals to assess for enlargement. Patients with small varices in a decompensated cirrhotic or who have red spots should be placed on nonselective β-blockers, which help decrease portal pressures to decrease variceal size and the risk of bleeding. Patients with medium and large varices can undergo endoscopic variceal ligation (EVL) or use nonselective β-blockers, depending on local expertise and patient preference.

Patients with cirrhosis who present with hematemesis or melena should be considered to have a variceal bleed, and treated accordingly, until endoscopic evaluation can occur. Patients require careful resuscitation, since overtransfusion can increase portal pressures and potentiate further bleeding. Somatostatin analogs (e.g., octreotide) have been shown to decrease portal pressures and improve the achievement of hemostasis when combined with EVL. Endoscopic assessment should be undertaken within 12 hours of admission. Patients with cirrhosis and GI bleeding are also at high risk of infectious complications, such as urinary tract infections, pneumonia, bacteremia, and SBP. Thus they should receive antimicrobial prophylaxis with a third-generation cephalosporin or fluoroquinolone. If

EVL cannot control bleeding, or if patients experience rebleeding, an emergent TIPS can decompress the portal system.

Hepatic Encephalopathy

As liver function decreases, ammonia and other toxins begin to accumulate in the blood and cause cerebral dysfunction. Encephalopathy is graded from I to IV using the West Haven criteria and ranges from subtle changes in behavior, cognition, and concentration to overt coma.

Asterixis may be present with grade I, but is marked in grades II to III, being absent once patients progress to a hepatic coma. The treatment is aimed at correcting any precipitating causes (e.g., infection, hypovolemia, renal failure) and then reducing the ammonia burden, regardless of blood concentration. The intestinal tract serves as a major site of ammonia production from numerous bacterial species. Laxatives (such as lactulose or polyethylene glycol) and the antibiotic rifaximin target the reduction of these species to decrease ammonia production.

CHAPTER 140

Sickle Cell Disease

VICTOR P. BILAN

INTRODUCTION

Sickle cell disease (SCD) comprises a group of hemo-globinopathies resulting from the inheritance of two mutant β-globin genes. The primary mutation, sickle hemoglobin (HbS), results from a single amino acid substitution that converts a glutamate residue at the sixth codon into valine (E6V). HbS undergoes abnormal polymerization under conditions of stress, hypoxemia, or dehydration, causing affected erythrocytes to adopt a rigid, sickle-shaped conformation. These sickled cells clog the microvasculature, injure the endothelium, and set off inflammatory cascades affecting every organ in the body. Management of SCD consists of early diagnosis through newborn screening, treatment of acute and chronic complications, and mitigation of the HbS burden through use of hydroxyurea and blood transfusions. Hematopoietic stem cell transplant is the only curative therapy.

PATHOPHYSIOLOGY

Normal adult hemoglobin (HbA) is a tetramer of four protein chains containing two α-subunits and two β-subunits. The high concentration of hemoglobin in erythrocytes requires a high degree of solubility to prevent polymerization and precipitation. The globin tertiary structure accordingly puts hydrophilic domains on the exterior for solubility, and hydrophobic domains in the interior of the protein, where the oxygen-carrying heme moieties reside.

In SCD, the E6V substitution in the β-globin subunit creates an exposed exterior hydrophobic region, which tends to polymerize reversibly with the corresponding region on another HbS molecule. Any stress leading to decreased blood oxygen (e.g., high altitude, smoking, sleep apnea) or dehydration (e.g., infection or physical exertion) can trigger polymerization of HbS into helical ropes, which deform the erythrocyte into a rigid curved shape

that lends its name to the disease (Fig. 140.1). A related mutation that converts the sixth position glutamate into lysine (E6K) forms the molecular basis of hemoglobin C, which itself does not cause sickling but leads to cuboid-shaped deposits known as hemoglobin C crystals, which may be visualized on a peripheral blood smear.

Polymerization of HbS happens most readily in regions of slow-flow and low-oxygen tension such as the spleen, bones, and pulmonary arterial circulation. The tendency to polymerize depends strongly on the concentration of HbS, and thus on erythrocyte volume. Inflexible sickled erythrocytes cannot traverse microvasculature, leading to thrombosis and tissue ischemia. The sickled red cells hemolyze readily, leading to chronic hemolytic anemia, and they are abnormally immunogenic and proinflammatory, leading to abnormal activation of platelets and neutrophils, cytokine release, and (eventually) multifold end-organ complications. Sickled red cells have an abnormally short lifespan of 2 to 21 days due to both extravascular and intravascular hemolysis. As such, patients with severe SCD require a **chronic reticulocytosis** of 5% to 8% to maintain a hemoglobin of 6 to 9 g/dL.

The sickle cell gene can appear in homozygous form (SS) or may be compound heterozygous with another β-globin variant (e.g., Sβ⁰-thalassemia, Sβ⁺-thalassemia, or SC), or heterozygous in combination with a normal β-globin gene (SA, or sickle cell trait). Overall, the most severe phenotype is seen in patients with SS or Sβ⁰-thalassemia. Sβ⁺-thalassemia and SC genotypes generally lead to a milder disease course, while patients with SA are largely asymptomatic.

RISK FACTORS

Sickle cell disease is an autosomal recessive disorder requiring two copies of the mutant HbS gene. The prevalence of SCD among African Americans is around

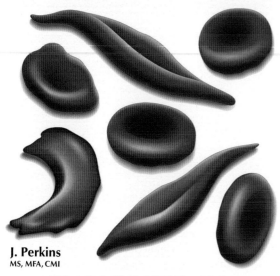

J. Perkins
MS, MFA, CMI

FIG. 140.1 Sickled Red Blood Cells.

1 in 600, with an incidence of 1 in 360 live births. The prevalence of SA trait is around 8% in African Americans.

SA trait confers a degree of protection against infection by the malaria parasites *Plasmodium falciparum* and *P. vivax*, as the erythrocytes infected by these organisms preferentially sickle and are destroyed by monocytes in the spleen. This is believed to confer a survival advantage of SA individuals in malaria-endemic regions and the persistence of the allele in the population despite the devastating consequences of the homozygous state. In support of this model, a striking overlap worldwide between malaria-endemic regions and regions of high HbS prevalence is observed, most strongly in West Africa.

PRESENTATION, EVALUATION, AND DIAGNOSIS

Since 2006, all 50 US states have adopted screening for congenital hemoglobinopathies, including SCD, as part of routine newborn screening. Traditionally, hemoglobin electrophoresis has been the test of choice for suspected hemoglobinopathies (and monitoring of the HbS burden for treatment purposes), with genotyping now available as well.

On average, patients with SS or Sβ⁰-thalassemia SCD have hemoglobin levels in the range of 6 to 9 g/dL, while those with Sβ⁺-thalassemia and SC variants have higher hemoglobin values of 9 to 14 g/dL. Hemoglobin can plunge precipitously during a hemolytic episode or an aplastic crisis triggered by a parvovirus infection. Baseline laboratory studies in SCD typically show chronic

hemolysis with low haptoglobin and high lactate dehydrogenase levels. Chronic reticulocytosis in the range of ≥5% is commonly observed and indicative of ongoing hemolysis. The peripheral smear in all patients with SCD demonstrates sickled erythrocytes irrespective of whether an acute SCD crisis is occurring. Platelets may be high owing to the chronic inflammatory milieu of SCD. Neutrophils are increasingly known to play an important role in the inflammatory cascades of SCD, with chronic neutrophilia emerging as a marker of poorer outcomes.

The most common complication of SCD is **vasoocclusive crisis (VOC),** where sickled erythrocytes lodge in capillary beds throughout the body, resulting in tissue ischemia and severe pain in the chest, large joints, and limbs. In children this may take the form of the **hand-foot syndrome** with painful, swollen fingers and toes (dactylitis). VOC may arise in the setting of infection, hypoxemia, dehydration, or other physiological stressors, although frequently there is no clear precipitant. Some patients may present with fever, leukocytosis, and increased hemolytic markers, although these signs need not be present.

Over time, repeated ischemic insults of VOC combined with the deleterious effects of chronic hemolytic anemia give rise to the manifold end-organ complications of SCD, which include:

- Neurological: Thrombosis and vasoocclusion lead to narrowing of cerebral arteries and an increased risk of stroke. Children with SCD are at risk of ischemic stroke, while adults tend to have hemorrhagic strokes. Both overt stroke and silent infarcts in SCD lead to cognitive delay and impaired school performance. Moyamoya of the cerebral vasculature may also develop in some patients.
- Ophthalmological: Local hypoxemia and retinal vascular occlusion induce neovascularization and proliferative retinopathy, leading to an increased risk of retinal detachment, glaucoma, and vitreous hemorrhage.
- Cardiac: Microvascular occlusion, iron overload, and a high cardiac output state lead to cardiomyopathy and congestive heart failure.
- Pulmonary: Pulmonary arterial hypertension is a common chronic complication and a strong predictor of mortality in SCD. It arises through multiple mechanisms, including chronic hypoxemia (from anemia), pulmonary vascular endothelial injury (induced by free hemoglobin, nitrous oxide depletion, and inflammatory mediators), and chronic pulmonary thromboembolism.
- Gastrointestinal: Many patients with SCD develop pigment gallstones and pancreatitis as a result of

chronic hemolysis. Repeat red blood cell transfusions, which many SCD patients receive, can lead to chronic liver disease and cirrhosis as a result of transfusion-related iron overload. Over time, autoinfarction of the spleen occurs, leading to **functional asplenia.**

- Renal: Papillary necrosis with infarction and destruction of the renal calyces leads to proteinuria and eventual isosthenuria in almost all patients.
- Genitourinary: **Priapism** is common in males with SCD and is due to occlusion of the penile vasculature.
- Skeletal: Repeated infarction leads to avascular necrosis of long bones such as the femur and humerus, often requiring orthopedic surgeries.
- Dermatological: SCD patients frequently develop leg ulcers due to vascular compromise.
- Hematological: Bone marrow suppression that would normally be transient and inconsequential (e.g., from drugs or viruses including parvovirus) leads to aplastic crisis in SCD patients due to the short lifespan of affected erythrocytes and a chronically taxed hematopoietic system.

Two life-threatening complications of SCD must always be kept in mind. One is overwhelming infection by encapsulated organisms due splenic infarction and the resultant functional asplenia in nearly all SCD patients. This was the main driver of childhood mortality in SCD before the establishment of antibiotic prophylaxis as a standard of care. A second is the **acute chest syndrome (ACS),** defined by the presence of a lung opacity on chest radiography in combination with any of several other clinical signs or symptoms, including fever, hypoxemia, tachypnea, chest pain, cough, wheezing, or other manifestations of cardiopulmonary compromise. In ACS, an insult such as a viral infection or fat embolism, combined with the inflammatory response induced by sickled red blood cells in the pulmonary vasculature, produces a vicious cycle of pulmonary inflammation, impaired oxygenation, and further sickling, culminating in acute respiratory distress syndrome with severe hypoxemia and lung infiltrates (see Chapter 91).

TREATMENT

If a diagnosis of SCD is established via newborn screening, management begins immediately with prophylactic penicillin at least until age 5 to reduce the risk of infection by encapsulated organisms. Such children are also subjected to expanded vaccination schedules, including pneumococcal vaccination. Together, these interventions have greatly improved the life expectancy of patients with SCD.

Routine monitoring of pediatric patients with transcranial Doppler ultrasound identifies patients at highest risk of stroke, who typically have abnormally high flow velocities through the cerebral arteries due to narrowing of the vasculature. Such patients are maintained on strict red cell transfusion regimens, often for life, which have proven to be effective in reducing stroke risk. Either exchange or simple transfusion can be used, the former to target a HbS concentration <30%, the latter to raise the hemoglobin to 10 g/dL. Compared to simple transfusions, red cell **exchange transfusions** lower HbS percentage much more rapidly and cause less hypervolemia and **iron overload;** the latter consideration is particularly important in patients who are chronically transfused, all of whom require monitoring for iron overload and chelation therapy if it develops. However, red cell exchange transfusions are also more expensive than simple transfusions, require placement of specialized intravenous (IV) lines and use of apheresis equipment, and have the potential to cause increased red cell alloimmunization from exposure to high numbers of red cell units. Such alloimmunization against minor erythrocyte antigens can lead to delayed transfusion reactions and difficulty in securing future compatible donor units and must be monitored carefully as well.

Management of the other complications of SCD is supportive. Treatment of VOC consists of parenteral opioids, judicious hydration with IV fluids, and investigation for an underlying trigger such as infection (although such a cause often is not found). ACS requires treatment with empirical antibiotics, bronchodilators, supplemental oxygen and, depending on the severity, immediate red cell exchange transfusion and lung protective ventilation in the event of respiratory failure. Adult SCD patients who undergo surgery with general anesthesia are generally treated with simple transfusion to bring their preoperative hemoglobin to 10 g/dL.

The mainstay of chronic treatment for both children and adults with SCD is **hydroxyurea,** a chemotherapeutic drug that stimulates an increase in the production of fetal hemoglobin (HbF) through mechanisms that are not entirely understood. HbF, due to its high affinity for oxygen, strongly inhibits the polymerization of HbS, and has been demonstrated to reduce the frequency of painful crises in SCD patients. Hydroxyurea is recommended for all children, regardless of symptoms, and for adults with three or more pain crises per year or any other life-limiting SCD symptoms. The dose is titrated to the maximum that is tolerated without causing severe leukopenia. A commonly raised concern about long-term hydroxyurea use is an increased risk of secondary malignancy, but epidemiological studies have not shown this to be the case.

A number of targeted therapies for SCD are under investigation but not yet widely available. Gene therapy to edit the defective beta-globin gene, or provide the patient with additional globin genes to increase the production of HbF or HbA2, is largely in the preclinical phase. The amino acid L-glutamine, as well as crizanlizumab, a monoclonal antibody directed against the endothelial adhesion molecule P-selectin, have been shown to reduce the binding of sickled cells to the endothelium and reduce the frequency of painful crises. Allosteric stabilizers of HbS such as voxelotor, which binds to the alpha-subunit and inhibits polymerization, also show promise in reducing the frequency of VOCs and increasing hemoglobin levels.

Hematopoietic stem cell transplant is curative in SCD and increasingly successful with the development of less morbid, nonmyeloablative conditioning regimens. Suitable patients must have a healthy human leukocyte antigen (HLA)–matched donor, preferably a sibling. Risks include engraftment failure and graft-vs-host disease, but in appropriately selected patients, these risks may be manageable.

CHAPTER 141

Thalassemia

VICTOR P. BILAN

INTRODUCTION

The **thalassemias** are a related group of inherited autosomal recessive anemias that arise from unbalanced production of the subunits of adult hemoglobin **(HbA)**, a tetramer of two α-globin chains and two β-globin chains ($\alpha_2\beta_2$). Failure to produce either of the two subunits at the normal rate leads to ineffective erythropoiesis, microcytic anemia with intramedullary hemolysis, and **iron overload**. The phenotypic severity of the thalassemias ranges from asymptomatic carrier states to death in utero, and patients with severe forms can be transfusion dependent from infancy.

The thalassemias are common throughout Africa, Southeast Asia, the Middle East, the Indian subcontinent, and the Mediterranean, and represent a significant public health burden. About 5% of the world's population are carriers for **α-thalassemia,** and 1.5% carry **β-thalassemia.** The tendency of thalassemia mutations to be most prevalent in malaria-endemic regions suggests a selective advantage in the form of resistance to severe *falciparum* malaria infection, which has been demonstrated in the carrier state and mild forms of disease. With the rare exception of cure through hematopoietic stem cell transplantation (SCT), management of the symptomatic forms is supportive. The mainstays of therapy are transfusion of red blood cells (RBCs) to compensate for ineffective erythropoiesis, and management of iron overload, which occurs both endogenously and iatrogenically as a result of transfusion.

PATHOPHYSIOLOGY

The gene encoding the α-chain is duplicated on chromosome 16, with four copies in each diploid cell, whereas the β-globin gene exists in one copy on chromosome 11, with two copies per cell. Under normal conditions, production of α-globin and β-globin is approximately equimolar. Thalassemia results when an inherited mutation or deletion of one or more of the globin genes causes relative underproduction of that chain, leading to ineffective erythropoiesis: α-Thalassemia arises from an inherited mutation in one or more α-globin genes, while β-thalassemia arises from a mutation in β-globin.

The morbidity of α-thalassemia and β-thalassemia arises from two mechanisms: anemia and iron overload. The anemia of thalassemia is **microcytic** and due to ineffective erythropoiesis: When α-globin and β-globin synthesis is mismatched, hemoglobin synthesis is impaired, and functional erythrocytes are not effectively produced, leading to a compensatory gross expansion of hematopoietic tissue in the bone marrow. Aggregates of the unaffected, unpaired globin chains accumulate in the membranes of the erythrocytes that are produced, leading to their removal from circulation by the spleen. In more severe cases, blood transfusions must be administered to support life. Eventually, iron overload and deposition of excess iron into the liver and other tissues arises both naturally (from the body's attempts to maximize gastrointestinal iron absorption far beyond normal levels to support erythropoiesis) and iatrogenically (as a consequence of blood transfusions) (Fig. 141.1).

The human genome contains genes for several hemoglobin subunits other than α and β that are expressed sequentially during gestation to produce embryonic hemoglobin and **fetal hemoglobin (HbF).** Embryonic hemoglobins Gower and Portland, composed of subunits ζ, ε, and α, are expressed first but disappear by 12 weeks of gestation and are replaced by HbF ($\alpha_2\gamma_2$), which is the predominant hemoglobin until it is replaced by HbA within 6 months after birth. Thus defects in α-chain synthesis that comprise α-thalassemia would, in principle, become apparent in utero, when the developing fetus depends on HbF for oxygen delivery (although, among the α-thalassemias, only hydrops fetalis noticeably affects the fetus in the form of in utero fetal demise). In contrast, defects of β-chain synthesis that cause β-thalassemia do not manifest until production of HbF wanes during the postpartum period, and the infant comes to depend on β chain containing HbA.

The α-thalassemias result from either deletions or inactivating mutations of one or more of the four α-globin genes (αα/αα). They are broadly categorized as:

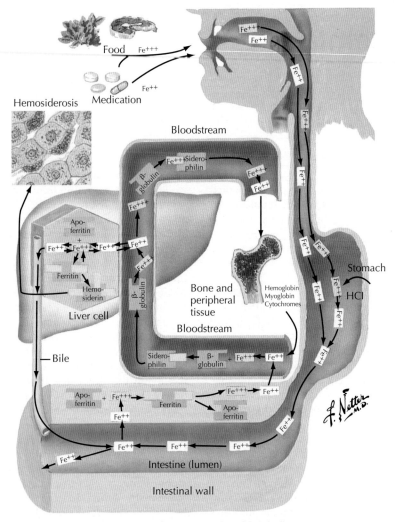

FIG. 141.1 **Overview of Iron Metabolism.**

- **α-thalassemia minima,** involving deletion or inactivation of only one of the four genes (-α/αα). This is clinically silent apart from mild microcytosis.
- **α-thalassemia minor** or **trait,** involving deletion or inactivation of two α-genes. These abnormalities can be either on the same chromosome (-/αα, or α-thalassemia-1 trait) or on different chromosomes (-α/-α, or α-thalassemia-2 trait). Patients with α-thalassemia minor or trait are typically asymptomatic, although laboratory studies may reveal microcytosis and minimal anemia.
- **HbH disease** (-α/-). This produces moderate anemia with hemoglobin values in the range of 9.5 to 10.5 g/dL and formation of HbH molecules containing four β-globin subunits (β_4).

- **Hydrops fetalis** (-/-). This is the most severe form of α-thalassemia, characterized by production of a γ_4 tetramer (i.e., hemoglobin Bart) resulting from attempts to synthesize HbF in the absence of α-chains. The hemoglobin Bart molecule is unable to deliver oxygen to the tissues due to an exceptionally high oxygen affinity, leading to fetal demise in utero or neonatal death shortly after birth.

In some cases, nondeletional α-globin mutants in an HbH pattern can cause symptomatic hemolytic anemia. An example is hemoglobin Constant Spring (HbCS), common in Southeast Asia, in which a native stop codon site is mutated, leading to generation of an additional 31 amino acids in the finished protein. The HbCS messenger ribonucleic acid (mRNA) is unstable, which results in decreased α-globin production. Patients with genotype -α/-α^{CS} have hemolysis, jaundice, and splenomegaly beyond what is observed in HbH disease (-α/−), thought to be due to additional erythrocyte membrane stress resulting from accumulation of the HbCS protein.

The β-thalassemias result from mutations in β-globin genes that lead to either reduced (mild) or absent β-globin synthesis from that locus. Hundreds of mutations are known, in both coding and regulatory regions, affecting all stages of transcription, translation, and posttranslational mRNA processing. The β-thalassemia syndromes are classified as:

- **β-thalassemia trait** or **minor.** This arises from the presence of a single β-globin mutation and leads to an asymptomatic carrier state with mild microcytic anemia.
- **β-thalassemia intermedia.** This arises from coinheritance of two mild β-globin mutations, or one mild and one severe mutation. The clinical course is variable, and patients may have mild-to-severe microcytic anemia with hemoglobin values generally ≥7 g/dL.
- **β-thalassemia major.** This arises when two severe β-globin mutations allow no β-globin synthesis. Patients with β-thalassemia major have severe microcytic anemia, require transfusional support for life, and die by 5 to 10 years of age without such supportive care.

Hemoglobin E (HbE) is a specific β-globin mutation common in Southeast Asia, which results in reduced levels of β-globin gene expression and a mildly unstable hemoglobin. When present in trait form (i.e., heterozygous β^E), the disease results in a mild microcytic anemia similar to β-thalassemia minor. In homozygous form (β^E/β^E), a more prominent microcytosis with mild anemia is seen. When combined with either α-thalassemia or β-thalassemia, a variable phenotype can result, and some patients with β-thalassemia/β^E have a clinical course similar to those with severe β-thalassemia intermedia.

β-thalassemia mutations can also coexist with the sickle cell β-globin mutation (β^S). Often, this combination results in a phenotype identical to sickle cell disease, with affected patients suffering from complications of venoocclusive disease, acute chest syndrome, and stroke (see Chapter 140 for further details).

PRESENTATION, EVALUATION, AND DIAGNOSIS

The distinguishing laboratory feature of the thalassemias is hypochromic, microcytic anemia that does not respond to iron supplementation. In many instances, thalassemia can be differentiated from iron deficiency on the basis of the **Mentzer index,** the ratio of mean corpuscular volume (MCV) to RBC count. The Mentzer index in thalassemia is usually low (<13) due to a very low MCV and a normal or increased RBC count, and high (>13) in iron deficiency due to a reduction in RBC count. The peripheral blood smear in thalassemia characteristically shows target RBCs arising from an abnormal red cell membrane-to-cytoplasm ratio secondary to defective hemoglobin synthesis, in contrast to the red cell morphology of iron deficiency, which is notable for anisopoikilocytosis.

Hemoglobin disorders such as thalassemia are often diagnosed at birth via routine newborn screening. Currently, all 50 states include electrophoretic screening for hemoglobinopathies as part of their routine panels. The typical hemoglobin electrophoresis pattern is normal in α-thalassemia minima, minor, or trait since ≥50% of the α-globin alleles are normal; in such patients, α-globin gene mutation analysis is required to confirm the diagnosis. By contrast, the hemoglobin electrophoresis in β-thalassemia characteristically shows elevations in **HbA2** ($\alpha_2\delta_2$), a minor hemoglobin variant comprising 2% to 3% of normal hemoglobin in adults, and, in more severe cases, HbF.

Patients with severe thalassemia have symptoms related to ineffective erythropoiesis, anemia, and iron overload. Ineffective erythropoiesis leads to **extramedullary expansion** of erythropoietic tissue in the spleen, liver, skull, and long bones. Bony expansion in the skull causes typical morphological features of frontal bossing and chipmunk facies due to hypertrophy of the maxillae, characteristically seen in the β-thalassemias; bone expansion in the long bones leads to instability and pathological fractures.

While most thalassemia patients are able to maintain hemoglobin concentrations of ≥7 g/dL on their own, those with more severe disease require red cell transfusion support for survival. Anemia is most extreme in the case of hydrops fetalis, where no functional hemoglobin is produced to support the growing fetus, which becomes grossly edematous with a massively hypertrophied placenta, resulting in fetal demise in utero or neonatal death shortly after delivery due to hypoxemia and high-output heart failure. Even in patients with less severe forms of thalassemia, heart failure due to anemia remains a problem in the absence of adequate transfusional support, along with developmental delays, growth retardation, and poor exercise tolerance.

Iron overload, both endogenous and iatrogenic due to transfusions, causes much of the morbidity of the thalassemias. Iron deposits preferentially in the liver, leading to liver failure and cirrhosis, and in the heart, leading to restrictive cardiomyopathy and heart failure. In the absence of iron chelation therapy, nearly every organ in the body can be affected, with untreated patients often having hypogonadism and infertility (due to iron deposition in the testes and ovaries) and diabetes (due to iron overload in the pancreas).

TREATMENT

The main treatment of the thalassemias is supportive care, consisting of red cell transfusions to manage anemia and iron chelation to manage iron overload. Transfusions are required primarily in β-thalassemia major and begin early in life to maintain hemoglobin levels in the range of 9 to 10 g/dL. Splenectomy has also historically been performed in many pediatric patients with β-thalassemia major to alleviate the severity of the hemolytic anemia and offer some transfusion independence, although the effect is short lived, with most splenectomized patients eventually requiring reinstatement of transfusion therapy later in life.

The goal of **iron chelation** therapy is to reduce ferritin levels to <2500 ng/mL, or <1000 ng/mL if possible. Several forms of iron chelation agents are available, the major ones being deferoxamine (available in intravenous or subcutaneous formulations), deferasirox (oral), and deferiprone (oral). Deferoxamine and deferasirox have side effects or retinal toxicity and ototoxicity, so patients on these agents require routine ophthalmological and audiological examination. Deferiprone can rarely cause agranulocytosis. Liver and cardiac MRI with specialized iron quantitation protocol is rapidly emerging as an accepted, noninvasive methodology to accurately gauge therapeutic response to iron chelation at the end-organ level.

As with other inherited disorders of hemoglobin, hematopoietic SCT is curative, but this requires the patient to have a human leukocyte antigen (HLA)–matched donor and accept the associated risks of myeloablation and transplant. As donors may be unavailable and the risks of SCT remain significant, gene therapy to substitute functional globin genes represents a promising therapeutic approach. A 2018 study of patients with transfusion-dependent β-thalassemia transduced native CD34 cells with a lentivirus encoding HbA and reinfused those cells into patients following myeloablative conditioning. All patients saw a reduced need for transfusions at 26 months.

CHAPTER 142

Microangiopathic Hemolytic Anemia (MAHA)

DEBBIE JIANG

INTRODUCTION

Microangiopathic hemolytic anemia (MAHA) results when red blood cells (RBCs) are sheared apart in obstructed small blood vessels. These cells, known as **schistocytes,** are the defining feature of MAHA and are readily identified on a peripheral blood smear (Fig. 142.1).

MAHA is distinguished from other subtypes of hemolytic anemia, where hemolysis occurs from intrinsic membrane defects (e.g., hereditary spherocytosis), faulty enzyme function (e.g., glucose-6-phosphate dehydrogenase [G6PD] deficiency), immune-mediated destruction (e.g., autoimmune hemolytic anemia), or mechanical trauma in the large vessels (e.g., prosthetic heart valves). An overview of the approach to hemolytic anemia is shown in Fig. 142.2.

When the microvasculature becomes occluded by thrombus, or when the endothelial lining of the microvasculature is damaged and contributes to MAHA, the pathological term **thrombotic microangiopathy (TMA)** is applied. The TMAs are diverse but characteristically present with MAHA, thrombocytopenia, and end-organ damage. Many different disease states can lead to the development of TMA, and the pathophysiology of TMA depends on the underlying condition. The most common cause is **disseminated intravascular coagulopathy (DIC).** In severe sepsis leading to DIC, overactivation of the coagulation cascade results in obstructing thrombi that break apart circulating RBCs (see Chapter 144 for a detailed discussion).

Other causes of include **thrombotic thrombocytopenic purpura (TTP),** Shiga-mediated **hemolytic uremic syndrome (HUS),** atypical HUS (aHUS), drug-induced TMA, **malignant hypertension, severe preeclampsia,** the **HELLP syndrome** (hemolysis, elevated liver enzymes, low platelets), catastrophic antiphospholipid syndrome, cancer, HIV infection, autoimmune disease, vasculitis, and cocaine use.

OVERVIEW OF PATHOPHYSIOLOGY AND EVALUATION

The primary pathology in the TMAs is the formation of platelet-rich microthrombi in the microvasculature. On pathological evaluation, the vessel walls are thickened with myointimal concentric proliferation (described as onion skinning), and swollen capillary endothelial cells may be observed detaching from the basement membrane. Although these pathological changes can occur in any microvascular bed, the renal vasculature is particularly susceptible and represents a preferred site for biopsy when a diagnosis of TMA must be established on pathological grounds.

Malignancy can cause TMA through DIC or through the production of micrometastases occluding the vasculature. Autoimmune diseases such as systemic sclerosis or systemic lupus erythematosus may result in microvascular damage and occlusion as a result of immune complex deposition on endothelial surfaces. Vasculitides, including polyarteritis nodosa and granulomatosis with polyangiitis, can also lead to TMA through vascular inflammation leading to endothelial injury.

MAHA/TMA figures prominently in the differential diagnosis of a patient with new-onset anemia and thrombocytopenia. When confronted with such findings, a peripheral smear is necessary to confirm the presence of schistocytes and thrombocytopenia, both of which are required for a diagnosis of TMA; generally, the finding of ≥ 2 schistocytes per 100× high-power field is consistent with MAHA. Supporting laboratory studies should demonstrate intravascular hemolysis with a markedly high lactate dehydrogenase (LDH), a low haptoglobin, indirect hyperbilirubinemia, and an elevated reticulocyte count. Since the hemolytic anemia in MAHA is mechanical rather than immune driven, Coombs testing is negative.

Once MAHA/TMA is confirmed, additional history and evaluation are crucial to determine the etiology.

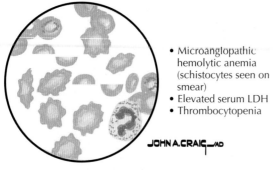

- Microangiopathic hemolytic anemia (schistocytes seen on smear)
- Elevated serum LDH
- Thrombocytopenia

JOHN A. CRAIG—MD

FIG. 142.1 **Schistocytes.** *LDH,* Lactate dehydrogenase.

As a general rule, the three major types of TMA that must always be ruled out are DIC, TTP, and HUS. DIC is characterized by a consumptive coagulopathy that results in abnormal coagulation tests (i.e., a prolongation of the prothrombin time and partial thromboplastin time, elevation of the D-dimer level, and a decrease in fibrinogen level). By contrast, these coagulation parameters in TTP and HUS are normal, since the pathology of these disorders arises from platelet-rich microthrombi or vascular obstruction without coagulopathic changes.

If the coagulation studies do not suggest DIC, then the general dogma is that patients with MAHA/TMA are

Site of RBC destruction	
Intravascular: blood vessels	**Extravascular: spleen**
↑↑↑ LDH ↓↓ haptoglobin ↑ reticulocyte response ↑ indirect bilirubin E.g.: cold autoimmune hemolytic anemia, thrombotic microangiopathy, disseminated intravascular coagulation	↑ LDH ↓ or normal haptoglobin ↑ reticulocyte response ↑ indirect bilirubin E.g.: warm autoimmune hemolytic anemia, hereditary spherocytosis, G6PD deficiency, sickle cell disease, thalassemia

Immune vs. nonimmune	
Immune	**Nonimmune**
Warm autoimmune hemolytic anemia • DAT: IgG+, C3+/– • Smear: RBC spherocytes • Causes: medications, autoimmune disease, lymphoma **Cold autoimmune hemolytic anemia** • DAT: IgG–, C3+ • Smear: RBC agglutination • Causes: EBV, Mycoplasma, lymphoma (esp. Waldenstrom macroglobulinemia)	Hereditary spherocytosis G6PD deficiency Sickle cell disease Thalassemia Thrombotic microangiopathy Disseminated intravascular coagulation

Intrinsic vs. extrinsic to RBC	
Intrinsic to RBC	**Extrinsic to RBC**
Hereditary spherocytosis G6PD deficiency Sickle cell disease Thalassemia	Warm autoimmune hemolytic anemia Cold autoimmune hemolytic anemia Thrombotic microangiopathy Disseminated intravascular coagulation

FIG. 142.2 **Hemolytic Anemia: Categorization Based on Site of Red Blood Cell** *(RBC)* **Destruction, Immune/Nonimmune, or Intrinsic/Extrinsic to RBC.** *DAT,* Direct antiglobulin test; *EBV,* Epstein-Barr virus; *G6PD,* glucose-6-phosphate dehydrogenase; *LDH,* lactate dehydrogenase.

considered to have TTP or HUS unless another cause of microangiopathy can be readily identified. The reason for this is that TTP/HUS are viewed as "can't-miss" diagnoses that must be acted upon immediately whenever they are encountered.

TREATMENT OVERVIEW AND SPECIFIC CLINICAL ENTITIES

The role of blood product transfusion in MAHA/TMA is primarily supportive. In patients with DIC, transfusions of packed RBCs, platelets, fresh frozen plasma, and cryoprecipitate are sometimes given to keep platelet counts, hemoglobin, coagulation studies, and fibrinogen at appropriate levels. In TTP, platelet transfusions have historically been contraindicated due to a concern that this might trigger a flare of TTP, although more recent data have challenged this assertion.

Disseminated Intravascular Coagulation

For patients with DIC, treatment is aimed at the underlying cause. The most common causes of DIC are sepsis and severe infection. Malignancy may also cause a chronic DIC picture. See Chapter 144 for further details.

Thrombotic Thrombocytopenic Purpura

In TTP, the originating defect results from a severe deficiency (<10%) in **ADAMTS13,** the metalloproteinase responsible for cleaving **von Willebrand factor** (vWF). This deficiency can be inherited, as occurs in Upshaw-Schulman syndrome, or (more commonly) acquired through the development of autoantibodies against ADAMTS13. A deficiency in ADAMTS13 leads to the development of unusually large vWF multimers, resulting in platelet aggregation, occluding the microvasculature and resulting in thrombocytopenia and MAHA (Fig. 142.3).

Approximately 2.9 in 1 million adults are diagnosed with TTP each year. Classically, the clinical presentation of TTP is described by a pentad of fever, anemia, thrombocytopenia, renal failure, and altered mental status. In reality, the classic pentad occurs in only 5% of patients; neurological findings are common (with one-third of patients having nonspecific findings such as headache or confusion, and one-third having focal abnormalities), while fever is rare and kidney injury usually absent or minimal. As such, in the modern era, the presence of schistocytes and thrombocytopenia without coagulopathy and without another established cause are sufficient for a putative diagnosis of TTP. In a patient with suspected TTP, an ADAMTS13 level should be sent in the acute setting; an ADAMTS13 <10% strongly

supports a diagnosis of TTP, while a complete absence of ADAMTS13 is 89% sensitive and 100% specific for TTP. However, some patients with TTP may have an ADAMTS13 level >10%, which can be iatrogenic from platelet transfusions or the result of interassay variation.

As indicated, patients with schistocytes, thrombocytopenia, and normal coagulation studies are considered to have TTP or HUS until proven otherwise. Upfront, such patients are usually empirically treated for TTP. The standard of care for treatment of TTP is **plasma exchange (PLEX),** which removes antibodies against ADAMTS13 and adds back normal ADAMTS13. PLEX is generally continued until the platelet count normalizes for 2 days. Some investigators follow ADAMTS13 levels after recovery from TTP based on emerging data that such levels might predict TTP relapse. Rituximab, a monoclonal antibody against CD20, may have a role in preventing and treating such relapses.

Hemolytic Uremic Syndrome (Shiga Mediated)

Shiga-mediated HUS, also known as classic HUS, is characteristically associated with *Escherichia coli* **O157:H7** infection, although *Shigella, Yersinia,* and other strains of *E. coli* have been implicated as well. The Shiga toxin directly damages and causes swelling of the endothelium, occluding the microvasculature. Shiga toxin may also induce secretion of abnormally large multimers of vWF.

Shiga-mediated HUS primarily affects children. The classic presentation is of a patient who is exposed to contaminated water or undercooked meats and then develops acute bloody diarrhea and abdominal pain. The development of HUS usually occurs about 5 to 10 days after onset of gastrointestinal symptoms. Acute kidney injury (AKI) is common, with as many as 50% of patients requiring temporary dialysis (Fig. 142.4). Neurological manifestations can be present in 30% to 60% of patients. Stool testing for Shiga toxin-producing bacteria such as *E. coli* O157:H7 is generally performed as part of the standard diagnostic workup.

Most patients with Shiga-mediated HUS make a full recovery with supportive care, including hydration and platelet transfusions for severe thrombocytopenia or active bleeding. Dialysis is sometimes used temporarily until renal function improves. Antibiotics are not given, as they usually do not improve outcomes and may increase HUS risk due to release of more Shiga toxin from intestinal bacteria.

Atypical Hemolytic Uremic Syndrome

aHUS is caused by derangements in the alternative complement pathway. About 60% of cases have an

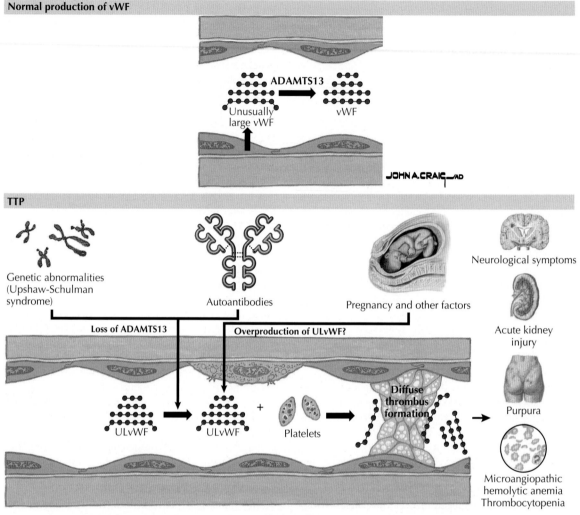

Normal production of vWF

ADAMTS13

Unusually large vWF

vWF

JOHN A.CRAIG—AD

TTP

Genetic abnormalities (Upshaw-Schulman syndrome)

Autoantibodies

Pregnancy and other factors

Neurological symptoms

Acute kidney injury

Loss of ADAMTS13

Overproduction of ULvWF?

ULvWF

ULvWF

+

Platelets

Diffuse thrombus formation

Purpura

Microangiopathic hemolytic anemia Thrombocytopenia

FIG. 142.3 **Thrombotic Thrombocytopenic Purpura** *(TTP)*. *ULvWF*, Ultra-large von Willebrand factor; *vWF*, von Willebrand factor.

identifiable mutation in a gene encoding an alternative complement factor (e.g., *C3*) or one of the regulatory factors in the alternative complement cascade (e.g., *MCP*, *CFB*, *CFH*, *CFI*, or *THBD*). The unregulated activation of alternative complement proteins throughout the body causes endothelial injury and platelet dysregulation and aggregation.

aHUS is a rare disease, afflicting 0.5 to 2 patients per million. It is more often seen in children than in adults, but the diagnosis should be considered in all patients who are putatively given a diagnosis of TTP but do not respond to standard TTP therapy, who have an ADAMTS13 level >10%, or in patients who do not

fit the typical presentation of TTP, HUS, or other forms of MAHA/TMA. In contrast to TTP, AKI is a common feature of aHUS.

Most patients with aHUS are initially treated for TTP with PLEX before a diagnosis of aHUS is made. Patients with MAHA/TMA whose platelet counts do not respond to PLEX, who have >10% ADAMTS13 activity, or who have significant renal dysfunction should be considered for targeted treatment of aHUS. Primary treatment of aHUS in the modern era is eculizumab, a terminal complement inhibitor, which alleviates hemolysis and leads to improved renal function and overall outcomes, albeit at the expense of an increase in infectious risk

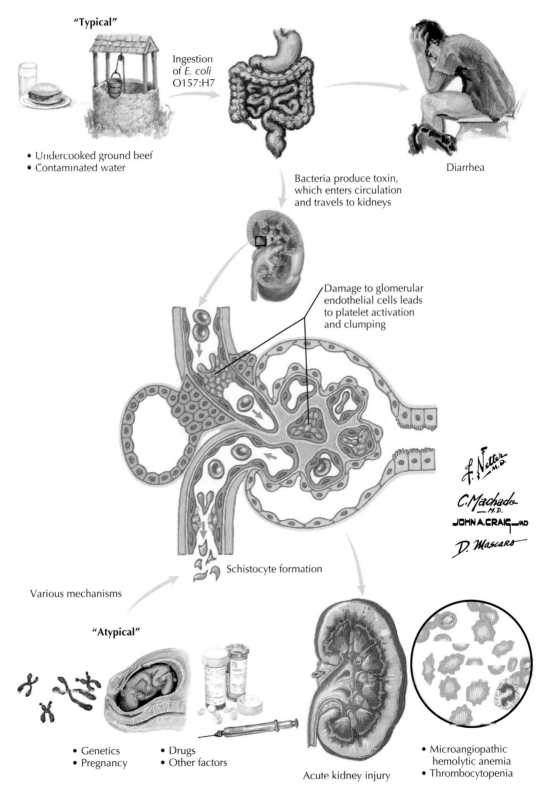

"Typical"

Ingestion
of *E. coli*
O157:H7

• Undercooked ground beef
• Contaminated water

Diarrhea

Bacteria produce toxin,
which enters circulation
and travels to kidneys

Damage to glomerular
endothelial cells leads
to platelet activation
and clumping

Schistocyte formation

Various mechanisms

"Atypical"

• Genetics
• Pregnancy
• Drugs
• Other factors

Acute kidney injury

• Microangiopathic
  hemolytic anemia
• Thrombocytopenia

FIG. 142.4 **Hemolytic Uremic Syndrome.**

from encapsulated bacteria. As such, patients who are being planned for eculizumab therapy must be vaccinated for meningococcus prior to initiation of this drug.

Drug-Induced Thrombotic Microangiopathy

Medications like calcineurin inhibitors and quinine have been implicated in drug-induced TMA. In the case of quinine, an immune-mediated response driven by quinine-dependent antibodies is thought to cause endothelial injury. These patients present with acute TMA after quinine exposure. On the other hand, calcineurin inhibitors have a direct, dose-dependent toxic effect on endothelial cells, leading to gradual microvascular occlusion and chronically worsening renal function. Withdrawal of the offending agent and supportive care are cornerstones of management.

Malignant Hypertension, Preeclampsia, HELLP

In malignant hypertension, preeclampsia, and HELLP syndrome, elevated blood pressure causes damage to arterioles, resulting in leakage of prothrombotic inflammatory factors such as fibrinogen into the lumen of the vessel. Direct endothelial cell injury and death occurs, giving rise to the term **fibrinoid necrosis** in describing the fibrin-staining necrosis seen on biopsy. There is also emerging literature supporting a role for complement dysregulation in preeclampsia and HELLP syndrome, similar to aHUS. Aggressive blood pressure control as in hypertensive emergency may be all that is required in malignant hypertension. Patients with preeclampsia and HELLP syndrome should receive blood pressure control and supportive care, and both conditions generally resolve following fetal delivery.

CHAPTER 143

Hemophilia

FAHAD FARUQI

INTRODUCTION

Hemophilia, from the Greek words *haima*, meaning "blood," and *philia*, meaning "to love," is a group of recessive genetic disorders of coagulation. Patients with hemophilia are prone to bleeding. Depending on the severity of the disease, some hemophilia patients bleed only after major trauma or surgery, while others bleed spontaneously. Three major types of hemophilia are recognized, each defined by an impairment of one coagulation factor: **hemophilia A** (factor VIII deficiency), **hemophilia B** (factor IX deficiency), and **hemophilia C** (factor XI deficiency). Famously, the royal families of Europe in the 18th and 19th centuries were afflicted with hemophilia B.

PATHOPHYSIOLOGY

Factor VIII, factor IX, and factor XI are part of the intrinsic pathway of the coagulation cascade (see Chapter 34). The coagulation cascade begins with the extrinsic pathway and activation of factor VII by tissue factor. Activated factor VIIa forms a tenase complex that converts factor X to activated factor Xa, generating a prothrombinase complex that converts prothrombin to activated thrombin, which in turn converts fibrinogen into fibrin. Thrombin also activates the intrinsic pathway, including factor VIII, which complexes with activated factor IX. The factor VIIIa/IXa complex activates thousands of factor X molecules, amplifying coagulation beyond the initial extrinsic pathway trigger, leading to hemostasis. Thrombin also activates factor XI, which activates factor IX, further augmenting the coagulation cascade. Without adequate levels of factors VIII, IX, and XI, the body's ability to form stable clots becomes impaired.

Hemophilia A demonstrates X-linked inheritance, as the gene for factor VIII, *F8*, resides on the X chromosome. The disease predominantly affects males and is seen at a frequency of about 1 in 5000 male births. A number of different mutations in *F8* have been described, the most common of which is an inversion of the long arm of the X chromosome found in 40% of patients with severe hemophilia A. Deletions and nonsense mutations may also give rise to severe hemophilia A, while missense mutations tend to cause mild disease.

Hemophilia B also demonstrates X-linked inheritance, as the gene for factor IX, *F9*, is located on the X chromosome. Hemophilia B is comparatively rare, affecting 1 in 30,000 male births. About one-third of affected individuals present as index cases with no family history of bleeding, possibly due to de novo mutations in *F8* or *F9*. Females with heterozygous *F8* or *F9* mutations are technically considered disease carriers but may display a mild hemophiliac phenotype owing to lyonization of one of the two X chromosomes, which further reduces factor VIII or IX levels.

Hemophilia C inheritance is autosomal recessive as the factor XI gene, *F11*, is located on chromosome 4. It is more common than the other two types of hemophilia and has a predilection for Ashkenazi Jews, about 10% of whom are carriers.

PRESENTATION, EVALUATION, AND DIAGNOSIS

In hemophilia A and B, the severity of bleeding correlates with factor VIII and IX activity, respectively. Patients with <1% factor VIII or IX activity have spontaneous bleeding and are classified as having **severe** hemophilia. Patients with a factor VIII or IX activity between 1% and 5% bleed mostly after minor injury or procedures and are classified as having **moderate** hemophilia. Patients with a factor VIII or IX activity between 5% and 20% tend to bleed only with procedures and are classified as having **mild** hemophilia.

The pattern of bleeding in hemophilia tends to be coagulopathic rather than mucosal (Fig. 143.1). In mucosal bleeding, as exemplified by von Willebrand disease and platelet function disorders, bleeding occurs immediately after trauma to the mucosal surfaces, and petechial skin lesions are common. In coagulopathic bleeding, as exemplified by the hemophilias, bleeding is

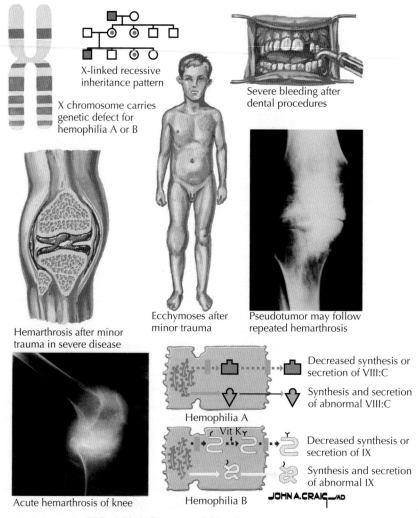

X-linked recessive
inheritance pattern

X chromosome carries
genetic defect for
hemophilia A or B

Severe bleeding after
dental procedures

Hemarthrosis after minor
trauma in severe disease

Ecchymoses after
minor trauma

Pseudotumor may follow
repeated hemarthrosis

Decreased synthesis or
secretion of VIII:C

Synthesis and secretion
of abnormal VIII:C

Hemophilia A

Vit K

Decreased synthesis or
secretion of IX

Synthesis and secretion
of abnormal IX

Hemophilia B

Acute hemarthrosis of knee

JOHN A.CRAIG—AD

FIG. 143.1 **Patterns of Bleeding in Hemophilia.**

often delayed in onset; deep bruising is common while petechiae are rare, and patients typically do not bleed excessively from minor skin injuries but have significant postsurgical bleeding. The differences in these bleeding patterns reflect distinctions between primary versus secondary hemostasis. However, considerable overlap between the two processes exists, and many patients with mucosal or coagulopathic defects have similar bleeding manifestations such as epistaxis, gastrointestinal bleeding, or hematuria (see Chapter 34).

The majority of patients with hemophilia A or B have severe disease and present within the first year of life. In severe hemophilia, bleeding occurs spontaneously, and bleeding sites mirror growth, development,

and physical activity. During the neonatal period, intracranial hemorrhage arising from delivery, and bleeding with circumcision, may occur. Infants and toddlers demonstrate spontaneous hemorrhage into joint spaces, termed **hemarthrosis,** which commonly involves the knees, elbows, ankles, hips, or shoulders, with certain target joints being preferentially affected more than others. Hemarthrosis usually begins as mild joint pain and tenderness but progresses rapidly over the course of hours to severe pain, warmth, swelling, and limited range of motion. Repeated episodes of untreated or undertreated hemarthrosis eventually give way to hemophilic arthropathy, characterized by chronic joint damage with persistent, severe limitations in range of motion, inflammation in the joint space, synovitis, and (eventually) joint space narrowing.

Patients with mild or moderate hemophilia A or B usually do not experience significant bleeding in the absence of trauma or procedures, although moderate hemophilia A and B patients still may experience recurrent hemarthrosis and develop hemophilic arthropathy. For patients with hemophilia C, bleeding risk is unpredictable and does not necessarily correlate with factor XI activity. Bleeding typically occurs after surgery, but spontaneous bleeding is unusual. Postsurgical bleeding is particularly prevalent in tissues with high fibrinolytic activity such as the teeth, tonsils, nose, and genitourinary tract. Menorrhagia, postpartum hemorrhage, and bleeding after circumcision are common.

All boys with unexplained bleeding manifestations should be evaluated for hemophilia. Laboratory testing for suspected hemophilia beings with measurements of the prothrombin time (PT) and the activated partial thromboplastin time (aPTT). In patients with hemophilia, the PT will be normal and the PTT prolonged due to defects in the intrinsic pathway of the coagulation cascade. If the PTT is prolonged, a 1:1 PTT mixing study should be performed and activities of factors VIII, IX, and XI obtained. The complete workup of an abnormal PTT is described in detail in Chapter 34. An isolated decrease in factor VIII, IX, or XI activity with an aPTT that corrects on a 1:1 mixing study will confer a diagnosis of hemophilia.

TREATMENT

Treatment of hemophilia A and B has evolved significantly in the last 50 years. In the past, fresh frozen plasma was used, which has relatively low concentrations of factors VIII and IX, necessitating that high volumes of plasma be given. Cryoprecipitate, derived from plasma and enriched in factor VIII, offered more robust delivery of factor VIII in treatment of hemophilia A. Purified factor VIII and IX products represented a major advance in the care of hemophilia A and B. However, the repeated administration of these blood products over time rendered patients at high risk for transfusion-related infection with HIV, hepatitis B, and hepatitis C. Screening for these conditions among blood donors dramatically reduced the risk of transfusion-related infections, but ultimately the advent of recombinant factor VIII and IX products revolutionized hemophilia care.

Patients with severe hemophilia A or B are usually treated with prophylactic intravenous infusions of recombinant factor VIII or IX to prevent hemarthroses and the subsequent development of hemophilic arthropathy. In some patients with severe hemophilia A or B, repeated administration of factor VIII or IX may lead to the generation of specific coagulation factor inhibitors that impair the efficacy of factor replacement; treatment of such patients can be enormously challenging, and strategies to address this must be individualized. Patients with mild or moderate hemophilia A or B usually do not require prophylactic factor replacement but may need hemostatic support for invasive procedures; for major procedures, factor VIII or IX replacement is often given beforehand and sometimes afterward, while for minor procedures, desmopressin, a hormone that stimulates the release of factor VIII and von Willebrand factor from endothelial cells, may be used. Antifibrinolytic agents such as tranexamic acid or aminocaproic acid may also be adjunctive measures to reduce bleeding risk. Gene therapy in hemophilia A and B is a topic of active research, with some encouraging studies in the literature.

Patients with severe hemophilia A or B also often suffer other long-term complications. Because bleeding problems and hemostatic interventions begin early in life, psychosocial difficulties are common, especially during the adolescent and young adult years. Obesity is common due to inactivity. Dental health is frequently poor owing to aversion to tooth brushing because of bleeding risk.

Hemophilia C is treated differently from hemophilia A and B. In hemophilia C, fresh frozen plasma is used for treatment and prevention of bleeding in the United States, while purified factor XI is available in the United Kingdom and is preferentially used there.

CHAPTER 144

Disseminated Intravascular Coagulation

FAHAD FARUQI

INTRODUCTION

Disseminated intravascular coagulation (DIC) is a systemic process characterized by uncontrolled activation of the **coagulation cascade** leading to the formation of thrombi in the microvasculature of one or more organs in the body. The excessive activation of the coagulation cascade consumes the body's supply of coagulation factors and leads to fibrinolysis, which in turn increases the risk of hemorrhage.

PATHOPHYSIOLOGY

Normal hemostasis requires a delicate balance between coagulation to prevent hemorrhage and fibrinolysis to facilitate tissue repair (see Chapter 34 for a discussion of normal coagulation). DIC disrupts this balance through massive activation of both coagulation and fibrinolysis. Some forms of DIC are characterized predominantly by excessive formation of fibrin-containing thrombi; in such cases, end-organ damage predominates as the primary cause of morbidity and mortality. In other instances of DIC, hyperfibrinolysis predominates, and bleeding becomes the major presenting symptom.

DIC is not a primary disorder but is instead triggered by another underlying pathological process such as infection, sepsis, trauma, pancreatitis, malignancy, an obstetrical complication, severe intravascular hemolysis (e.g., from a hemolytic blood transfusion reaction), or envenomation (Fig. 144.1). The initiating event in DIC is activation of intravascular coagulation through exposure to procoagulant molecules, particularly tissue factor (TF). Increased levels of TF may arise through a number of different mechanisms, including endothelial cell damage (as occurs in trauma), lipopolysaccharide exposure (as seen in sepsis), cancer (with TF being produced by some cancer cell types), or monocyte activation (as occurs during a hemolytic transfusion reaction). Damage-associated molecular patterns (DAMPs) such as cell-free deoxyribonucleic acid (DNA), extracellular

histones, and high-mobility group box 1 (HMGB1) protein are thought to mediate central roles in DIC. These DAMPs assemble in neutrophil extracellular traps (NETs) that arise through NETosis, in which dying neutrophils release their intracellular contents and form extracellular webs of chromatin, histones, and other materials, which together activate coagulation. Inflammatory cytokines such as interleukin-6 and tumor necrosis factor-α exert changes on a number of procoagulant and anticoagulant proteins, leading to a hypercoagulable state.

Unlike normal thrombogenesis, coagulation in DIC is not limited to a specific site of vasculature injury; instead, fibrin formation occurs throughout the circulatory system and especially in the microvasculature. These thrombi cause shearing of red blood cells as they traverse the microvasculature, resulting in a **microangiopathic hemolytic anemia** (i.e., **thrombotic microangiopathy [TMA]**; see Chapter 142). Due to excessive coagulation, platelets are consumed, leading to thrombocytopenia. The excessive clot burden activates fibrinolysis; tissue plasminogen activator is released, which converts plasminogen to plasmin, degrading fibrin and other coagulation factors. Levels of natural anticoagulant proteins such as antithrombin, protein C, and protein S decrease, perpetuating the formation of microthrombi and triggering further activation of coagulation and fibrinolysis cascades.

PRESENTATION, EVALUATION, AND DIAGNOSIS

DIC should be suspected in any patient with abnormal bleeding or clotting manifestations, as these may be indicators of dysregulated hemostasis. Since DIC is typically a secondary phenomenon, an underlying cause must be evaluated, and the presentation of DIC will differ accordingly. Clinically, DIC may be an acute or chronic process. Acute DIC is commonly seen in severe infection, trauma, or obstetrical complications. Chronic

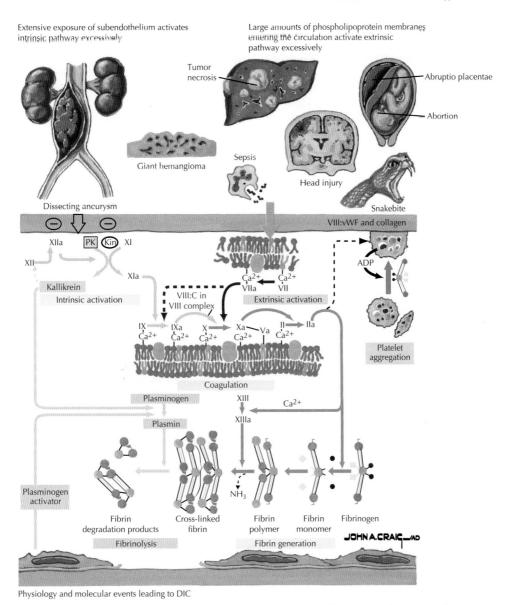

Extensive exposure of subendothelium activates intrinsic pathway excessively

Large amounts of phospholipoprotein membranes entering the circulation activate extrinsic pathway excessively

Tumor necrosis

Abruptio placentae

Abortion

Giant hemangioma

Sepsis

Head injury

Dissecting aneurysm

Snakebite

VIII:vWF and collagen

XIIa   PK Kin   XI

XII

ADP

Kallikrein

Intrinsic activation

Xa
VIIa   Ca2+   Ca2+
VII

Extrinsic activation

VIII:C in
VIII complex

IX   IXa   X   Xa   Va   II   IIa
Ca2+   Ca2+   Ca2+   Ca2+   Ca2+

Platelet aggregation

Coagulation

Plasminogen

XIII   Ca2+

Plasmin

XIIIa

Plasminogen activator

NH3

Fibrin
degradation products   Cross-linked fibrin   Fibrin polymer   Fibrin monomer   Fibrinogen

JOHN A. CRAIG—AD

Fibrinolysis

Fibrin generation

Physiology and molecular events leading to DIC

FIG. 144.1 Some Causes of and Molecular Events Leading to Disseminated Intravascular Coagulation (DIC). *ADP,* Adenosine 5′-diphosphate.

DIC is characteristically associated with malignancy—an exception being **acute promyelocytic leukemia** (APL), which causes acute DIC with life-threatening hemorrhage if not treated promptly.

Acute DIC patients often have petechiae, purpura, and other bleeding symptoms as a result of **consumptive coagulopathy**. They may demonstrate oozing from catheter insertion sites, wounds, and mucosal surfaces. In more severe cases, hemorrhagic skin necrosis and diffuse purpura in a reticular pattern may be seen, and major hemorrhage, including gastrointestinal bleeding or intracranial hemorrhage, may occur. End-organ damage from microthrombi can lead to acute kidney injury and oliguria, and jaundice from liver injury and TMA is also common. Thrombi within the cerebral vascular beds can cause seizures, focal neurological deficits, and altered mental status. The following laboratory findings are characteristically seen:

1. Prolongation of the prothrombin time (PT) and/or activated partial thromboplastin time (aPTT), which arises as a consequence of depleting coagulation factors
2. A reduced platelet count, which arises due to platelet consumption
3. A low **fibrinogen** level, which results from consumption of fibrinogen
4. An increase in **D-dimer** or fibrin-split products, which results from increased fibrin clot formation and fibrinolysis

Chronic DIC patients may be asymptomatic. PT, PTT, fibrinogen, and platelet counts may be normal, although D-dimer levels will invariably be high.

Because of TMA, both acute and chronic DIC patients typically have abnormal hemolytic markers, including an increase in lactate dehydrogenase (LDH) and reduction in haptoglobin. The peripheral blood smear in DIC will often show schistocytes due to TMA, although these may be seen in any TMA process and are not specific to DIC.

A common differential diagnosis encountered in clinical medicine is DIC versus the coagulopathy of advanced liver disease. The liver is the major site of production for almost all coagulation factors except factor VIII, which is produced by endothelial cells. Patients with cirrhosis or advanced liver disease often have prolonged PT and/or PTT values and low fibrinogen levels. On laboratory testing, the two can be distinguished by measuring a factor VIII level, which is typically elevated in advanced liver disease but low in DIC.

TREATMENT

The mainstay of DIC management is to treat the underlying cause. However, even if the underlying cause of DIC is promptly treated, endothelial damage will take time to repair, and patients may remain in DIC well after their underlying clinical syndrome has resolved. As a result, transfusion support is often indicated in treatment of acute DIC to prevent bleeding complications. The exact parameters for transfusion are not universally agreed upon, but most investigators believe that packed red blood cells may be transfused to maintain hemoglobin levels >7 g/dL and that platelets may be administered to maintain the platelet count >10,000 to 20,000/μL in the absence of bleeding or 50,000/μL if there is significant bleeding. In some instances, fresh frozen plasma may be transfused to normalize PT and PTT values. **Cryoprecipitate** (which is enriched in fibrinogen, von Willebrand factor, factor VIII, and factor XIII) may be transfused to maintain the fibrinogen level above a certain threshold, usually 50 to 150 mg/dL, if there is active bleeding.

Patients with acute DIC due to APL require urgent treatment of APL, usually with all-trans retinoic acid–containing and/or arsenic trioxide–containing regimens, in addition to transfusion support. In APL, platelets and cryoprecipitate are transfused to maintain platelet counts and fibrinogen levels at higher levels than in other forms of DIC due to an extremely high risk of bleeding. The prognosis of APL with DIC is excellent as long as treatment is initiated early and transfusion support is aggressively maintained. By contrast, chronic DIC in the setting of other types of malignancy does not require transfusion support and generally does not alter the management of patients with cancer, although it is viewed as an adverse prognostic marker.

CHAPTER 145

Hypercoagulable States and Deep Venous Thrombosis

MIA DJULBEGOVIC

INTRODUCTION

Hypercoagulable states are characterized by an increased tendency to form blood clots. The typical manifestation is **venous thromboembolism (VTE)**, defined as **deep venous thrombosis (DVT)** or **pulmonary embolism (PE)**. DVT refers to thrombosis of the deep veins in the leg or pelvis (iliac, femoral, popliteal, or calf veins), or in the arm (subclavian, axillary, brachial, or brachiocephalic). DVT is distinct from **superficial thrombophlebitis,** which refers to thrombosis of the peroneal or saphenous vein of the leg or the cephalic vein in the arm. A common misconception is the classification of the superficial femoral vein, which is in fact a deep vein. Annually in the United States, up to 900,000 people will develop VTE, to which up to 100,000 deaths are attributed.

PATHOPHYSIOLOGY AND RISK FACTORS

In the 1800s, German physician Rudolph Virchow proposed three factors to explain VTE, known as **Virchow triad:** vessel wall injury, stasis of blood flow, and hypercoagulability. Classically, platelets were thought to play a minor role in venous thrombosis, whereas arterial thrombosis was viewed as a predominantly platelet-rich clot. Thrombophilia, defined as a hypercoagulable state due to a disorder of plasma coagulation, was observed to more commonly manifest as venous, rather than arterial, thrombosis.

A number of reversible factors may increase the risk of developing VTE (Table 145.1). In addition, five major heritable thrombophilias have been identified that underlie ~20% of VTE cases:

- **Factor V Leiden (FVL):** This is the most common heritable thrombophilia, affecting ~5% of whites but fewer (<1%) blacks (or African Americans) or Asians. The molecular basis is a point mutation in the factor V gene, which converts an arginine at position 506 to glutamine (R506Q), rendering the factor V protein resistant to cleavage by the activated protein C (APC)

complex, which normally functions in termination of the coagulation cascade by cleaving activated factors Va and VIIIa. The risk of VTE in patients with FVL is enormously magnified in the presence of estrogen, as both conditions cause APC resistance.

- **Prothrombin gene mutation:** This is the second most common heritable thrombophilia, affecting 1% to 5% of whites but far fewer (≤0.2%) blacks (or African Americans) or Asians. The molecular basis is a point mutation that converts guanine nucleotide into adenosine at position 20210 in the 3′ untranslated region of the factor II gene (G20210A), leading to increased prothrombin gene expression.

- **Antithrombin deficiency:** This is a rare thrombophilia, affecting 0.2% to 0.4% of the population. The phenotype arises from a deficiency in antithrombin, which normally functions to cleave and inactivate multiple activated coagulation factors in the intrinsic and common coagulation cascade (e.g., factors XIIa, XIa, IXa, Xa, and IIa), particularly in the presence of heparin.

- **Protein C deficiency:** This thrombophilia, affecting 0.2% to 0.5% of the population, arises from a deficiency in protein C, part of the APC complex that cleaves and inactivates factors Va and VIIIa.

- **Protein S deficiency:** This thrombophilia, affecting 0.1% of all patients, arises from a deficiency in protein S, part of the APC complex.

Patients who are heterozygous for one of the heritable thrombophilias already mentioned have a fourfold to tenfold increase in VTE risk compared to the general population. However, for those with homozygous or compound heterozygous thrombophilia mutations, the risk of VTE in some instances is higher. That said, the majority of patients with a heritable thrombophilia do not develop VTE, owing to incomplete penetrance of the thrombophilia genes and a number of epigenetic and environmental factors that further modulate VTE risk. The risk of VTE is higher with the factor deficiencies (antithrombin, protein C, and protein S deficiency) than

TABLE 145.1
Risk Factors for Venous Thromboembolism

High Risk	Moderate Risk	Low Risk
Fracture of the hip/leg	Prior VTE	Travel (>4 hours)
Total hip/knee replacement	Thrombophilia (inherited or acquired)	Bedrest (>3 days)
Major thoracic or abdominal surgery (>30 min of anesthesia)	Cancer	Tobacco use
	Foreign body (e.g., central venous catheter)	
	Hormone therapy (OCPs, estrogen, testosterone)	
	Pregnancy or postpartum state	

OCPs, Oral contraceptive pills; *VTE,* venous thromboembolism.
Modified from Anderson FA, Spencer FA: Risk factors for venous thromboembolism, *Circulation* 107(23 suppl 1):I-9–I-16, 2003.

with FVL or prothrombin gene mutation, but the latter two are more prevalent.

Several acquired thrombophilias have been described. Some of the most important are:

- **Antiphospholipid syndrome (APS):** This is a disorder characterized by the development of antiphospholipid antibodies that lead to venous or arterial thrombosis or, in women, recurrent pregnancy morbidity. The condition has clinical overlap with systemic lupus erythematosus and immune thrombocytopenia, with many patients having all three conditions.
- Cancer: The hypercoagulable state of malignancy was first described in the 1860s by French physician Armand Trousseau, who noted migratory superficial thrombophlebitis in several cancer patients (including, later on, himself). Termed **Trousseau syndrome,** the hypercoagulability of malignancy was eventually observed to encompass not only superficial vein thrombosis but also DVT, PE, and other types of venous and arterial thrombotic events. It was historically described as a feature of mucin-producing solid tumor malignancies such as pancreatic, gastric, or lung cancer, although later studies identified an increased risk of thrombosis in numerous other types of cancers, including lymphoma and other hematological malignancies. Several mechanisms have been described that underlie this phenomenon, including production of tissue factor by cancer cells, release of tumor microparticles containing tissue factor and other hypercoagulable factors, increased expression of cell adhesion molecules and proinflammatory cytokines, and activation of platelets in cancer.
- **Heparin-induced thrombocytopenia (HIT):** This is a condition characterized by the development of venous or arterial thrombosis following exposure to heparin. The pathogenic basis is the generation of antibodies against complexes of platelet factor 4 (a component of α-granules in platelets) and heparin,

leading to platelet activation, thrombocytopenia, and thrombosis. It generally occurs ≥4 days after exposure to unfractionated heparin or, less commonly, low molecular weight heparin.

PRESENTATION, EVALUATION, AND DIAGNOSIS

DVT typically presents with pain, edema, and erythema in the affected leg (Fig. 145.1). PE may present as tachypnea, tachycardia, hypoxia, shortness of breath, cough, hemoptysis, and/or chest pain (see Chapter 89 for further information). Given the broad differential diagnoses for patients presenting with these symptoms (e.g., cellulitis and DVT can present similarly, as can acute coronary syndrome, pericarditis, and PE), scoring systems can help determine the clinical probability of VTE and need for additional diagnostic testing. The **Wells score for DVT or PE** can calculate the pretest probability of DVT or PE, respectively, and can help guide further workup. A commonly used blood test is the **D-dimer** level, a breakdown product of fibrinolysis and laboratory marker of acute thrombosis. If the pretest probability of VTE by Wells score is low and a D-dimer level is negative, then VTE is unlikely; by contrast, patients with a low pretest probability of VTE and a positive D-dimer test, or those with moderate-to-high pretest probability by Wells score, should undergo imaging studies. For evaluation of DVT, venous compression Doppler ultrasound is the diagnostic test of choice (Fig. 145.2). The preferred test for diagnosis of PE is CT angiography. When intravenous contrast is contraindicated (such as in renal disease or pregnancy), ventilation/perfusion scanning is a safe alternative.

Once VTE is diagnosed, the next step is to categorize it as **provoked, unprovoked,** or **cancer associated.** This distinction will determine the risk of VTE recurrence and will guide duration of anticoagulation. A provoked VTE arises as a result of a major, reversible thrombotic risk

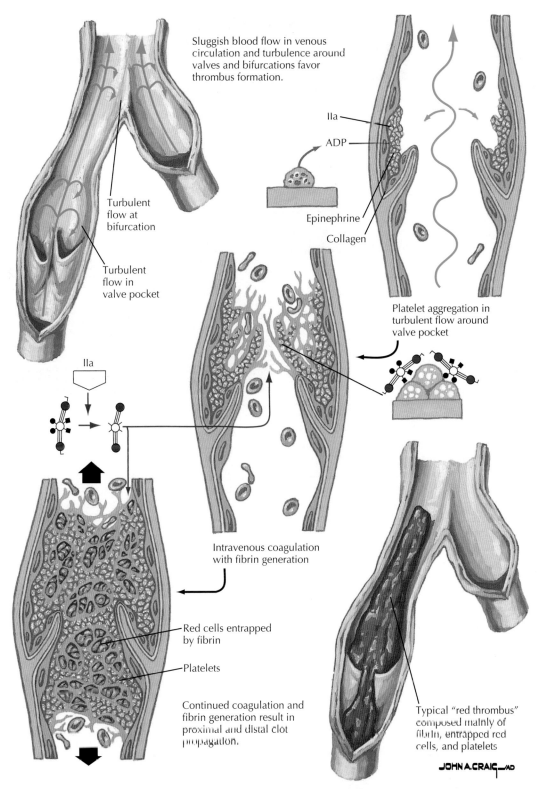

Sluggish blood flow in venous circulation and turbulence around valves and bifurcations favor thrombus formation.

IIa

ADP

Epinephrine

Collagen

Turbulent flow at bifurcation

Turbulent flow in valve pocket

Platelet aggregation in turbulent flow around valve pocket

IIa

Intravenous coagulation with fibrin generation

Red cells entrapped by fibrin

Platelets

Continued coagulation and fibrin generation result in proximal and distal clot propagation.

Typical "red thrombus" composed mainly of fibrin, entrapped red cells, and platelets

JOHN A. CRAIG—AD

FIG. 145.1 **Formation of a Deep Venous Thrombosis.** *ADP,* Adenosine diphosphate.

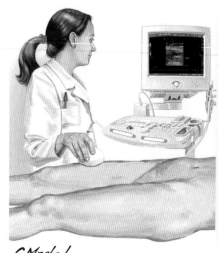

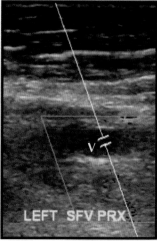

Duplex ultrasound. Notice lack of blood flow (no color or flow wave pattern) in occluded, left superficial femoral vein (*V*).

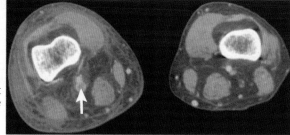

CT venography. CT exam through the legs shows a clot in the right femoral vein (*arrow*). Overall increased size of right thigh compared with left thigh with increased soft tissue swelling and edema is visible.

FIG. 145.2 Ultrasound and CT Diagnosis of Deep Venous Thrombosis.

factor such as major general surgery or major trauma, or prolonged immobility. An unprovoked VTE arises in the absence of a reversible thrombotic risk factor. The literature indicates that among patients with provoked VTE who complete an initial period of anticoagulation, the risk of VTE recurrence after anticoagulation is stopped is very low, while for those with unprovoked VTE, the risk of clot recurrence after cessation of anticoagulation is higher. Many patients have minor thrombotic risk factors, the spectrum of which is detailed in Table 145.1; for such patients, the risk of VTE recurrence is intermediate between wholly provoked and unprovoked VTE.

Cancer-associated VTE arises as a result of cancer or cancer therapy and has a higher risk of clot recurrence as long as the cancer remains active. About 5% to 10% of patients with unprovoked VTE will be diagnosed with cancer 1 year later; as a result, it is advised that all patients with unprovoked VTE have symptom-directed and age-appropriate cancer screening.

The possibility of thrombophilia as a contributor to VTE risk is often considered in young patients with VTE, or those with family histories of first-degree relatives with VTE. At least half of all cases of VTE have a genetic basis, as the presence of a first-degree relative with VTE increases the risk of a first VTE event, even if no inherited thrombophilia is detectable. However, to date, no study has definitively demonstrated that thrombophilia testing impacts medical management of VTE insofar as duration or intensity of anticoagulation is concerned. As such, thrombophilia testing should not be done in patients with provoked VTE, as the results do not impact medical management, and the utility of thrombophilia testing in evaluation of unprovoked VTE is uncertain, although many patients and providers favor pursuing it for informative purposes. When performed, thrombophilia testing should not be obtained during an acute thrombotic event or during anticoagulation since either can influence test results. Specific tests to work up the major heritable thrombophilias are as follows:

- FVL: The screening test for this is APC resistance test, which measures resistance of the factor V protein to APC cleavage. If the APC resistance test is abnormal, then this should be followed by a genetic test, which examines for the presence of the FVL mutation.
- Genetic testing for the prothrombin gene mutation G20210A.

- Antithrombin deficiency: This is evaluated by measuring antithrombin antigen and activity levels. A low antigen and activity level characterize type I antithrombin deficiency (a quantitative deficiency in amount of protein). A normal antigen and low activity characterize type II antithrombin deficiency (a qualitative deficiency due to an impairment in protein function).
- Protein C deficiency: Like antithrombin deficiency, protein C deficiency is evaluated by measuring protein C antigen and activity levels, which characterize type I (quantitative) from type II (qualitative) deficiencies. It is important to note that warfarin will decrease protein C and protein S levels and therefore impact these test results.
- Protein S deficiency: This is evaluated by measuring protein S functional (a measure of protein S activity), protein S total antigen, and protein S free antigen. A reduction in all three characterizes type I protein S deficiency, while a reduction in protein S functional with normal total and free antigen defines type II deficiency. Type III deficiency is characterized by low functional and free antigen levels.

Among the acquired thrombophilias, APS deserves special mention, owing to some unique clinical and laboratory features. APS is an acquired thrombophilia due to autoantibodies against phospholipid-associated proteins. APS can be primary (due to an unknown cause) or secondary (in the setting of rheumatological disease, malignancy, or drugs). The diagnosis requires:

- Clinical criteria: These include a history of prior venous or arterial thrombosis, unexplained pregnancy complication, or unexplained pregnancy loss (i.e., three first-trimester miscarriages or one late miscarriage).
- Laboratory criteria: These include three tests, known as **lupus anticoagulant, anticardiolipin antibodies,** and **anti-β$_2$-glycoprotein antibodies.** False-positive lupus anticoagulant results may occur in the setting of acute thrombosis or concomitant anticoagulation. It is also worth noting that patients with positive lupus anticoagulant often have prolongation of coagulation factor tests, particularly the partial thromboplastin time (PTT). The reason for this is that the PTT reaction used to measure the PTT value is dependent on the presence of free phospholipids, which are titrated in the presence of antiphospholipid antibodies leading to prolongation of clotting times in vitro, even though the clinical phenotype is an increased risk of thrombosis rather than bleeding.
- To establish a diagnosis of APS, patients must meet clinical criteria and must have at least one laboratory test positive on two occasions, 12 weeks apart.

TREATMENT
Acute Management

Patients presenting with acute VTE require therapeutic anticoagulation to prevent thrombus extension, embolization, and recurrence. **Direct oral anticoagulants (DOACs)** have comparable efficacy to **vitamin K antagonists (VKA)** and may even demonstrate lower bleeding according to some studies. DOACs include factor Xa inhibitors (rivaroxaban, apixaban, and edoxaban) and the direct thrombin inhibitor dabigatran. **Low molecular weight heparin (LMWH), intravenous unfractionated heparin (UFH),** and fondaparinux are alternatives, or can be used as bridging to warfarin when non-VKA are contraindicated (such as mechanical heart valve). Bridging refers to overlapping a non-VKA with warfarin until the INR is ≥2 (typically at least 5 days), which may be necessary when using a VKA due to comparatively earlier inhibition of protein C and protein S than factors II, VII, IX, and X by VKA, leading to increased thrombogenesis when a VKA is first initiated. Pregnant patients presenting with acute VTE should be treated with LMWH, since DOACs and VKA are contraindicated in pregnancy. LMWH is also the preferred anticoagulant in cancer-associated VTE. The treatment of isolated DVT of the distal leg veins (which includes the paired peroneal, posterior tibial, and anterior tibial veins) is controversial given the lower risk of proximal thrombus extension and embolization.

Inferior vena caval filters (IVCF) are only indicated when the risk of bleeding outweighs the benefits of anticoagulation in the acute setting. Since IVCF are thrombogenic and increase the risk of recurrent VTE, anticoagulation should be started as soon as bleeding risk permits, and retrievable IVCF should be removed as soon as possible. Patients presenting with hemodynamic instability due to massive PE should receive systemic thrombolysis (preferred over catheter-directed thrombolysis). High-risk patients, including those with a higher bleeding risk, or patients with submassive PE who may eventually require systemic thrombolysis, should be treated with UFH due to ease of reversibility. See Chapter 89 for further details on classification and treatment of PE.

When possible, risk factor avoidance or modification is essential to acute VTE management. Estrogen therapy and estrogen-containing contraceptives are contraindications in the setting of new or prior VTE and should be discontinued. Progestins generally do not confer hypercoagulability, and low-dose progestin-only contraceptives in pill form or intrauterine devices can be used after adequate anticoagulation; the thrombogenicity of depot progestin remains controversial.

Duration of Anticoagulation

Patients presenting with a provoked VTE event should discontinue anticoagulation after 3 months of treatment. The duration of anticoagulation is a more complex decision in unprovoked VTE. Since patients with unprovoked VTE have a higher risk of recurrence after discontinuation of anticoagulation, long-term anticoagulation should be considered. Factors associated with a higher risk of VTE recurrence include male gender, younger age, and a positive D-dimer 1 month after discontinuing anticoagulation. The role for surveillance compression ultrasonography to guide treatment in patients with prior DVT is unclear and currently not considered the standard of care. Prediction models such as the DASH score (<u>D</u>-dimer, <u>a</u>ge, <u>s</u>ex, <u>h</u>ormones) and Vienna model can be useful in identifying patients at a higher risk of VTE recurrence who may benefit from extended anticoagulation. Active malignancy (defined as receiving treatment within the last 6 months) carries the highest risk for VTE recurrence, and patients should continue anticoagulation as long as the cancer is active. The need for extended anticoagulation based on VTE recurrence risk should be balanced with each patient's comorbidities (e.g., need for antiplatelet therapy), bleeding risk, and personal preferences. Patients with a high risk of VTE recurrence who choose to discontinue full-dose, therapeutic anticoagulation may benefit from secondary prevention with low-dose warfarin, apixaban, rivaroxaban, or aspirin.

Bleeding Risks and Reversibility

DOACs have at least similar and perhaps favorable bleeding risk in comparison to VKA, with less intracranial hemorrhage and generally similar risks of gastrointestinal bleeding, though dabigatran and rivaroxaban might carry higher risks of gastrointestinal bleed than warfarin. One advantage of anticoagulation with VKA or UFH is easy reversibility. Coagulopathy from VKA can be reversed with vitamin K, **fresh frozen plasma,** or **prothrombin complex concentrate,** whereas protamine can be used for UFH. Among the DOACs, dabigatran can be reserved with idarucizumab, while andexanet-α is approved for reversal of life-threatening hemorrhage in patients on rivaroxaban or apixaban.

CHAPTER 146

Multiple Myeloma

MATTHEW K. LABRIOLA

INTRODUCTION

Multiple myeloma (MM) is a type of hematological malignancy known as a **plasma cell dyscrasia,** defined by a proliferation of malignant plasma cells. It is the second most common hematological malignancy after non-Hodgkin lymphoma, accounting for ~1% of all cancers. The median age for MM is 62 years in men and 61 years in women. MM is two times more likely to occur in African Americans than Caucasians and has a male-to-female ratio of 1.4:1. The defining clinical features of symptomatic MM are known as the **CRAB criteria** and include hypercalcemia, renal impairment, anemia, and bone disease.

PATHOPHYSIOLOGY

MM arises from malignant transformation of plasma cells of postgerminal center derivation. The disease typically originates as a premalignant condition called **monoclonal gammopathy of undetermined significance (MGUS),** which develops through the acquisition of cytogenetic abnormalities that result from antigenic stimulation. Additional genetic changes and alterations in the bone marrow microenvironment then facilitate the transformation of MGUS into MM (Fig. 146.1).

MM cells demonstrate altered expression of adhesion molecules, leading to increased interactions with the bone marrow microenvironment. These interactions stimulate cytokine secretion and the production of growth factors such as vascular endothelial growth factor, enhancing malignant plasma cell growth and triggering antiapoptotic signals that result in increased tumor cell survival. MM cells further inhibit osteoblasts and activate osteoclasts within the bony matrix itself, leading to the development of hypercalcemia and characteristic osteopenia and bone lytic lesions seen in active disease (Fig. 146.2).

The malignant plasma cells of MM produce a **monoclonal (M) immunoglobulin (Ig) protein** composed of either a κ or λ light chain, which, in the majority of cases, is complexed with a heavy chain of IgG, IgA, IgM, or IgD isotype. Because all the malignant plasma cells in MM produce the same M protein, MM may be classified by the type of light and heavy chains produced—the most common being IgG, which comprises 60% to 70% of MM cases, followed by IgA (20%) and light-chain MM (15%–20%).

M proteins cause end-organ damage through several mechanisms. The most frequent site of organ damage is the kidney in the form of light-chain cast nephropathy (i.e., MM kidney). Under normal circumstances, light chains are freely filtered across the glomerulus and are mostly reabsorbed in the proximal tubule. In MM, light-chain production exceeds tubular reabsorption, and the light chains bind to a protein called uromodulin in the nephron and form intratubular casts that cause inflammation and fibrosis. Direct reabsorption of filtered light chains in the proximal tubule also causes direct tubular injury.

In some instances, light-chain proteins themselves deposit in the glomeruli and cause glomerular damage, leading to a specific type of renal pathology known as **light-chain deposition disease (LCDD).** Light chains can also form amyloid fibrils, resulting in AL amyloidosis, which causes glomerular damage leading to nephrotic syndrome and hefty albuminuria. LCDD and amyloidosis can be distinguished on the basis of Congo red stain, which is negative in the former and positive in the latter (see Chapter 147 for a more detailed discussion).

PRESENTATION, EVALUATION, AND DIAGNOSIS

MGUS and MM are distinguished by a number of different clinical and laboratory criteria. MM itself can be further categorized as smoldering or symptomatic depending on the absence or presence, respectively, of CRAB criteria. These defining criteria are presented in Table 146.1.

MGUS is common and its prevalence a function of age. It is present in ~3% of the population in patients age >50 years and ~7.5% of the population in patients age >85 years.

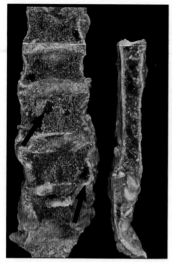

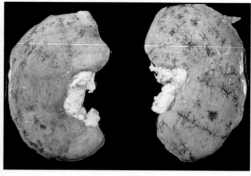

"**Myeloma kidney.**" Form of protein nephrosis caused by excessive proteinuria. Note pale color and swelling of kidneys.

Multiple myeloma infiltration of bone marrow. Causing multiple osteolytic lesions *(arrows).*

FIG. 146.1 **Multiple Myeloma.** (Reused with permission from Buja ML, Krueger GRF: *Netter's illustrated human pathology updated edition,* Philadelphia, 2013, Elsevier.)

TABLE 146.1
Diagnostic Criteria of MGUS, Asymptomatic MM, and Symptomatic MM

	MGUS	MM	
		Smoldering	Symptomatic
M protein concentration	<3 g/dL	≥3 g/dL	≥3 g/dL[a]
Bone marrow clonal plasma cells	<10%	≥10%	≥10%[b]
CRAB	No	No	Yes

[a]Serum free light chain (κ/λ or λ/κ) ratio ≥100 is defined as symptomatic MM.
[b]Bone marrow clonal plasma cells ≥60% is defined as symptomatic MM.
CRAB, Hypercalcemia, renal impairment, anemia, bone disease; *MGUS,* monoclonal gammopathy of undetermined significance; *MM,* multiple myeloma.
Data from Rajkumar SV, Dimopoulos MA, Palumbo A, et al: International Myeloma Working Group updated criteria for the diagnosis of multiple myeloma, *Lancet Oncol* 15:e538, 2014.

The major clinical features of symptomatic MM are the CRAB criteria, as defined by:

- Hypercalcemia (serum calcium >11.5 mg/dL), due to increased osteoclast activity
- Renal impairment (serum creatinine >2 mg/dL), due to toxic effects of filtered light chains leading to cast nephropathy, LCDD, AL amyloidosis, or hypercalcemia
- Anemia (hemoglobin <10 g/dL), due to bone marrow disease, anemia of renal disease, or anemia of inflammation
- Bone disease, including lytic lesions, severe osteopenia, or pathological fracture

Constitutional symptoms such as fatigue, weakness, and weight loss are common in MM. Recurrent infections can occur from suppression of normal immunoglobulins by the malignant plasma cell clone (a phenomenon known as immunoparesis) and leukopenia from proliferation of clonal myeloma cells within bone marrow. Neuropathy due to monoclonal gammopathy can also occur as a result of several mechanisms (see Chapter 148 for a brief discussion on Waldenstrom macroglobulinemia).

The initial workup of patients with suspected MM includes:

- Complete blood count (CBC), to evaluate for anemia. Note that the peripheral blood smear in MM commonly demonstrates **rouleaux** formation due to a high protein concentration.
- Basic metabolic panel, to evaluate kidney function and calcium level. Of note, the anion gap in MM is

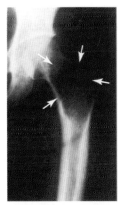

Anteroposterior view of proximal femur. Vague radiolucent lesion *(arrows)*.

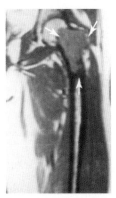

Coronal MRI. Lesion (same as above) has gray signal *(arrows)* in contrast to brighter signal of marrow fat.

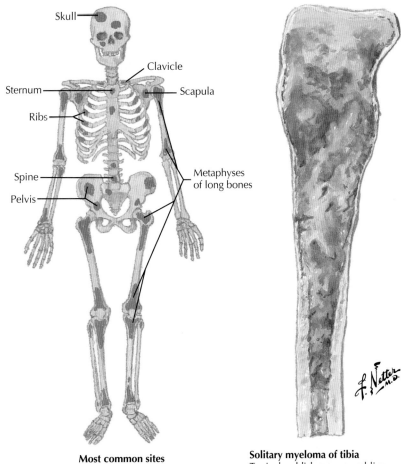

Skull

Clavicle

Sternum

Scapula

Ribs

Spine

Metaphyses of long bones

Pelvis

Most common sites of involvement

Solitary myeloma of tibia
Typical reddish gray, crumbling, soft, neoplastic tissue replaces cortices and marrow spaces. In this case, no invasion of soft tissue.

FIG. 146.2 **Bony Involvement of Multiple Myeloma.**

usually decreased due to a net positive ionic charge conferred by the excess abnormal immunoglobulin.

- Serum and urine protein electrophoresis (SPEP and UPEP, respectively). SPEP and UPEP fractionate serum and urine proteins, respectively, into albumin and the various globulin fractions (i.e., α1, α2, β, and γ), allowing for visualization of M proteins that appear as monoclonal spikes in the γ-globulin fraction. The SPEP will detect both immunoglobulin and heavy-chain M proteins and is positive in ~80% of patients. The UPEP is more sensitive for light-chain M proteins and may be positive in many instances where the SPEP is negative.

- Serum and urine immunofixation electrophoresis (SIFE and UIFE, respectively). SIFE and UIFE allow

for identification of specific immunoglobulin and heavy-chain M proteins identified on abnormal SPEP and UPEP studies.

- Serum and urine free light chains (FLC). The FLC assay is among the most sensitive tests to evaluate for M protein. Abnormal κ/λ ratios are suggestive of monoclonal gammopathy. In patients with an established diagnosis of MM, FLC may also be followed to gauge treatment response.

- Quantitative immunoglobulins. This assay measures the concentrations of IgG, IgM, and IgA heavy chains and is the most accurate means of quantitating the amount of heavy-chain protein.

- Bone marrow biopsy with cytogenetic analysis and fluorescence in situ hybridization (FISH). A bone marrow biopsy is required to quantitate the percentage of plasma cells in the marrow. Cytogenetic and FISH analyses confer important prognostic and therapeutic information.

- Skeletal survey, to evaluate for lytic bone lesions. The skeletal survey is essentially a whole-body x-ray study and is the major radiological exam to look for lytic bone lesions in MM, although more recently, MRI has emerged as a more sensitive imaging modality. If a patient with suspected MM has focal pain without lesion seen on x-ray, then CT or MRI should be obtained. Bone scan is not sensitive for detecting lytic lesion and is not routinely utilized in the workup of suspected MM.

Once a diagnosis of MM is established, the **International Staging System (ISS)** is used to further characterize the disease. The ISS is based on two laboratory markers, β_2 microglobulin and albumin, both measured from the serum, as follows:

- Stage I, defined as β_2 microglobulin <3.5 mg/L and albumin ≥3.5 g/dL. The median overall survival of ISS stage I MM is 62 months.
- Stage II, defined as β_2 microglobulin <3.5 mg/L and albumin <3.5 g/dL, OR β_2 microglobulin 3.5 to 5.5 mg/L. Median survival of stage II MM is 44 months.
- Stage III, defined as β_2 microglobulin ≥5.5 mg/L. Median survival of stage III MM is 29 months.

TREATMENT

Patients with MGUS and smoldering MM can be observed but carry a risk for progression to symptomatic MM. The rate of such progression for MGUS is 1% per year with a lifetime risk of 25%, while the rate of progression for SMM is considerably higher at 10% per year for the first several years. Once a diagnosis of MGUS is established, close observation is necessary with measurements of blood counts, renal function, calcium, and M protein tests within 6 months of the initial diagnosis and then annually if the tests are stable. The initial management of SMM is similar to MGUS except that the interval for repeat testing is shorter, although there are some emerging data in support of treatment of select SMM patients with high-risk features.

Patients with symptomatic MM require immediate treatment. MM is a very steroid-responsive disease, so all treatment approaches utilize steroids in the form of dexamethasone or prednisone. Historically, the mainstay of MM treatment was autologous stem cell transplant (ASCT) using a conditioning regimen of high-dose melphalan (a myeloablative alkylating agent) and steroids. ASCT resets the disease back by several years and may be considered for patients <70 years of age with good performance status and without severe comorbidities such as congestive heart failure or end-stage renal disease. Unfortunately, many MM patients are transplant ineligible, and in the past, therapies for such patients were limited.

Over the past few decades, the therapeutic landscape in MM has been dramatically transformed by the development of numerous targeted agents, including proteasome inhibitors (e.g., bortezomib or carfilzomib), immunomodulatory drugs (e.g., thalidomide, lenalidomide, or pomalidomide), and newer agents such as elotuzumab (an inhibitor of CD319) and daratumumab (an inhibitor of CD38). The explosion of these therapeutic options in MM, most of which are very well tolerated and have excellent responses when given in combination with each other and with steroids, have revolutionized the treatment of MM, essentially converting it from an acutely lethal malignancy into a chronic disease in the vast majority of patients. Toxicities with these agents are generally manageable and include thrombocytopenia and thromboembolic disease with lenalidomide, peripheral neuropathy and zoster reactivation with bortezomib, and heart failure with carfilzomib. Presently it is unclear what the optimal role of ASCT is in the context of these multiple, targeted therapeutic options in MM.

Treatment of MM also entails symptomatic management. To protect patients from further bone disease, bisphosphonates should be initiated and local radiation should be utilized if the patient has a known bony lesion. Denosumab, a receptor activator of nuclear factor κB (RANK) ligand inhibitor, may also be used. Patients with cast nephropathy require intravenous fluids and immediate initiation of antineoplastic therapy to decrease their light-chain load.

CHAPTER 147

Amyloidosis

WAQAS A. MALICK

INTRODUCTION

Amyloidosis is a group of protein folding disorders characterized by the extracellular deposition of insoluble protein **fibrils**. The protein fibrils are composed of misfolded protein subunits that assume a common antiparallel, β-pleated sheet-rich structural conformation leading to the formation of higher-order oligomers. Amyloid diseases are classified according to whether they are systemic or localized, acquired or inherited, and their clinical patterns. There are several types of systemic amyloid disorders, named by the convention "A" followed by an abbreviation of the misfolded protein, which include the following:

- **AL amyloid** (previously known as primary systemic amyloidosis): This is the most commonly encountered type of amyloidosis, in which the amyloid protein is comprised of immunoglobulin light chains from a plasma cell dyscrasia.
- **AA amyloidosis** (previously referred to as **secondary amyloidosis**): This is characterized by amyloid protein formed from serum amyloid A (SAA), an acute phase reactant produced by the liver.
- **AF amyloid** (previously referred to as **familial amyloidosis**): This is mostly due to heritable mutations in the *ATTR* gene, which encodes prealbumin.
- **Senile systemic amyloidosis:** This has significant overlap with familial amyloidosis in that it arises from the ATTR protein, but in senile systemic amyloidosis the ATTR protein is wild type, and hence the disease is acquired.
- **AB$_2$M amyloidosis** (also known as dialysis-related amyloidosis): This arises from deposition of β$_2$-microglobulin, whose levels accumulate in patients with end-stage renal disease and dialysis.

This chapter will provide a brief overview of these disorders, including pathophysiology, clinical presentation and evaluation, and treatment.

PATHOPHYSIOLOGY AND EPIDEMIOLOGY

In general, amyloidosis results from extracellular tissue deposition of amyloid fibrils, which are insoluble polymers comprised of low molecular weight subunit proteins. Fibrils form when mutations lead to disruption of protein folding mechanisms, recycling, or disposal mechanisms. The effect of these mutations is compounded by the presence of a disorder leading to increased production of precursor amyloidogenic proteins, such as a plasma cell dyscrasia or chronic inflammation.

AL amyloidosis is due to the deposition of protein derived from immunoglobulin light-chain fragments produced in plasma cell dyscrasias, most commonly multiple myeloma (see Chapter 146), although Waldenstrom macroglobulinemia/lymphoplasmacytic lymphoma and other non-Hodgkin lymphomas can also rarely give rise to this. AL amyloidosis is the most common type of systemic amyloidosis in North America with an estimated incidence of 4.5 cases per 100,000.

AA amyloidosis is typically due to the increased production of the precursor protein SAA, which is produced in the liver as an acute phase reactant and serves as a chemoattractant for monocytes and lymphocytes and an inducer of cytokine release. Elevated levels of SAA have been found in rheumatoid synovium. Chronic inflammation causes elevation of SAA levels, which leads to fibril formation and deposition.

AF amyloidosis encompasses a vast array of autosomal dominant diseases. The most common form of AF amyloidosis is due to mutations in the *TTR* (**transthyretin**) **gene** (referred to as ATTR amyloidosis), which encodes prealbumin. There are over 100 TTR mutations associated with ATTR amyloidosis. TTR deposits composed of wild type, unmutated TTR fibrils also occur with aging, leading to senile amyloidosis. This type of amyloidosis is rare, with an estimated incidence of <1 per 100,000 cases in the United States. However, the incidence of inherited cardiac amyloidosis due to TTR mutations may be as high as 3% to 4% in African Americans in the United States.

Dialysis-related amyloidosis is seen in patients with end-stage renal disease who have been on hemodialysis for a prolonged period of time. Patients on dialysis are unable to clear circulating β$_2$-microglobulin, which leads to increased deposition of β$_2$-microglobulin amyloid.

However, it is believed improvements in dialysis membranes are likely leading to a decrease in the incidence of dialysis-related amyloidosis.

PRESENTATION, EVALUATION, AND DIAGNOSIS

The presentation of amyloidosis largely depends on the amount of amyloid deposition and the organs in which amyloid is deposited. Most commonly, amyloidosis involves the heart, kidneys, gastrointestinal (GI) tract, nervous system, and musculoskeletal system (Fig. 147.1). The diagnosis of amyloidosis requires tissue sampling of affected organs, which displays a characteristic apple-green birefringence on **Congo red staining**. Mass spectrometry is typically done to confirm the specific type of amyloid protein.

Amyloid cardiomyopathy is common in AL and TTR amyloidosis. A restrictive cardiomyopathy can develop due to the deposition of amyloid in cardiac muscle, leading to both systolic and diastolic dysfunction and presenting symptoms of heart failure, presyncope, or angina. Characteristic electrocardiographic findings include low-voltage QRS complexes, a pseudoinfarction pattern with pathological Q waves, and—in some instances—heart block. A transthoracic echocardiogram will show increased left ventricular wall thickness and diastolic dysfunction in the earliest stages, whereas more advanced disease may have right ventricular diastolic dysfunction as well; a classic starry-sky pattern to the myocardium is no longer considered specific to amyloidosis, owing to advances in echocardiographic techniques in general. Brain natriuretic peptide levels are often markedly elevated in cardiac amyloidosis. Cardiac MRI and technetium-pyrophosphate nuclear imaging offer quite specific modalities for noninvasive testing for amyloidosis. A right heart catheterization with endomyocardial biopsy should follow all of these tests to confirm the diagnosis.

Renal amyloidosis typically occurs with AL and AA amyloidosis. The clinical manifestations will vary depending on the site of deposition of amyloid in the kidneys (Fig. 147.2). Most commonly, amyloid is deposited in the glomeruli, and patients present with asymptomatic proteinuria that progresses to nephrotic syndrome. A urinalysis typically shows proteinuria while the urine

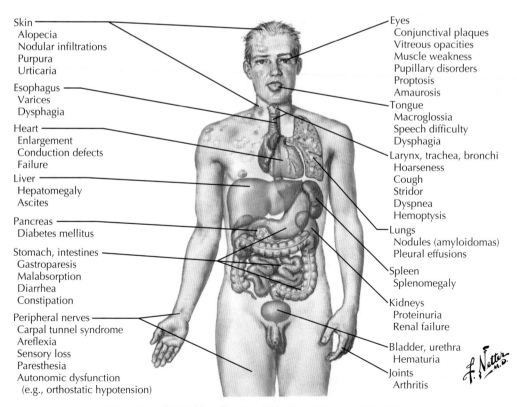

FIG. 147.1 **Deposition Sites and Manifestations of Amyloidosis.**

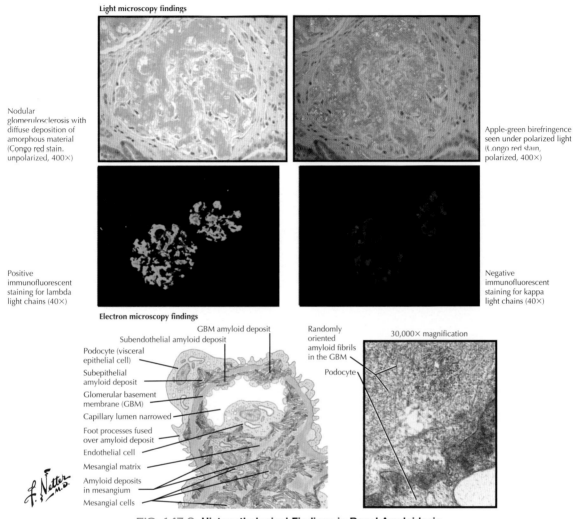

Light microscopy findings

Nodular glomerulosclerosis with diffuse deposition of amorphous material (Congo red stain, unpolarized, 400×)

Apple-green birefringence seen under polarized light (Congo red stain, polarized, 400×)

Positive immunofluorescent staining for lambda light chains (40×)

Negative immunofluorescent staining for kappa light chains (40×)

Electron microscopy findings

GBM amyloid deposit
Subendothelial amyloid deposit
Podocyte (visceral epithelial cell)
Subepithelial amyloid deposit
Glomerular basement membrane (GBM)
Capillary lumen narrowed
Foot processes fused over amyloid deposit
Endothelial cell
Mesangial matrix
Amyloid deposits in mesangium
Mesangial cells

Randomly oriented amyloid fibrils in the GBM
Podocyte
30,000× magnification

FIG. 147.2 **Histopathological Findings in Renal Amyloidosis.**

sediment is bland. A diagnosis of renal amyloidosis can be confirmed with renal biopsy.

Other sites of amyloid deposition include the GI tract, nervous system, and musculoskeletal system. Depending on the site of deposition in the GI system, patients can present with hepatomegaly, splenomegaly, gastroparesis, constipation, or intestinal dysmotility. For neurological presentations, patients can present with abnormalities in the peripheral nervous system, autonomic nervous system (with orthostatic hypotension being a classic manifestation), and (rarely) central nervous system. Amyloid can also deposit in the joints, periarticular soft tissues, and muscles, leading to symptoms of muscle swelling

and carpal tunnel syndrome. Patients with amyloidosis may also have coagulopathy, most commonly acquired factor X deficiency leading to bleeding, bruising, and prolongation of the prothrombin time and the activated partial thromboplastin time.

Diagnosis of systemic amyloidosis requires tissue biopsy in a patient with high suspicion for amyloidosis. Biopsies can be obtained from either site of clinical involvement (kidneys, GI tract, heart) or uninvolved sites such as fat pads, salivary glands, or rectal mucosa. An abdominal fat pad aspiration and biopsy represent a common diagnostic method, but the sensitivity of this is low.

TREATMENT

The treatment of amyloidosis is targeted at the underlying diseases leading to amyloidosis. For patients with AL amyloidosis, therapy targeting the underlying plasma cell dyscrasia is indicated (typically a combination of cyclophosphamide, bortezomib, and dexamethasone, or, in patients who fail this combination, the CD38 inhibitor daratumumab). Treatments to alleviate manifestations of organs affected by amyloid deposition should also be pursued, such as diuretics for heart failure management in patients with cardiac amyloidosis. Some forms of hereditary amyloidosis due to proteins produced in the liver can be treated with liver transplantation, preferably if early in the disease course. Research is ongoing into potential treatments that interfere with precursor protein production or inhibit fibril formation (e.g., tafamidis for ATTR).

CHAPTER 148

Lymphoma

MICHAEL J. GRANT

INTRODUCTION

Neoplasms of the lymphoid cell lines are divided into leukemias and lymphomas. Typically, the lymphoid leukemias are characterized by circulating malignant lymphoid cells in the blood and bone marrow, while lymphomas present as a malignant lymph node mass. The distinction between the two, however, is often blurred, as many lymphoid leukemias have lymph node involvement, and many lymphomas have circulating malignant B cells or bone marrow infiltration. This section will focus on lymphomas.

Lymphomas may be derived from precursor or mature B cells, precursor or mature T cells, or natural killer cells. Classically, lymphomas are separated into two broad categories: **Hodgkin lymphoma (HL)** and **non-Hodgkin lymphoma (NHL).**

HODGKIN LYMPHOMA

HL is an uncommon malignancy, comprising 10% of all lymphomas worldwide, with ~8500 new cases diagnosed in the United States each year. Two major types of HL have been described, with distinct clinical presentations and biology: classical Hodgkin lymphoma (cHL) and nodular lymphocyte predominant Hodgkin lymphoma (NLPHL); of these, cHL is much more common and is the focus of this chapter.

Epidemiologically, HL has a slight male predominance and a bimodal age distribution, with peaks in the early 20s and in the seventh decade and beyond. Risk factors for HL include prior infection with Epstein-Barr virus (EBV, the primary causative agent of infectious mononucleosis) or HIV, use of immune suppression agents (e.g., in transplant patients or those with autoimmune diseases), or familial factors that are less well defined.

The most common presenting symptom is **lymphadenopathy,** which is typically painless and affects the cervical or supraclavicular nodes. "B" symptoms, defined as fever, drenching night sweats, or unintended weight loss, may be present for weeks to months preceding the diagnosis; a recurring fever with a predictable periodicity, known as the Pel-Ebstein fever, is rare but characteristic of the disease. Many patients have a mediastinal mass or mediastinal enlargement from lymphadenopathy noted on chest x-ray, but cardiopulmonary symptoms such as chest discomfort, dyspnea, or cough are unusual. Pruritus is fairly common. A rare but pathognomonic feature is pain at involved lymph node sites following alcohol ingestion.

The defining pathological feature of cHL is the **Reed-Sternberg (RS) cell,** which represents the malignant cell of cHL. RS cells are large, with characteristic bilobed owl's eye nuclei (Fig. 148.1). They are of B-cell origin but lack CD19, CD20, and other common B-cell surface markers and instead are usually positive for CD15 and CD30 on immunohistochemistry. The involved lymph nodes in HL typically have few RS cells and instead have a large inflammatory infiltrate containing eosinophils, plasma cells, monocytes, histiocytes, and other lymphocytes. Four histological subtypes of cHL have been described, based on the type of inflammatory infiltrate present: nodular sclerosis (the most common subtype, characterized by bands of fibrous, sclerotic tissue separating clusters of inflammatory cells), lymphocyte rich (containing a preponderance of lymphocytes), lymphocyte depletion (containing few lymphocytes), and mixed cellularity (containing a broad mixture of cell types).

cHL first develops at central lymph node regions in the upper body, then progresses anatomically in linear fashion through contiguous lymph node chains. The physical exam in patients with cHL should therefore evaluate all lymph node chains, particularly in the cervical and supraclavicular regions. Hepatosplenomegaly is sometimes present in advanced stage disease.

A definitive diagnosis of HL can only be established by pathological evaluation of involved tissue. Excisional biopsy of a malignant node is the preferred diagnostic test, as this allows for a complete pathological evaluation of RS cells and lymph node architecture. Core needle biopsy and fine-needle aspiration are often inadequate in the evaluation of cHL due to the paucity of RS cells

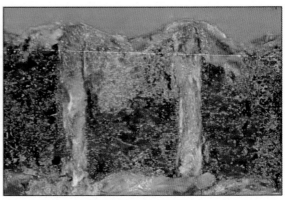

Gross infiltration of spleen in Hodgkin disease

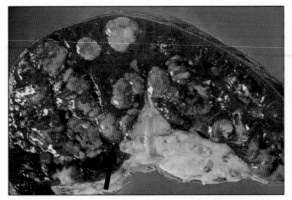

Gross infiltration of spine in Hodgkin disease

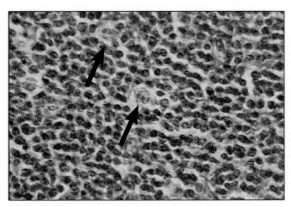

Lymphocyte-predominant type of Hodgkin disease. With only occasional Hodgkin and Reed-Sternberg cells (arrows)

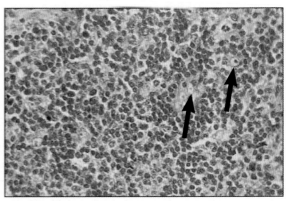

Mixed cellularity type of Hodgkin disease. With mixed population of lymphocytes, histiocytes (which may show epithelioid features), eosinophils, Hodgkin and Reed-Sternberg cells (arrows)

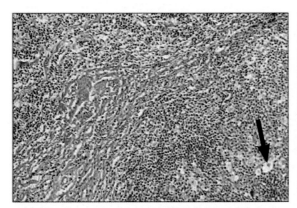

Nodular sclerosis type (C1) of Hodgkin disease. With paracortical atrophy, fibrosis, and typical lacunar-type Hodgkin and Reed-Sternberg cells (arrow)

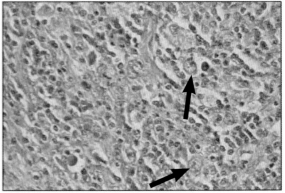

Lymphocyte-depleted type (C2) of Hodgkin disease. Showing predominance of atypical histioid blasts with many Hodgkin and Reed-Sternberg cells (arrows)

FIG. 148.1 **Gross and Microscopic Pathology of Hodgkin Lymphoma.** (Reused with permission from Buja ML, Krueger GRF: *Netter's illustrated human pathology updated edition,* Philadelphia, 2013, Elsevier.)

and the preponderance of inflammatory cells in affected lymph nodes.

As part of the workup of cHL, clinicians should obtain basic labs, including measurements of renal and liver function, albumin, and a complete blood count (CBC) with a white blood cell (WBC) differential to examine the lymphocyte count, which has prognostic significance in advanced stage cHL. HIV screening should be done. The erythrocyte sedimentation rate (ESR) has prognostic significance in early stage cHL and is routinely measured as well. Lactate dehydrogenase (LDH), though important in evaluation of NHL (as discussed later), is of little clinical relevance in cHL. All patients with a new diagnosis of cHL require a combination positron emission tomography (PET)/CT scan for staging and for monitoring disease response to therapy; CT scan alone is insufficient for the initial workup of this disease. Staging of cHL is determined by the **modified Ann Arbor staging system.**

The modified Ann Arbor staging system is a reliable gauge of anatomical progression of cHL (although the same staging system is used in NHL, as well). The prognosis of limited stage cHL depends on ESR value, the number and bulkiness of involved lymph node sites, and possibly other factors. Historically, the prognosis of advanced stage cHL was measured by the international prognostic score, containing several distinct clinical and laboratory variables (WALMASH: <u>W</u>BC count, <u>a</u>ge, <u>l</u>ymphocyte count, <u>m</u>ale gender, <u>a</u>lbumin, <u>s</u>tage, <u>h</u>emoglobin), although in recent years, interim PET/CT scans checked in the middle of therapy have proven to be useful in determining prognosis and guiding overall treatment plans.

In the past, radiation was the mainstay of treatment for cHL. Mantle radiation (i.e., radiation in a mantle or cloaklike distribution) led to cures in most patients, but almost all developed late-onset toxicities in the exposed neck and mediastinal organs (e.g., thyroid disease, breast or lung cancer, structural heart disease, early-onset coronary artery disease, or lung disease). Secondary malignancies as a result of prior intensive chemotherapy and radiation treatments exceeded the total number of deaths from cHL itself. Over time, efforts to limit radiation field exposure and to incorporate abbreviated chemotherapy regimens with low toxicity significantly improved outcomes, and in the modern era, ≥90% of patients with cHL will be cured of their disease.

For patients with limited stage cHL, the standard of care is a combination of a limited number of cycles of a chemotherapy regimen known as ABVD: <u>A</u>driamycin (<u>d</u>oxorubicin), <u>b</u>leomycin, <u>v</u>inblastine, <u>d</u>acarbazine, followed by involved-field radiation therapy (IFRT). For patients with advanced stage cHL, several cycles of ABVD are usually given; IFRT may be added in patients with bulky disease. Interim PET/CT scans performed in the middle of therapy and end-of-treatment PET/CT scans performed on completion of therapy have high predictive value for progression-free survival. In patients who relapsed after primary therapy, salvage high-dose chemotherapy and autologous stem cell transplantation are usually performed. Other salvage regimens, such as brentuximab vedotin, programmed death-1 pathway inhibitors, or allogenic stem cell transplantation, may also be used with encouraging outcomes.

NON-HODGKIN LYMPHOMA

NHL is the most common hematological malignancy, representing 90% of lymphomas worldwide, with almost 70,000 new cases diagnosed in the United States each year. There are >70 subtypes of NHL according to the World Health Organization classification system. This review will focus on the most common NHL subtypes.

Similar to cHL, the most common presentation of NHL is painless lymphadenopathy, although the distribution of lymph node involvement in NHL is variable depending on the specific subtype. Roughly one-third of NHL patients have constitutional or B symptoms.

As with cHL, excisional biopsy of an enlarged lymph node is the standard diagnostic test for evaluation of NHL. The morphological evaluation of an excised lymph node focuses on cell morphology and architecture, in addition to the proliferative index of the malignant cells, which is usually measured by a specific stain called the Ki67 index. Flow cytometry and deoxyribonucleic acid (DNA) studies such as karyotype, fluorescence in situ hybridization (FISH), and polymerase chain reaction (PCR) may aid in the diagnosis. Bone marrow biopsy is usually performed to assess marrow involvement. If central nervous system (CNS) involvement is suspected, a lumbar puncture with flow cytometry and cytopathology is required. Staging in most instances is based on the modified Ann Arbor staging system used for cHL; an updated version called the Lugano classification was formulated in 2011, which may have greater clinical relevance in NHL.

Several laboratory tests are routine in the evaluation of NHL. All patients should have basic laboratory tests of renal and liver function and a CBC with WBC differential. LDH and β_2-microglobulin measured at the time of initial diagnosis have prognostic significance. PET/CT scan is part of the standard staging of **highly aggressive** and **aggressive NHL** and may be used in some instances of **indolent NHL** to rule out localized sites of disease transformation.

To facilitate an understanding of NHL, it is useful to categorize the different types of NHL according to their clinical behavior. Highly aggressive NHLs display a very rapid onset of presentation and progression; generally, these lymphomas will lead to death within weeks if left untreated but respond well to chemotherapy. Aggressive NHLs will lead to death within months if left untreated but also respond well to chemotherapy. Indolent NHLs have a lengthy clinical course, with a survival on the order of years if left untreated, but responses to chemotherapy treatments are generally only transient, and most affected patients end up dying from complications related to their disease.

Treatment of NHL depends on the specific subtype. For highly aggressive and aggressive NHL, treatment must begin immediately and generally consists of combination chemotherapy or chemoimmunotherapy. For indolent NHL, in the absence of symptoms, cytopenias, or end-organ involvement, observation is generally preferred. Treatment outcomes in B-cell NHL have been greatly improved by the incorporation of rituximab, a monoclonal murine antibody against the CD20 antigen located on the surfaces of most B cells.

Highly Aggressive Non-Hodgkin Lymphoma

The prototypical highly aggressive NHL is **Burkitt lymphoma (BL)**, a B-cell NHL. Almost all cases of BL contain a translocation involving the c-*myc* protooncogene on chromosome 8; the most common translocation, t(8;14), places the c-*myc* gene next to the immunoglobulin variable region heavy-chain gene on chromosome 14. Histologically, BL is characterized by sheets of malignant B cells peppered with spots of macrophages actively phagocytosing apoptotic, necrotic cells, giving rise to a starry-sky pattern (Fig. 148.2); the malignant cells have a very high proliferation rate (Ki67 index ∼95%–100%). The disease is strongly associated with EBV infection. Three forms of BL are recognized: **endemic BL**, which occurs in Africa, afflicts pediatric patients, and is characterized by the development of large jaw tumors that are 100% positive for EBV; **sporadic BL**, occurring in Western nations and associated with EBV in about half of cases; and **immunodeficiency-associated BL**, occurring in HIV-positive patients and also associated with EBV in about half of cases. Prognosis is generally favorable with intensive combination chemotherapy regimens incorporating rituximab.

Aggressive Non-Hodgkin Lymphoma

The prototypical aggressive NHL is **diffuse large B-cell lymphoma (DLBCL)**, the most common subtype of NHL, which typically affects patients in their seventh decade of life. Pathologically, DLBCL is characterized by the presence of large, malignant B cells that disrupt normal lymph node architecture and have an intermediate proliferation rate (Ki67 index ∼60%–70%). Prognosis is gauged by the International Prognostic Index (IPI), which incorporates five variables (APLES: age, performance status, LDH, extranodal disease, stage), although other molecular features can affect this, including germinal center versus activated B-cell derivation of the tumor cells (as established by immunohistochemistry) and the presence or absence of c-*myc* and other gene rearrangements. The standard treatment of DLBCL is RCHOP: rituximab, cyclophosphamide, hydroxydaunorubicin (doxorubicin), Oncovin (vincristine), and prednisone, which generally leads to favorable outcomes.

Indolent Non-Hodgkin Lymphoma

Several types of indolent NHL have been described:

- **Follicular lymphoma (FL).** This is the most common indolent NHL. It presents at a median age of 60 years and has a slight female predominance. Pathologically, FL is characterized by the presence of small malignant B cells with preservation of normal lymph node architecture. The malignant B cells all contain a t(14;18) translocation involving the *BCL2* antiapoptotic gene on chromosome 18. Rituximab-containing chemoimmunotherapy regimens are often used to treat patients with symptomatic disease.

- **Marginal zone lymphoma (MZL).** MZL may arise in a number of different tissues, both nodal and extranodal. The disease develops as a result of localized immunological stimuli. The most common form is extranodal MZL of the gastrointestinal mucosa-associated lymphoid tissue (MALT), or MALToma, which typically occurs in the stomach as a result of *Helicobacter pylori* infection and can be cured with antimicrobial therapy directed against *H. pylori* (see Chapter 129 for details). Another important form is splenic MZL, which is characterized by the development of massive splenomegaly, is associated with hepatitis C infection, and can be treated effectively with rituximab or splenectomy.

- **Mantle cell lymphoma (MCL).** MCL is a disease of older men. The lymphoma cells are characterized by the presence of a t(11;14) translocation involving the cyclin D1 gene on chromosome 11. Clinically, a subset of patients may present with lymphomatous polyposis involving the gastrointestinal tract. While some cases of MCL have an indolent course, in many instances MCL behaves like an aggressive NHL, requiring treatment with intensive rituximab-containing chemoimmunotherapy regimens in conjunction with autologous stem cell transplant, often with poor outcomes.

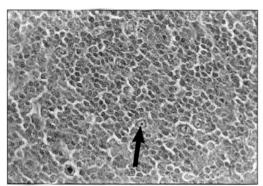

Lymphoplasmacytoid non-Hodgkin lymphoma (**NHL**). Showing a mixture of lymphocytes, plasmacytoid cells and occasional immunoblast (arrow; Giemsa stain)

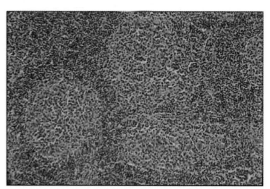

Follicular non-Hodgkin lymphoma (**FCC**) (follicular center cell lymphoma). Showing nodular, partly follicular, structure with a mixed small and large cell population (Giemsa stain)

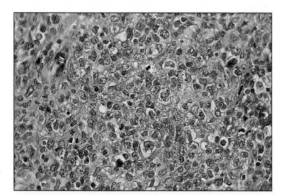

Follicular center cell lymphoma. With predominant large cells. The follicular may be still discernible or completely lost (H & E stain)

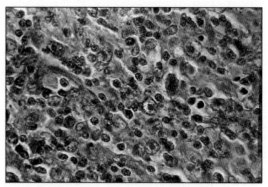

Large cell immunoblastic NHL. Showing predominance of immunoblasts (arrow) with some plasmacytoid features (PAS stain)

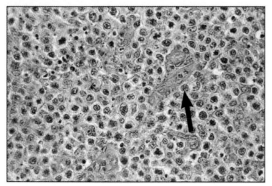

Immunoblastic T-cell–type large cell lymphoma. Showing histiocytoid cells and prominent (partly infiltrated) postcapillary venules (arrow)

FIG. 148.2 Microscopic Pathology of Selected Non-Hodgkin Lymphoma *H&E,* Hematoxylin and eosin. (Reused with permission from Buja ML, Krueger GRF: *Netter's illustrated human pathology updated edition,* Philadelphia, 2013, Elsevier.)

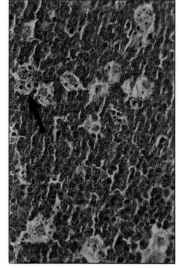

Burkitt-type NHL (here classical Burkitt lymphoma). Showing densely packed lymphoblasts with scattered histiocytes containing nuclear debris (starry sky pattern; arrow)

- **Hairy cell leukemia (HCL).** HCL is characterized by the presence of malignant B cells with hairy cytoplasmic projections. The disease typically results in a triad of pancytopenia, splenomegaly, and an inability to obtain a bone marrow aspirate sample due to the presence of fibrosis in the marrow. Purine analogs such as cladribine or pentostatin are the major therapies used and lead to favorable outcomes and long-term remission, although in many patients, the disease eventually recurs.
- **Lymphoplasmacytic lymphoma/Waldenstrom macroglobulinemia (LPL/WM).** LPL/WM is characterized by the presence of malignant B lymphocytes, plasma cells, and lymphoplasmacytic cells (the latter demonstrating a morphology intermediate between lymphocytes and plasma cells), which characteristically result in excess production of IgM immunoglobulin protein (Fig. 148.3). The high levels of IgM lead to **hyperviscosity syndrome** with symptoms of visual blurring, epistaxis, sinus disease, bleeding, and other small-vessel pathology. Plasmapheresis can be used in patients who present with severe hyperviscosity symptoms.
- **Chronic lymphocytic leukemia/small lymphocytic lymphoma.** This is discussed separately in Chapter 149.

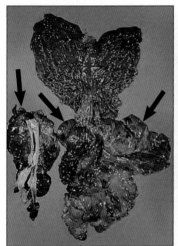

Waldenström disease. Prominent enlargement of paragastric, parapancreatic, and paraaortic lymph nodes caused by atypical lymphoplasmacytoid infiltration in the disease (*arrows*)

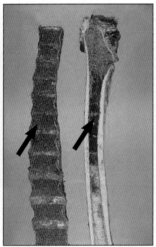

Waldenström disease. Diffuse infiltration of bone marrow. Note pale color of bone marrow and reduction of trabecular bone (*arrows*)

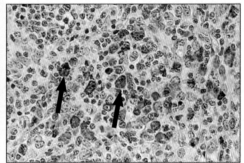

Waldenström disease. Microscopy of atypical mixed lymphoplasmacytoid cell population (immunostain: brown cells containing monoclonal immunoglobulin; *arrows*)

FIG. 148.3 **Waldenstrom Disease.** (Reused with permission from Buja ML, Krueger GRF: *Netter's illustrated human pathology updated edition,* Philadelphia, 2013, Elsevier.)

CHAPTER 149

Chronic Lymphocytic Leukemia (CLL)

ABHIRAMI VIVEKANANDARAJAH

INTRODUCTION

Chronic lymphocytic leukemia (CLL) is the most common acute adult leukemia in Western countries, accounting for nearly 30% of all leukemias in the United States. CLL demonstrates a male predominance and is largely a disease of the elderly, with a median age of diagnosis of ~70 years, although younger patients may rarely be affected. There are no known risk factors for CLL, but about 10% to 15% of cases may be familial.

PATHOPHYSIOLOGY

CLL is due to proliferation of a malignant B-lymphocyte clone. This malignant clone is thought to arise from a variety of mechanisms, including antigenic stimulation, interactions with the microenvironment, and genetic mutations. These processes give rise to a CLL precursor state known as monoclonal B-cell lymphocytosis (MBL), characterized by a low-level expansion of monoclonal B lymphocytes with immunophenotypic features identical to CLL cells. Over time, the MBL clone grows and accumulates more genetic mutations, ultimately giving rise to CLL (Fig. 149.1).

CLL is biologically identical to **small lymphocytic lymphoma (SLL)**, an indolent non-Hodgkin lymphoma. The primary difference between the two is that in CLL, the malignant B cells circulate in the blood at high levels, whereas in SLL, the malignant cells partition largely in the lymph nodes.

PRESENTATION, EVALUATION, AND DIAGNOSIS

CLL is usually discovered incidentally on routine blood work demonstrating **lymphocytosis**. Most CLL patients are asymptomatic at initial presentation. As the disease progresses, patients can develop lymphadenopathy, constitutional or "B" symptoms (e.g., fevers, drenching night sweats, or unintended weight loss), splenomegaly, or progressive anemia or thrombocytopenia.

The differential diagnosis of CLL includes both neoplastic and nonneoplastic conditions that result in peripheral blood lymphocytosis. The neoplastic conditions include MBL, mantle cell lymphoma (MCL), prolymphocytic leukemia (PLL), follicular lymphoma, splenic marginal zone lymphoma, hairy cell leukemia, or lymphoplasmacytic lymphoma. The most common nonneoplastic cause of lymphocytosis is viral infection.

The diagnosis of CLL is established on the basis of a complete blood count (CBC) showing lymphocytosis and a peripheral blood flow cytometry study showing clonal B cells with an immunophenotype characteristic of CLL. The National Cancer Institute and World Health Organization define CLL according to the following criteria:

1. An absolute lymphocyte count ≥5000/μL in the peripheral blood
2. Flow cytometry with clonal B cells expressing B-cell antigens CD19, CD20 (often dim), and CD23; the T-cell antigen CD5; either κ or λ light chain; and very low levels of surface immunoglobulin

A bone marrow examination is not necessary for diagnosis of CLL.

MBL is characterized by the presence of CLL cells with a circulating absolute lymphocyte count <5000/μL, without lymphadenopathy, splenomegaly, anemia, or thrombocytopenia. SLL is diagnosed on the basis of a lymph node containing CLL cells, with a circulating absolute B-cell count <5000/μL and absence of anemia or thrombocytopenia.

Several genetic abnormalities may be seen in CLL, which are of prognostic significance. Patients with CLL should have fluorescence in situ hybridization (FISH) performed on the peripheral blood to identify these abnormalities (Table 149.1).

The presence of immunoglobulin heavy-chain variable region (IGHV) genes without somatic hypermutation (i.e., nonmutated IGHV), expression of the *ZAP70* tyrosine kinase gene product, and expression of CD38 on CLL cells are also associated with adverse outcomes.

TABLE 149.1
Prognostic Implication and Frequency of Genetic Abnormalities in CLL

Genetic Abnormality	Frequency in CLL	Overall Survival
Deletion, long arm of chromosome 13 (del[13q14])	55% of cases	If sole marker, confers favorable prognosis with decades-long survival
Trisomy-12	15%–20% of cases	Intermediate risk factor
Deletion, long arm of chromosome 11 (del[11q23])	15% of cases	Poor prognosis
Deletion, short arm of chromosome 17 (del[17p13]); encodes TP53	15% of cases	Poorest prognosis in CLL

CLL, Chronic lymphocytic leukemia.
Modified from Wilhelm K, Yang D: A review of pharmacologic options for previously untreated chronic lymphocytic leukemia, *J Oncol Pharm Pract* 17(2):91–103, 2011.

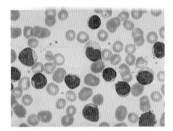

FIG. 149.1 **Chronic Lymphocytic Leukemia.**

CLL is commonly associated with a number of classic features of immune dysfunction. These are independent of the stage or prognosis of CLL itself and include:

- Hypogammaglobulinemia, which renders CLL patients susceptible to a number of infections, including *Streptococcus pneumoniae, Staphylococcus aureus,* and *Haemophilus influenzae*
- Autoimmune hemolytic anemia (AIHA), which occurs in 5% to 10% of CLL patients
- Immune thrombocytopenia (ITP), which occurs in 1% to 5% of CLL

Lastly, a small percentage of CLL patients may develop transformation into aggressive diffuse large B-cell lymphoma (DLBCL), known as **Richter transformation.** Richter transformation is mostly seen in CLL patients who have been previously treated for chronic leukemia. Unlike de novo DLBCL, Richter transformation carries a poor prognosis.

STAGING

The Rai staging system is the most commonly used staging system for CLL in the United States. It consists of five stages (Table 149.2).

TABLE 149.2
Rai Staging System

Stage	Features	Median Survival
0	Lymphocytosis	>12.5 years
1	Lymphocytosis with lymphadenopathy	8.5 years
2	Lymphocytosis with splenomegaly +/− hepatomegaly	6 years
3	Lymphocytosis with anemia	1.5 years
4	Lymphocytosis with thrombocytopenia	1.5 years

Based on original article from Rai KR, Sawitsky A, Cronkite EP, et al: Clinical staging of chronic lymphocytic leukemia, *Blood* 46(2):219–234, 1975.

TREATMENT

Most patients with newly diagnosed CLL are initially managed by observation, as the disease is usually discovered incidentally. Treatment is indicated in progressive CLL if there are symptoms such as fatigue or "B" symptoms, or if there is worsening lymphadenopathy, hepatosplenomegaly, anemia, thrombocytopenia, end-organ dysfunction as a result of CLL, or a rapid doubling time in the absolute lymphocyte count.

Conventional systemic therapy in CLL generally does not achieve cure but can lead to remission. In CLL patients who require treatment, several different options are available. Historically, chlorambucil (an alkylating agent) was the standard of care and led to remissions in about half of treated patients, with minimal toxicity. In the 2000s, chlorambucil was replaced by fludarabine (a purine analog) as studies demonstrated superior efficacy of the latter, albeit at the expense of much greater infectious risk due to myelosuppression and profound CD4 lymphopenia lasting 1 year after completion of therapy. Fludarabine has also been associated with the development of AIHA and ITP.

In the modern era, younger CLL patients are most commonly treated with a combination known as FCR, consisting of fludarabine, cyclophosphamide (an alkylating agent), and rituximab (murine anti-CD20 monoclonal antibody). FCR has an overall response rate of ~70% and may lead to sustained remissions in a small percentage of patients. Side effects include profound myelosuppression, lymphopenia, and immunosuppression. A small percentage of patients treated with FCR may later develop myelodysplastic syndrome.

In older CLL patients, a common regimen is BR, consisting of bendamustine (an alkylating agent with purine analog-like properties) and rituximab. This regimen has lower response rates than FCR but is much more tolerable and therefore preferred over FCR in elderly patients.

The most important advance in the treatment of CLL is the development of inhibitors to **Bruton tyrosine kinase (BTK)**, a critical protein for expansion of CLL clones. Ibrutinib, an oral agent, was the first BTK inhibitor approved by the US Food and Drug Administration (FDA) for use in newly diagnosed or previously treated CLL. Ibrutinib has outstanding response rates in CLL and is one of the few agents with demonstrable efficacy in the subset of CLL patients who have del(17p). Ibrutinib is generally well tolerated but has some important side effects, which include diarrhea, dyspnea, atrial fibrillation, and bleeding due to platelet dysfunction.

Other newer CLL treatment regimens include idelalisib (oral inhibitor of phosphatidylinositol-3 kinase), ofatumumab (humanized anti-CD20 monoclonal antibody) plus chlorambucil, obinutuzumab (another humanized anti-CD20 monoclonal antibody) plus either chlorambucil or bendamustine, alemtuzumab (anti-CD52 monoclonal antibody), or venetoclax (BCL2 inhibitor).

Few treatments in CLL have been known to cure patients of the disease. One is reduced intensity conditioning allogeneic **stem cell transplant,** which is not commonly done in CLL. The second is chimeric antigen receptor (CAR) T-cell therapy, which is presently available only on an experimental basis.

For CLL patients who develop AIHA or ITP, the standard of care is identical to those with AIHA or ITP who do not have CLL. Such treatments typically include prednisone with or without rituximab. Interestingly, there is some emerging data that ibrutinib may help to control AIHA in CLL patients, as well.

CHAPTER 150

Chronic Myelogenous Leukemia (CML)

MANISHA BHATTACHARYA

INTRODUCTION

Chronic myelogenous leukemia (CML) is a myeloid neoplasm characterized by abnormal proliferation of myeloid cells. The median survival of untreated CML is on the order of several years. Among all hematological malignancies, CML is unique in that it arises from one genetic abnormality known as the **Philadelphia chromosome** (Ph), characterized by a reciprocal translocation between the ABL1 tyrosine kinase gene *(ABL1)* on chromosome 9 and the breakpoint cluster region *(BCR)* gene on chromosome 22 (t[9;22]), giving rise to a **BCR-ABL1** fusion product. This hybrid BCR-ABL1 tyrosine kinase is exquisitely sensitive to treatment with a class of targeted drugs known as **tyrosine kinase inhibitors (TKIs)**. The development of TKIs heralded the era of molecular therapeutics in cancer.

PATHOPHYSIOLOGY AND RISK FACTORS

According to the World Health Organization classification, CML is categorized as a myeloproliferative neoplasm (MPN)—the others being polycythemia vera, essential thrombocytosis, and primary myelofibrosis (see Chapter 153 for details). Unlike other MPNs, CML is distinguished on the basis of the Ph. The presence of the BCR-ABL1 fusion protein is believed to confer a growth advantage on myeloid cells via increased activation of proliferative pathways due to constitutive activation of the fusion tyrosine kinase, which leads to decreased cell apoptosis and abnormal proliferation patterns.

The annual incidence of CML is 1.5 per 100,000 people, with a slight male predominance. The two major risk factors for developing CML are age and exposure to ionizing radiation, the latter peaking at 5 to 10 years postexposure. There are no well-characterized familial genetic susceptibilities associated with development of CML, although some instances of family members with multiple types of MPNs, including CML, have been observed. It is very uncommon for CML to develop as a secondary malignancy after comprehensive cancer treatment for another malignancy.

PRESENTATION, EVALUATION, AND DIAGNOSIS

The median age of diagnosis of CML is 50 to 60 years. Most patients have vague symptoms at initial presentation, such as fatigue, weight loss, or easy bruising or bleeding. The physical examination may reveal hepatosplenomegaly; lymphadenopathy is not common, owing to the myeloid, rather than lymphoid, origin of the disease. A routine complete blood count typically demonstrates leukocytosis. The white blood cell differential and peripheral blood smear usually show circulating myeloid precursor cells at all stages of differentiation (i.e., mature neutrophils, bands, metamyelocytes, myelocytes, promyelocytes, and blasts); basophilia, anemia, and thrombocytosis may also be seen (Fig. 150.1). Other labs may show hyperuricemia and/or an elevated cyanocobalamin level. The diagnosis of CML is based on the presence of the BCR-ABL1 translocation, leukocytosis in the peripheral blood, and the abovementioned characteristic smear features.

The differential diagnosis of CML includes other MPNs, acute myeloid leukemia, leukemoid reactions, and other conditions giving rise to reactive leukocytosis. A low leukocyte alkaline phosphatase level can distinguish CML from a leukemoid reaction or other reactive leukocytosis.

There are three phases of CML:

- **Chronic phase.** This is the most common phase at initial presentation and is characterized by a fairly indolent course, with a typical duration of several years if left untreated. Patients with chronic phase CML have <10% blasts in the bone marrow and blood.
- **Accelerated phase.** This arises after chronic phase and represents an intermediate period of leukemic transformation en route to blast crisis. Patients with accelerated phase CML have between 10% and 20% blasts in the bone marrow or blood, or other high-risk features such as profound basophilia, thrombocytopenia, progressive splenomegaly, or clonal evolution (i.e., acquisition of new genetic abnormalities other than the Ph).

- **Blast crisis.** This is characterized by acute myeloid (or, less commonly, acute lymphoblastic) leukemia. It is diagnosed on the basis of having >20% blasts in the bone marrow or blood.

Patients with suspected CML should have molecular and/or cytogenetic testing from the blood to confirm the

presence of the Ph. Such testing can be accomplished via polymerase chain reaction (PCR), fluorescence in-situ hybridization (FISH), or karyotype, with PCR being the most sensitive. A bone marrow biopsy is also usually done for accurate analysis of molecular features, evaluation of other cytogenetic abnormalities, and evaluation of features of accelerated phase or blast crisis. Once a diagnosis of CML is established, BCR ABL1 titers from the blood and/or bone marrow must be obtained as these levels are used to follow response to treatment

TREATMENT

Historically, CML was treated with interferon-α and cytarabine (a cytosine analog) to slow progression, although many patients eventually required hematopoietic stem cell transplantation for an attempt at cure. In the 1990s, the molecular revolution in cancer was spurred by the development of **imatinib**, a TKI with activity against the BCR-ABL1 kinase. Imatinib and other TKIs block the usually constitutive activity of the BCR-ABL1 fusion protein (Fig. 150.2). For patients with chronic phase CML, lifelong administration of TKIs maintains the

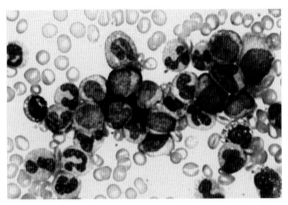

FIG. 150.1 **Chronic Myelogenous Leukemia: Blood Smear.**

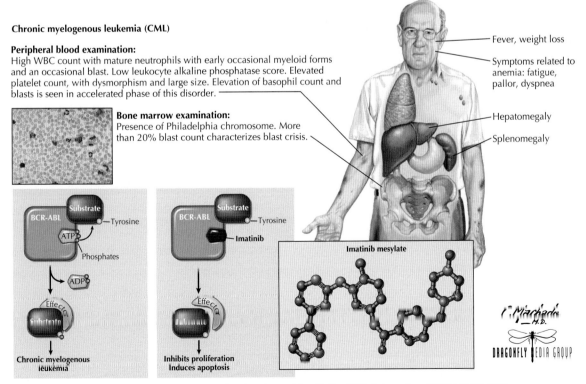

FIG. 150.2 **Chronic Myelogenous Leukemia and Imatinib.** *ADP,* Adenosine diphosphate; *ATP,* adenosine triphosphate; *WBC,* white blood cell.

disease in a dormant state, such that transplant can be deferred. The durable response rate of chronic phase CML to TKIs is ~90%, with the vast majority of patients achieving long-term remission and attaining an almost normal life span. Treatment responses are assessed by peripheral blood BCR-ABL1 quantitative PCR every 3 months for at least the first year, with periodic bone marrow surveillance.

Common side effects of TKIs include nausea, vomiting, diarrhea, constipation, muscle cramps, bone pain, leg edema, and weight gain. The side effect profiles of second-generation TKIs (e.g., dasatinib and nilotinib) are more favorable, except for a few complications specific to each of these medications—dasatinib can lead to pleural effusion and pulmonary hypertension, while nilotinib can lead to cardiac arrhythmias due to QTc prolongation. In clinical trials, there have been no differences in overall survival when comparing imatinib with second-generation TKIs, although the second-generation TKIs may be associated with faster and deeper molecular responses and lower rates of transformation from chronic to accelerated or blast phase.

During treatment with TKIs, at times, an increase in BCR-ABL1 titer may be observed. The most common cause of this is nonadherence with the TKI regimen, and usually disease control can be restored with complete medication adherence. In some cases, a serial rise in BCR-ABL1 titer may be observed despite treatment adherence; such an occurrence is concerning for the development of TKI resistance and impending treatment failure, which can lead to accelerated phase and blast crisis. TKI resistance can arise as a result of various mutations in the BCR-ABL1 fusion protein; in such cases, a change in TKI therapy can often overcome this resistance.

For CML patients who present in accelerated phase or blast crisis, the prognosis is much poorer than in chronic phase. Upfront TKI therapy and an evaluation for possible hematopoietic stem cell transplantation are indicated. The poor prognosis of accelerated phase and blast crisis CML, and the fact that TKI treatment during chronic phase can prevent progression to accelerated phase or blast crisis, underscores the importance of early TKI treatment and maintenance of disease remission in CML.

CHAPTER 151

Acute Myeloid Leukemia (AML)

NATALIE F. UY • KINJAN PARIKH

INTRODUCTION

Acute myeloid leukemia (AML) is a hematopoietic neoplasm that develops from myeloid precursor cells. Under normal conditions, the myeloid hematopoietic stem cell gives rise to granulocytes, monocytes, erythrocytes, and megakaryocytes. AML arises when myeloid precursor cells acquire genetic mutations that lead to clonal proliferation and a reduced ability of the precursor cells to differentiate into mature cells, resulting in accumulation of abnormal myeloid **blasts,** which represent the leukemic cells. Despite advances in molecular prognostic factors, allogeneic hematopoietic cell transplantation, and new drug development over the past few decades, a majority of patients still relapse and die from the disease.

PATHOPHYSIOLOGY AND RISK FACTORS

AML results from aberrant differentiation of myeloid progenitor cells. During leukemogenesis, an accumulation of genetic changes in myeloid stem cells leads to a population of rapidly proliferating myeloid precursors, known as myeloid blasts, which have reduced capacity to mature. The presence of myeloid blasts representing $\geq 20\%$ the cellularity in the bone marrow or in the blood is the defining pathological feature of AML. As these blasts infiltrate the bone marrow, other differentiated cell lines, such as platelets, red blood cells, and mature granulocytes, become relatively diminished and are ultimately unable to perform their normal functions.

AML is a rare cancer, with 10,500 new cases diagnosed annually, accounting for 1.2% of cancer deaths in the United States. Geographically, the highest incidence of AML is seen in North America and Europe. The median age of diagnosis is ~67 years, although the incidence increases with age. The male-to-female ratio is approximately 5:3 and remains constant over different races. A number of genetic and environmental factors are associated with an increased risk of developing AML, including radiation exposure, various chemicals (e.g., chemotherapy agents, benzene, and other aromatic organic solvents), and genetic abnormalities (e.g.,

trisomy 21 and Fanconi anemia). **Secondary AML** may arise out of other preexisting hematological diseases, such as myelodysplastic syndrome or myeloproliferative neoplasms.

PRESENTATION, EVALUATION, AND DIAGNOSIS

AML patients frequently present with fatigue, pallor, or weakness as a result of anemia. Bleeding or hemorrhagic findings, such as gingival bleeding, ecchymoses, epistaxis, or menorrhagia, may occur due to thrombocytopenia. Fever may arise as a result of the leukemic blasts themselves or from occult infection due to leukopenia or immunological impairment resulting from the leukemia itself. Rarely, **leukostasis** can occur as a consequence of blast crisis, when the number of circulating myeloblasts is $\geq 100,000/\mu L$; characteristic signs and symptoms of leukostasis include respiratory failure, visual problems, and central nervous system abnormalities.

Physical exam findings in AML may include gingival bleeding or hypertrophy, oral thrush, or skin manifestations such as leukemia cutis (i.e., infiltration of the skin by leukemic blasts) or Sweet syndrome (neutrophilic dermatosis, typically seen in association with AML and other myeloid malignancies). Hepatomegaly and splenomegaly are present in ~10% of cases. Palpable lymphadenopathy and significant lymph node enlargement are uncommon, reflecting the myeloid, rather than lymphoid, derivation of the leukemic blasts. AML patients sometimes present with symmetric or migratory polyarthritis or arthralgias.

In terms of laboratory evaluation of AML:
- The complete blood count (CBC) in patients with AML often shows an elevated white blood cell (WBC) count with circulating myeloid blasts, although some patients may have a low WBC (sometimes referred to as aleukemic leukemia). The CBC also typically demonstrates anemia and thrombocytopenia, reflecting infiltration of the bone marrow by leukemic blasts.

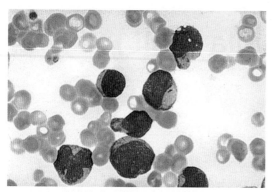

FIG. 151.1 **Blasts in Acute Myeloid Leukemia.**

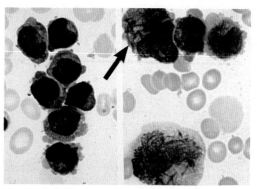

Blood smear of acute promyelocytic leukemia (APL), showing myeloblasts and promyelocytes with Auer rods and bundles *(arrow)*

FIG. 151.2 **Auer Rods.**

- Patients with suspected AML should be evaluated for metabolic and electrolyte abnormalities, particularly **tumor lysis syndrome,** which can lead to hyperuricemia, hyperkalemia, hyperphosphatemia, acute kidney injury, and metabolic acidosis. Basic chemistries, uric acid, phosphorus, and lactate dehydrogenase should therefore be routinely checked in all patients with suspected AML.
- Disseminated intravascular coagulation (DIC) is also common, particularly in the subtype of AML known as **acute promyelocytic leukemia** (APL). As a result, basic coagulation studies (prothrombin time [PT], international normalized ratio [INR], activated partial thromboplastin time [aPTT]), and a fibrinogen level should be obtained in all patients undergoing evaluation for AML.
- The peripheral blood smear in AML may show myeloid blasts, which appear as immature cells with large nuclei, prominent nucleoli, and pale blue cytoplasm (Fig. 151.1). These cells may also contain Auer rods (pink, granular structures in a linear shape, located in the cytoplasm), which are pathognomonic of myeloblasts and characteristic of the APL subtype of AML (Fig. 151.2).
- Flow cytometry from the peripheral blood may aid in the diagnosis of AML. This technique uses immunofluorescence to stain for specific cell proteins that may be unique to myeloid blasts. In AML patients, peripheral blood flow cytometry commonly reveals circulating myeloid blasts with an abnormal cellular immunophenotype.
- Bone marrow aspiration and biopsy is central to the diagnosis of AML, as the disease is defined by the presence of myeloid blasts accounting for ≥20% of the bone marrow or blood. Typically, the bone marrow will be hypercellular secondary to the replacement of

normal marrow space by blasts. Other pathological features, such as dysplasia or fibrosis, also sometimes may be seen.

PROGNOSIS AND STAGING

All AML patients should undergo cytogenetic analysis of their bone marrow biopsy to determine any cytogenetic abnormalities, which are seen in 50% of patients. The World Health Organization classification categorizes AML based on underlying cytogenetic or molecular genetic abnormalities.
- **Favorable-risk AML:** Certain cytogenetic abnormalities, such as the (15;17) translocation in APL, the (8;21) translocation, or an inversion in chromosome 16, are associated with a favorable prognosis in AML.
- **Intermediate-risk AML:** A normal cytogenetic profile is associated with an intermediate-risk prognosis in AML.
- **High-risk AML:** Monosomy-5, monosomy-7, a deletion in the short arm of chromosome 11, or complex cytogenetics (i.e., three or more cytogenetic abnormalities) are associated with an unfavorable prognosis in AML.

In addition to cytogenetic analysis, molecular studies can further discern prognosis in AML. Patients with AML and normal cytogenetics who also have a point mutation in the *NPM1* (nucleophosmin) gene are considered to be in a favorable risk group. AML patients with normal cytogenetics and an internal tandem duplication in the *FLT3* tyrosine kinase gene are viewed as having high-risk disease.

Independent of DNA abnormalities, other patient-specific and disease-specific risk factors are of prognostic importance in AML. Advanced age is the most important patient-specific adverse risk factor in AML. Patients with secondary AML arising out of myelodysplastic syndrome or a myeloproliferative neoplasm also typically have high-risk disease, which in some cases may be a direct result of complex cytogenetic and molecular abnormalities.

TREATMENT

Treatment of AML depends on patient-specific factors such as age, performance status, and other comorbidities, and AML-specific factors such as cytogenetic and molecular studies and the presence or absence of myelodysplastic syndrome. Risk stratification into favorable-risk, intermediate-risk, or high-risk disease is crucial for management of AML.

Primary treatment of AML consists of two phases of chemotherapy and consideration of allogeneic hematopoietic stem cell transplant (HSCT):

- **Induction chemotherapy:** The goal of induction therapy is to achieve complete remission, defined by the presence of <5% myeloblasts on a bone marrow biopsy performed 1 month after the first day of induction. The standard induction chemotherapy, referred to as 7+3, combines 7 days of continuous cytarabine with an anthracycline on days 1 to 3. Approximately 70% of patients will achieve complete remission on this protocol, but the remissions are usually not sustained. The induction chemotherapy regimen results in severe pancytopenia in all patients, requiring most patients to remain hospitalized for ~1 month after the start of induction, until the absolute neutrophil count recovers to acceptable levels; granulocyte colony-stimulating factors are not used routinely in AML patients undergoing induction chemotherapy as the data for this have been inconclusive. Platelet and packed red blood cell transfusions are routinely administered. The use of prophylactic antibiotics and antifungals to prevent febrile neutropenia varies by institution depending on the local flora and resistance patterns.

- **Consolidation chemotherapy:** Following attainment of complete remission, AML patients usually proceed with consolidation chemotherapy, where the goal is to eliminate or further reduce any residual disease burden in the bone marrow. Consolidation chemotherapy is less intensive than induction chemotherapy and has a lower early mortality rate. The standard consolidation regimen is high-dose cytarabine (HiDAC), which, like induction chemotherapy, can lead to prolonged cytopenias and is also associated

with two specific complications, keratoconjunctivitis (for which prophylactic dexamethasone eye drops are typically administered) and cerebellar toxicity. For younger AML patients with favorable-risk disease who have achieved complete remission after induction chemotherapy, three to four cycles of consolidation chemotherapy are typically the standard of care, which results in cures in ~60% of treated patients.

- **Allogeneic HSCT:** For eligible AML patients with high-risk disease, or those who either do not achieve remission or relapse after therapy, allogeneic HSCT from an HLA-matched donor is the treatment of choice. Allogeneic HSCT in such patients has the lowest rate of relapse and best chance of cure due to a potential graft-vs-tumor effect, but benefits are limited by treatment-related mortality due to infection and graft-vs-host disease.

Targeted therapy has become increasingly introduced into AML treatment at various stages of therapy. Such agents may be used in patients with specific molecular abnormalities, such as NPM1 or FLT3 internal tandem duplications, although the use of these agents is still largely investigational.

Older AML patients are a challenge to treat due to comorbidities that limit treatment dosing and options and a higher incidence of unfavorable AML subtypes resistant to chemotherapy. For healthy older patients, standard induction is recommended. For those with comorbidities or poor performance status, **hypomethylating agents** such as 5-azacitidine or decitabine can induce remissions and prolong survival in some patients. The small subset of older patients who do achieve remission often will receive some mild form of postremission therapy, but such patients are prone to treatment-related toxicity; HiDAC consolidation and allogeneic HSCT are generally not tolerable in these patients, but hypomethylating agents or targeted therapy may be options. Unfortunately, the prognosis for elderly AML patients or those with relapsed/refractory disease remains dismal.

Lastly, treatment of APL differs from other forms of AML in that it is based on the use of two agents: all-trans retinoic acid (ATRA) and arsenic trioxide. APL is strongly associated with DIC, which is the major source of mortality in untreated patients. For patients with suspected AML who have Auer rods on their peripheral blood smear, ATRA may be started for empiric treatment of APL even before a diagnosis of AML is confirmed, as early use of ATRA decreases the risk of APL induced DIC and mortality. APL patients who survive the initial treatment phase enjoy a favorable cure rate of >85%.

CHAPTER 152

Myelodysplastic Syndromes (MDS)

MAXIMILIAN STAHL • MARTIN S. TALLMAN

INTRODUCTION

Myelodysplastic syndromes (MDS) comprise a group of malignant hematopoietic stem cell disorders featuring dysplastic, ineffective blood cell production and variable risk of transformation to **acute myeloid leukemia (AML)**. The defining feature of MDS is **dysplasia** of the hematopoietic cells in the bone marrow (i.e., an abnormal appearance of the hematopoietic cells, often signaling a precancerous state).

The precise incidence of de novo MDS is not known because nonspecific symptoms may evade detection in early stages of the disease. However, conservative estimates propose that there are ~10,000 cases diagnosed annually in the United States.

MDS is a heterogeneous disease entity ranging from **low-risk MDS (LR-MDS)** to **high-risk MDS (HR-MDS).** Life expectancy of MDS ranges from several years for LR-MDS patients to months for very HR-MDS patients due to high risk of transformation to AML. Therefore accurate prognostication is vital to choosing the appropriate treatment plan. While HR-MDS is managed by aggressive treatment approaches with the goal of cure, the focus in LR-MDS is on symptom control and prevention of progression to AML.

PATHOPHYSIOLOGY

The pathogenesis of MDS is incompletely understood. MDS arises from hematopoietic stem or progenitor cells, which acquire multiple mutations, resulting in a clonal process at the expense of normal hematopoiesis. More recently, many MDS-causing mutations have been discovered, such as mutations in genes implicated in epigenetic deoxyribonucleic acid (DNA) modification and chromatin regulation, cell signaling, and pre–messenger ribonucleic acid (pre-mRNA) splicing. These mutations may accumulate in hematopoietic cells long before the development of histological dysplasia. LR-MDS and HR-MDS represent a dichotomy of disease pathology involving combinations of these mutations.

In LR-MDS, ineffective erythropoiesis is caused by increased apoptosis in the bone marrow, leading to anemia or, in some cases, pancytopenia. In contrast, decreased apoptosis in HR-MDS results in an increase in immature **blasts** in the bone marrow, thus increasing the chance of transformation to AML that is characteristic of HR-MDS. Thus, while LR-MDS shares similarities with aplastic anemia, HR-MDS is much closer to AML in terms of its pathophysiology, prognosis, and treatment.

RISK FACTORS

Age is an independent risk factor for MDS, as older hematopoietic stem cells accumulate mutations, which may lead to dysplasia. The median age of MDS diagnosis is ≥65 years. Prior treatment with chemotherapy is an important risk factor for MDS, especially exposure to certain chemotherapy drugs such as cyclophosphamide (an alkylating agent), etoposide (a topoisomerase II inhibitor), or doxorubicin (a DNA intercalator that also inhibits topoisomerase II). Environmental risk factors, such as radiation (e.g., radiotherapy, nuclear reactor accident), certain chemicals (particularly benzene), and heavy metals have also been linked to increased risk for MDS.

PRESENTATION, EVALUATION, AND DIAGNOSIS

The clinical presentation of MDS is nonspecific, and patients are often asymptomatic at presentation. Frequently, abnormalities noted on routine blood work (e.g., anemia, leukopenia, thrombocytopenia, or pancytopenia) may prompt further workup; unexplained macrocytic anemia is commonly observed, and a classic presentation in MDS is of an older patient with long-standing, unexplained macrocytic anemia. If symptoms are present, they can be explained as a result of associated cytopenias (e.g., fatigue and pallor in patients with anemia, increased susceptibility for infections in

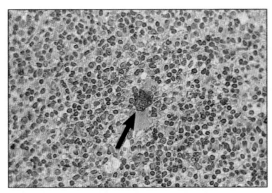

Myelodysplastic syndrome. Bone marrow biopsy specimen showing diffuse marrow hyperplasia with predominance of erythroblasts and dysplastic megakaryocytes *(arrow)*

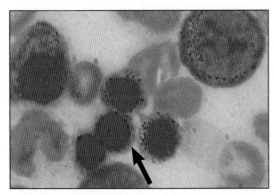

Myelodysplastic syndrome. Typical ring sideroblasts in blood smear *(arrow)*

FIG. 152.1 **Potential Findings in Myelodysplastic Syndromes.** (Reused with permission from Buja ML, Krueger GRF: *Netter's illustrated human pathology updated edition*, Philadelphia, 2014, Elsevier, p 356.)

patients with leukoneutropenia, or bleeding in patients with thrombocytopenia).

The diagnosis of MDS is made by the demonstration of cytopenia(s), dysplasia in the peripheral blood and/or bone marrow, and exclusion of AML. A bone marrow biopsy is required to make a definite diagnosis (Fig. 152.1). Importantly, patients with a blast count of ≥20% of the total cells of the bone marrow aspirate, or with certain genetic abnormalities typical for AML (e.g., t[8;21], inv[16], or t[15;17]) regardless of blast proportion, are considered to have AML.

Importantly, conditions other than MDS can give rise to dysplasia of the hematopoietic cells and need to be excluded before a diagnosis of MDS can be made; these include medications and toxins (including

chemotherapy and alcohol), viral infections (e.g., HIV, hepatitis, cytomegalovirus [CMV], and Epstein-Barr virus [EBV]), poor nutritional status (particularly deficiencies of vitamin B$_{12}$, folate, and copper), immune-mediated cytopenias (e.g., aplastic anemia, large granular lymphocyte leukemia), and autoimmune diseases such as lupus. It is also important to exclude myeloproliferative neoplasms, as these can often demonstrate morphological dysplasia, as well (see Chapter 153 for further details).

Based on the World Health Organization (WHO), MDS may be classified into six entities differentiated by morphology, immunophenotype, blast percentage, and cytogenetics:

- MDS with single lineage dysplasia
- MDS with multilineage dysplasia
- MDS with ringed sideroblasts
- Excess blasts (MDS-EB), which can be subcategorized by blast percentage in bone marrow:
  - MDS-EB1 (5%–9% blasts)
  - MDS-EB2 (10%–19% blasts)
- MDS with isolated loss of the long arm of chromosome 5 (5q minus or 5q- syndrome)
- MDS unclassifiable

Patients with MDS arising as a result of prior exposures to chemotherapy agents, radiation, or other toxic exposures have historically often been described as having secondary or therapy-related MDS (t-MDS). In the WHO classification, such patients, and those with AML arising from similar chemotherapy exposures, are categorized together as having therapy-related myeloid neoplasms.

TREATMENT

Treatment of MDS depends on prognosis (Fig. 152.2). The most commonly used risk assessment tool to gauge prognosis is the **Revised International Prognostic Scoring System (IPSS-R)**. It consists of five different variables:

- Blast percentage in the marrow
- Hemoglobin
- Platelet count
- Absolute neutrophil count
- Cytogenetic profile

Patients are divided into five risk groups based on this score. These may be conceptualized into two categories: those with lower risk MDS and those with higher risk disease. Patients with lower risk MDS are typically treated with supportive care or low-intensity therapies, while those with higher risk disease require immediate treatment due to the high chance of transformation to AML. Patients with secondary or t-MDS arising as a result of

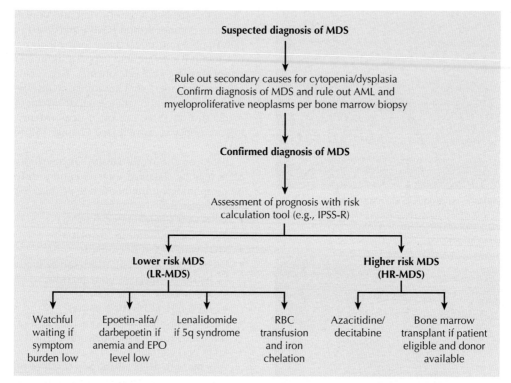

Suspected diagnosis of MDS

↓

Rule out secondary causes for cytopenia/dysplasia
Confirm diagnosis of MDS and rule out AML and
myeloproliferative neoplasms per bone marrow biopsy

↓

Confirmed diagnosis of MDS

↓

Assessment of prognosis with risk
calculation tool (e.g., IPSS-R)

**Lower risk MDS
(LR-MDS)**

| Watchful waiting if symptom burden low | Epoetin-alfa/darbepoetin if anemia and EPO level low | Lenalidomide if 5q syndrome | RBC transfusion and iron chelation |

**Higher risk MDS
(HR-MDS)**

| Azacitidine/decitabine | Bone marrow transplant if patient eligible and donor available |

FIG. 152.2 Diagnostic and Treatment Algorithm for Myelodysplastic Syndromes. *AML,* Acute myeloid leukemia; *EPO,* erythropoietin; *IPSS-R,* Revised International Prognostic Score; *MDS,* myelodysplastic syndrome; *RBC,* red blood cell.

prior drug, chemotherapy, or other exposures often have unfavorable cytogenetic profiles and a worse prognosis than those with de novo MDS.

Lower Risk Myelodysplastic Syndromes

Patients with lower risk MDS who have chronic, symptomatic anemia often may receive **erythropoiesis-stimulating agents (ESAs),** such as epoetin-α and darbepoetin, if baseline erythropoietin levels are low. Patients with deletion of the long arm of chromosome 5 (5q- syndrome) are typically treated with lenalidomide, an immunomodulatory agent with a broad range of effects in other hematological malignancies (e.g., multiple myeloma or lymphoma) as well. Many lower risk MDS patients eventually require chronic transfusions, which can lead to **iron overload.** Iron chelation therapy may be utilized to prevent cardiac and liver dysfunction secondary to iron overload in case of prolonged transfusion requirements (e.g., more than 20 to 30 transfusions) or if there is laboratory evidence of iron overload (ferritin >1000 μg/L). The hypomethylating agents azacitidine and decitabine can be used in select lower risk MDS patients

who fail to respond to ESAs or other treatments, but it is preferred to reserve these agents for patients with higher risk MDS, as the disease can become resistant to these agents.

Higher Risk Myelodysplastic Syndromes

The hypomethylating agents azacitidine and decitabine represent cornerstones of treatment for higher risk MDS; these agents reduce transfusion dependence and improve overall survival in patients with higher risk MDS. Some patients with higher risk MDS may be treated similarly to those with AML and given intensive induction chemotherapy. The only definitive cure for higher risk MDS is **hematopoietic stem cell transplantation,** which may be an option if a donor is available and if the patient is a suitable transplant candidate, although the latter may be less likely given the typical age of onset of this disease. Importantly, if patients experience a loss of response to hypomethylating agents, their median overall survival is <6 months. Multiple promising novel agents such as Luspatercept, a TGF-β ligand trap, and APR-246, a p53-activating drug, are in clinical trial development.

CHAPTER 163

Myeloproliferative Neoplasms

MAXIMILIAN STAHL • MARTIN S. TALLMAN

INTRODUCTION

Myeloproliferative neoplasms (MPN), as their name implies, are a group of clonal disorders characterized by deregulated production of one or several myeloid-lineage cells, including erythrocytes, leukocytes, and platelets. Broadly, they can be divided into Philadelphia chromosome (Ph)–positive and Ph-negative MPN. The major Ph-positive MPN is chronic myeloid leukemia (see Chapter 150 for further details). The major Ph-negative neoplasms are **polycythemia vera (PV), essential thrombocythemia (ET),** and **myelofibrosis (MF).**

PV and ET are characterized by high erythrocyte and platelet counts, respectively, and an increased risk for arterial and venous thrombosis; survival rates for many patients with these disorders are not much lower than in the general population. MF can be either primary (PMF) or secondary to PV (post-PV MF) or to ET (post-ET MF). Patients with MF can have debilitating symptoms, cytopenias, and splenomegaly and bare a significant risk of transformation into leukemia and a reduced life expectancy. The therapeutic spectrum in MPN ranges from watchful waiting and medical therapy to stem cell transplantation. Medical therapy for MPN has been revolutionized with the development of the **Janus kinase (JAK) inhibitor ruxolitinib.**

PATHOPHYSIOLOGY

PV, ET, and PMF are thought to represent different spectra along a continuum of disease. PV is character-ized by increased clonal production of red blood cells, platelets, and (in some instances) leukocytes. ET leads to the isolated clonal production of platelets and (in some instances) leukocytes. PMF is defined by fibrotic remodeling of the bone marrow leading to decreased blood cell production in the marrow and extramedullary hematopoiesis in the spleen.

At least three distinct, acquired genetic mutations can be found in the majority of patients with PV, ET, or PMF. The V617F mutation in exon 14 of JAK2 (*JAK2*

V617F) is present in 95% of PV, 55% of ET, and 65% of PMF patients; this mutation impairs a negative auto-regulatory mechanism in the JAK2 protein, resulting in constitutive hyperactivation of the JAK-STAT pathway. A second mutation in exon 14 of *JAK2* can be found in a small percentage of PV patients who lack *JAK2* V617F. Mutations in *CALR* (which encodes a calcium-binding protein involved in protein retention in the endoplasmic reticulum) and thrmbopoeitin receptor *MPL* are also present in ET and PMF at varying frequencies; *CALR* mutations lead to hyperactivation of the JAK-STAT pathway, while *MPL* mutations lead to constitutive activation of the thrombopoietin receptor.

PRESENTATION, EVALUATION, AND DIAGNOSIS

Most symptoms in MPN are nonspecific and include constitutional symptoms (e.g., fatigue and inactivity, night sweats, weight loss, and fever) as well as abdominal discomfort and early satiety due to splenomegaly. Classic symptoms are aquagenic pruritus (i.e., itching after a warm shower) due to erythrocytosis, and erythromelalgia (i.e., burning redness of the palms or soles) due to micro-vascular occlusion. Many patients may also experience bone pain due to excess bone marrow proliferation in the long bones. Patients with PV may have hyperviscosity secondary to erythrocytosis, of which symptoms include headache, blurred vision, and plethora.

The most common complication of the MPNs is thrombosis, which affects 35% of PV, 20% of ET, and 10% of PMF patients. Thrombosis in MPN character-istically occurs in the splanchnic vasculature (i.e., the portal, splenic, or mesenteric veins, or the hepatic vein in the form of Budd-Chiari syndrome), although any venous or arterial bed may be involved. The white blood cell (WBC) count and the presence of the *JAK2* V617F mutation are major predictors of thrombosis in all MPNs; other predictors of thrombosis include the hemoglobin or hematocrit in PV, or the platelet count in

ET. Conversely, ET patients with extreme thrombocytosis (defined as a platelet count >1,000,000/μL) can develop acquired **von Willebrand disease** due to adsorption of large von Willebrand factor multimers on the abnormal platelets. All MPNs carry a risk of transformation into acute myeloid leukemia (AML), although such risk is much higher in MF (6%–18% after 15 years) than in PV (5.5%) or ET (2%). In addition, both PV and ET can progress to post-PV or post-ET MF.

A patient's symptom burden in MPN can be assessed by several patient-reported outcome tools (e.g., MPN10, which rates 10 different symptoms on a scale of 0–10). Some patients come to a physician's attention by routine blood work showing abnormal cell counts; a classic (albeit not specific) finding in MPNs is basophilia. The diagnostic workup for MPN consists of excluding secondary causes for each disease category and obtaining confirmatory studies either in the form of molecular or mutational studies *(JAK2, CALR, MPL)* or a bone marrow biopsy. A brief overview of the approach to working up each of the major MPNs is as follows:

- PV: Patients with PV have erythrocytosis as defined by an elevation in red blood cell mass, hemoglobin (>16.5 g/dL in men or >16 g/dL in women), or hematocrit (>49% in men or >48% in women). The first step in the evaluation is to determine whether the erythrocytosis is spurious (i.e., due to low plasma volume), primary (i.e., EPO independent, due to a bone marrow problem such as PV), or secondary (i.e., EPO dependent, due to factors exogenous to the bone marrow). Secondary causes are most common and include cigarette smoking, chronic hypoxemia (e.g., due to obstructive sleep apnea, chronic lung disease, high-altitude exposure, or cardiopulmonary shunt), medications (e.g., androgens, anabolic steroids, or exogenous EPO), or EPO-secreting solid tumors (e.g., renal cell cancer or hepatocellular cancer). Measurements of EPO can distinguish between secondary erythrocytosis, where EPO levels are high, and primary erythrocytosis, where EPO production is suppressed. In patients with primary erythrocytosis and a low EPO level, the diagnosis of PV can be established on the basis of the *JAK2* V617F (or a *JAK2* exon 14) mutation, with the bone marrow characteristically showing hypercellularity, trilineage growth, and prominent erythroid, granulocytic, and megakaryocytic proliferation (Fig. 153.1).

- ET: Patients with ET have thrombocytosis as defined by an elevation in the platelet count ≥450,000/μL. Similar to PV, the first step in the evaluation is to determine whether the thrombocytosis is primary or secondary. Secondary causes of thrombocytosis

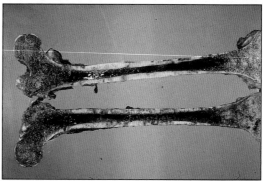

Polycythemia vera.
Hematopoietic hyperplasia of bone marrow, femur

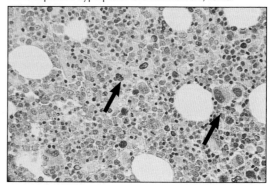

Polycythemia vera.
Bone marrow biopsy showing hematopoietic hyperplasia, reduced trilinear maturation, and increased immature megakaryocytes *(arrows)*

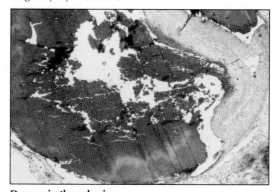

Deep vein thrombosis.
Complication of polycythemia vera

FIG. 153.1 **Polycythemia Vera.** (Reused with permission from Buja ML, Krueger GRF: *Netter's illustrated human pathology updated edition*, Philadelphia, 2013, Elsevier.)

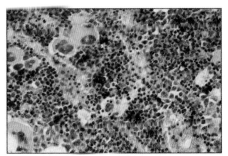

Bone marrow biopsy of essential thrombocythemia (ET). With diffuse marrow hyperplasia and increased partly immature megakaryocytes (red cells = myelopoiesis)

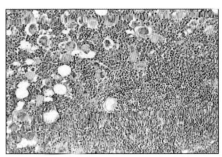

Bone marrow biopsy of ET. Showing hyperplastic hematopoiesis with increased numbers of megakaryocytes, yet no increased fibroplasia (reticulin stain)

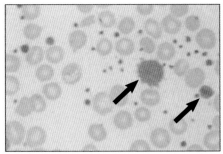

Blood smear of ET. Showing increased number of immature and giant platelets (*arrows*)

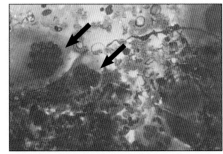

Bone marrow smear of ET. Showing unusual clotting and increased number of immature giant megakaryocytes (*arrows*)

FIG. 153.2 **Essential Thrombocythemia.** (Reused with permission from Buja ML, Krueger GRF: *Netter's illustrated human pathology updated edition*, Philadelphia, 2013, Elsevier.)

include infection, inflammation, iron deficiency, acute blood loss, surgery, trauma, other malignancy, and splenectomy. A diagnosis of ET is established by excluding secondary causes of thrombocytosis (based on history and on select laboratory tests such as erythrocyte sedimentation rate, C-reactive protein, and iron studies), and by the presence of a clonal MPN mutation (*JAK2* V617F or a mutation in *CALR* or *MPL*) and/or bone marrow findings of increased megakaryocyte proliferation with megakaryocyte atypia (Fig. 153.2).

- PMF: Patients with PMF commonly present with symptoms of splenomegaly and/or anemia. Splenomegaly is explained by extramedullary hematopoiesis in the spleen, and impressively large spleen sizes can frequently be seen on physical examination. The peripheral blood smear characteristically shows teardrop red blood cells and leukoerythroblastosis (i.e., the presence of early, left-shifted granulocytes, nucleated red blood cells, and blasts), which are representative of fibrosis in the marrow (see Chapter 40 for details). The diagnosis of PMF is established

on the basis of several criteria that include the finding of reticulin or collagen fibrosis in the marrow with megakaryocyte atypia, and the presence of a *JAK2*, *CALR*, or *MPL* mutation or another clonal marker.

TREATMENT

Determining the symptom burden (e.g., per MPN10) and prognosis of the disease is critical before a decision about MPN treatment can be made. Several prognostication tools exist, which are specific for PV, ET, and MF and are based on patient age, blood counts, thrombosis history, and in some cases cytogenetic or molecular analysis.

- PV and ET: The main goal of treatment of PV is to reduce thrombotic complications. All patients should be on low-dose aspirin and maintain a hematocrit <45%. For patients <60 years of age with no thrombotic history, **phlebotomy** is the mainstay of therapy, while for patients age >60 years or with a current or past history of thrombosis, hydroxyurea is typically added as cytoreductive therapy. The JAK inhibitor ruxolitinib may be used in PV patients who are intolerant to or have a suboptimal hematological response to hydroxyurea.

- ET: As with PV, the main goal of treatment of ET is to reduce thrombosis. Patients <60 years of age with no thrombotic history can be treated with aspirin alone. Patients age >60 years or with a current or past history of thrombosis should be maintained on aspirin plus cytoreductive therapy, typically with hydroxyurea. Anagrelide, an inhibitor of megakaryocyte maturation, is sometimes used as an alternate platelet-lowering drug, although the side effect profile and efficacy are less favorable than with hydroxyurea. Positive data for ruxolitinib in ET are also emerging.
- PMF: The treatment of PMF varies according to the severity of the disease. In patients with mild anemia, EPO or danazol (an androgen) may be beneficial.

For patients with symptomatic splenomegaly the JAK2 inhibitors *or* ruxolitinib or fedratinib may be used. Select PMF patients with high-risk features may be eligible for stem cell transplantation, which can reverse the fibrotic process in the marrow but is associated with many toxicities.

In light of the favorable experience of ruxolitinib in PV, ET, and PMF, numerous other JAK inhibitors are under development. Importantly, the activity of ruxolitinib is not dependent on the presence or absence of a *JAK2* mutation, as the activity of the JAK-STAT pathway is considered to be upregulated in Ph-negative MPNs independent of whether JAK2 is mutated or not. Another therapeutic option in MPNs is pegylated interferon-alfa-2a, which may be a disease-modifying agent in PV and ET as gauged by reductions in *JAK2* V617F titer.

CHAPTER 154

Aplastic Anemia (AA)

BALAKUMAR KRISHNARASA

INTRODUCTION

Aplastic anemia (AA) refers to a disease state of diminished or absent hematopoietic precursors in the bone marrow, leading to pancytopenia. It can be congenital or acquired. It is rare in the United States, with an incidence of three to six cases per million population per year, although the incidence in Southeast Asia and Mexico is much higher. The age at onset of the disease is typically between 15 and 25 years, with a second peak after age 60. The major known causes of AA include exposure to chemicals, drugs, viruses, and ionizing radiation, but most cases in the United States are idiopathic.

PATHOPHYSIOLOGY

Under normal circumstances, the pluripotent hematopoietic stem cell gives rise to committed progenitor cells, which in turn differentiate into the various myeloid, lymphoid, erythroid, and megakaryocytic cell lines. AA arises as a consequence of destruction or failure of the pluripotent stem cell, leading to a bone marrow failure state.

AA may be inherited or acquired. Inherited AA, or **inherited bone marrow failure syndromes (IBMFS)**, are a heterogeneous group of congenital disorders, some of which include:

- **Fanconi anemia.** This arises from mutations in any of a number of different genes involved in deoxyribonucleic acid (DNA) repair. Characteristic features include pancytopenia and dysmorphic features, such as short stature, malformed thumbs, or other end-organ defects.
- Dyskeratosis congenita (DKC). This is a telomere disorder in which affected individuals have pancytopenia and often display oral leukoplakia and changes of the skin and nails.
- Shwachman-Diamond syndrome. This usually leads to congenital neutropenia.
- Diamond-Blackfan anemia. This arises from mutations in ribosomal ribonucleic acid (RNA) genes, leading to anemia with a number of dysmorphic features,

such as short stature, microcephaly, wide-set eyes, cleft palate, or micrognathia.

Acquired causes of AA are more common than IBMFS. Acquired AA is believed to arise from T-lymphocyte–mediated destruction of pluripotent stem cells. The major causes of acquired AA include:

- Drugs and medications, such as NSAIDs (indomethacin, diclofenac), anticonvulsants (carbamazepine, phenytoin), chloramphenicol, gold, arsenic, and allopurinol
- Cytotoxic chemotherapy
- Toxic chemicals, particularly benzene and industrial solvents
- Ionizing radiation
- Viral infections, including viral hepatitis, HIV, parvovirus, Epstein-Barr virus (EBV), and cytomegalovirus (CMV)
- Autoimmune diseases
- Pregnancy

It should be noted that severe deficiencies of vitamin B_{12} and folic acid can also lead to pancytopenia, although the bone marrow in these cases shows megaloblastic erythropoiesis rather than the hypocellularity seen in AA. Also, anorexia nervosa can lead to cytopenias with a hypocellular marrow due to gelatinous degeneration of the marrow contents.

PRESENTATION, EVALUATION, AND DIAGNOSIS

Patients with AA present with clinical manifestations due to pancytopenia. Anemia may lead to fatigue, pallor, or weakness. Thrombocytopenia can lead to gingival bleeding, ecchymosis, petechiae, or (in women) menorrhagia. Neutropenia can result in increased infection risk, leading to various bacterial or fungal infections.

The physical exam in patients with AA may reveal petechiae, mucosal bleeding, or pallor. Hepatosplenomegaly and lymphadenopathy are generally not present. IBMFS may be suspected in young patients with personal and family histories of pancytopenia; short stature,

Histopathology of normal and abnormal marrow states

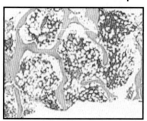 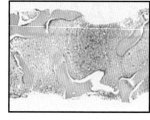 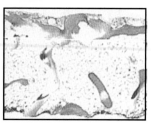

Normocellular marrow   Hypercellular marrow   Hypocellular marrow

FIG. 154.1 **Evaluation of Bone Marrow.**

dysmorphic features, musculoskeletal abnormalities, or nail or skin abnormalities also may point to an IBMFS.

In terms of laboratory evaluation of AA:

- The complete blood count (CBC) in patients with AA shows low white blood cell (WBC) counts, low hemoglobin, and low platelet counts. The mean corpuscular volume (MCV) may sometimes be high, although this may often be seen in bone marrow disorders other than AA.

- The reticulocyte count in AA is typically low, consistent with a state of reduced bone marrow hematopoietic activity.

- A bone marrow biopsy is required to establish a diagnosis of AA, which is defined by a reduction in bone marrow cellularity. In a normal patient, the percentage of hematopoietic cells to fat cells in the marrow space is equal to about 100% minus the patient's age. The bone marrow biopsy in AA, however, shows hypocellularity, with a percentage of hematopoietic cells lower than what would otherwise be expected for the patient's age (Fig. 154.1).

- Adjunctive lab tests routinely checked in the workup of AA include viral hepatitis serologies, HIV testing, parvovirus serologies, EBV and CMV viral load, vitamin B_{12} and folate levels, antinuclear antibodies, and flow cytometry to evaluate for large granular lymphocytes (a form of T or NK cell whose clonal production can lead to pancytopenia).

- Peripheral flow cytometry to evaluate for **paroxysmal nocturnal hemoglobinuria (PNH)** is also routinely checked due to an association of AA with PNH.

The major alternate diagnosis to consider in evaluation of a potential case of AA is a rare variant of myelodysplastic syndrome (MDS) known as hypoplastic MDS, in which the bone marrow demonstrates both dysplastic features and hypocellularity. The distinction between AA and hypoplastic MDS can be challenging, as the low cellularity of the marrow may preclude adequate evaluation for dysplastic changes in the absence of clonal cytogenetic abnormalities.

AA can be classified into categories based on the severity of the neutropenia. Severe AA is classified as having bone marrow cellularity <30% and two of these criteria: absolute neutrophil count <500/µL, platelet count <20,000/µL × 10^9/L, or absolute reticulocyte count <40,000/µL. Very severe AA includes all of these criteria with absolute neutrophil count <200/µL.

TREATMENT

Without treatment, patients with severe or very severe AA develop infectious and hemorrhagic complications, which can be fatal. Allogeneic bone marrow transplant is the treatment of choice for children, adolescents, and adults <40 years of age with severe AA in whom transplant-related morbidity and mortality is low and life expectancy is long. All transplant-eligible patients should be HLA typed at the time of diagnosis of AA to identify potential related donors. Bone marrow donor grafts are preferred over peripheral blood stem cells due to a higher success rate with the former in severe AA. Outcomes in patients <20 years of age are better than in older patients. The majority of AA patients who survive 2 years after bone marrow transplantation attain normal blood counts and have normal life spans.

In older AA patients or those who are not transplant eligible, immunosuppressive therapy consisting of antithymocyte globulin (ATG) and cyclosporine is the mainstay of treatment and yields overall response rates of 60% to 80% about 3 months after the start of therapy. Relapse rates are high, and about 35% of patients previously treated successfully with ATG and cyclosporine develop relapsed AA 5 years later. Long-term outcomes of AA patients treated with immunosuppressive therapy are further clouded by an increased risk of developing MDS or acute myeloid leukemia.

All patients with severe or very severe AA require supportive care in the form of blood product transfusions. These products should be irradiated and leukocyte depleted; CMV-negative products should be used in patients who are CMV negative. Historically, in transplant-eligible patients, blood transfusions were kept to a minimum out of concern that such transfusions might lead to alloimmunization and transplant failure, but such concerns are no longer the case.

CHAPTER 155

Breast Cancer

KARISHMA K. MEHRA

INTRODUCTION

Among women in the United States, **breast cancer** is the most frequent cancer and the second leading cause of cancer mortality. In 2016, there were ~250,000 new cases and 40,000 related deaths. Mortality rates have been declining since the early 1990s due to improved screening, decreased use of hormone replacement therapy, and newer treatments. Nonetheless, breast cancer continues to be a major public health problem, with an estimated 2.8 million women in the United States living with a current or past diagnosis.

PATHOPHYSIOLOGY

The female breast is composed of glandular and stromal tissues. The glandular tissue, which accounts for 10% to 15% of the breast mass, contains lobules and ducts that are responsible for milk production. The stroma consists primarily of fat, the amount of which is directly responsible for the size of the breast. Several known and unknown environmental, hormonal, and genetic factors can prompt a normal glandular cell to transform into a malignant cell. It is believed that early in carcinogenesis, these malignant cells proliferate to form **lobular** or **ductal carcinoma in situ** (LCIS or DCIS, respectively), depending on the cell of origin. Later, these tumors invade through the basement membrane, becoming invasive lobular or ductal carcinomas.

The **estrogen receptor (ER)** is overexpressed in many breast cancers. In ER-positive breast cancers, estrogen is believed to play a role in carcinogenesis by causing cellular proliferation and induction of aneuploidy. The **progesterone receptor (PR)** also frequently is seen in breast cancer and is a good prognostic marker, although the role of progesterone in carcinogenesis is not as well defined. *HER2/neu* is a protooncogene that is often overexpressed in breast cancer. The mechanism of carcinogenesis is unknown; however, cancers with *HER2/neu* overexpression are more aggressive, with rapid tumor proliferation, resistance to standard chemotherapy, and early recurrences. Fortunately, use of targeted therapies has allowed HER2 overexpression to morph into a more favorable prognostic marker.

RISK FACTORS

Numerous factors are associated with an increased risk of breast cancer. Female gender, older age, obesity, and a history of atypical hyperplasia (high-risk, benign lesion caused by proliferation of dysplastic cells in the breast) are known risk factors. Other factors can be broadly classified as follows:

- **Inherited:** Individuals with first-degree relatives with breast cancer (mother, sibling) are at slightly increased risk, likely due to a combination of undiscovered genetic defects and shared exposures. There are also known germline mutations linked to breast cancer. The most important are mutations in *BRCA1* and *BRCA2* genes. Carriers of *BRCA* mutations have a 30% to 80% lifetime risk of developing breast cancer. The incidence of BRCA1 mutations is highest in Ashkenazi Jews. Other known germline mutations include Li-Fraumeni syndrome (mutation in *TP53*) and Cowden syndrome (mutation in *PTEN*).
- **Hormonal:** Increased estrogen exposure is also an established risk factor. Early menarche (age <12 years), nulliparity, late age of first pregnancy (age >35 years), late age of menopause (age >55 years), and use of hormone replacement therapy all increase the risk of breast cancer.
- **Lifestyle:** Increased alcohol consumption (≥5 g/day based on epidemiological studies) and smoking both increase the risk of breast cancer.
- **Environmental:** Exposure to ionizing radiation, especially among patients who have received therapeutic irradiation to the chest (e.g., survivors of lymphoma), also increases breast cancer risk.

SCREENING

There are varying opinions regarding the appropriate age and frequency of screening among individuals with average risk. The American Cancer Society recommends a discussion about screening starting at age 40 years, with annual mammograms starting at age 45. The frequency may be reduced to every other year at age 55. Screening should continue as long as expected survival exceeds 10 years. The US Preventive Services Task Force recommends biennial mammograms from 50 to 74 years, and a discussion about screening starting at age 40. Clinical and self-breast examinations are no longer recommended. There are specific screening criteria for patients with higher risk (i.e., those with extensive family history or inherited germline mutations).

PRESENTATION, EVALUATION, AND DIAGNOSIS

Patients most frequently present with abnormalities on screening mammograms. Patients or their physicians may also notice a breast or axillary mass, changes in the skin overlying the breast, nipple inversion/flattening,

or bloody nipple discharge (Fig. 155.1). Breast pain is uncommon. The classical **peau d'orange** or orange-peel skin occurs when tumor cells infiltrate the skin and cutaneous lymphatic system. More systemic signs and findings (e.g., fatigue, weight loss, pain, elevated liver enzymes) may be present when a patient presents with metastatic disease.

Diagnostic mammograms and ultrasound (US) are performed to confirm an abnormality and to differentiate between cystic and solid lesions, respectively. Core needle biopsies are preferred over fine-needle aspirations (FNA), since the tissue obtained by FNA is scant and cannot distinguish between in situ and invasive carcinoma. Further tissue characterization determines histological grade as well as ER, PR, and HER2 status. Breast MRI may be required in patients with dense breast tissue to evaluate tumor size and detect other lesions.

Breast cancer is staged using the TNM classification. The T designation corresponds to the size of the tumor. Tis indicates in situ carcinoma, T1 tumors are ≤2 cm, T2 tumors are between 2 and 5 cm, T3 tumors are ≥5 cm, and T4 tumors are those that involve the chest wall or skin. The N designation indicates the number of lymph

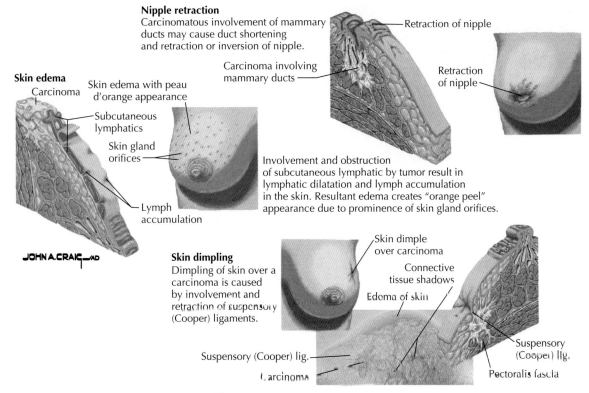

Nipple retraction
Carcinomatous involvement of mammary ducts may cause duct shortening and retraction or inversion of nipple.

Retraction of nipple

Carcinoma involving mammary ducts

Retraction of nipple

Skin edema
Carcinoma

Skin edema with peau d'orange appearance

Subcutaneous lymphatics

Skin gland orifices

Lymph accumulation

Involvement and obstruction of subcutaneous lymphatic by tumor result in lymphatic dilatation and lymph accumulation in the skin. Resultant edema creates "orange peel" appearance due to prominence of skin gland orifices.

JOHN A. CRAIG—MD

Skin dimpling
Dimpling of skin over a carcinoma is caused by involvement and retraction of suspensory (Cooper) ligaments.

Skin dimple over carcinoma

Connective tissue shadows

Edema of skin

Suspensory (Cooper) lig.

Carcinoma

Suspensory (Cooper) lig.

Pectoralis fascia

FIG. 155.1 Breast Cancer: Clinical Presentation.

nodes involved. N0 indicates no lymph node involvement, N1 is 1 to 3 axillary node involvement and/or in internal mammary nodes with metastases detected by sentinel lymph node biopsy; N2 is 4 to 9 axillary node involvement, or in clinically detected internal mammary lymph nodes in the absence of axillary node metastases; N3 is ≥10 axillary node involvement, or infraclavicular or ipsilateral internal mammary nodes in the presence of positive axillary nodes or in ipsilateral supraclavicular lymph nodes. Presence of distant metastatic disease is classified at M1. As per the National Comprehensive Cancer Network (NCCN), no further imaging is required for stages I and II unless specific signs or symptoms are present that suggest potential metastasis. For patients with

stage III disease, CT scan of chest, abdomen, and pelvis, along with a nuclear medicine bone scan or a positron emission tomography (PET)/CT scan, is recommended to rule out metastatic disease.

TREATMENT

The treatment of stage I to III breast cancer requires a multidisciplinary team, including surgeons, radiation oncologists, and medical oncologists.

The surgical options include modified radical mastectomy and breast conservation surgery (BCS), also called **lumpectomy** or partial mastectomy (Figs. 155.2 and 155.3). The decision of which therapy to

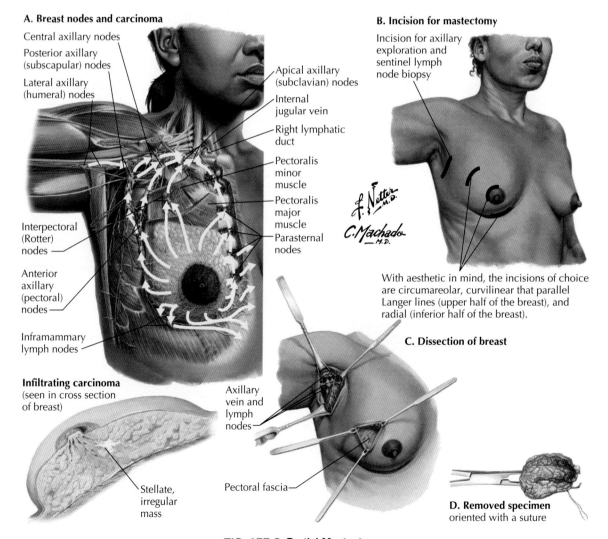

A. Breast nodes and carcinoma

Central axillary nodes
Posterior axillary (subscapular) nodes
Lateral axillary (humeral) nodes
Apical axillary (subclavian) nodes
Internal jugular vein
Right lymphatic duct
Pectoralis minor muscle
Pectoralis major muscle
Parasternal nodes
Interpectoral (Rotter) nodes
Anterior axillary (pectoral) nodes
Inframammary lymph nodes

Infiltrating carcinoma (seen in cross section of breast)
Stellate, irregular mass

B. Incision for mastectomy

Incision for axillary exploration and sentinel lymph node biopsy

With aesthetic in mind, the incisions of choice are circumareolar, curvilinear that parallel Langer lines (upper half of the breast), and radial (inferior half of the breast).

C. Dissection of breast

Axillary vein and lymph nodes
Pectoral fascia

D. Removed specimen oriented with a suture

FIG. 155.2 **Partial Mastectomy.**

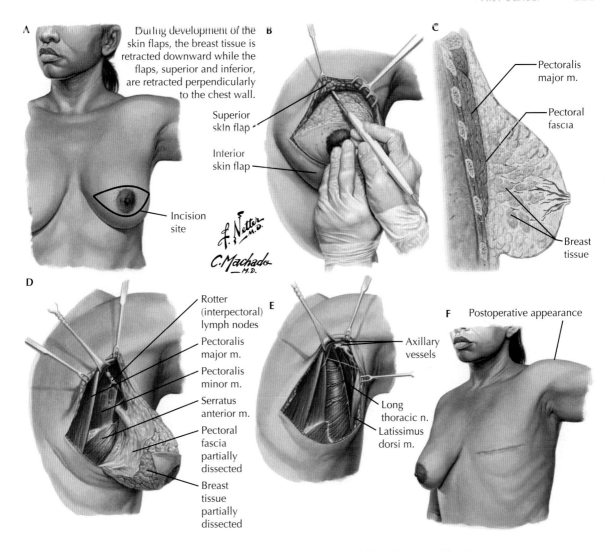

A

During development of the skin flaps, the breast tissue is retracted downward while the flaps, superior and inferior, are retracted perpendicularly to the chest wall.

B

C

Superior
skin flap

Inferior
skin flap

Incision
site

Pectoralis
major m.

Pectoral
fascia

Breast
tissue

D

Rotter
(interpectoral)
lymph nodes

Pectoralis
major m.

Pectoralis
minor m.

Serratus
anterior m.

Pectoral
fascia
partially
dissected

Breast
tissue
partially
dissected

E

Axillary
vessels

Long
thoracic n.

Latissimus
dorsi m.

F

Postoperative appearance

FIG. 155.3 **Total Mastectomy With Modified Radical Technique.** *m.*, Muscle; *n.*, nerve.

undergo is based on factors that include size of tumor, multifocality of disease, and patient preference. Adjuvant radiation usually is indicated in patients who undergo BCS, have positive lymph nodes, positive margins, and/or large tumors. Multiple trials have shown no long-term survival difference in patients with early stage breast cancer who underwent mastectomy versus BCS and adjuvant radiation. In addition to excision of the primary tumor, in patients who do not have clinical/radiological evidence of axillary lymph node involvement, a **sentinel lymph node biopsy (SLNB)** is performed. The sentinel nodes are defined as the first lymph nodes that receive lymphatic drainage from the primary tumor and are identified intraoperatively by

injecting a dye and radiolabeled isotope around the primary tumor. In some circumstances, if the sentinel lymph nodes are positive for metastatic disease, an axillary lymph node dissection (ALND) may be performed. This method decreases the morbidity associated with ALND, including lymphedema, pain, wound infection, and decreased shoulder mobility. Multiple studies have shown no difference in overall survival in clinically node-negative patients who underwent a SLNB to a prophylactic ALND.

Patients with high-risk disease (node-positive, ER/PR/Her2-negative cancers) should receive multidrug adjuvant chemotherapy regimens that include anthracyclines and/or taxanes. A prognostic multigene test (21-gene assay) can be sent for patients with lymph node–negative and ER/PR-positive tumor ≥0.5 cm in size to assess if they would benefit from adjuvant chemotherapy. Patients are divided into low, intermediate, and high risk for recurrence based on the results of this assay. It has been shown that patients with low-risk disease do not benefit from chemotherapy and will have a good prognosis with endocrine therapy alone, while high-risk patients have a definite overall survival benefit with adjuvant chemotherapy. There is an ongoing trial to assess the absolute benefit of chemotherapy in patients in the intermediate-risk group, and the decision is currently based on clinical factors and patient preference. Patients with HER2/neu amplification are treated with antibodies targeting HER2; at present, the approved agents are trastuzumab and pertuzumab, which are administered along with cytotoxic chemotherapy.

Both chemotherapy and HER2-directed therapy can be administered prior to surgery (neoadjuvant) in selected patients with high-risk cancers; however, there is no clear survival benefit over adjuvant treatment.

All patients with ER/PR-positive breast cancer benefit from adjuvant endocrine therapy. Tamoxifen, a **selective estrogen receptor modulator (SERM),** is used in premenopausal women. **Aromatase inhibitors** (letrozole, anastrozole, exemestane) are used in postmenopausal women or in premenopausal women with additional ovarian suppression (both medically and surgically induced). Aromatase inhibitors prevent the conversion of androgen to estrogen in peripheral tissues by blocking the enzyme aromatase; however, this does not affect estrogen produced by the ovaries, and therefore these agents cannot be used in premenopausal women

with functional ovaries without ovarian suppression. Endocrine therapy is initiated after the completion of chemotherapy and radiation. The current recommendation is that treatment continue for 5 years; however, recent data demonstrated a benefit for continuing therapy for up to 10 years.

Patients with stage IV breast cancer receive systemic therapy (i.e., endocrine therapy or chemotherapy) to control disease and palliate symptoms. For ER/PR-positive tumors, sequential endocrine therapy is given until evidence of resistance to these agents is seen. For hormone-negative or endocrine therapy–resistant tumors, sequential single agent chemotherapy is used. Many agents have been approved for these patients, and choice of agent depends on various factors, including patient comorbidities, performance status, and side effect profiles. Palliative surgery and radiation can be used to improve quality of life.

SURVIVORSHIP

Breast cancer survivors must have routine follow-up with clinical exams and breast imaging. Routine blood work and imaging is not indicated. Side effects of chemotherapy and endocrine therapy, such as neuropathy, cardiac toxicity, sexual side effects, infertility, osteoporosis, and menopausal symptoms, must be monitored and addressed. Patients should be educated about leading a healthy lifestyle and its association with decreased risk of breast cancer recurrence. The NCCN recommends a low-fat, plant-based diet and moderate intensity physical activity for 150 minutes per week in survivors.

CHAPTER 156

Thyroid Cancer and Thyroid Nodules

TYLER F. STEWART • RACHEL ARAKAWA

THYROID CANCER

Introduction

Thyroid cancer accounts for >95% of all new endocrine cancers in the United States, with an estimated 64,300 new cases and nearly 2000 deaths in 2016. It is the fifth most common cancer in women, in whom 75% of new cases are diagnosed. The incidence has increased by 240% over the last three decades, in large part because of increased use of diagnostic imaging and the detection of earlier stage cancers.

At the time of presentation, 68% of thyroid cancers remain confined to the thyroid (i.e., localized disease), 27% have spread to regional lymph nodes (i.e., regional disease), and 4% have distant metastases. The 5-year overall survival rates are 99.9% and 97.8% for local and regional disease, respectively, but only 54.1% for distant disease.

The presentation, clinical course, and treatment options differ significantly based on specific pathology. Thyroid cancer is broken into three categories: **differentiated, anaplastic,** or **medullary.**

Differentiated Thyroid Cancer

Differentiated thyroid carcinomas (DTCs) arise from follicular thyroid cells and make up >90% of thyroid cancers. Subtypes include **papillary** (Fig. 156.1), **follicular** (including Hürthle cell), and poorly differentiated, which account for 85%, 12%, and <3% of cases, respectively. About 5% of DTCs are associated with familial syndromes, including familial adenomatous polyposis and Cowden syndrome. Radiation exposure, particularly in the first decade of life (e.g., radiotherapy for childhood malignancies), is also a major risk factor.

Patients often present after an incidental thyroid nodule is detected on physical exam or imaging. A fine-needle aspiration (FNA) confirms the diagnosis. Preoperative neck ultrasound (US) is performed to evaluate the extent of the primary tumor and involvement of cervical lymph nodes. A neck CT can also be helpful, particularly if patients present with bulky lymphadenopathy. If suspicious lymph nodes are identified, additional FNAs may be performed. Chest CT is indicated if there appears to be caudal extension of the primary tumor into the mediastinum or symptoms to suggest metastatic disease.

Observation may be considered for patients with very small (<1 cm), low-risk DTCs. However, for the vast majority of patients with DTC, surgery is the initial treatment, even in the setting of metastatic disease. Patients with tumors <1 cm, no extrathyroidal extension, and no evidence of lymph node disease may be candidates for thyroid lobectomy. Those with tumors >4 cm, evidence of extrathyroidal extension, or lymph node disease should undergo total **thyroidectomy.** The approach to patients with tumors that are 1 to 4 cm is determined on an individual basis. Neck dissection is indicated when cervical nodes are positive for disease. When tumors are >4 cm, there is a potential role for prophylactic neck dissection even in the absence of cervical disease.

The American Thyroid Association (ATA) guidelines stratify DTCs into three risk groups: low, intermediate, and high. Low-risk disease is defined as disease confined to the thyroid gland, completely resected at surgery, and lacking vascular invasion or aggressive histological features (i.e., tall cell, columnar cell, or hobnail variants). Intermediate-risk features include cervical lymph node disease, microscopic extrathyroidal extension, aggressive histological features, and vascular invasion. High-risk features include gross extrathyroidal extension, incomplete tumor resection, distant metastases, and elevated thyroglobulin (Tg) serum levels 6 to 12 weeks after surgery.

Postoperatively, the two main risk reduction strategies for DTCs are **radioactive iodine (RAI) therapy** and thyroid-stimulating hormone (TSH) suppression with levothyroxine. DTCs often concentrate iodine, and RAI therapy with ^{131}I is generally effective for remnant thyroid ablation or treatment of distant disease. Postsurgical RAI therapy is generally recommended unless the disease is limited to the thyroid or the patient is <45 years of age without distant metastatic disease. As DTC tumors

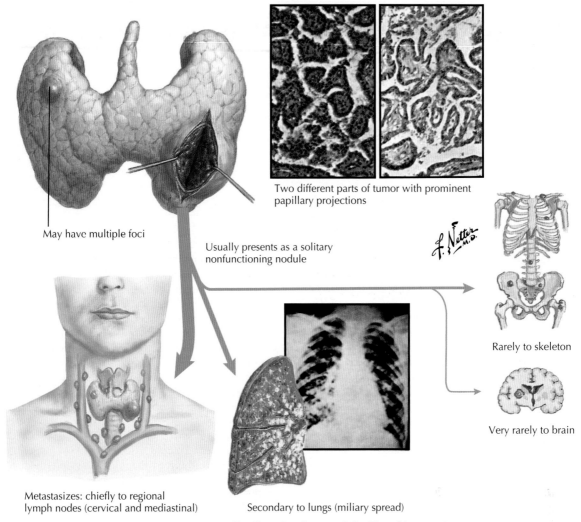

May have multiple foci

Two different parts of tumor with prominent papillary projections

Usually presents as a solitary nonfunctioning nodule

Rarely to skeleton

Very rarely to brain

Metastasizes: chiefly to regional lymph nodes (cervical and mediastinal)

Secondary to lungs (miliary spread)

FIG. 156.1 **Papillary Carcinoma of the Thyroid.**

are sensitive to TSH stimulation, TSH suppression with levothyroxine therapy is also an essential part of postoperative treatment. For high-risk individuals, an initial TSH suppression goal is <0.1 mU/L. For intermediate-risk and low-risk individuals, the goals are generally 0.1 to 0.5 mU/L and 0.5 to 2 mU/L, respectively. Patients should be monitored for recurrence using serum TSH levels, serum Tg and Tg antibody levels, and neck US generally every 6 months. Patients with high-risk disease may benefit from ^{131}I whole body scans.

The management of local recurrence or distant disease depends on the site, symptoms, and rate of progression. DTCs are often very slow-growing cancers, and recurrences (even distant metastases) often do not require immediate

treatment. If patients are asymptomatic, they can often be observed with serial imaging. Limited disease can be treated locally with surgery or radiation (with or without chemotherapy).

Metastatic DTC is often sensitive to RAI therapy, which should be used as first-line treatment. The disease is considered RAI refractory if it does not concentrate RAI, concentrates RAI in some but not all sites, or progresses despite adequate RAI concentration. The approach to such disease has changed significantly in the last decade. Cytotoxic chemotherapy with classical agents has been largely disappointing, and its use has been superseded by the emergence of oral tyrosine kinase inhibitors (TKIs). Sorafenib, a multitargeted TKI, was approved for DTC in 2013 after studies showed improved progression-free survival (PFS) of 10.8 months compared to 5.8 months with placebo. Lenvatinib, another oral TKI, was approved in 2015 following studies showing improved PFS of 18.3 months compared to 3.6 months with placebo. More recently, molecular testing has become standard for advanced DTC to identify potentially targetable alterations in genes such as *BRAF, NTRK, RET,* or in the *PI3K/AKT/MTOR* pathway.

Anaplastic Thyroid Cancer

Anaplastic thyroid carcinoma (ATC) is a very aggressive form of thyroid cancer with a median survival of ~6 months. These undifferentiated cancers are also derived from follicular cells and constitute 1% of all thyroid cancers. Unlike with DTC, patients often present in the seventh or eighth decade of life with a rapidly enlarging neck mass. Ninety percent of patients present with regional or distant spread at the time of diagnosis.

ATC is commonly associated with either a concurrent diagnosis or a previous history of DTC, suggesting an etiology either from dedifferentiated DTC or shared risk factors. Due to their aggressive nature, all ATCs are considered stage IV at time of diagnosis. The morbidity and mortality generally result from progression of local disease, such as respiratory failure from destruction of the upper airway, rather than from metastatic disease. Surgery, if possible, is the mainstay of treatment. RAI is ineffective. The combination of doxorubicin and a platinum-based agent is the preferred chemotherapy regimen but is often ineffective. Combined surgery and chemoradiation appears to be more effective than any single modality. Similar to DTC, molecular testing has become essential to identify targetable mutations in ATC. In 2018, the combination of dabrafenib and trametinib was approved for ATC after demonstrating a response rate of 57% in BRAF V600E mutation-positive ATC. Trials of novel targeted agents, multitargeted TKIs, and immunotherapy are ongoing.

Medullary Thyroid Cancer

Medullary thyroid carcinomas (MTCs) arise from neuroendocrine-derived **parafollicular cells (C cells)** of the thyroid gland, which produce calcitonin. MTCs constitute 5% of all thyroid cancers. Most MTCs are sporadic, but ~25% are associated with hereditary syndromes, such as the multiple endocrine neoplasia (MEN2A and MEN2B) syndromes. The *RET* protooncogene is mutated in these syndromes and plays a key role in the development of MTC. Patients with MTC should be offered screening for germline mutations in *RET* to determine the need to screen family members. Those

with confirmed mutations may be offered prophylactic total thyroidectomy.

Most patients with sporadic MTC present with a painless thyroid mass, though patients with bulky or metastatic disease may present with diarrhea from high calcitonin levels. Individuals with familial MTC present at a younger age (15–25 years compared to 40–45 years). The prognosis depends greatly on the stage of the disease. Patients with disease confined to the thyroid have an overall survival of 99% and 96% at 5 and 10 years, respectively. For those with regional disease (i.e., involvement of cervical nodes), the rates are 91% and 77%, respectively. The 5-year and 10-year survival rates fall to 51% and 44%, respectively, for distant disease (Fig. 156.2).

The workup for MTC should include neck US, calcitonin and carcinoembryonic antigen (CEA) levels, genetic testing, and evaluation for conditions that occur in MEN (e.g., pheochromocytoma, hyperparathyroidism). Calcitonin levels correlate with disease burden at diagnosis, response to therapy, and relapse. In patients with extensive neck disease or calcitonin levels >500 pg/mL, imaging studies (CT neck/chest/liver and bone scintigraphy) are recommended to assess for metastatic disease.

Those with local or regional disease should undergo total thyroidectomy with neck dissection. Patients with metastatic disease may benefit from surgical intervention for local disease control and symptom palliation. The efficacy of chemotherapy and radiation has been disappointing. At present, the most effective therapies are TKIs. Vandetanib, a TKI that targets RET, EGFR, and VEGFR kinases, was approved in 2011 after a trial showed a predicted PFS of 30.5 months compared to 19.3 months with placebo. Cabozantinib, a TKI that targets RET, c-MET, and VEGFR, was approved in 2012 after a trial demonstrated a PFS of 11.2 months compared to 4 months with placebo.

THYROID NODULES
Introduction

Thyroid nodules are a common clinical problem typified by abnormal growths of thyroid tissue that are radiologically distinct from the surrounding thyroid gland. They can present as palpable masses on exam or incidentally on imaging obtained for other indications. Most are benign, but evaluation is always targeted to exclude thyroid cancer, with close attention paid to risk factors for malignancy. **Serum thyrotropin** (TSH) and thyroid US are valuable tools for diagnosis. FNA is the most sensitive and cost-effective means of characterizing

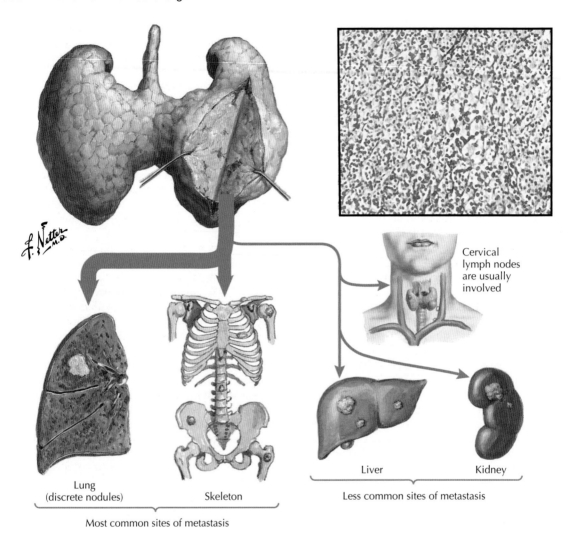

Cervical
lymph nodes
are usually
involved

Lung
(discrete nodules)

Skeleton

Liver   Kidney

Less common sites of metastasis

Most common sites of metastasis

FIG. 156.2 **Medullary Carcinoma of the Thyroid.**

nodules and the need for surgery. Benign nodules can be followed serially with US and are associated with a positive clinical course and negligible mortality risk.

Epidemiology and Risk Factors

The annual incidence of thyroid nodules is estimated to be 0.1% per year in the United States, and the lifetime probability for developing a thyroid nodule is 10%. Palpable nodules occur in only 4% to 7% of patient, and US is markedly more sensitive, able to detect nodules in 19% to 67% of asymptomatic patients. Thus nodules are often discovered incidentally on radiographic studies obtained for other reasons and lack a corresponding palpable thyroid lesion. Such incidentalomas carry the same risk of malignancy as palpable nodules of the same size. Thyroid nodules are four times more common in women. Nodule growth, also observed in pregnancy and multiparity, is thought to be influenced by estrogen and progesterone. Other risk factors include elderly age, low iodine intake, and exposure to ionizing radiation.

Despite the age-related increase, thyroid cancer is found in only 3% to 15% of all nodules. Over the past 40 years, thyroid cancer incidence has tripled, with an estimated 14.3 per 100,000 cases in 2009, thought driven primarily by increased detection of incidental nodules due to increased imaging for other medical indications.

Patients should be asked about their risk factors for thyroid cancer, such as prior head and neck radiation and a family history of thyroid cancer (see earlier discussion for further information). The risk of papillary thyroid cancer (PTC) increases by up to sixfold if present in a first-degree relative. Other familial thyroid cancer syndromes include Cowden syndrome (of the PTEN hamartoma tumor syndrome), familial adenomatous polyposis, and MEN in which MTC occurs. Other risk factors for thyroid cancer include extremes of age (<20 and >70 years) and male sex.

Presentation, Evaluation, and Diagnosis

Initial assessment focuses on the location, size, and growth of the neck mass. Rapid growth of the nodule, suggestive of underlying cancer, can cause dysphagia, neck discomfort, or hoarseness due to compression of the recurrent laryngeal nerve. Rapid growth can also arise from hemorrhage into a benign nodule or a cyst. Nonthyroidal conditions that may confer a nodular appearance include metastatic tumors, parathyroid cysts, lipomas, paragangliomas, and infiltrative disorders such as hemochromatosis. Patients should be asked about symptoms of hypothyroidism and hyperthyroidism, as nodules can be associated with overt thyroid dysfunction.

Nodules have various characteristics on palpation, ranging from soft and mobile to firm and fixed, the latter two being suggestive of cancer. Patients may be directed to swallow, moving the gland up from the sternal notch or overlying sternocleidomastoid muscle, to improve the definition of the gland against the palpating hand. Gland texture, mobility, tenderness, and size should be assessed. An enlarged thyroid can be palpable and visible on inspection, but the size of the gland alone does not represent thyroid function. Physical exam also should assess for regional lymph node enlargement that may represent local metastasis from thyroid cancer.

Initial laboratory studies include a serum thyrotropin (TSH) level to determine if the nodule is functioning, or producing thyroid hormone, which leads to a low TSH. Subsequent **radionuclide scan with** ^{123}**I** may show a "hot nodule" that has high radioiodine uptake due to autonomous production of thyroid hormone. Hyperfunctioning nodules with a low or undetectable TSH are almost always benign, and biopsy is almost never necessary. However, "cold nodules" (low to normal uptake on radionuclide scan) should be biopsied, as they confer a 5% to 15% risk for cancer. Patients with clinically apparent hyperthyroidism warrant further investigation with serum antibody testing, as the presence of cold or warm nodules does not preclude a concomitant diagnosis of Graves disease (see Chapter 73 for details).

In contrast, a normal or high TSH level increases the likelihood of malignancy. Higher levels of TSH have been shown to correlate with an increased risk of malignancy, but other serum markers, including calcitonin and Tg, lack the evidence for clinical use in diagnosis. Patients with thyroid nodules and normal/high TSH should undergo thyroid US to detect the number, size, and structure of nodules. US characteristics associated with malignancy include microcalcifications, irregular borders, hypoechogenicity, taller-than-wide shape, and increased vascularity. Multiple malignant features increase the specificity for diagnosing thyroid carcinoma, but US alone cannot be used to differentiate benign from malignant nodules. Patients with incidentally discovered nodules should be referred for US, as other imaging modalities lack the sensitivity to guide management.

FNA is the most accurate method of diagnosing thyroid nodules. FNA is indicated when nodules are ≥1 cm in greatest dimension with an intermediate to high suspicion pattern on US, 1.5 cm with a low suspicion pattern, and 2 cm or larger with a very low suspicion pattern. FNA of subcentimeter nodules with multiple suspicious features should be done but has not been associated with improved clinical outcomes.

FNA samples are classified into one of five categories under the **Bethesda system:** 70% of nodules have benign cytology, including colloid nodules, macrofollicular adenomas, and lymphocytic thyroiditis; 5% are classified as malignant and confer a 94% to 100% chance of representing a true malignancy; the remaining 25% are classified as indeterminate lesions and should be considered for molecular analysis to aid in diagnosis and the decision to pursue surgery. Mutational analysis can identify genes associated with thyroid cancer, such as *BRAF* and *RAS* mutations, which have a high positive predictive value (84%–100%), specificity (86%–100%), and generally are thought to be an effective rule-in test for those with high clinical or radiographic suspicion for cancer. Long-term data are currently lacking regarding the association between molecular testing and clinical outcomes but is currently being investigated.

Treatment

Patients with benign nodules have an excellent prognosis; FNA has a low false-negative rate, and long-term follow-up studies have not documented many deaths attributable to thyroid cancer. Benign nodules without suspicious clinical or US findings can be followed with repeat US in 1 to 2 years, which can be spaced to every 3 to 5 years if the nodule has not grown on serial US. Repeat FNA is recommended if the nodule has grown >50% in volume or increased by >20% in at least two dimensions with an increase of >2 mm. Nodules with high suspicion pattern on repeat US should receive repeat imaging and possible FNA within 12 months.

Indeterminate nodules with cytology of undetermined significance can be rebiopsied with molecular testing. If inconclusive, the nodule can be monitored or surgically resected. Patients may elect to undergo surgical resection, as opposed to watchful waiting, if they desire an immediate diagnosis. Indeterminate nodules with cytology classified as follicular neoplasms (or suspicious for neoplasm) should be referred for hemithyroidectomy or subtotal thyroidectomy.

Thyroidectomy is indicated if the FNA cytology is malignant or suspicious for malignancy. The presence of oncogenes on mutational analysis, such as the *BRAF* mutation, should also prompt surgery given its high predictive value for cancer. Other indications for thyroidectomy include bilateral nodules with a need for surgery in at least one nodule, a history of radiation to the head or neck, a family history of thyroid cancer, a nodule >4 cm in diameter, or benign nodules with compressive symptoms. Hemithyroidectomy can be considered based on anatomical presentation and anticipated success of surgery. Postoperative complications include hypoparathyroidism and recurrent laryngeal nerve paralysis, but these can be minimized by selection of an experienced thyroid surgeon.

Secondary treatments have limited roles. Radioiodine (^{131}I) ablation may be used to treat toxic nodular goiters but should not be the first-line therapy if compressive symptoms are present or for large nodules that may require high doses of radioiodine. Percutaneous ethanol injection (PEI) involves injection of sterile 100% alcohol into a tumor cavity to dehydrate cells and denature cellular proteins. It can be used for thyroid cysts or nodules with a large fluid component to decrease recurrence rates. Levothyroxine is not recommended for routine use to suppress nodule growth.

CHAPTER 157

Lung Cancer

JEFFREY MUFSON

INTRODUCTION

Lung cancer is responsible for more deaths worldwide than any other type of cancer, and it is the second most common cancer after prostate cancer in men, and breast cancer in women. The 5-year survival rate remains low, at ~18%, primarily because of the typically advanced stage at diagnosis.

The vast majority of lung cancers are subdivided into four major histological subtypes: adenocarcinoma, squamous cell carcinoma, large cell carcinoma, and **small cell carcinoma;** another tumor subtype, known as carcinoid, is much rarer (Fig. 157.1). Adenocarcinoma, squamous cell, and large cell carcinoma together constitute the **non–small cell lung cancers (NSCLCs),** the most common group overall.

PATHOPHYSIOLOGY

Mutations in specific genes have been identified in different types of lung cancer, providing insight into pathogenesis and offering novel therapeutic targets. In particular, mutations in **EGFR, ALK,** and ROS1 found in NSCLCs are the most clinically significant because they can be targeted using novel receptor tyrosine kinase inhibitors.

EGFR, the gene encoding the epidermal growth factor receptor, is one of the most commonly mutated protooncogenes in NSCLCs. EGFR is a receptor tyrosine kinase that promotes cellular proliferation and survival, and thus activating mutations result in tumor growth. EGFR mutations are more prevalent in NSCLCs arising in women and never smokers.

Likewise, fusion of ALK with EML4 activates a receptor tyrosine kinase and causes uncontrolled cellular proliferation. Such mutations are also more common in NSCLCs in never smokers, and they occur in about 3% to 7% of lung adenocarcinomas overall. Finally, chromosomal rearrangements in the ROS1 gene, which encodes another receptor tyrosine kinase, are also present in about 1% to 2% of NSCLCs.

KRAS gene mutations occur in about 25% of all lung adenocarcinomas and predict poorer overall survival. The identification of a KRAS mutation usually obviates the need for further molecular typing, as there is generally no overlap between the presence of a KRAS mutation and the presence of a EGFR, ALK, or ROS1 mutation. Currently, no targeted therapy exists for KRAS mutations.

RISK FACTORS

Cigarette smoking is the largest and most important risk factor, responsible for 90% of lung cancers. Cigar and pipe smoking are also associated with lung cancer, though the association is weaker. Second-hand exposure also increases the risk of lung cancer, with the relative risk equal to 1.4 in one large study. The main carcinogenic substances in cigarette smoke are polycyclic aromatic hydrocarbons and N-nitrosamines, which irreversibly bind to deoxyribonucleic acid (DNA) and cause replication errors. Of note, although most cases of lung cancer are attributable to tobacco use, most heavy smokers do not develop lung cancer, highlighting the importance of additional, poorly understood genetic factors.

Other environmental risk factors include exposure to arsenic, chromium, nickel, radiation, radon, air pollution, and asbestos.

PRESENTATION, EVALUATION, AND DIAGNOSIS

The majority of lung cancers are discovered at a late stage, which contributes to the high mortality of the disease. Current recommendations are for adults aged 55 to 80 who have a >30 pack-year smoking history, who continue to smoke or who quit <15 years ago, to undergo annual low dose chest CT. Candidates for screening should be carefully selected based on their fitness and willingness to undergo a local treatment for early lung cancer (i.e., surgery) and other comorbidities.

Squamous cell	Small cell	Adenocarcinoma	Large cell

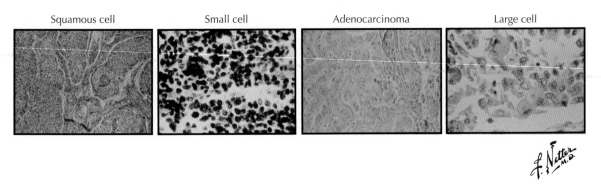

FIG. 157.1 **Major Histological Classifications of Lung Cancer.**

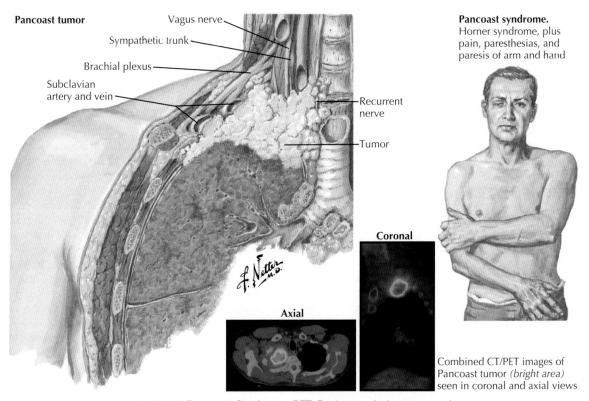

Pancoast tumor

Vagus nerve

Sympathetic trunk

Brachial plexus

Subclavian artery and vein

Recurrent nerve

Tumor

Pancoast syndrome.
Horner syndrome, plus pain, paresthesias, and paresis of arm and hand

Coronal

Axial

Combined CT/PET images of Pancoast tumor *(bright area)* seen in coronal and axial views

FIG. 157.2 **Pancoast Syndrome.** *PET,* Positron emission tomography.

The most common symptoms of lung cancer are cough, shortness of breath, fatigue, weight loss, and fevers; additional symptoms include hemoptysis and hoarseness. If brain metastases have occurred, then headache, seizure, and/or focal neurological deficits may also be present. The **Horner syndrome** (miosis, ptosis, anhidrosis) may be present in the case of a superior sulcus tumor, also known as a **Pancoast tumor,** compressing the sympathetic trunk (Fig. 157.2). Paraneoplastic syndromes (e.g., **Lambert-Eaton myasthenic syndrome,** Cushing syndrome, and syndrome of inappropriate antidiuretic hormone secretion [SIADH]) may occur with small cell lung cancers.

Most patients undergo chest radiography as the initial diagnostic test, followed by a CT scan if there is any abnormality or the clinical suspicion remains elevated.

If a lung cancer is identified, patients should undergo complete imaging, with CT of the abdomen/pelvis or a positron emission tomography (PET)/CT scan. Brain MRI should be pursued in all small cell lung cancer patients, given the high risk of metastasis, and in all patients with stage III or higher non–small cell lung cancer.

Distant lesions should be preferentially sampled to both diagnose and properly stage the cancer. If a solitary lung mass is seen, patients should undergo bronchoscopy with endobronchial ultrasound for lymph node evaluation. If the lymph nodes are normal, biopsy or resection of the primary mass should be pursued.

The staging for non–small cell lung cancer follows the tumor-node-metastasis (TNM) system. Staging for small cell lung cancer utilizes the Veterans Administration Lung Group system, which categorizes disease as limited or extensive. Limited disease is confined to one hemithorax and can be encompassed in one radiation field.

TREATMENT

The treatment of lung cancer depends on the histological classification and stage. All smokers should be encouraged to pursue and be assisted with smoking cessation as part of the treatment plan.

Non–Small Cell Lung Cancer
Stages I and II

Early-stage NSCLCs are surgically resected with curative intent. Lobectomy (or greater) is preferred over wedge resection when tolerable. In patients who cannot tolerate surgery, radiotherapy (RT) is an alternative. Patients who receive postoperative RT, however, have decreased survival, and thus RT is not recommended as a standard adjunct to surgery. If positive surgical margins are present and additional resection would not be tolerated, however, adjuvant RT can be considered.

Adjuvant chemotherapy is not advised for stage Ia disease but is standard for stage II disease. In stage Ib disease, the decision depends on the presence or absence of high-risk features, such as poor differentiation, vascular invasion, visceral pleural involvement, size, unknown lymph node status (Nx), and wedge resection.

Stage III

The treatment of stage III disease is complex, and a full discussion is beyond the scope of this chapter. Stage III patients are typically subdivided into two groups of patients: those with incidentally discovered N2 disease at surgery and those with known N2/N3 disease. Patients found to have N2 disease at surgery receive adjuvant chemotherapy with or without RT, depending on the concern for local recurrence. Patients with known N2 disease are either treated with preoperative chemotherapy followed by surgery or with definitive chemoradiotherapy. Patients with infiltrating stage IIIa disease or IIIb disease (contralateral or multistation mediastinal, supraclavicular, or multiple visible nodes on imaging) are typically treated with definitive chemoradiotherapy if their performance status is adequate.

Stage IV

The treatment of metastatic disease begins with an assessment of a variety of molecular markers and immunostains. Current guidelines recommend that these tests only be obtained in stage IV disease, as targeted therapy and **immunotherapy** are only approved in the metastatic setting, though they are increasingly being performed with earlier stage disease to assist with long-term treatment planning should these patients relapse. Patients should undergo *EGFR, ALK,* and *ROS1* testing; *KRAS* testing is also usually included as part of a broad molecular panel that seeks to uncover rarer driver mutations, which may be targetable in a clinical trial. Patients with *EGFR* mutations should receive osimertinib. Patients with an *ALK* should be treated with alectinib, and *ROS1* translocation should be treated with crizotinib.

Immunotherapy is a rapidly evolving realm of therapeutic intervention, and tissue should be stained to assess for PD-L1 expression. PD-L1 is a ligand for the program death-1 receptor (PD1) expressed on activated T cells. PD-L1 binding suppresses T-cell function, but monoclonal antibodies have been developed that bind to both PD1 (nivolumab) and PD-L1 (pembrolizumab) to block their interaction, thereby increasing T-cell function and cancer cell destruction. Thus if high levels of PDL1 (>50%) expression are found, patients can receive immune checkpoint blockade therapy with pembrolizumab in the first-line setting. Patients with >1% PD-L1 staining would be candidates for pembrolizumab as a second-line agent, and if PD-L1 staining is absent, they may receive nivolumab after progression on chemotherapy.

Immunotherapy can lead to generalized inflammation, but on occasion can progress to severe and life-threatening reactions, including myocarditis, colitis, and pneumonitis. Neuropsychiatric syndromes may be the result of an encephalitis. Corticosteroids can be given to suppress most of these reactions, though life-threatening complications may require treatment with tumor necrosis factor-α inhibitors. Typically, low-dose steroids for mild complications such as arthritis are not thought to abrogate the effectiveness of immunotherapy, but debate is ongoing regarding the effect of high doses of steroids on efficacy of immunotherapy. Severe side effects necessitating high-dose steroids should prompt consideration for therapy discontinuation.

If genetic and molecular testing are unremarkable, patients should receive traditional chemotherapy, with selection of agents based on histology. For adenocarcinoma, a common regimen is a platinum-based agent plus pemetrexed (commonly known as a platinum doublet). For squamous cell carcinomas, gemcitabine is used in lieu of pemetrexed. Bevacizumab, a monoclonal antibody targeting vascular endothelial growth factor (VEGF), can be used in combination with chemotherapy for nonsquamous cell carcinomas (adenocarcinoma and large cell).

Once patients achieve a response with first-line chemotherapy, maintenance chemotherapy is initiated to delay disease progression and control symptoms. Once patients progress on chemotherapy, immune therapy is the second-line choice. Palliative care consultation should also be requested for all patients with metastatic lung cancer, as a randomized trial of patients with

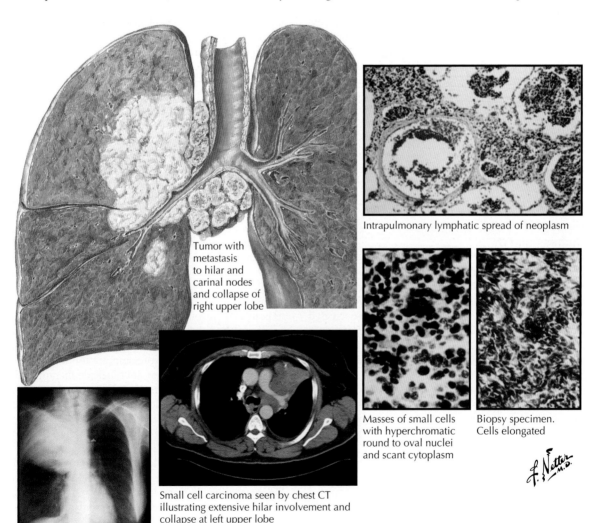

Tumor with metastasis to hilar and carinal nodes and collapse of right upper lobe

Intrapulmonary lymphatic spread of neoplasm

Masses of small cells with hyperchromatic round to oval nuclei and scant cytoplasm

Biopsy specimen. Cells elongated

Small cell carcinoma seen by chest CT illustrating extensive hilar involvement and collapse at left upper lobe

Chest radiograph demonstrating right upper lobe collapse from an infiltrating small cell carcinoma

FIG. 157.3 **Small Cell Carcinoma of the Lung.**

stage IV NSCLC found that early palliative care led to improved quality of life, fewer depressive symptoms, and a significantly improved overall survival (11.6 months compared to 8.9 months).

Small Cell Lung Cancer
Limited stage
The mainstay of treatment is combined chemotherapy (cisplatin and etoposide) and radiation. Although response rates are high (70%–90%), relapse rates are also high, and the median overall survival even with treatment is 14 to 20 months. Once the patient recovers from chemoradiation, prophylactic cranial irradiation is performed to reduce the risk of central nervous system metastases.

Extensive stage
The prognosis for extensive stage disease is dismal, with a 2-year overall survival rate of ~12% (Fig. 157.3). Patients are treated with a platinum doublet that includes either etoposide or irinotecan. When brain metastases are present, whole brain radiation is used following chemotherapy (or more urgently, if neurological symptoms are present).

Relapsed/refractory disease
Most patients with small cell lung cancer will relapse after first-line treatment. Palliative chemotherapy with topotecan is standard, but several agents can be used, including combination immunotherapy with ipilimumab/nivolumab.

CHAPTER 158

Esophageal Cancer

EMILY N. KINSEY

INTRODUCTION

Esophageal cancer is the eighth most common cancer worldwide and sixth most common cause of cancer death. The worldwide distribution of esophageal cancer varies, with the highest prevalence seen in the so-called Asian esophageal cancer belt, which stretches from China to the Middle East. Symptoms typically occur late in the course of the disease, so most patients have advanced disease at the time of diagnosis. Developments in treatment have improved survival, but the overall 5-year survival rate is still <20%.

ANATOMY AND HISTOLOGY

The esophageal wall is composed of five distinct layers. From the lumen outward, the layers are the superficial mucosa, lamina propria, submucosa, muscularis propria, and adventitia. All parts of the gastrointestinal tract other than the esophagus have an outermost layer called the serosa; the lack of this layer in the esophagus may be part of the reason esophageal cancers are more likely to spread locally.

The cell types that line the esophageal lumen vary based on anatomical location. Squamous epithelial cells are found in the proximal and middle thirds of the esophagus, while glandular cells are found in the distal third and gastroesophageal junction. Accordingly, **squamous cell carcinomas** are typically located in the middle third of the esophagus, while **adenocarcinomas** are found in the distal third and gastroesophageal junction. Very rare types of esophageal cancers include small cell carcinoma, lymphoma, and leiomyoma.

RISK FACTORS

Squamous cell carcinomas and adenocarcinomas of the esophagus have similar survival rates but distinct risk factors and geographic distribution. Male gender and smoking are risk factors for both, though the male predominance is stronger for adenocarcinoma, while smoking is a stronger risk factor for squamous cell carcinoma.

Alcohol use increases the risk of squamous cell carcinoma, and the effect is synergistic with smoking. The consumption of very hot beverages also increases the risk, while a diet rich in fruits and vegetables may be protective.

Central obesity, gastroesophageal reflux disease (GERD), and higher body mass index all increase the risk of adenocarcinoma. **Barrett esophagus,** a complication of GERD, is a precursor to dysplasia and adenocarcinoma (see Chapter 128).

In the past, squamous cell carcinomas were more common in the United States than adenocarcinomas; however, as rates of obesity have increased, adenocarcinomas have become more common. A similar pattern has occurred in other developed nations. In contrast, developing nations typically have a higher prevalence of squamous cell carcinomas.

PRESENTATION

Esophageal cancers are generally asymptomatic until they become obstructive or near obstructive, form a stricture, or metastasize (Fig. 158.1). A common symptom is **dysphagia** for solids but not liquids. Other symptoms include regurgitation, chest pain, and heartburn. Involvement of the recurrent laryngeal nerve may cause hoarseness. If the tumor bleeds, hematemesis or melena may occur. Weight loss or other constitutional symptoms may also be present.

DIAGNOSIS AND STAGING

Patients who report dysphagia, regurgitation, or melena should undergo upper endoscopy with biopsy and endoscopic ultrasound, which can establish a definitive diagnosis of esophageal cancer that includes grade, depth of invasion, and histology. Patients with confirmed cancers should also undergo a positron emission tomography (PET)/CT scan to assess local extension and search for

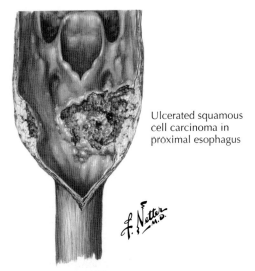

Ulcerated squamous cell carcinoma in proximal esophagus

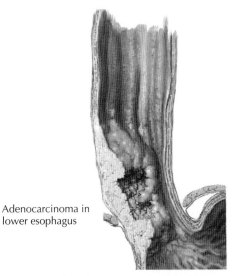

Adenocarcinoma in lower esophagus

Tapering of esophageal lumen at site of carcinoma

Thickening of esophageal wall at site of carcinoma

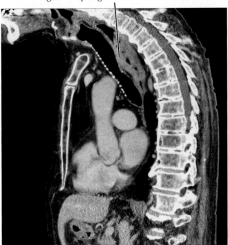

Barium esophagram

CT scan

FIG. 158.1 **Esophageal Cancer.**

remote metastases. If the esophageal tumor is located above the carina, a bronchoscopy should be performed to rule out airway invasion.

The staging of esophageal cancers is based on the TNM classification. The depth of tumor invasion is the T designation. T1 tumors have invaded the lamina propria (T1a) or submucosa (T1b), T2 tumors the muscularis, T3 the adventitia, and T4 adjacent structures. T4 can be further subclassified to distinguish between invasion of the pericardium, pleura, and diaphragm (T4a) and further

invasion into the heart, trachea, great vessels, or aorta (T4b). Nodal designation is an important branchpoint in the treatment algorithm: Once the cancer has spread to the lymph nodes, surgery alone is no longer sufficient. The number of positive lymph nodes is also an important prognostic indicator. N1 indicates disease in 1 or 2 regional lymph nodes, N2 in 3 to 6 nodes, and N3 in >7 nodes. The presence of a distant metastasis, or M1 disease, is another important branchpoint because surgery is no longer appropriate.

Previously, squamous cell carcinoma and adenocarcinoma were staged together, but now two distinct staging systems exist. The histological grade is incorporated into the staging of node-negative cancers of either type. Grade 1 refers to well differentiated, 2 to moderately differentiated, 3 to poorly differentiated, and 4 to undifferentiated. Location is only important for early-stage squamous cell carcinomas.

TREATMENT

The treatment of esophageal cancer usually includes surgery, chemotherapy, and radiation. The exceptions are very early-stage cancers, for which surgery alone is curative, and late-stage cancers, for which surgery is not indicated.

T1 disease without nodal invasion can be cured with surgery alone. T1a squamous cell or adenocarcinoma can be treated with **esophagectomy**, endoscopic resection, or endoscopic resection followed by ablation. T1b tumors are typically treated with esophagectomy; however, superficial T1b adenocarcinomas are an exception and can be treated with endoscopic therapies, like T1a tumors. For all T1 tumors, systemic therapy is not needed postoperatively.

If lymph nodes are involved, preoperative (neoadjuvant) systemic therapy is recommended. The evidence for treating potentially resectable esophageal cancers with preoperative chemoradiation comes from the CROSS trial, which showed a significant increase in overall survival when patients were treated with chemoradiation and surgery versus surgery alone (49.4 months compared to 24 months). Postoperative management varies from observation to more systemic treatment (i.e., chemoradiation or additional chemotherapy), depending on the tumor histology, resection margins, and the node status at surgery.

For some patients, surgical resection is either unfeasible or inappropriate. Such patients include those with tumors in the cervical esophagus (<5 cm from the cricopharyngeus muscle, due to the high morbidity of surgery), with metastases (stage IV disease), and with T4b tumors (i.e., invasion into critical thoracic structures). Such patients receive definitive chemoradiation with the same regimens used in preoperative chemoradiation, though a higher dose of radiation is required.

For patients with metastatic disease, a typical front-line chemotherapy regimen includes a fluoropyrimidine and a platinum. All patients with metastatic adenocarcinoma should be tested for HER2. If patients are HER2 positive, then the monoclonal antibody directed at HER2 (trastuzumab) should be added to the initial treatment regimen. The addition of trastuzumab to front-line chemotherapy is based on the survival advantage seen in the ToGA trial. Immunotherapy with pembrolizumab is a recent addition to the treatment arsenal. All patients with metastatic disease should be tested for PDL1 expression using the Combined Positive Score (CPS), as this score currently determines their eligibility for pembrolizumab.

CHAPTER 159

Gastric Cancer

EVAN ROSENBAUM

INTRODUCTION

Gastric cancer accounts for ~10% of cancer deaths and is the third most common cause of cancer-related death worldwide. More than half of gastric cancers are diagnosed at a late stage, and consequently the prognosis is often poor. The estimated 5-year overall survival (OS) rate for gastric cancer is 28.3%.

Nearly all stomach cancers are adenocarcinomas, and they are categorized as proximal or distal. Proximal tumors, which are more common in Western countries, include those in the proximal lesser curvature, cardia, and gastroesophageal junction (GEJ). Distal tumors are more common in many Asian countries, parts of Central and South America, and in the former Soviet Union.

The incidence of gastric cancer is greatest in Eastern countries, such as China and Japan. The incidence has decreased in the United States in recent decades, related to fewer distal tumors. At the same time, however, the incidence of proximal tumors, which tend to be more aggressive and treatment resistant, has increased.

PATHOPHYSIOLOGY

Gastric adenocarcinomas are classified based on histopathological findings as intestinal or diffuse subtypes. The intestinal subtype tends to be well differentiated. Approximately half of intestinal subtype cancers are associated with *Helicobacter pylori* infection. The pathogenesis involves a multistep progression from gastritis to intestinal metaplasia to invasive carcinoma (see Chapter 129 for details).

The diffuse subtype is more undifferentiated, more likely to be proximal, and more likely to invade and metastasize. All layers of the stomach can become infiltrated and diffusely thickened, causing a loss of distensibility and a leather-bottle appearance known as linitis plastica (Fig. 159.1). The mechanism of carcinogenesis is similar to that of esophageal and GEJ adenocarcinomas. The loss of E-cadherin protein expression, normally encoded by the cadherin-1 (*CDH1*) gene, leads to a loss of cell adhesion molecules and subsequent cell proliferation and tumor invasion. *CDH1*

mutations also occur in hereditary diffuse gastric cancer (HDGC), a rare autosomal dominant genetic disorder with a high risk of gastric cancer.

The epidermal growth factor receptor family, including HER1 and HER2, is overexpressed in many gastric cancers, as is vascular endothelial growth factor (VEGF) and its receptor. In some tumors, overexpression of c-MET, a tyrosine kinase receptor, leads to constitutive activation of HER2 and contributes to oncogenesis. Monoclonal antibodies and small molecule inhibitors are being developed to target these proteins and inhibit their downstream signaling pathways.

RISK FACTORS

Numerous environmental risk factors have been associated with gastric adenocarcinoma. Such factors include frequent consumption of nitrates (found in processed meats, pickled vegetables, and salted or smoked fish); infrequent consumption of fruits and vegetables; occupational exposure to coal, nickel, rubber, or timber; cigarette smoking; prior gastric surgery; *H. pylori* infection; Epstein-Barr virus (EBV) infection; and radiation exposure.

Inherited risk factors include African, Hispanic, and Native American ancestry as well as several genetic syndromes, which account for a total of 3% to 5% of gastric cancers. Such syndromes include HDGC (hereditary diffuse gastric cancer), Lynch syndrome, juvenile polyposis syndrome, Peutz-Jeghers syndrome, familial adenomatous polyposis, and Li-Fraumeni syndrome.

PRESENTATION, EVALUATION, AND DIAGNOSIS

Patients with gastric cancer may be asymptomatic. If present, symptoms are usually vague and nonspecific, including night sweats, weight loss, early satiety, fatigue, abdominal pain, nausea, dysphagia, and/or gastrointestinal bleeding.

Screening is only performed in endemic regions, such as in Japan, where patients are risk stratified based on

Polypoid Adenocarcinoma

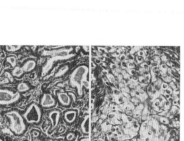

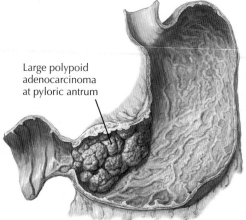

Large polypoid adenocarcinoma at pyloric antrum

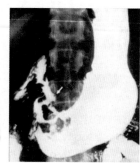

Adenocarcinoma   Colloid carcinoma

Radiographic appearance of polypoid adenocarcinoma

Scirrhous Carcinoma

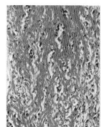

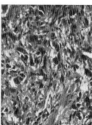

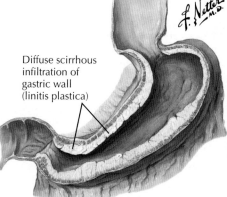

Diffuse scirrhous infiltration of gastric wall (linitis plastica)

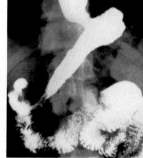

Linitis plastica   Scirrhous carcinoma

Radiographic appearance of linitis plastica

FIG. 159.1 **Carcinomas of the Stomach.**

the results of *H. pylori* serologic testing, measurement of pepsinogen levels, and endoscopy. The serum levels of carcinoembryonic antigen (CEA); human chronic gonadotropin-β; and cancer antigens 19-9 (CA19-9), CA125, CA72-4, and CA50 may also be elevated, though their sensitivity as diagnostic markers is poor.

The American Joint Committee on Cancer (AJCC) recommends the use of the TNM (tumor, nodal, metastasis) classification system for the staging of gastric cancer. Gastric cancer tends to spread locally and to local and regional lymph nodes, though hematogenous spread can also occur. Tumors can spread intramurally in a radial fashion, or they can penetrate through the serosal layer of the stomach into adjacent organs. The majority of tumors have serosal invasion and lymphatic involvement at diagnosis. Metastasis typically occurs to the esophagus, duodenum, omentum, spleen, adrenal glands, diaphragm, liver, pancreas, or colon. If the cancer spreads via

intrathoracic lymph nodes, clinical manifestations may include left supraclavicular lymphadenopathy, known as Virchow node, or left axillary lymphadenopathy, also called Irish node. Meanwhile, involvement of the lymphatic chain in the falciform ligament can lead to a Sister Mary Joseph node, manifesting as a subcutaneous periumbilical tumor.

Both esophagogastroduodenoscopy (EGD) and CT scan are used for the diagnosis and staging of gastric cancer. EGD permits direct visualization and biopsy of the primary tumor. Endoscopic ultrasound (EUS) is used for perioperative staging because it accurately assesses tumor invasion depth and regional lymph node involvement. Staging laparoscopy with peritoneal lavage allows direct visualization of regional lymph nodes and surrounding organs and the examination of peritoneal cytology; it increases the likelihood of detecting metastatic disease and is recommended when other noninvasive imaging modalities demonstrate localized, resectable disease. ¹⁸F-fluorodeoxyglucose (FDG)/positron emission tomography (PET) plays a limited role in the primary staging of gastric cancer because of poor FDG uptake by diffuse subtype tumors.

TREATMENT

Surgery is the primary treatment for resectable, nonmetastatic gastric adenocarcinomas; it is typically accompanied by preoperative, perioperative, or adjuvant chemotherapy, with or without radiation. Surgery is essential for obtaining an accurate pathological stage and may be curative if negative margins are achieved.

The surgical approach and extent depend on the location, size, and characteristics of the tumor. Stage I, or early gastric cancers, that are well differentiated, superficial, and small (<3 cm) can potentially be removed via endoscopic mucosal resection or limited surgical resection (gastrotomy with excision, as opposed to gastrectomy). Stage I cancers with poor tumor characteristics, as well as stage II and III tumors, require gastrectomy with lymph node resection. The goal of surgical resection is to eliminate any evidence of macroscopic or microscopic residual tumor. Proximal, large midgastric, or linitis plastica tumors usually require total gastrectomies, while distal tumors can often be removed with a partial gastrectomy (Fig. 159.2).

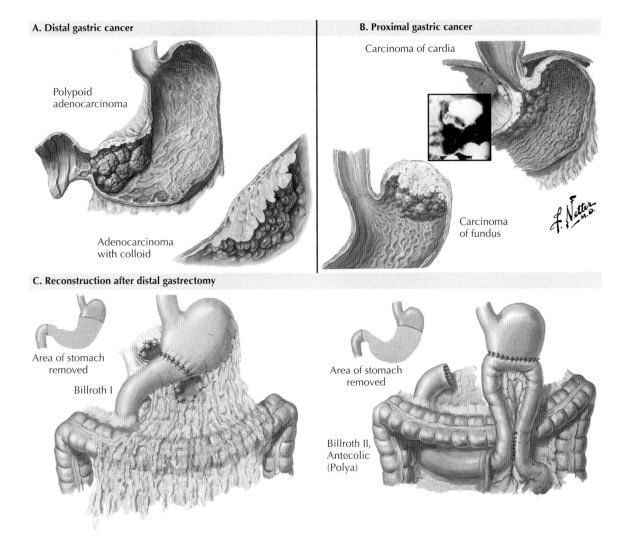

A. Distal gastric cancer

Polypoid adenocarcinoma

Adenocarcinoma with colloid

B. Proximal gastric cancer

Carcinoma of cardia

Carcinoma of fundus

C. Reconstruction after distal gastrectomy

Area of stomach removed

Billroth I

Area of stomach removed

Billroth II, Antocolic (Polya)

FIG. 159.2 **Distal and Proximal Gastric Cancer and Reconstruction.**

An essential component of surgical staging is extensive resection of lymph nodes, with 15 nodes being the accepted minimum. Studies in Japan have found that a nodal resection extending along the left gastric, common hepatic, celiac, and splenic arteries leads to an increase in OS and decreased locoregional recurrence. Studies in the United States have been less definitive, instead finding an increase in morbidity and mortality with extensive resections.

In addition to surgery, chemotherapy in both the perioperative and adjuvant settings increases OS in locally advanced gastric cancer. The addition of radiotherapy to either perioperative or adjuvant chemotherapy may further increase pathological response rates and improve OS. Chemotherapies with demonstrated benefit include pyrimidine analogs, platinum analogs, anthracyclines, taxanes, and camptothecins. Multiagent regimens have a greater effect on OS than single agent regimens, though adverse effects are also increased. Some of these regimens include cisplatin and fluorouracil (CF); fluorouracil, leucovorin, and oxaliplatin (FOLFOX); and epirubicin, cisplatin, and fluorouracil (ECF).

Patients with metastatic gastric cancer are treated both to palliate symptoms and to improve survival. The decision to treat with systemic therapy depends on patient and tumor characteristics and must take into account the risk versus benefit of treatment over supportive care alone. In the past decade, a number of drugs have become available to treat metastatic gastric cancer. Fluorouracil plus a platinum analog continues to be a commonly used first-line treatment regimen. Trastuzumab, a monoclonal antibody targeting HER2, increases OS when added to first-line chemotherapy in patients with HER2-positive tumors. Ramucirumab is a monoclonal antibody targeting the VEGF receptor 2 that increases survival when combined with paclitaxel, a taxane, in the second-line setting. The drug pembrolizumab, an antibody that blocks the immune checkpoint protein PD-1, is approved for use in the third-line setting in patients who express the programmed death-ligand 1 (PD-L1) protein. Research is ongoing to identify novel targeted agents with efficacy in gastric cancer. Local interventions that may aid in symptom palliation include radiotherapy, endoscopic stent placement, percutaneous gastrostomy or jejunostomy tube placement, and palliative surgical resection.

CHAPTER 160

Colorectal Cancer (CRC)

JESSICA YANG

INTRODUCTION

Colorectal cancer (CRC) is the fourth most common cancer in the United States. Though mortality has been progressively declining since 1990, CRC remains the second leading cause of cancer-related death, after lung cancer.

The majority of CRCs are carcinomas, with >90% being adenocarcinomas. Specific morphological variants of adenocarcinoma, known as *signet ring* and *mucinous*, are associated with a poorer prognosis. Other types of colon cancer, such as neuroendocrine or mesenchymal tumors, are uncommon and will not be further discussed in this chapter.

RISK FACTORS

Several factors are associated with an increased risk of CRC, including inflammatory bowel disease, prior polyps or colon cancer, a first-degree relative diagnosed at <50 years of age, low-fiber diet, alcohol, obesity, and diabetes. Interestingly, the long-term use of aspirin may have a protective effect against CRC, particularly for patients with a genetic predisposition (Fig. 160.1).

The two known inherited forms of CRC are **hereditary nonpolyposis CRC (HNPCC, or Lynch syndrome)** and **familial adenomatous polyposis (FAP)**. FAP is caused by an inherited, inactivating mutation in the *APC* tumor suppressor gene, which leads to loss of β-catenin regulation and the formation of hundreds to thousands of colonic polyps. Although FAP causes only 0.5% to 1% of all CRCs, mutations in *APC* are also found in the majority of sporadic tumors.

Lynch syndrome is an inherited autosomal dominant disease characterized by microsatellite instability (MSI) arising from mutations in deoxyribonucleic acid (DNA) mismatch repair (MMR) proteins (*MSH2, MSH6, MLH1, PMS1,* and *PMS2*). Patients are also at risk for developing breast, ovarian, endometrial, pancreas, biliary, gastric, small bowel, and genitourinary cancers. The Amsterdam criteria, also known as the 3-2-1 rule, are used to determine the likelihood of Lynch syndrome:

three or more family members with CRC, at least two of whom are first-degree relatives; two successive generations affected; one family member with diagnosis before age 50. Mutations in MMR proteins are also found in 10% to 15% of sporadic CRCs. In describing such tumors, MSI-high (MSI-H) is equivalent to deficient MMR, and microsatellite stable (MSS) is equivalent to proficient MMR.

PRESENTATION

Patients with early-stage colon cancer may be asymptomatic and diagnosed as a result of screening, but most cases are diagnosed after the onset of symptoms. The most common symptoms and findings include abdominal pain, hematochezia, a change in bowel habits, and unexplained iron-deficiency anemia. Patients may rarely present with symptoms of bowel obstruction or even perforation.

Right-sided cancers generally manifest as occult blood loss and iron deficiency. Left-sided cancers more often present with constipation, owing to stool being more formed and the lumen being smaller. Rectosigmoid cancers often present with hematochezia, with rectal cancers also associated with rectal pain, tenesmus, and decreased stool caliber (Fig. 160.2).

About one in four patients will have metastatic disease at the time of presentation, with the most common sites being regional lymph nodes, liver, lungs, and peritoneum. Such patients may present with right upper quadrant pain, abdominal distention/ascites, and supraclavicular and/or periumbilical lymphadenopathy.

DIAGNOSIS AND STAGING

In general, older individuals (age >50) presenting with hematochezia or unexplained iron-deficiency anemia should proceed to a colonoscopy/flexible sigmoidoscopy as early as possible. If a tumor is identified, biopsies are obtained to establish a tissue diagnosis. The biopsy and imaging findings are used to determine the clinical

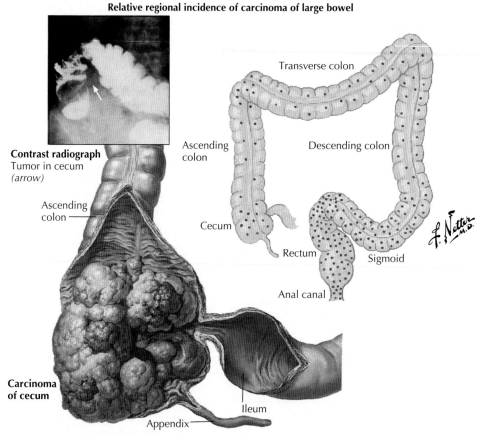

Relative regional incidence of carcinoma of large bowel

Contrast radiograph
Tumor in cecum
(arrow)

Ascending
colon

Transverse colon

Descending colon

Ascending
colon

Cecum

Rectum

Sigmoid

Anal canal

**Carcinoma
of cecum**

Ileum

Appendix

Characteristic	Description
Site	98% adenocarcinomas: 25% in cecum-ascending colon, 25% in sigmoid colon, 25% in rectum, 25% elsewhere
Prevalence	Highest in United States, Canada, Australia, New Zealand, Denmark, Sweden; males affected 20% more than females
Age	Peak incidence at 60–70 years
Risk factors	Heredity, high-fat diet, increasing age, inflammatory bowel disease, polyps

FIG. 160.1 **Malignant Tumors of the Large Intestine.**

stage, which is the most important indicator of outcome and determines treatment approach.

The TNM staging system of the American Joint Committee on Cancer is the preferred system. Current guidelines recommend that all patients undergo contrast-enhanced CT scans of the chest, abdomen, and pelvis to assess for lymph node involvement and distant metastases. A liver-phase MRI may better elucidate hepatic lesions if CT findings are not definitive or resection is being considered. Positron emission tomography (PET) scans are not routinely used for initial staging but can be useful in monitoring for recurrences (Fig. 160.3).

Serum carcinoembryonic antigen (CEA) should not be used as a screening or diagnostic test because of its limited sensitivity and specificity; however, preoperative levels have prognostic value, and postoperative levels are useful in evaluating persistent or recurrent disease.

TREATMENT
Colon Cancer

Patients with stage 0 (carcinoma in situ or intramucosal cancer) or stage I disease are generally cured with endoscopic or surgical resection alone. Most patients with stage II disease can also be cured with surgery, but those with more locally advanced tumors or certain high-risk clinicopathological features (e.g., T4 primary tumor, high-grade or poorly differentiated histology with mucinous

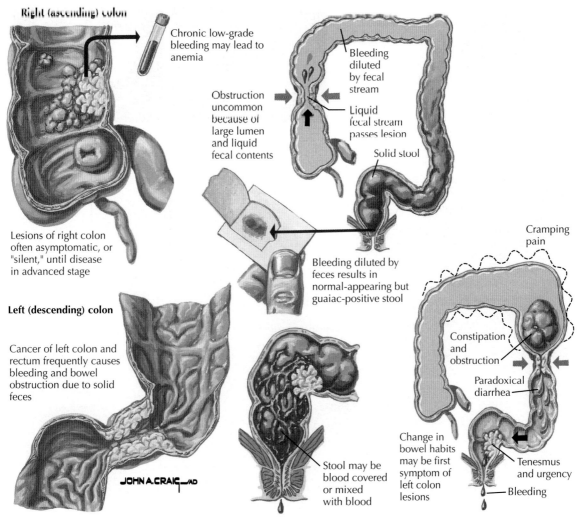

Right (ascending) colon

Chronic low-grade bleeding may lead to anemia

Obstruction uncommon because of large lumen and liquid fecal contents

Bleeding diluted by fecal stream

Liquid fecal stream passes lesion

Solid stool

Lesions of right colon often asymptomatic, or "silent," until disease in advanced stage

Bleeding diluted by feces results in normal-appearing but guaiac-positive stool

Cramping pain

Left (descending) colon

Cancer of left colon and rectum frequently causes bleeding and bowel obstruction due to solid feces

Constipation and obstruction

Paradoxical diarrhea

Change in bowel habits may be first symptom of left colon lesions

Stool may be blood covered or mixed with blood

Tenesmus and urgency

Bleeding

JOHN A.CRAIG—AD

FIG. 160.2 **Clinical Manifestations of Colorectal Cancer.**

or signet ring features, evidence of lymphovascular or perineural invasion, close/indeterminate/positive surgical margins, inadequately sampled lymph nodes, bowel obstruction/perforation, or high preoperative CEA) may benefit from adjuvant systemic therapy. The overall impact on survival, however, is not clear. In one large randomized trial, adjuvant therapy was associated with a significant 22% reduction in risk of disease recurrence compared to observation among patients with stage II disease, but there was only a nonsignificant trend toward better survival. Of note, the prognosis among patients with stage II disease is better with MSI-H tumors than with MSS tumors, possibly due to the accumulation

of genetic mutations and activation of the immune system.

Patients with stage III (node-positive) disease should receive surgery and adjuvant chemotherapy. Fluorouracil (5FU) in combination with leucovorin (LV) was historically the standard regimen, but two pivotal trials clearly demonstrated that the addition of oxaliplatin to 5FU and LV (FOLFOX) improved disease-free and overall survival compared to 5FU/LV alone. Both trials included patients with stage II and III disease, but only those with stage III disease experienced a survival benefit. 5FU may be replaced with capecitabine, an oral prodrug that is metabolized to 5FU. Thus approved regimens include

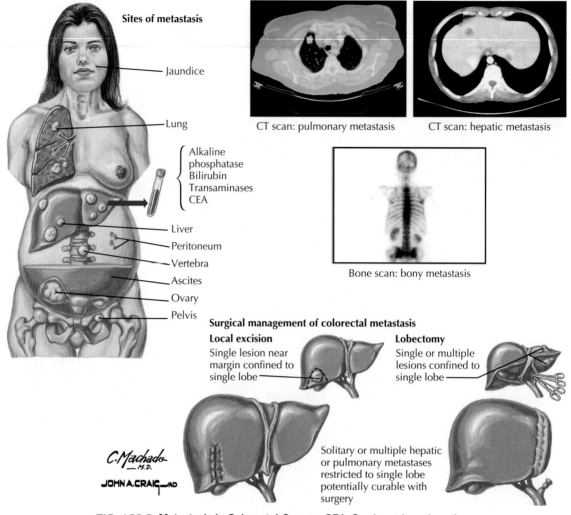

Sites of metastasis

Jaundice

Lung

Alkaline phosphatase
Bilirubin
Transaminases
CEA

Liver
Peritoneum
Vertebra
Ascites
Ovary
Pelvis

CT scan: pulmonary metastasis

CT scan: hepatic metastasis

Bone scan: bony metastasis

Surgical management of colorectal metastasis

Local excision
Single lesion near margin confined to single lobe

Lobectomy
Single or multiple lesions confined to single lobe

Solitary or multiple hepatic or pulmonary metastases restricted to single lobe potentially curable with surgery

C. Machado
—M.D.

JOHN A. CRAIG—AD

FIG. 160.3 **Metastasis in Colorectal Cancer.** *CEA,* Carcinoembryonic antigen.

FOLFOX or XELOX (capecitabine plus oxaliplatin) for 6 months.

Patients with stage IV metastatic disease are usually treated with chemotherapy alone, though surgery may be required in cases of uncontrollable gastrointestinal (GI) bleeding, obstruction, or perforation. A small subset of patients with isolated pulmonary or hepatic metastasis may also be potentially cured with a combination of systemic treatment and resection. For decades, standard first-line therapy consisted of 5FU/LV, but the introduction of irinotecan, oxaliplatin, and biological agents targeting angiogenesis and epidermal growth factor receptor (EGFR) have significantly improved survival. The current first-line options include FOLFOX, XELOX,

and FOLFIRI (irinotecan plus 5FU and LV). FOLFOXIRI, a more intensive regimen combining all three active agents (5FU, oxaliplatin, and irinotecan) is generally reserved for fit patients with potentially resectable disease.

Bevacizumab, a monoclonal antibody targeting VEGF-A, has been shown to enhance the efficacy of irinotecan-based and oxaliplatin-based regimens; however, its use is associated with complications such as uncontrolled hypertension, GI perforation, severe hemorrhage, wound healing complications, and arterial thromboembolism. Careful patient selection is therefore necessary to minimize harm.

The anti-EGFR antibodies cetuximab and panitumumab have demonstrated efficacy as single agents and in combination with chemotherapy for patients with *KRAS* wild type tumors. *KRAS* is a phosphorylated signal transducer that is part of the EGFR signaling pathway, and thus *KRAS* mutations lead to constitutive activation regardless of therapeutic EGFR inhibition. Mutations in *NRAS* and *BRAF* also predict a lack of response to anti-EGFR therapy.

Regorafenib and TAS-102 (trifluridine-tipiracil) are FDA-approved oral agents for treatment of metastatic disease after progression on the aforementioned therapies. Immune checkpoint inhibition with pembrolizumab, a programmed death-1 (PD1) inhibitor, also has demonstrated activity in patients with MMR-deficient tumors.

Rectal Cancer

Rectal cancers have a higher overall risk of recurrence compared to similarly staged colon cancers. Surgery is the primary curative treatment. Total mesorectal excision is the preferred technique, with local excision reserved only for patients with T1 tumors. Resection alone is adequate for stage I disease, but neoadjuvant chemoradiotherapy with a sensitizing fluoropyrimidine (5FU or capecitabine) is the standard of care for stage II and III disease. The treatment of metastatic rectal cancer is the same as that for metastatic colon cancer.

Colorectal Cancer Screening

Screening has been shown to decrease CRC mortality. Several modalities are available: guaiac-based fecal occult blood testing annually, fecal immunochemical test (FIT) annually (detects occult blood via reaction to human hemoglobin protein), Cologuard every 3 years (composite test, including FIT and molecular assays for mutations and biomarkers), flexible sigmoidoscopy every 5 years, CT colonography (virtual colonoscopy) every 5 years, flexible sigmoidoscopy every 10 years plus FIT annually, and colonoscopy every 10 years. In general, stool-based tests help detect early-stage disease, but endoscopic tests can also prevent cancer by detecting and removing polyps prior to malignant transformation. A shared decision-making approach is recommended. Average-risk patients should begin screening at age 50. Those with genetic syndromes such as FAP or Lynch syndrome require early intensive screening. Patients with a positive family history (first-degree relative <60 years old with CRC or adenoma) should begin screening at age 40, or 10 years earlier than the youngest age at diagnosis, whichever is earlier.

CHAPTER 161

Pancreatic Cancer

JEREMY B. JACOX

INTRODUCTION

Pancreatic cancer accounts for just over 3% of all new cancer diagnoses in the United States. It is now the third leading cause of cancer mortality with a 5-year survival rate of just 9.3%. The poor outcomes result, in part, from the typically late presentation at diagnosis, with only 10% of tumors still localized, and the vast majority already having regional lymphatic (29%) or metastatic (53%) spread. Pancreatic cancer most commonly afflicts those older adults, with a median age of 70 years at diagnosis. Less than 3% of patients are <45 years of age at the time of diagnosis.

PATHOPHYSIOLOGY

Pancreatic ductal adenocarcinoma (PDAC) is the major subtype (90%) of pancreatic cancer and the focus of this chapter. Pancreatic neuroendocrine tumor (PNET), another uncommon type of pancreatic cancer (<10%), derives from hormone-secreting cells (islet cells). The physiological consequences of dysregulated secretion of insulin, glucagon, somatostatin, and other potent secretagogues accounts for functional variants of PNETs (Fig. 161.1).

PDAC is a mucin-secreting, gland-forming tumor of the ductal epithelium of the exocrine pancreas. Like most solid tumors, PDAC is driven by an accumulation of single, missense point mutations in critical oncogenes and tumor suppressor pathways. Most early lesions contain mutations in *KRAS2* (a GTPase in the mitogen-activated protein [MAP] kinase pathway central to cell proliferation) and *CDKN2A* (also known as *p16INK4a*, involved in G1/S phase cell cycle control), while later lesions often have mutations in *SMAD4* (part of the transforming growth factor-β [TGF-β] signaling pathway) and *TP53* (deoxyribonucleic acid [DNA] damage control). These mutations may be driven by chronic inflammatory insults to pancreatic epithelial cells (e.g., chronic pancreatitis, tobacco use), which may be accelerated by germline defects in DNA damage repair pathways.

PDACs progress sequentially from premalignant lesions of pancreatic intraepithelial neoplasia (PIN Ia/Ib) to more advanced, proliferative lesions (PIN II/III) that become malignant, invasive, and ultimately metastatic. As this process typically requires 10 to 20 years, there is significant interest in early detection. A small proportion of PDACs derive from cystic lesions, such as **intraductal papillary mucinous neoplasms (IPMNs)** and mucinous cystic neoplasms (MCNs). IPMNS are mucinous cysts that derive from ductal epithelial stem cells. Main duct IPMNs have a high likelihood (70%) of developing PDAC compared to branch duct IPMNs (20%). MCNs also have malignant potential (30%) but are rarer, typically present in women, and do not involve pancreatic ducts; they are often large, viscous cysts with ovarian-type mucinous stroma.

RISK FACTORS

The major risk factors for PDAC are tobacco use, male gender, African American race, and advanced age. Additional modifiable risk factors include diabetes mellitus, obesity, chronic alcohol abuse, and chronic pancreatitis. Several familial syndromes are associated with increased risk of PDAC, including Peutz-Jeghers syndrome, Lynch syndrome, hereditary breast/ovarian cancer (*BRCA2* mutations), and familial adenomatous polyposis. Finally, syndromes that increase the risk of chronic pancreatitis also increase the risk of pancreatic cancer, such as hereditary pancreatitis and cystic fibrosis.

PRESENTATION, EVALUATION, AND DIAGNOSIS

A common presentation of pancreatic cancer is the insidious onset of **painless jaundice** in an elderly patient due to **common bile duct (CBD) obstruction,** typically from a large proximal pancreatic mass (Fig. 161.2). A pancreatic head PDAC may have a favorable prognosis, due to earlier clinical presentation of obstructive jaundice,

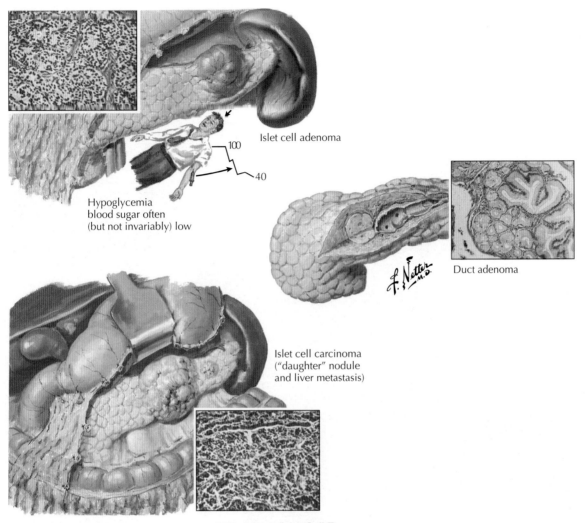

Islet cell adenoma

100
40

Hypoglycemia
blood sugar often
(but not invariably) low

Duct adenoma

Islet cell carcinoma
("daughter" nodule
and liver metastasis)

FIG. 161.1 **Islet Cell Tumors.**

than a pancreatic tail PDAC, which is more likely to present with occult metastases at the time of presentation.

Additional symptoms reflect the chronic processes of inflammation, cachexia, pancreatic insufficiency, and locoregional infiltration; the most common include weight loss, anorexia, lethargy, depression, diabetes mellitus, nausea/vomiting, bloating, steatorrhea, pruritis, and epigastric/shoulder/back pain. The constellation of new-onset back pain, lethargy, and diabetes mellitus is relatively specific to pancreatic cancer.

Although several circulating tumor antigens (most notably CA19-9) exist, there is no clinically validated blood or imaging test to screen for pancreatic cancer. Several recent studies, however, have found that

glypican-1+ exosomes (a proteoglycan signal–containing extracellular vesicle) and circulating DNA and miRNAs are secreted specifically in the blood in early PDAC and may become future screening biomarkers.

If there is clinical concern for pancreatic cancer, the initial workup should consist of a triple-phase contrast-enhanced abdominal CT to assess for pancreatic mass lesions, ductal dilation, and any involvement of critical adjacent structures (including vasculature). CT has optimal sensitivity for detection of primary lesions, though MRI is more sensitive for detecting liver metastases and pancreatic cystic tumors. Recent trials suggest ^{19}F-fluorodeoxyglucose (19-FDG) positron emission tomography (PET)/CT scanning offers incremental

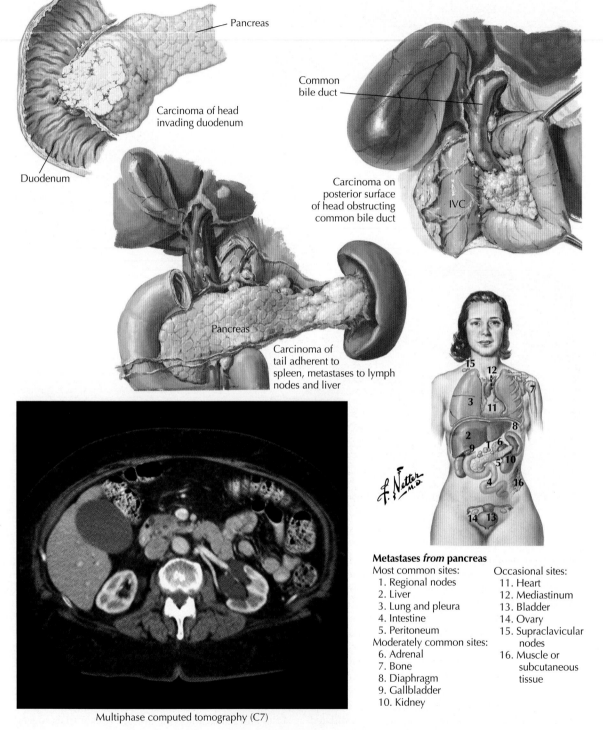

Pancreas

Carcinoma of head
invading duodenum

Duodenum

Common
bile duct

Carcinoma on
posterior surface
of head obstructing
common bile duct

IVC

Pancreas

Carcinoma of
tail adherent to
spleen, metastases to lymph
nodes and liver

Metastases *from* pancreas

Most common sites:
1. Regional nodes
2. Liver
3. Lung and pleura
4. Intestine
5. Peritoneum

Moderately common sites:
6. Adrenal
7. Bone
8. Diaphragm
9. Gallbladder
10. Kidney

Occasional sites:
11. Heart
12. Mediastinum
13. Bladder
14. Ovary
15. Supraclavicular
    nodes
16. Muscle or
    subcutaneous
    tissue

Multiphase computed tomography (C7)

FIG. 161.2 **Clinical Features of Pancreatic Cancer.** *IVC,* Inferior vena cava.

improvement for diagnosis and staging, particularly for sensing small, nonhepatic metastases, but its value is still being determined.

The current nonsurgical gold standard for the tissue diagnosis of pancreatic cancer is **endoscopic ultrasound (EUS),** with fine-needle aspiration (FNA) or core needle biopsy (CNB) of any mass lesions. Endoscopic retrograde cholangiopancreatography (with potential biliary stenting or limited brush biopsy) or magnetic resonance cholangiopancreatography (MRCP) are often valuable adjunct diagnostic imaging methods, can be less invasive (MRCP) or therapeutic (ERCP, as for stenting), and elucidate pancreatobiliary anatomy, but they are less sensitive for PDAC.

Based on findings from biopsy and imaging, PDAC can be staged according to the American Joint Committee on Cancer (AJCC) TNM (tumor, node, metastasis) system.

TREATMENT

The therapeutic approach to PDAC depends on whether disease is surgically resectable, borderline resectable, locally advanced or metastatic. Successful surgical candidates typically have excellent performance status, small mass (<25-mm diameter), no evidence of regional lymphatic spread (nodal involvement) or peritoneal/hepatic implantation, <180-degree encasement of vascular structures (the celiac axis and superior mesenteric artery [SMA]), and high likelihood of negative margins. Unfortunately, <10% of patients meet these criteria, as most already have stage IIb/III or higher PDAC with nodal, vascular, or metastatic disease and are therefore nonresectable.

Surgical resection permits definitive pathological evaluation and yields the optimal prognosis (70-month median overall survival [OS]). The most common surgery for PDAC in the pancreatic head, uncinate process, and neck is **pancreaticoduodenectomy (the Whipple procedure),** which involves resection of the pancreatic head, partial gastric pylorus/antrum, and duodenum, with reanastomoses of the gastric body, remnant biliary duct, and pancreatic body and duct to the jejunum. To minimize postoperative problems with gastric emptying and bile-reflux gastritis, the modified Whipple may be pylorus sparing. Other surgical options include distal pancreatectomy with splenectomy, more typically for pancreatic tail lesions without biliary invasion. Total pancreatectomy is rarely indicated. Staging laparoscopy often precedes the full resection procedure, to evaluate for peritoneal seeding or liver implants that may not have been diagnosed on imaging. In 10% to 15% of cases, this evaluation upstages the cancer, and full resection is generally aborted.

The role of chemotherapy varies by the ability to surgically resect a tumor following diagnosis. Resectable tumors are traditionally treated with upfront resection, but neoadjuvant chemotherapy may be considered for patients with high risk features. Borderline resectable tumors with limited vascular involvement are given neoadjuvant chemotherapy followed by pancreatectomy. Locally advanced (extensive vascular involvement) are treated with chemotherapy or chemoradiation, though the benefit may be only marginal; only a small subset undergo pancreatectomy. Of note, patients who undergo pancreatectomy should be considered for postoperative chemotherapy, particularly if not given chemotherapy preoperatively. Adjuvant modified FOLFIRINOX (oxaliplatin, dose-reduced irinotecan, 5-FU, and leucovorin) in these high-risk patients (most stage IIB or lower) confers a significant OS benefit over gemcitabine, from a median OS 35 months to 54.4 (based on PRODIGE-24).

Patients with metastatic disease at presentation are candidates for chemotherapy alone. Similarly, modified FOLFIRINOX has largely replaced gemcitabine as the first-line regimen (11-month median OS, compared to 6.8 months for gemcitabine, per the PRODIGE-4 trial). Gemcitabine with nanoparticle albumin-bound paclitaxel (nab-paclitaxel) has also emerged as an effective alternative first-line option (8.5-month median OS). Both treatments require patients to have high-performance status.

Novel T-cell checkpoint (anti-CTLA4/PD1/PDL1) inhibitors have been trialed in metastatic PDAC but with disappointing results, unlike with melanoma and non–small cell lung cancer. It is currently believed that such poor responses result from PDAC being an immune desert, with a dense stromal desmoplastic reaction and high interstitial pressure that excludes T cells. Recent trials of antifibrotic agents have also been negative.

Finally, it is essential to consider the overall well-being of the patient. Many patients are elderly, have other comorbidities, present with advanced disease, and have chronic pain and/or poor performance status. Thus the toxicities of the available therapies and burden of an extensive workup need to be assessed with regard to patient and caregiver preferences. The treatment plan should include a discussion of palliative measures (radiation to metastatic lesions, debulking therapy, stenting of the bile ducts or duodenum, celiac plexus block, and oral and transdermal pain medication), hospice care, and end-of-life decision making.

CHAPTER 162

Hepatocellular Carcinoma (HCC)

JASON M. BECKTA

INTRODUCTION

Hepatocellular carcinoma (HCC) is the fifth most common cancer in men and the seventh most common cancer in women. It is also the third leading cause of cancer-related death. There is significant variation in the distribution of morbidity and mortality of the disease, with the greatest burden in parts of Africa and East Asia. In the United States, the incidence of HCC has risen from 1.4 per 100,000 in 1975–1977 to 4.8 per 100,000 in 2005–2007.

PATHOPHYSIOLOGY

The pathophysiology of HCC begins with the development of dysplastic foci, or <1-mm clusters of abnormal hepatocytes. Once these clusters reach ≥1 mm, they are termed **dysplastic nodules** and are considered precancerous lesions with malignant potential. Dysplastic nodules are termed HCC once they demonstrate stromal invasion within the liver architecture. HCC can be further subdivided into early and progressed stages, with early tumors generally smaller (<2 cm) and better differentiated than progressed tumors. As with most malignancies, early HCC generally carries a more favorable long-term prognosis (Fig. 162.1).

The most common genetic abnormality in HCC is a mutation in the promoter region for an enzymatic subunit of telomerase *(TERT)*, which allows HCC cells to inappropriately maintain the length of their telomeres and avoid senescence/apoptosis. *TERT* promoter mutations are estimated to occur in 30% to 60% of HCC cases. HCC often features mutations in the *p53* gene as well. Many studies have described inappropriate histone modifications, microribonucleic acid (microRNA) expression, and chromatin remodeling as epigenetic changes that can also stimulate the development of HCC. The current literature on the pathophysiology of HCC describes an extraordinary range of molecular mechanisms for its development. As a result, it has been difficult to develop effective, targeted therapies.

RISK FACTORS

The most important risk factors for HCC are chronic liver disease and **cirrhosis,** most often resulting from infection with **hepatitis B** or **C** viruses (HBV or HCV, respectively) or excessive alcohol intake. HBV accounts for about one in two HCC cases worldwide, while HCV accounts for one in four. HBV carriers have a 10% to 25% lifetime risk of developing HCC. The widespread use of the HBV vaccine has significantly decreased the burden of HBV-related HCC around much of the world; however, rates of infection remain high throughout large parts of Africa and Asia, contributing to their disproportionate share of HCC incidence.

Alcohol abuse accounts for fewer cases of HCC worldwide but is a much more common risk factor in the United States. Studies have found a 16% increase in HCC risk with three or more drinks per day, and a 22% increase with six or more drinks per day.

Additional risk factors for HCC include diabetes mellitus, obesity, chronic aflatoxin exposure, nonalcoholic fatty liver disease (NAFLD) (see Chapter 137), and genetic diseases such as hemochromatosis, porphyria cutanea tarda, α1-antitrypsin deficiency, stage IV primary biliary cirrhosis, Wilson disease, and tyrosinemia. Aflatoxin is derived from *Aspergillus flavus,* which frequently contaminates food stores in Asia and Africa; long-standing exposure of hepatocytes to aflatoxin can result in *p53* mutations. The carcinogenic effect of aflatoxin is synergistic with that of HBV and HCV.

PRESENTATION AND DIAGNOSIS

In most patients, HCC is asymptomatic. When overt signs and symptoms occur, they are generally nonspecific findings related to chronic liver disease, such as jaundice, right upper quadrant pain, abdominal distension, weakness, and unintentional weight loss.

As with all cancers, early detection and treatment generally improve outcomes. Thus it is recommended that at-risk populations, including those with cirrhosis,

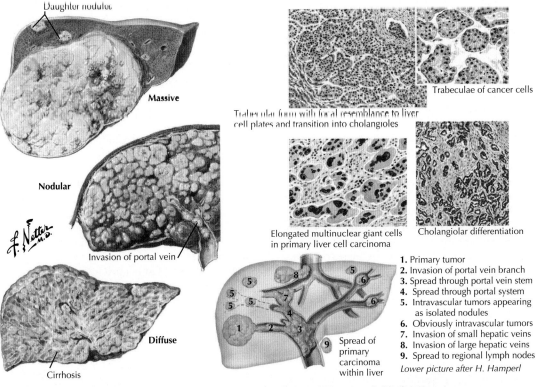

Daughter nodule

Massive

Nodular

Invasion of portal vein

Diffuse

Cirrhosis

Trabecular form with focal resemblance to liver cell plates and transition into cholangioles

Trabeculae of cancer cells

Elongated multinuclear giant cells in primary liver cell carcinoma

Cholangiolar differentiation

1. Primary tumor
2. Invasion of portal vein branch
3. Spread through portal vein stem
4. Spread through portal system
5. Intravascular tumors appearing as isolated nodules
6. Obviously intravascular tumors
7. Invasion of small hepatic veins
8. Invasion of large hepatic veins
9. Spread to regional lymph nodes

Spread of primary carcinoma within liver

Lower picture after H. Hamperl

FIG. 162.1 Gross and Microscopic Features of Hepatocellular Carcinoma.

a positive test for hepatitis B surface antigen, or a family history of HCC, undergo surveillance screening with ultrasound every 6 months. Although the measurement of blood **α-fetoprotein (AFP)** levels had been used as a screening test for nearly 60 years, liver ultrasound has been the preferred screening modality since the early 1980s.

Once detected, lesions <1 cm should be screened every 3 months via ultrasound, as it is usually difficult to discern whether these lesions are cancerous or regenerative nodules at this size. Meanwhile, lesions >1 cm should warrant further workup with liver phase, contrast enhanced CT, or MRI. Relative to normal liver tissue, HCC typically shows greater enhancement in the arterial phase (as it has predominantly arterial vascularization) and then loses enhancement in the venous phase. Liver biopsy is required only when imaging findings are equivocal.

Once HCC is diagnosed, CT scans of the chest, abdomen, and pelvis, and bone scan if skeletal symptoms are present, should be obtained to detect metastatic disease and help guide therapy. Extrahepatic metastasis of HCC most commonly occurs in the lung, abdominal lymph nodes, and bone.

No universal staging system exists within HCC; indeed, although a classic TNM staging system has been used in HCC, other systems include a variety of other factors, including status of underlying liver disease. The National Comprehensive Cancer Network (NCCN) stratifies patients into four categories based on the potential for surgical management:

- Potentially resectable or transplantable
- Unresectable
- Inoperable by performance status or comorbidity (local disease)
- Metastatic disease

Patients with HCC and underlying cirrhosis who may be candidates for liver transplantation, the only potential cure if not locally resectable, can be staged utilizing the **Milan criteria.** Staging systems for underlying cirrhosis, including MELD-Na scoring and the **Child-Pugh score,** may also help prognosticate in a diagnosis of HCC.

TREATMENT

The treatment of HCC depends on patient characteristics and the disease stage. Patients with single nodules, no underlying cirrhosis, and good liver function (as measured by the Child-Pugh score) can generally undergo curative resection of local disease.

Unfortunately, due to the asymptomatic nature of early-stage HCC, most tumors are too advanced for resection by the time of diagnosis. In these patients, liver transplantation may be considered, though there tends to be a high recurrence rate, and 5-year survival rates average <50%. These discouraging statistics are likely the result of poor patient selection. Liver transplantation should therefore only be considered in patients with early-stage disease, ideally using the Milan criteria (single HCC node <5 cm, or up to three separate nodules <3 cm with no evidence of vascular invasion/metastasis). When these criteria are applied, 5-year survival rates are >70%.

Patients who are not candidates for resection or transplantation can undergo percutaneous ablation. Common techniques are **radiofrequency ablation (RFA)** or **percutaneous ethanol injection (PEI).** Under radiologic or ultrasound guidance, needles are advanced into the tumor bulk, and either radiofrequency-derived thermal lesions or injected ethanol induce tumor necrosis. RFA is preferred over PEI, as it requires fewer treatment sessions and provides higher long-term survival rates. In smaller tumors, RFA may even be considered instead of surgical resection. As the waiting list for liver transplant can span several months, these ablative techniques can also be used to keep transplant candidates from progressing outside of the Milan criteria.

As HCC relies primarily on arterial, rather than portal, blood for circulation, transarterial embolization procedures offer another strategy for the control of nonresectable disease. **Transarterial chemoembolization (TACE)** involves particle embolization of the supplying artery combined with locally deployed chemotherapy (Fig. 162.2).

HCC is one of the most chemotherapy-resistant malignancies, and no systemic chemotherapies were recommended for advanced-stage patients until 2008. Randomized, controlled trials demonstrated that sorafenib,

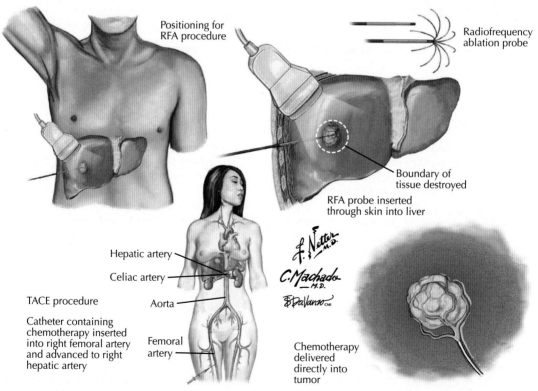

FIG. 162.2 **Radiofrequency Ablation *(RFA)* and Transarterial Chemoembolization *(TACE)* for Hepatocellular Carcinoma.**

an orally bioavailable tyrosine kinase inhibitor (TKI), increased median survival from 7.9 months to 10.7 months; potential side effects include diarrhea, hand and foot skin reaction, and weight loss. Regorafenib is a multikinase inhibitor with US Food and Drug Administration (FDA) approval for second-line therapy. Nivolumab, a programmed cell death 1 (PD1) inhibitor, was granted accelerated approval for patients who progress or do not tolerate sorafenib. In patients with HCC for whom no therapeutic options exist, the best supportive care should include measures to decrease

the incidence of cholangitis and acute hepatic failure via biliary decompression, and to control pain caused by bone metastasis or increasing tumor volume.

Despite technical advancements in the treatment of HCC, it remains an aggressive disease with a high mortality rate. As such, efforts directed toward prevention of the disease would have a significantly greater and more rapid impact. Vaccinations against HBV, alcohol cessation treatment, and treatment of metabolic syndromes have the highest potential for reducing the incidence of HCC and many other malignancies.

CHAPTER 163

Renal Cell Carcinoma (RCC)

JULIA E. MCGUINNESS

INTRODUCTION

Renal cell carcinoma (RCC), a primary malignancy of the kidney, is the seventh most common cancer worldwide. Its incidence has been rising by 3% to 4% annually since the 1970s, likely from increased incidental detection on abdominal imaging. Over 350,000 people worldwide were diagnosed with RCC in 2013, and 140,000 people die from it each year.

RCC is classified into subtypes based on cell morphology and histology. The majority (~70%) of RCC cases are termed **clear cell**, after the malignant cells' clear cytoplasm. Less common histological variants are papillary, which has a basophilic cytoplasm; chromophobe, which has an empty cytoplasm and a low mitotic rate that makes it less likely to metastasize; and collecting duct.

PATHOPHYSIOLOGY

Of all the subtypes, clear cell RCC has the best defined pathophysiology. Mutations or alterations to the **von Hippel-Lindau** gene, a tumor suppressor gene, have been implicated in >80% of clear cell cancers, including both sporadic and hereditary cases. These mutations lead to a loss of function of the VHL gene, responsible for the degradation of hypoxia-inducible factor-1 (HIF1), a key component in cell growth pathways and erythrogenesis. With the loss of this checkpoint, there is upregulation of platelet-derived growth factor (PDGF) and vascular endothelial growth factor (VEGF), leading to angiogenesis and promotion of cell proliferation, growth, and migration.

RISK FACTORS

The incidence of RCC peaks between the ages of 60 and 70 years. For unclear reasons, the incidence of RCC is higher in developed than in developing countries, and is also higher in males, with a male-to-female ratio of 1.5 : 1. Tobacco, obesity, and hypertension are all associated with increased risk of RCC. Toxins and medications such as trichloroethylene (a cleaning agent), NSAIDs, and alcohol also are possible risk factors. Diuretic use has been proposed as a risk factor, but it is unclear if hypertension is a confounder.

Although most RCCs are sporadic, several hereditary syndromes are associated with increased risk. The most notable is von Hippel-Lindau syndrome, which accounts for 1.6% of RCCs overall. This autosomal dominant disorder features loss of the VHL gene at the 3p25 locus, which causes RCC in 25% to 60% of patients along with other vascular tumors (including retinal hemangiomas and central nervous system hemangioblastomas), pancreatic cysts, islet cell tumors, and pheochromocytomas. Unfortunately, VHL-related RCC tends to be bilateral, multifocal, and present at a younger age, making metastatic RCC the most common cause of death in these patients.

Additional rare hereditary forms of RCC include hereditary papillary RCC, resulting from activating mutations in the MET protooncogene; hereditary leiomyomatosis RCC, from mutations in the fumarate hydratase gene involved in the Krebs cycle; and Birt-Hogg-Dubé syndrome, from mutations in *FLCN*, a tumor suppressor that interacts with the mTOR pathway. All of these syndromes also have autosomal dominant inheritance.

PRESENTATION, EVALUATION, AND DIAGNOSIS

Only 30% of patients with RCC are diagnosed on the basis of symptoms. Most cases are instead diagnosed incidentally when patients undergo abdominal imaging for other indications. Among those who do experience RCC-related symptoms, the most common are flank pain and gross hematuria. Less common symptoms are a palpable abdominal mass or a varicocele (from obstruction of a gonadal vein by the tumor).

Several paraneoplastic disorders have been associated with RCC and can occur at any stage. Hypertension often results from increased production of renin by the tumor and/or renal artery compression. Cachexia, weight

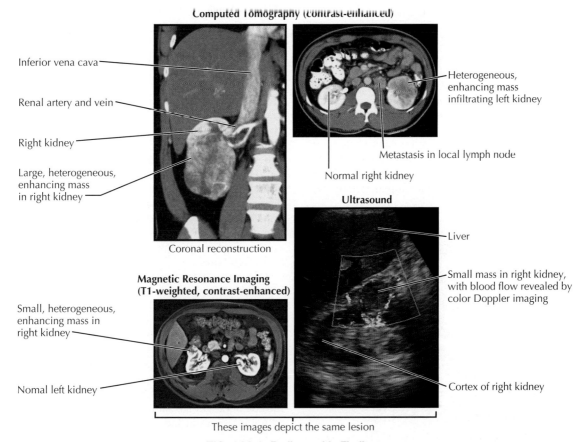

FIG. 163.1 Radiographic Findings.

loss, and fevers can all result from abnormal production of cytokines and prostaglandins. Hypercalcemia may result from production of parathyroid hormone–related protein (PTHrP), while polycythemia may result from increased production of erythropoietin. Stauffer syndrome is characterized by elevated hepatic enzymes in the absence of liver metastasis, resulting from elevated levels of interleukin-6 (IL-6) that promote lymphocytic infiltration of the liver parenchyma.

Although definitive diagnosis of RCC requires pathological confirmation, abdominal radiography has been the main modality used to determine if renal tumors are likely to be benign and malignant. The best imaging modalities to characterize renal tumors are precontrast and postcontrast CT or MRI of the abdomen and pelvis, which also identify venous involvement, tumor extension, and metastases (Fig. 163.1). The Bosniak criteria are used to determine the likelihood that renal cysts are malignant; characteristics favoring malignancy include a solid component, size >3 cm, multiple septations, septum irregularity or heterogeneity, wall or septum enhancement with contrast, gross calcifications, and heterogeneous cyst contents. An emerging imaging modality uses an iodine-labeled antibody against carbonic anhydrase IX, expressed in >90% of clear cell RCCs but not in normal kidney cells.

Biopsy was previously associated with cases of tumor seeding, but with modern techniques this is no longer considered a significant risk. As a result, percutaneous renal biopsy is now being used more frequently to establish the diagnosis of RCC in radiologically indeterminate masses. Complications occur in 0.3% to 5.3% of biopsies and can include bleeding, infection, and arteriovenous fistula formation.

The staging of RCC is based on the TNM system. For RCC, the T category is determined by tumor size, extension of the tumor into the associated renal vasculature, and invasion of Gerota fascia, the connective tissue surrounding the kidneys and adrenal glands. The most common sites of metastasis are the lungs, bone, and brain, but the adrenal glands, contralateral kidney, and liver can also be involved (Fig. 163.2). Patients with localizing clinical symptoms, renal tumors >7 cm in diameter, adenopathy, renal vein involvement, or adjacent organ involvement on imaging should have a chest CT, head CT or MRI, and bone scan for complete staging. At diagnosis, approximately one-third of patients have metastatic disease, and an additional 40% of patients who present with local disease develop metastases over the course of their lives.

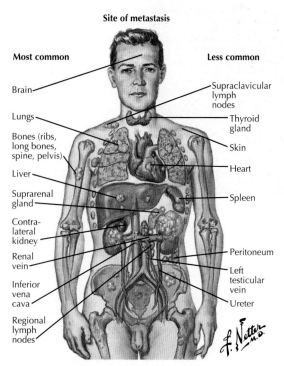

Site of metastasis

FIG. 163.2 **Common Sites of Metastasis.**

TREATMENT

The mainstay of treatment for all stages is surgical resection. RCCs are not responsive to traditional chemotherapeutic agents, and thus systemic therapies are reserved for metastatic or very advanced local disease.

Previously, radical nephrectomy was the standard surgical therapy for RCC; however, nephron-sparing surgery (local resection of tumor with sparing of as much healthy kidney as possible) is increasingly being used for smaller tumors and in patients with contraindications to radical nephrectomy (Fig. 163.3). The strongest indication for nephron-sparing surgery over radical nephrectomy is the presence of only one functional kidney; a relative indication is the presence of a disorder that may impair the contralateral kidney's future function. Other minimally invasive treatments include radiofrequency ablation and cryotherapy, but their long-term efficacy is not well known.

Of note, in patients who are elderly or have comorbidities that are associated with increased surgical risk, active surveillance with serial imaging is a viable option if tumors are small, particularly since 20% to 30% of small renal tumors are benign.

Patients with advanced or metastatic disease require systemic therapy. Over the past decade, therapies targeting agents involved in the pathogenesis of RCC (VEGF, PDGF, and mTOR) were the standard of care. VEGF antagonists include bevacizumab, sunitinib, sorafenib, and others. mTOR inhibitors include everolimus and temsirolimus.

Recent advances in the treatment of metastatic RCC have expanded the available options to include newer-generation VEGF antagonists such as cabozantinib and immunotherapy. Programmed cell death 1 (PD1) is a receptor present on T cells, and the interaction of PD1 with its ligand (PD-L1) on cancer cells prevents activation of the immune system to attack the cancer. Anti-PD1 agents such as pembrolizumab and nivolumab are now used alone or in combination with VEGF antagonists to treat metastatic RCC, and the combination can result in median overall survival of over 18 months.

Laparoscopic Partial Nephrectomy: Transperitoneal Approach

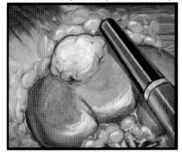

1. The tumor is identified and characterized using laparoscopic ultrasound.

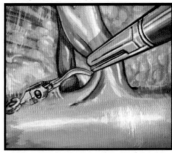

2. The renal artery is clamped.

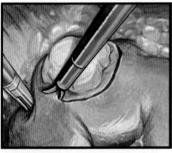

3. Using laparoscopic scissors, incision of the tumor (with a rim of normal parenchyma) begins.

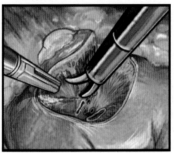

4. Dissection continues until the tumor is completely detached from the kidney.

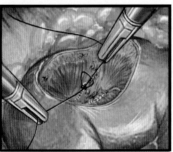

5. The collecting system is repaired using reabsorbable sutures.

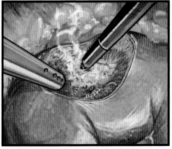

6. Electrocautery or argon beam device is used to coagulate the cortical aspects of the defect.

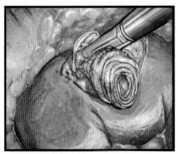

7. Hemostatic agents are placed in the defect.

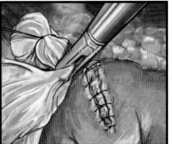

8. The defect in the renal parenchyma is closed, and the tumor is removed intact in an entrapment bag.

FIG. 163.3 Nephron Sparing Surgery.

CHAPTER 164

Bladder Cancer

MEGAN M. DUPUIS

INTRODUCTION

Bladder cancer is the sixth most common cancer in the United States, representing nearly 5% of all cancer diagnoses each year. The 5-year overall survival has stagnated for decades at around 77.5%; however, there has been a slight decrease in the incidence in recent years, likely because of lower rates of cigarette smoking.

The overwhelming majority of bladder cancers are **transitional cell carcinomas,** also known as **urothelial carcinomas** of the bladder, and are the focus of this chapter. Less than 10% of bladder cancers are adenocarcinomas or squamous cell carcinomas. For the remainder of this chapter, the term bladder cancer will refer to transitional cell carcinomas.

PATHOPHYSIOLOGY

The cellular layer that lines the bladder lumen is known as the mucosa and consists of transitional epithelial (urothelial) cells. The next layer is the lamina propria, a submucosal connective tissue layer. Beyond the lamina propria lies the muscularis layer, with three sheets of muscle collectively referred to as the detrusor. Finally, the muscularis is covered with adventitia, a loose connective tissue layer that helps fix the bladder in place.

Bladder cancer arises as a clonal defect in the transitional urothelium. Morphologically, bladder tumors are classified as flat and papillary. **Flat carcinomas** do not grow into the lumen of the bladder but rather spread over the surface of the mucosal layer. **Papillary carcinomas,** in contrast, develop into stalklike projections that grow into the lumen. If they are confined to the urothelial layer and have low-grade microscopic features, such tumors are termed either flat carcinoma in situ (CIS) or papillary urothelial neoplasm of low malignancy potential (PUNLMPs), respectively. If either a flat or papillary tumor grows into the muscularis layer, however, it is then considered a **muscle-invasive urothelial carcinoma** (Fig. 164.1).

As with other solid tumors, a variety of accumulated genetic defects contribute to bladder cancer and determine its invasiveness. For example, invasive bladder cancers frequently have mutations of the p53 tumor suppressor gene, whereas noninvasive papillary tumors typically do not. The antiapoptotic molecule survivin has been overexpressed in both noninvasive and muscle-invasive tumors, and high levels are associated with more severe disease and a greater risk of recurrence. Other common genetic alterations, such as of *FGFR* or *RAS*, may also contribute to bladder cancer development or progression.

RISK FACTORS

Bladder cancer is more prevalent in men, Caucasians, and the elderly. The most significant modifiable risk factor is cigarette smoking. Other environmental risk factors include chronic urinary tract infections, schistosomiasis, and exposure to aniline dye (common among textile and rubber factory workers). Several genetic syndromes have also been associated with bladder cancer. For example, **Lynch syndrome** (also referred to as **hereditary nonpolyposis colon cancer [HNPCC]),** is an inherited disease characterized by a defect in mismatch repair genes that leads to a variety of malignancies, including bladder cancer.

PRESENTATION, EVALUATION, AND DIAGNOSIS

The most common symptom of bladder cancer is painless hematuria. Although patients can present with either gross or microscopic hematuria, the likelihood of bladder cancer is much greater with gross hematuria. Patients may also present with regional bladder or pelvic pain, or with voiding issues such dysuria, dribbling, or increased frequency. The presence of constitutional symptoms such as fevers, weight loss, or remote sites of pain suggests late-stage, metastatic disease.

Any patient with unexplained hematuria, either gross or microscopic, warrants a workup that includes a clinic-based **cystoscopy** with direct visualization of the urethra and bladder. If any suspicious lesion is seen, a follow-up intraoperative procedure should be performed to allow for direct biopsy of the tumor, including the

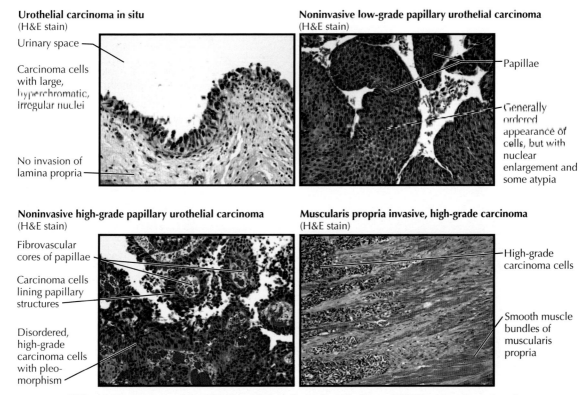

Urothelial carcinoma in situ
(H&E stain)

Urinary space

Carcinoma cells with large, hyperchromatic, irregular nuclei

No invasion of lamina propria

Noninvasive low-grade papillary urothelial carcinoma
(H&E stain)

Papillae

Generally ordered appearance of cells, but with nuclear enlargement and some atypia

Noninvasive high-grade papillary urothelial carcinoma
(H&E stain)

Fibrovascular cores of papillae

Carcinoma cells lining papillary structures

Disordered, high-grade carcinoma cells with pleomorphism

Muscularis propria invasive, high-grade carcinoma
(H&E stain)

High-grade carcinoma cells

Smooth muscle bundles of muscularis propria

FIG. 164.1 **Tumors of the Bladder: Histopathological Findings.** *H&E,* Hematoxylin and eosin.

muscularis layer, to characterize the presence or absence of tumor invasion. Urine cytology can also be obtained around the time of cystoscopy.

Staging

Bladder cancer is staged using the TNM classification system and is assigned an overall stage. Accurate staging requires cystoscopy and biopsy, as described earlier, as well as imaging studies to assess for locoregional or distant metastases. Suspicious lymph nodes or distant metastases may require biopsy to confirm extrapelvic disease.

CT urography (CT abdomen and pelvis, with and without contrast with excretory imaging) is recommended to evaluate the upper urinary tract, which cannot be adequately assessed by cystoscopy alone. Patients who are unable to tolerate iodinated contrast may instead be candidates for MRI. Unfortunately, both CT and MRI have high false-negative rates for nodal disease.

To evaluate for distant disease, chest x-rays are recommended for evaluation of lung lesions, although these are not sensitive for lesions <1 cm. Positron emission tomography (PET) scans are also useful for the evaluation of distant disease, although local recurrence is difficult

to detect as fluorodeoxyglucose (FDG) is excreted in the urine.

Treatment Based on Stage

For stage 0 and I bladder cancers, the standard of care is transurethral resection of the bladder tumor (TURBT), with repeat cystoscopy at 3 months (Fig. 164.2). As up to 70% of these superficial tumors recur, and 20% progress to invasive disease, close monitoring for residual tumor and/or tumor reseeding is essential. Guidelines recommend repeat cystoscopy and urine cytology every 3 to 6 months for the first 4 years following TURBT, then annually. During the TURBT procedure, it is recommended the patient receive a dose of intravesicular adjuvant chemotherapy, such as mitomycin or bacillus Calmette-Guerin (BCG), to prevent any remaining tumor cells from reseeding the bladder mucosa. If the pathology reveals a low-grade lesion, no further treatment is necessary. However, if the lesion is a high-grade tumor, the patient should receive multiple BCG treatments; current recommendations support administration every 3 weeks for 1 to 3 years. If the tumor has more aggressive features such as multiple sites of implantation,

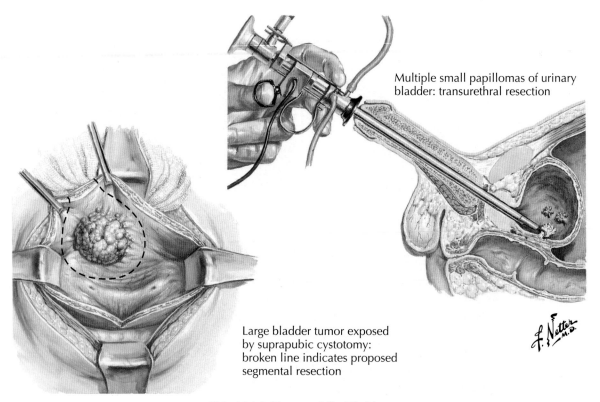

Multiple small papillomas of urinary bladder: transurethral resection

Large bladder tumor exposed by suprapubic cystotomy: broken line indicates proposed segmental resection

FIG. 164.2 **Tumors of the Bladder.**

a repeat TURBT is often required to ensure complete removal.

For stage II to III bladder cancers, patients should receive cisplatin-based neoadjuvant chemotherapy treatment prior to definitive surgical management. Less than 5% of cases of bladder cancer will occur in a location that is amenable to partial cystectomy, and therefore the typical surgical management includes removal of the entire bladder. For men, the recommended surgery is radical cystoprostatectomy, wherein the urinary bladder and prostate gland are removed. For women, it is pelvic exenteration, which involves removal of the urinary bladder, urethra, uterus, ovaries, vagina, and rectum, requiring the creation of a permanent colostomy and urinary diversion. For both sexes, these surgeries also include pelvic lymph node dissection and urinary diversion via an ileal conduit. Although adjuvant radiation has not been validated for all patients, it is reasonable to consider this treatment option in patients who had positive surgical margins, high grade disease, and/or positive lymph nodes.

In patients with stage IVA disease (cT4b, any N, any M; or M1a disease), the treatment consists of systemic therapy with a cisplatin-based chemotherapy regimen or concurrent chemoradiotherapy. If patients have a good response to therapy, completion of treatment with definitive radiation therapy is recommended. Typically, patients with stage IVA, M0 disease are not felt to be surgical candidates; however, if there is an excellent response to treatment and the tumor may be downstaged, then cystectomy can be considered.

For patients with stage IVB, M1 disease, front-line therapy is typically a cisplatin-based chemotherapy regimen. However, the immune checkpoint inhibitors pembrolizumab (anti–programmed cell death-1 [anti-PD1]) and atezolizumab (anti-PD-L1) have recently been approved in the front-line setting if patients have high PD-L1 expression levels. Additionally, these agents may also be used in the front line if the patient is platinum ineligible, regardless of PD-L1 levels. Checkpoint inhibitors have also been approved as second-line therapy after platinum-based therapy in the metastatic setting. In addition, for patients who have *FGFR2* or *FGFR3* genetic alterations, the fibroblast growth factor receptor–targeting drug erdafitinib has been recently approved in the second-line setting after failing platinum-based therapy.

CHAPTER 165

Melanoma

HAO XIE

INTRODUCTION

Melanoma is the most aggressive form of skin cancer. Cutaneous melanoma is the most common form and is the primary focus of this chapter. Subtypes include superficial spreading, nodular, **lentigo maligna,** and acral lentiginous subtypes. Noncutaneous forms of melanoma include mucosal, uveal, and desmoplastic, and will be briefly discussed.

PATHOGENESIS AND RISK FACTORS

Different subtypes of melanoma are associated with relatively unique oncogenic mutations. Point mutations of *BRAF*, especially *BRAF^{V600E}* or *BRAF^{V600K}*, are present in 45% of newly diagnosed cutaneous melanomas, resulting in constitutive activation of the RAS pathway and uncontrolled cellular proliferation. *NRAS* mutations are present in an additional 20% of cutaneous melanomas and are mutually exclusive of *BRAF^{V600E}* mutations. In contradistinction, *KIT* mutations and amplifications are present in 25% of mucosal and acral melanomas. *GNAQ* or *GNA11* mutations are present in 85% of uveal melanomas, leading to the activation of prosurvival signaling pathways.

The primary risk factors include exposure to **ultraviolet light** (which is dose dependent) (Fig. 165.1), personal history of melanoma, familial atypical multiple mole and melanoma syndrome, dysplastic nevus syndrome, increased number of nevi, dysplastic nevi, large congenital nevi, immunosuppression, and melanocortin-1 receptor variants (associated with fair skin, red hair, and freckles). First-degree relatives with melanoma confer a >50% increase in the chance of a patient developing melanoma. Familial melanomas are associated with mutations in *CDKN2A* and *CDK4*, and patients with a familial melanoma syndrome must be monitored for the development of dysplastic nevi.

PRESENTATION AND SCREENING

Several tools have been created to help identify early cutaneous melanomas. The most widely used criteria,

known as the **ABCDE rule,** identify features that increase the likelihood of disease and need for biopsy: A refers to asymmetry, B to irregular border, C to color variation, D to diameter ≥6 mm, and E to evolution or change in an existing nevus or development of a new lesion (Fig. 165.2).

There is no clear consensus among major expert groups regarding routine screening for melanoma. Total body skin examination may be performed to screen for cutaneous melanoma in patients with risk factors. Small suspicious lesions require full-thickness excisional biopsies, with normal skin margins of 1 to 2 mm. Shave biopsies are often performed but should be avoided. Wider diameter lesions can be addressed with a full-thickness incisional biopsy through an area of the greatest tumor thickness.

STAGING

The tumor-node-metastasis (TNM) criteria are used to stage cutaneous melanoma. **Breslow thickness** is a critical prognostic factor of melanoma and is measured as the distance between the upper layer of the epidermis and the deepest point of tumor penetration. If the Breslow thickness of the primary tumor is >1 mm, sentinel lymph node biopsy should be performed at the time of complete excision. Furthermore, if the primary tumor is >0.76 to 1 mm thick and possesses ulceration and/or has a mitotic rate ≥1/mm², a sentinel lymph node biopsy should also be performed. If sentinel lymph nodes are positive for metastatic disease, imaging (CT chest/abdomen/pelvis, brain MRI, and/or positron emission tomography [PET]/CT) to provide baseline staging should be considered. If metastases are present, a serum lactate dehydrogenase (LDH) concentration should also be measured (Fig. 165.3).

TREATMENT

The primary treatment of cutaneous melanoma is surgery with wide local excision and/or sentinel lymph node biopsy. The margin of excision is based on the Breslow

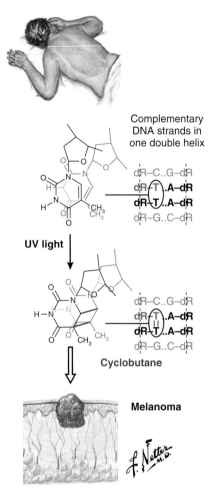

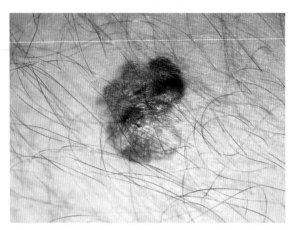

FIG. 165.2 **Melanoma, Exhibiting Asymmetry, Border Irregularity, Color Variation, Diameter ≥6 mm, and Evolution—Components of the ABCDE Rule.**

FIG. 165.1 **Deoxyribonucleic Acid *(DNA)* Alterations in the Presence of Ultraviolet *(UV)* Light.**

thickness of the primary tumor. The recommended margins are 0.5 to 1 cm for Tis tumors, 1 cm for T1 tumors, 1 to 2 cm for T2 tumors, and 2 cm for T3/4 tumors. Margins may be modified in anatomically restricted areas such as the face or ear. Sentinel lymph node biopsies should be performed in circumstances as previously mentioned. If a positive sentinel node is identified, a completion lymphadenectomy should be discussed and strongly considered. If a patient presents with clinical lymphadenopathy, a fine-needle aspiration should be performed of the suspicious node, and a completion lymphadenectomy should be performed in conjunction with a wide local excision if there are no distant metastases.

For stage IIB, IIC, and III disease, adjuvant therapy is considered to reduce the risk of lymph node recurrence.

Adjuvant high-dose interferon or pegylated interferon improve progression-free survival but not overall survival, and treatment-related toxicities from interferon include flulike symptoms, leukopenia, thrombocytopenia, transaminitis, and depression. In recent clinical trials, the use of **checkpoint inhibitors,** such as ipilimumab, nivolumab, and dabrafenib plus trametinib for BRAF-mutated melanoma, significantly improved survival.

For stage IV disease, the treatment options were historically limited, although recent advances in targeted therapies and immunotherapies have led to improved outcomes. Dacarbazine was the previous agent of choice but had only a 10% response rate and a usually short-lived response. Vemurafenib and dabrafenib are novel, mutant-selective BRAF inhibitors for patients with *BRAF^{V600}* mutations, and they have been associated with 50% overall response rate and prolonged overall survival compared with dacarbazine.

Unfortunately, patients with *BRAF^{V600}* mutant melanoma usually develop resistance ~6 months after starting vemurafenib or dabrafenib. Common resistance mechanisms include amplifications and splice variants of *BRAF^{V600}* mutation and the development of *NRAS* and *MEK1/2* mutations. Trametinib and cobimetinib are MEK1/2 inhibitors that were introduced to overcome these resistance mechanisms. Indeed, the combination of dabrafenib and trametinib, or of vemurafenib and cobimetinib, was associated with 76% response rate and significantly improved progression-free survival in BRAF-inhibitor naïve patients; however, the response rate dropped to 15% for patients with prior resistance to BRAF inhibitors. Trametinib has been associated with rare

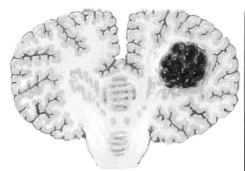

Cerebellar metastasis from cutaneous melanoma

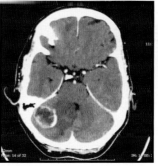

CT with contrast enhancement shows a similar large metastasis in the right cerebellum with effacement of the fourth ventricle

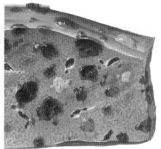

Malignant melanoma metastases to the liver

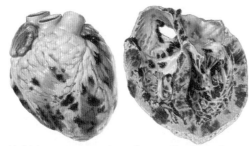

Multiple metastases to heart from malignant melanoma

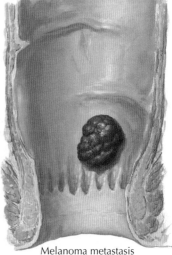

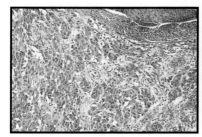

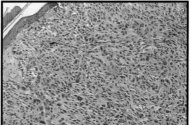

Sheets of bizarre-appearing melanocytes

Large nodular melanoma

Melanoma metastasis to the large intestine

FIG. 165.3 Metastatic Melanoma.

but severe ocular side effects, including blurred vision, retinal detachment, and retinal vein occlusion.

Melanoma has a high mutation load and is thus thought to be a very immunogenic tumor. Therapies that augment the immune response to the tumor have been used to improve response rates and survival. High-dose interleukin-2 (IL2) was the first approved immunotherapy for metastatic melanoma, and it achieved a 16% response rate and durable response for >10 years in complete responders. The addition of the gp100 cancer vaccine to high-dose IL2 improved the response rate and progression-free survival.

Novel immunotherapies have led to further improvements in overall survival. Cytotoxic T-lymphocyte–associated antigen 4 (CTLA4) is an inhibitory immune checkpoint protein on the surface of activated and regulatory T lymphocytes. Ipilimumab, an anti-CTLA4 antibody, is associated with only a 10% to 15% response rate, but the response is durable and led to improved survival. The programmed cell death-1 (PD1) receptor is another T-cell receptor that suppresses the immune response. Pembrolizumab and nivolumab are anti-PD1 antibodies that demonstrated ~30% response rate, durable response, and significantly prolonged survival. The combination of ipilimumab and nivolumab further increased the overall response rate, though approximately half of the patients who received this combination therapy developed serious adverse events related to systemic inflammation (e.g., colitis, pneumonitis), which require treatment with steroids.

CHAPTER 166

Prostate Cancer

KELLY J. FITZGERALD

INTRODUCTION

Adenocarcinoma of the prostate is the most common cancer in American males, with nearly 175,000 new cases projected for 2019. Although the high prevalence makes prostate cancer the second leading cause of cancer death among men, only 1 in 41 diagnosed patients will die of prostate cancer. This discrepancy reflects the indolent nature of many cases that are identified in earlier stages.

The treatment of low-risk cancers that would otherwise not have caused morbidity or mortality unnecessarily exposes patients to adverse treatment effects, such as incontinence and impotence, and increases overall health care costs. Unfortunately, the factors that determine the progression from low-grade, localized tumors to metastatic disease are still largely unknown. Therefore it remains challenging to identify patients with early-stage disease in whom the benefits of diagnosis and treatment outweigh the potential harms.

RISK FACTORS, CLINICAL PRESENTATION, AND SCREENING

The major risk factors include having a first-degree relative with prostate cancer and African American race. The use of 5α-reductase inhibitors to treat benign prostatic hyperplasia (BPH) is known to lower both **prostate-specific antigen** (PSA) score and the risk of developing prostate cancer, though there is no demonstrable mortality benefit.

Most men with early-stage prostate cancer are asymptomatic, though some experience symptoms of urinary obstruction (such as frequency, hesitancy, and urgency) and hematuria. Because symptoms are so infrequent, screening tests are generally required to identify patients in need of further work-up. The two available screening tests are measurement of serum PSA concentrations and digital rectal examination (DRE).

The American Cancer Society recommends that patients and doctors discuss screening in the context of individual risk factors, weighing the possible benefit of early detection against the risk of false positives and further testing. Men aged 45 to 75 years are potential candidates for screening, since prostate cancer is extremely rare in younger men. Although the incidence rises with age, prostate cancer is unlikely to cause death in men age >75 years given its indolent nature, so screening in this group is not recommended. Younger men with a life expectancy <10 years are also unlikely to benefit.

PSA Testing

PSA is a protease secreted by the prostate to increase semen fluidity. Prostate cancer increases serum PSA concentrations both because of increased production and disruption of local microvasculature. PSA is not a cancer-specific marker, however, and nonneoplastic etiologies (such as BPH, prostatitis, and prostate injury) can also elevate levels.

PSA values >10 ng/mL are strongly suggestive of cancer, but lower values are less specific. Using a PSA test threshold of 4 ng/mL, the sensitivity and specificity for detecting prostate cancer are 21% and 91%, respectively. Unfortunately, the positive predictive value (PPV) of a PSA >4 ng/mL is only 30%. Some studies have used a lower cutoff value of 3 ng/mL to improve sensitivity, at the cost of a further reduction in specificity and PPV.

Two large randomized trials have examined whether PSA screening confers a prostate cancer–specific mortality benefit. The European Randomized Study of Screening for Prostate Cancer (ERSPC) found a 21% reduction in mortality among patients offered PSA screening compared to a control group; however, absolute rates of death were low, and 781 men had to be screened to prevent one death over the span of 13 years.

In contrast, the US Prostate, Lung, Colorectal, and Ovarian (PLCO) study found no difference in mortality at 13 years among men assigned to annual PSA screening compared to a control group. The trial was complicated by significant crossover, however, with up to 90% of the men in the control arm receiving at least one PSA test.

The overall impression was that routine, nonselective PSA screening would expose a large number of men to unnecessary further testing and treatment without a significant impact on mortality. Accordingly, the US

Preventive Services Task Force recommended against routine PSA screening in 2012.

Digital Rectal Exam

DRE can sometimes detect prostate nodularity or masses; however, no randomized control studies have found that the routine performance of this test results in a mortality benefit. The DRE is usually positive in the presence of larger tumors (volumes >0.5 cm³) and tumors that have spread beyond the prostate.

EVALUATION, DIAGNOSIS, AND STAGING

An elevated serum PSA level or abnormal DRE often prompts a transrectal ultrasound-guided prostate biopsy (Fig. 166.1). The current standard of care is to collect at least 12 biopsy cores (extended pattern)—6 from the lateral-peripheral zone and 6 from the center—as well as extra cores from any identifiable prostate lesions. A pathologist then evaluates each core and assigns a **Gleason score** ranging from 2 to 10, with ≤6 representing well differentiated carcinoma and 10 indicating anaplastic growth. The Gleason score is determined by adding up two subscores (ranging from 1–5) that characterize the first and second most common histopathological patterns on the biopsies. Gleason scores will thus often be written in an $x + y$ format, such as $4 + 3 = 7$ (Fig. 166.2).

Along with the Gleason score, prostate cancers are also classified based on the TNM (tumor, node, metastasis) staging system. Beyond the ultrasound used to guide

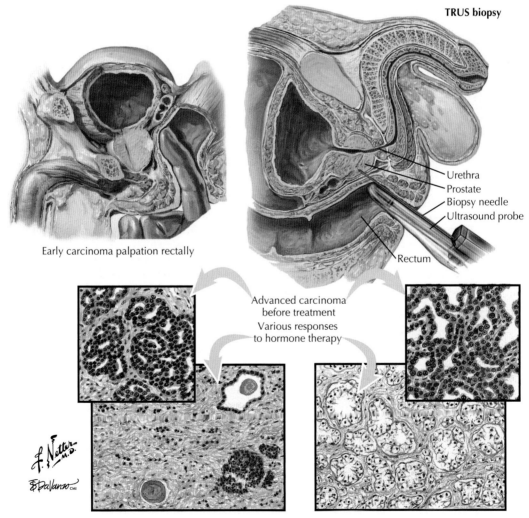

TRUS biopsy

Early carcinoma palpation rectally

Urethra
Prostate
Biopsy needle
Ultrasound probe
Rectum

Advanced carcinoma before treatment
Various responses to hormone therapy

FIG 166.1 Transrectal Ultrasound (TRUS)-Guided Prostate Biopsy.

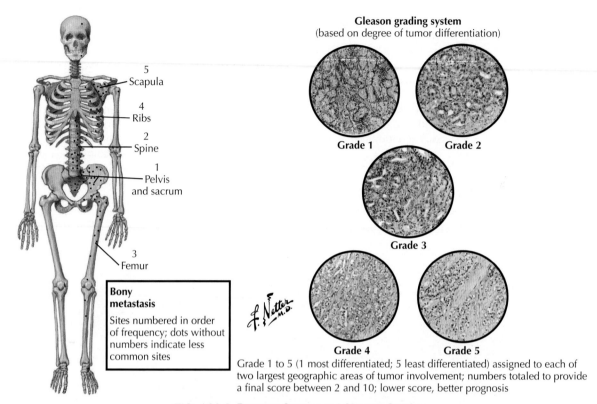

Gleason grading system
(based on degree of tumor differentiation)

5
Scapula
4
Ribs
2
Spine
1
Pelvis
and sacrum

3
Femur

Bony metastasis

Sites numbered in order of frequency; dots without numbers indicate less common sites

Grade 1   Grade 2

Grade 3

Grade 4   Grade 5

Grade 1 to 5 (1 most differentiated; 5 least differentiated) assigned to each of two largest geographic areas of tumor involvement; numbers totaled to provide a final score between 2 and 10; lower score, better prognosis

FIG. 166.2 **Prostate Cancer and Gleason Scoring.**

the transrectal ultrasound, additional imaging (pelvic CT, MRI, or bone scan) can be considered if the PSA is >10 ng/mL, the Gleason score is ≥8, large lesions (T3 or T4) are present, or the patient complains of bone pain (especially in the back, a frequent site of metastases).

TREATMENT

Localized Disease

Patients are first stratified into risk groups based on several characteristics (size, Gleason score, PSA level, number of cancer-positive biopsy cores), then treatment decisions are further refined based on expected lifespan, which depends on age, comorbidities, and functional status.

Patients with lower-risk disease (T1–2a tumor size, Gleason score ≤6, PSA <10 ng/mL, and <3 biopsy cores positive) and life expectancy <10 years should undergo observation. If disease burden becomes symptomatic, palliative treatment can then be initiated. **Active surveillance,** in contrast to regular observation, usually involves repeat prostate biopsies, with the goal of curative treatment if PSA levels or Gleason scores increase. In

one study, 66% of men avoided surgery, radiation, and/ or chemotherapy for 5 years using active surveillance. Currently, there are no clear parameters that define the ideal time to switch from active surveillance to treatment.

Patients with localized, low-risk to moderate-risk cancer (T1–2c tumor size, Gleason score ≤7, PSA ≤20 ng/mL) and >10 years life expectancy should receive surgery or radiation. **Radical prostatectomy** can be performed using open technique (retropubic or perianal approach) or laparoscopic technique, the latter with or without robotic assistance (Fig. 166.3). All three approaches have comparable outcomes in the hands of experienced surgeons at high-volume centers. Radical prostatectomy reduced the absolute risk of death from prostate cancer by 11% when compared to active surveillance in men with localized tumors and predicted lifespans >10 years. The potential complications of surgery include incontinence, impotence, and postoperative events (such as deep venous thromboses during convalescence).

Radiation therapy can be administered as **external beam** (EBRT) or as **brachytherapy** (implantation of short-range radioactive seeds in the prostate). The two techniques can also be used together. Potential

A. Laparoscopic robot-assisted radical prostatectomy

Robotic radical prostatectomy

B. Anatomical position of the prostate. The prostate is located within the pelvis between the bladder and urethra, adjacent to the rectum, surrounded by a venous plexus and neurovascular bundles.

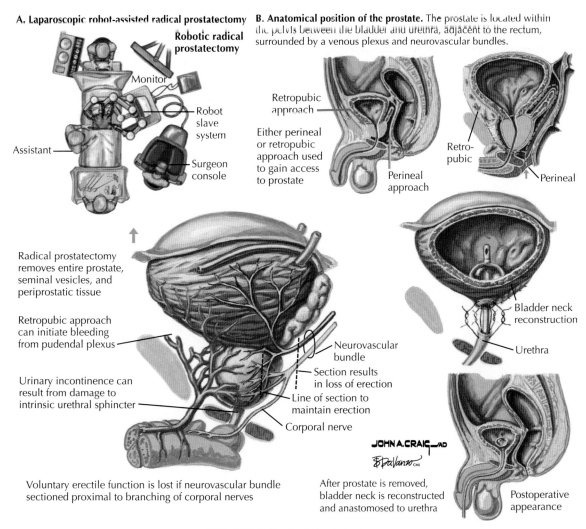

Monitor

Robot slave system

Assistant

Surgeon console

Retropubic approach

Either perineal or retropubic approach used to gain access to prostate

Perineal approach

Retropubic

Perineal

Radical prostatectomy removes entire prostate, seminal vesicles, and periprostatic tissue

Retropubic approach can initiate bleeding from pudendal plexus

Urinary incontinence can result from damage to intrinsic urethral sphincter

Neurovascular bundle

Section results in loss of erection

Line of section to maintain erection

Corporal nerve

Bladder neck reconstruction

Urethra

JOHN A. CRAIG AD

Voluntary erectile function is lost if neurovascular bundle sectioned proximal to branching of corporal nerves

After prostate is removed, bladder neck is reconstructed and anastomosed to urethra

Postoperative appearance

FIG. 166.3 Radical Prostatectomy.

complications of radiation therapy include radiation proctitis, erectile dysfunction, and temporary bowel and bladder dysfunction. The Prostate Cancer Outcomes Study demonstrated equivalent mortality outcomes between surgery and EBRT in early-stage prostate cancer.

Advanced Disease

The treatment for more advanced disease (T3 or higher tumor, Gleason 8–10, PSA >20 ng/mL) without metastases begins with **androgen deprivation therapy** (ADT). Since prostate cancer often begins as a hormone-sensitive tumor, castration through either orchiectomy or the use of a luteinizing hormone–releasing hormone (LHRH) agonist or antagonist often achieves adequate tumor

control. The addition of other antiandrogens (such as the androgen receptor antagonist apalutamide) is under active investigation, but recent trials provide evidence for improved overall survival when used in combination with ADT. The side effects of ADT include osteoporosis, increased risk of cardiovascular disease and diabetes, loss of libido, and impotence. Because the side effect profile leads to high rates of treatment cessation, an intermittent (as opposed to continuous) dosing schedule is being examined as a means of potentially reducing adverse effects without compromising efficacy.

In the setting of metastatic disease, systemic agents from multiple drug classes are also initiated. These include docetaxel (a microtubule binder), abiraterone (an androgen synthesis inhibitor), and antiandrogens such as enzalutamide (an inhibitor of androgen receptor binding and signaling). One additional treatment with a particularly interesting mechanism is sipuleucel-T. This therapy requires harvest of a patient's dendritic cells, treatment of the cells with a fusion protein of prostatic acid phosphatase and granulocyte-macrophage colony-stimulating factor, and then reinfusion of the modified cells into the patient with the goal of triggering the immune system to attack the tumor. Because prostate cancer most commonly metastasizes to bone, osteoclast-inhibiting agents (such as zoledronic acid and denosumab), or direct cancer cytotoxic agents that concentrate in bone (such as radium-223), may also be helpful.

Index

Page number followed by t, f, or b indicates table, figure, or box, respectively.